W9-BCV-117

Gerontological Nurse Practitioner Review and Resource Manual 2nd Edition

Maren S. Mayhew, MS, ANP, GNP

Marilyn W. Edmunds, PhD, ANP, GNP

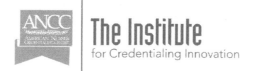

Library of Congress Cataloging-in-Publication Data

Mayhew, Maren Stewart.
  Gerontological nurse practitioner review and resource manual / Maren S. Mayhew, Marilyn W. Edmunds.-- 2nd ed.
    p. ; cm.
  Includes bibliographical references and index.
  ISBN-13: 978-0-9768213-0-4
  ISBN-10: 0-9768213-0-3
  1. Geriatric nursing—Examinations, questions, etc. 2. Nurse practitioners—Examinations, questions, etc. 3. Nurses—Licenses—United States—Examinations—Study guides.
  [DNLM: 1. Geriatric Nursing—Examination Questions. 2. Nurse Practitioners—Examination Questions. WY 18.2 M469g 2005] I. Edmunds, Marilyn W. II. Title.

  RC954.M39 2005
  618.97'023—dc22

                    2005017402

Published by
American Nurses Credentialing Center
Institute for Credentialing Innovation
8515 Georgia Ave., Suite 400
Silver Spring, MD 20910-3492
800-284-2378
email: revmanuals@ana.org
www.nursecredentialing.org

ISBN 10: 0-9768213-0-3
     13: 978-0-9768213-0-4

**The Gerontological Nurse Practitioner Review and Resource Manual Project
was completed by Nurse Practitioner Alternatives, Inc.**

**Columbia, Maryland
March 2005**

Please direct your comments and/or queries to:
revmanuals@ana.org

The health care services delivery system is a volatile marketplace demanding superior knowledge, clinical skills, and competencies from all registered nurses. Nursing autonomy of practice, and nurse career marketability and mobility in the new century hinge on affirming the profession's formative philosophy which places a priority on a lifelong commitment to the principles of education and professional development. The knowledge base of nursing theory and practice is expanding, and while care has been taken to ensure the accuracy and timeliness of the information presented in the *Gerontological Nurse Practitioner Review Manual,* clinicians are advised to always verify the most current national treatment guidelines and recommendations and to practice in accordance with professional standards of care used with regard to the unique circumstances that apply in each practice situation. In addition, every effort has been made in this text to insure accuracy and, in particular to confirm that drug selections and dosages are in accordance with current recommendations and practice, including the ongoing research, changes to government regulations and the developments in product information provided by pharmaceutical manufacturers. However, it is the responsibility of each nurse practitioner to verify drug product information and to practice in accordance with professional standards of care. In addition, the editors wish to note that provision of information in this text does not imply an endorsement of any particular products, procedures or services. As a review text, this content is provided at a level that describes what a GNP should know upon entry into practice. NPs may object, for religious or other reasons, to the provisions of certain services. That decision, too, must be left to the individual NP.

Therefore, the authors, editors, American Nurses Association (ANA), American Nurses Association's Publishing (ANP), American Nurses Credentialing Center (ANCC), and the Institute for Credentialing Innovation cannot accept responsibility for errors or omissions, or for any consequences or liability, injury and/or damages to persons or property from application of the information in this manual and make no warranty, express or implied, with respect to the contents of the *Gerontological Nurse Practitioner Review and Resource Manual.*

Introduction to the Continuing Education (CE) Contact Hour Application Process for Gerontological Nurse Practitioner Review and Resource Manual, 2nd Edition

The Institute for Credentialing Innovation now offers the continuing education contact hours for this manual online at www.NursingWorld.org, the American Nurses Association's Web site. This process involves answering approximately 50 questions that test knowledge of the information contained within this manual. The continuing education contact hours can be completed at any time and a certificate can be printed from the Web site immediately upon successful completion of the test.

The *Gerontological Nurse Practitioner Review and Resource Manual* is designed to meet the following objectives:

1. Analyze history and physical examination findings for signs and symptoms of common diseases experienced by geriatric patients.
2. Develop comprehensive treatment plans for common diseases and disorders experienced by the geriatric patient, including laboratory testing, radiological examination and pharmacological management.
3. Discuss issues related to advance practice that influence the role of the nurse practitioner.

Upon completion of this manual *and* the online CE test, a nurse can receive a total of 40 (forty) continuing education contact hours. **The entire process—online test and evaluation form—must be completed by December 31, 2007 in order to receive credit.**

To begin the process, please e-mail revmanuals@ana.org *or* go to the ANCC website at www.nursecredentialing.org for specific instructions.

Your patience with this new process is greatly appreciated.

Inquiries or Comments

If you have any questions about the CE contact hours, please e-mail The Institute at: revmanuals@ana.org. You may also mail any comments to Barbara Burnham, RN, BSN, MA, Editor/Project Manager, at the address listed below.

Duplicate CE Certificates

Once you have successfully passed the CE test on NursingWorld, you may go back and re-print your certificate as often as you wish.

The Institute for Credentialing Innovation
American Nurses Credentialing Center
Attn: Editor/Project Manager
8515 Georgia Avenue, Suite 400
Silver Spring, MD 20910-3492
Fax: (301) 628-5342

The American Nurses Association is accredited as a provider of continuing nursing education by the American Nurses Credentialing Center's Commission on Accreditation and approved by the California Board of Registered Nursing, Provider Number CEP6178.

INTRODUCTION

Welcome to the 2nd edition of the *Gerontological Nurse Practitioner Review and Resource Manual*. This manual is designed as a review text for the American Nurses Credentialing Center's Gerontological Nurse Practitioner Certification Examination. As such, it is designed to describe the information required for a geriatric nurse practitioner as they enter practice.

This text as a whole was constructed to help the reader meet three objectives:

1. To analyze history and physical examination findings for signs and symptoms of common disease experienced by geriatric patients
2. To develop comprehensive treatment plans for common diseases and disorders experienced by the geriatric patient, including laboratory testing, radiological examination, and pharmacologic management
3. To discuss issues of advance practice that influence the role of the geriatric nurse practitioner

Consistent with these objectives, the revised edition has been updated with all of the latest practice guidelines and medications. The information is written in a consistent format to facilitate information retrieval. In a text of this nature, only the most important information can be included. Each chapter has case studies that will help readers determine how well they have mastered the content and a specific bibliography for the section to aid NPs who determine they need more information. At the conclusion of the book, a 100-item practice test has been included as a separate section. This test is composed of items that are similar to and in some cases drawn from a previous GNP ANCC test pool. Answers to all the questions on the practice test are included in a separate chapter.

This manual is not intended to teach new material or to substitute for a sound educational program that provides sufficient clinical experience to allow the student to master skills. It should, however, help students identify areas in which they may wish to focus additional study.

In order to facilitate learning, some content is grouped together to help the learner. At the conclusion of Chapter One, Taking the Certification Examination, the NP should be able to list seven specific steps to help them in preparing for the examination; describe specific test taking skills used in multiple-choice examinations; and discuss the different features of the GNP certifying examination.

Chapter Two discusses the dimensions of the NP role in general and the GNP role in specific. At the conclusion of this chapter, the NP should be able to list specific historical factors that were important in the development of the role; to compare the different mechanisms that confirm legal authority for practice through state rules and regulations; and to identify the items that constitute medical malpractice.

Health Care Issues in Chapter Three is an especially important chapter for the GNP to master. At the conclusion of this chapter, the GNP should be able to define the basic concepts of epidemiology, identify modifications required in history taking, physical assessment, diagnostic testing and drug therapy for geriatric patients, and evaluate geriatric health maintenance recommendations including diet, exercise, immunization, and screening.

The remaining chapters constitute a system by system review of important content from which the GNP should be able to develop a differential diagnosis of common problems experienced by older adults from the relevant history and physical examination; to construct a logical diagnostic plan, including laboratory, radiologic, and other examinations; and within their scope of practice, to initiate a comprehensive treatment plan including nonpharmacologic and pharmacologic management.

Becoming a GNP allows the nurse a greater opportunity to continue to care for patients in traditional ways in which they have always excelled: teaching, counseling and patient advocacy. The GNP role is truly a new role, with a marriage between previous nursing knowledge and skills and new diagnostic and treatment authority. It is this blend of behaviors that have ensured that the GNP role has not only grown but has been accepted and appreciated in the health care community.

EDITORS FOR THE SECOND EDITION

Maren S. Mayhew, MSN, ANP/GNP
Suburban Hospital
Bethesda, MD

Marilyn W. Edmunds, PhD, ANP/GNP
NP Alternatives in Education, Inc.
Elliott City, MD

REVIEWERS FOR THE SECOND EDITION

Victoria L. Anderson, MSN, FNP
Nurse Practitioner
Laboratory of Host Defenses
National Institutes of Allergy and
Infectious Diseases
National Institutes of Health
Bethesda, MD

Eve Heemann Byrd, MSN, MPH, FNP
Associate Director
Fuqua Center for Late-Life Depression
Dept. of Psychiatry, Emory University
Atlanta, GA

Christy L. Crowther, MS, CRNP
Clinical Instructor
Department of Family Medicine
University of Maryland
School of Medicine
Baltimore, MD
Private Orthopedic Surgery Practice
Glen Burnie, MD

Susan D. McConnell, MSN, ANP/GNP
Research Nurse Practitioner
Emory University School of Medicine
Division of Rheumatology
Atlanta, GA

Justine Preis, MSN, ANP/GNP
Oak Crest Village
Baltimore, MD

Barbara Resnick, PhD, CRNP
Associate Professor
University of Maryland
School of Nursing
Baltimore, MD

Janine Smith, MS, ANP
Suburban Hospital
Bethesda, MD
Community Care Management

V. Inez Wendel, MS, ANP, GNP
Clinical Instructor
School of Nursing
GNP, School of Medicine
Division of Geriatric Medicine
and Gerontology
Johns Hopkins University
Baltimore, MD

Contributors to the First Edition

This book is the part of a series of NP Review Manuals developed for the American Nurses Credentialing Center and updated as a second edition. The Editors wish to thank the authors and reviewers of the Geriatric Review Manual Edition 1 and the Adult Review Manual Edition 1 and 2 for the outstanding clinical summaries developed for those books that are interwoven throughout this new book. Their excellent scholarship and research provided the basic content foundation and design for this book.

Victoria L. Anderson, MSN, FNP
Nurse Practitioner
Laboratory of Host Defenses
National Institutes of Allergy and
Infectious Diseases
National Institute of Health
Bethesda, MD
Hematology Disorders

Kathie C. Bronson, MS, ANP/GNP
Frederick Medical & Pulmonary Associates
Frederick, MD
Respiratory Disorders

Christy L. Crowther, MS, CRNP
Clinical Instructor
Department of Family Medicine
University of Maryland
School of Medicine
Baltimore, MD
Private Orthopedic Surgery Practice
Glen Burnie, MD
Musculoskeletal Disorders

Marilyn W. Edmunds, PhD, ANP/GNP
Private Practice
Nurse Practitioner Alternatives, Inc.
Columbia, MD
Dimensions of the GNP Role
Health Care Issues

Laurie Kennedy-Malone PhD, CS
Associate Professor
Director Adult/Gerontological
Nurse Practitioner Program
School of Nursing
University North Carolina Greensboro
Greensboro, NC
Dimensions of the GNP Role

Tracy L. MacGregor, MSN, CANP
National Institutes of Health
Internal Medicine Consultation
Service
Bethesda, MD
Gastrointestinal Disorders

Maren S. Mayhew, MS, ANP/GNP
Private Practice
Bethesda, MD
Faculty, NP Alternatives, Inc.
Columbia, MD
Musculoskeletal Disorders
Multisystem Syndromes
Gynecological Disorders
Renal Disorders
Infectious Diseases
Cardiovascular Disorders
Male Reproductive System Disorders
Taking the Certification Examination

Susan D. McConnell, MSN, ANP/GNP
Research Nurse Practitioner
Emory University School of Medicine
Department of Medicine
Atlanta, GA
Infectious Diseases

Sandra Bauer Melville, MSN, ANP
Milton, MA
Eyes, Ears, Nose and Throat Disorders

Candis Morrison, PhD, ANP
Associate Professor
School of Nursing
Johns Hopkins University
Baltimore, MD
Renal Disorders

Justine Preis, MSN, ANP/GNP
Oak Crest Village
Baltimore, MD
Dermatologic Disorders

Carolyn Rainey CRNP-F, MSN
Home and Community Care Program
Veterans Administration Medical Center
Washington, DC
Endocrine Disorders

Marsha K. Rauch, PhD, ARNP
Geriatric Nurse Practitioner
Medical & Educational Director, Florida Nurse
Practitioner Services, Inc.
Orlando, FL
Cardiovascular Disorders

Anne Reb, MS, NP
Nurse Practitioner, Instructor Medicine
Lombardi Cancer Center
Georgetown University Hospital
Washington, DC
Multisystem Syndromes
Gynecologic Disorders

Barbara Resnick, PhD, CRNP
Associate Professor
University of Maryland
School of Nursing
Baltimore, MD
Health Care Issues

Denise Sciullo, MSEd, MSN, NP, ND
Director of Intramural Research
Projects Neuro-Endocrinology
National Institutes of Health
Bethesda, MD
Psychiatric and Mental Health Disorders

Laura E. Shay, MS, ANP
National Institutes of Health
Advance Practice Consultant
Bethesda, MD
Gastrointestinal Disorders

V. Inez Wendel, MS, GNP
Clinical Instructor
School of Nursing
GNP, School of Medicine
Division of Geriatric Medicine
and Gerontology
Johns Hopkins University
Baltimore, MD
Co-Editor to First Edition
Endocrine
Hematology
Multisystem Syndromes
Neurologic Disorders

TABLE OF CONTENTS

Chapter 15 Neurologic Disorders 365

Chapter 16 Hematologic Disorders 393

Chapter 17 Endocrine Disorders 413

Chapter 18 Psychiatric-Mental Health Disorders   431

Appendix A Discussion of Case Studies   455

Appendix B Sample GNP Test   481

Appendix C Discussion of Multiple Choice Questions/Answers   489

Bibliography   499

Index   501

TAKING THE
CERTIFICATION EXAMINATION

1

PLEASE REMEMBER!

When you sign up to take a national certification exam you will receive a packet of information from the testing agency. Review it carefully and keep it where you can refer to it frequently. This packet will contain critical information to review carefully and will give good insight into the nature of the test. The agency will also send you an entry ticket or materials authorizing your entry into the exam that you must keep in a safe place until needed.

GENERAL SUGGESTIONS FOR PREPARING FOR THE EXAM
Step One: Control Your Anxiety

Everyone experiences anxiety when faced with the nurse practitioner certification exam.
- This exam will probably be the hardest evaluation you have ever taken. However, your program has been designed with taking this exam as one of its final goals.
- Your instructors took a similar exam to become nurse practitioners, and they no doubt talked to former students who have taken the exams, so they know how to help you prepare.

Step Two: Do Not Listen to Gossip About the Exam

There is a large volume of "information" about the tests based on reports from people who have taken the exams in the past.
- Because this information is based on the imperfect memory of people in a very stressful situation, it may not be very accurate.
- Information you hear from others is not verifiable.
- Because information from the testing facilities is limited, it is hard not to listen to the gossip.
- Individuals tend to remember the questions that they did not know in an exam.
- Some of this "common information" will be reflected in this chapter.
- Some of the review courses discuss this "information."
- A good deal of the lore discussed by students is from the many people who have taken the American Nurses Credentialing Center exam. However, this exam is now a computerized exam, and so experiences with the written tests may not be relevant.
- The questions on the NP exams change. A *Role Delineation Study of Nurse Practitioners* was completed for ANCC in 2003. This study provided statistical validity for the entry-level content of items included in the test.

Step Three: Set Reasonable Expectations for Yourself

- Do not expect to know everything.
- You do not need a perfect score in order to pass the exam.
- Do not try to know everything in great detail.
- The exam is designed for the NP at entry into practice.
- The most likely diagnoses will be on the exam; there will not be questions on rare diseases or atypical cases.
- Learn the general rules, not the exceptions.
- Think about the most likely presentation and most common therapy.

Step Four: Prepare Mentally and Physically

- While you are getting ready to take the exam, take good physical care of yourself.
- Get plenty of sleep, exercise, and eat well while preparing for the exam.
- These things are especially important while you are studying and immediately before the exam.

Step Five: Assess Current Knowledge

General Content

You will be given a list of general topics that will be on the exam when you register to take the exam. In addition, examine the table of contents of this book.

- What content do you need to know?
- How well do you know these subjects?

Take a Review Course

- Taking a review course is an excellent method of assessing your knowledge of the content that will be included in the exam.
- If you plan to take a review course, take it well before the exam so you will have plenty of time to master any areas of weakness the course uncovers.
- If you are prepared for the exam, you will not hear anything new in the course. You will be familiar with everything that is taught.
- If there are topics in the review course that are new to you, these will be the topics you will need to concentrate on in your studies.

Depth of Knowledge

How much do you need to know about a subject?

- You must come to some decisions about the depth of knowledge you believe is required for entry-level performance as an NP.
- You cannot know everything about a topic.
- Judge depth of knowledge by studying the information sent to you from the testing agency, what you were taught in school, what is covered in this text, and the general guidelines given in this chapter.
- Consult your class notes or clinical diagnosis and management textbook for the major points about a disease.
- Look at practice tests but make sure they are designed for the NP exam.
- For example, with regard to medications, know the drug categories and the major medications in each. Assume all drugs in a category are generally alike, and then focus on the differences between common drugs. Know the most important indications, contraindications, and side effects. Emphasize safety. The questions usually do not require you to know the exact dosage of a drug.

Step Six: Institute a Systematic Study Plan

Develop Your Study Plan
- Write up a formal plan of study.
  - Include topics for study, timetable, resources, and methods of study that work for you.
  - You may want to organize a study group, or you may decide you work better alone.
  - Schedule regular times to study.
- Identify resources to use for studying.
- To prepare for the examination, on your shelf you should have:
  - A good pathophysiology text
  - This review book
  - A physical assessment text
  - Your class notes
  - Other important sources include information from the testing facility, *Guide to Clinical Preventive Services*, a clinical diagnosis textbook, favorite journal articles, notes from a review course, and practice tests.
  - Know the important national standards of care for major illnesses, such as The Expert Panel Report 2: Guidelines for the Diagnosis and Management of Asthma.
  - Many treatment and assessment guidelines are available. Consult www.guideline.gov.
- Study the body systems from head to toe.
- The exams emphasize assessment, differential diagnosis, and plan of care for common problems seen in primary care, including common behavioral concerns.
- You will need to know facts and be able to interpret and analyze this information utilizing critical thinking.

Personalize Your Study Plan
- How do you learn best?
  - If you learn best by reading, follow some of the strategies that are listed.
  - If you learn best by hearing or talking, attend a review course or discuss topics with a colleague.
- Read everything the test facility sends you as soon as you receive it and several times during your preparation period. It will give you valuable information that will help guide your studying.
- Have a specific place with good lighting set aside for studying. Find a place with no noise or distractions. Assemble your study material.

Implement Your Study Plan
- Refer to your study plan regularly.
- Stick to your schedule.
- Allow for breaks when you get tired.
- When you start procrastinating, get help from a friend or reorganize your study plan.
- It is not necessary to follow your plan rigidly. Adjust as you learn where you need to spend more time.

> **You must have basic content knowledge. In addition, you must be able to use this information critically to think and make decisions about facts.**

- Memorize the basics of the things you will be required to know, such as the cranial nerves.
- Understand physiology. For example, every exam so far has had questions about the cardiac cycle and characteristics of different murmurs. Learn to draw one complete cardiac cycle, and then answer questions about murmurs from the diagram. Reason answers out rather than memorizing information about a particular murmur.
- In recent years, NP exams have asked many questions about health promotion. This information is covered well in *Guide to Clinical Preventive Services* (3rd ed.). The Guide, issued by the Department

of Health and Human Services, US Preventive Services Task Force (USPSTF) can be accessed online at http://www.ahrq.gov/clinic/prevnew.htm. Understand risk factors, screening and diagnostic tests, and primary, secondary, and tertiary prevention.

- Every year there also have been questions that require basic knowledge of anatomy, physiology, and assessment. This type of content is best reviewed using the assessment book you used in school.
- Diagnosis, management, and drug treatment specifics are best reviewed in class notes, a clinical diagnosis textbook, and journal articles. These types of questions often require analysis of data and critical thinking.

Focus on General Material

- Most of what you need to know is basic material that does not require constant updating.
- You do not need to worry about the latest information being published as you are studying for the exam. Remember, it may take 6 to 12 months for new information to be incorporated into test questions.

Pace Your Studying

- Stop your studying for the examination when you are starting to feel overwhelmed, and look at what is bothering you. Then make changes.
- Break overwhelming tasks into doable tasks.
- Stop and take breaks while studying.

Work With Others

- Talk with classmates about your preparation for the exam.
- Keep in touch with classmates, and help each other stick to your study plans.
- However, if your classmates start having anxiety attacks, walk away and do not let their anxiety infect you.
- Do not believe all the bad stories you hear about other people's experiences with the previous exams.
- Remember, you know as much as anyone about what will be on the next exam!

Consider a Study Group

- Study groups can provide practice in analyzing cases, interpreting questions, and critical thinking.
- You can discuss a topic and take turns presenting cases to have the group analyze the case.
- Study groups can also provide moral support and help you meet your study goals.

Step Seven: Strategies Immediately Before the Exam

Final Preparation Suggestions

- Use practice exams when studying to get accustomed to the exam format and time restrictions.
  - Many books that are labeled NP review books are simply a collection of examination questions.
  - If you have test anxiety, practice tests may help alleviate the anxiety.
  - Practice tests are helpful for you to learn to judge the time you take during an exam.
  - Practice tests are useful for gaining experience in analyzing questions.
  - However, books of questions may not uncover the gaps in your knowledge that a more systematic content review text will reveal.
- Know your test-taking style.
  - Do you rush through the exam without reading the questions?
  - Do you get stuck and dwell on a question for a long time?
  - You should spend about 45 to 60 seconds per question and finish with time to review questions of which you were not sure.

The Night Before the Exam

- Be prepared to get to the exam on time.
  - Know the test site location and how long it takes to get there.

- Take a practice drive of how to get to the testing site beforehand, if necessary.
- Get a good night's sleep.
- Eat sensibly.
- Avoid alcohol the night before.
- Assemble the required material—two IDs, admission card, pencil, and watch. Bring Kleenex, Tums, hard candy, and anything else you might want in your pocket.
- Know the exam room rules.
  - You will be provided with scratch paper, which will be collected at the end of the exam.
  - Nothing else is allowed in the exam room.
  - You will be required to put papers, backpacks, and other personal belongings in a corner of the room or in a locker.
  - No water or food will be allowed.
  - You will be allowed to walk to a water fountain and go to the bathroom one at a time.

The Day of the Exam
- Get there early. If you are late, you may not be admitted.
- Think positively.
- Remember your anxiety reduction strategies.
- Knowledge that you have studied hard and are well prepared will help with a positive attitude.

Specific Tips for Dealing With Anxiety
- Test-taking anxiety is a specific type of anxiety. Symptoms include upset stomach, sweaty palms, tachycardia, trouble concentrating, and a feeling of dread. But there are ways to cope with test anxiety.
  - There is no substitute for being well prepared.
  - Practice relaxation techniques.
  - Take a few deep breaths and concentrate on the task at hand.
  - Avoid alcohol, excess coffee, caffeine, or any new medications that might oversedate you or dull your senses or cause you to feel agitation.

FOCUS ON SPECIFIC TEST-TAKING SKILLS

In order to do well on the exam, you need good test-taking skills in addition to knowledge of the content and ability to use critical thinking.

All NP Certification Exams Are Multiple Choice
- Multiple-choice tests have specific rules inherent in the test construction.
- A multiple-choice question consists of three parts: the information (or stem), the question, and the four possible answers (one correct and three distractors).
- Careful analysis of each part is necessary. Read the entire question before answering.
- Practice your test-taking skills by analyzing the practice questions at the end of this book.

Analyze the Information Given
- Do not assume you have more information than is given.
- Do not overanalyze.
- Remember, the writer of the question assumes this is all of the pertinent information needed to answer the question.
- Do not make the question more complicated than it is.

What Kind of Question Is Asked?
- Are you supposed to recall a fact, apply facts to a situation, or understand and differentiate between options?
  - Read the question, thinking about what the question writer is asking. The test question writers are NPs, often faculty, who are asking questions about what they think is important.

- Look for key words or phrases that lead you. These help determine what kind of answer the question requires.

Examples of Key Words and Phrases:
- avoid
- best
- except
- not
- initial
- first
- contributing to
- appropriate
- most
- significant
- likely
- of the following
- most consistent with

Read All the Answers
- *If you are absolutely certain that answer A is correct as you read it, mark it, but continue to read the rest of the question so you do not trick yourself.*
- *If you are absolutely sure answer A is wrong, cross it off and continue reading the question.*
- After reading the entire question, go back, analyze the question, and select the most appropriate answer.
- Don't jump ahead.
- If you have a chief complaint, get more history. If you have a complete history, do the exam, etc.
- If the answers include two options that are the opposite of each other, one of the two is probably the correct answer.
- When numeric answers cover a wide range, a number in the middle is more likely to be correct.
- Statistics has shown that if you do not know the answer, c is a likely guess.
- Watch out for distracters, which are correct but don't answer the question, combine true and false information, or contain a word or phrase that is similar to the correct answer.
- Err on the side of caution.

Only One Answer Can Be Correct
- When more than one suggested answer is correct, you must identify the one answer that best answers the question asked.
- If you cannot choose between two answers, you have a 50% chance of getting it right if you guess.

Avoid Changing Answers
- Make changes only if you have a compelling reason to change an answer, such as remembering something additional or understanding the question better on rereading it.
- People more often change to a wrong answer than to a right answer.

Time Yourself to Complete the Whole Exam
- Do not spend a large amount of time on one question.
- If you cannot answer a question quickly, mark it and continue the exam.
- If time is left at the end, return to the difficult questions.
- Make educated guesses by eliminating the obviously wrong answers and choosing a likely answer even if you are not positive.
- Trust your instinct.
- Answer every question. There is no penalty for a wrong answer.
- Occasionally a question will remind you of something that helps you with a question earlier in the test. Look back at that question to see if what you are remembering affects how you would answer that question.

ABOUT THE GNP CERTIFICATION EXAM

The ANCC Computerized Exam
- The ANCC examination is now given only as a computer exam.
- Periodically, the ANCC does an extensive analysis of what NPs do and what they need to know, which serves as the foundation for the exam.

- ANCC test item writers are constantly updating and modifying the content to reflect what they think is current practice.
- Writers are also constantly revising the test questions based on how well they are answered.

Each Exam Is Different
- At any given exam site, there will be five different exams that may be given.
- The order of the test questions for every test is scrambled, so even if two people are taking the same exam, the questions will be in a different order.
- Remember this when you are talking to friends after the exam.

The Exam Consists of 175 Multiple-Choice Questions
- One hundred-fifty questions are part of the test, and how you answer will count toward your score.
- Twenty five are included to test and refine questions and will not be scored.
- You will not know which ones will count, so treat all questions the same.
- Total exam time is 3 hours.

Before the ANCC Exam, You May Take a 20- to 30-Minute Computerized Tutorial to Show You How to Take the Computer Test
- You will need to know how to use a mouse, scroll by either clicking arrows on the scroll bar or by using the up and down arrow keys, and perform other basic commands.
- The exam does not require computer expertise; however, if you are not comfortable with use of a computer, you should practice using a mouse and computer beforehand so you do not spend needless time on the mechanics of using the computer.

The Testing Process
- Each ANCC test question is independent of the other test questions.
  - For each case study, there is only one question.
  - This means a correct answer on any question does not depend on the correct answer to any other question.
  - Also, each question has four possible answers. There are no questions asking for combinations of correct answers or multiple-multiples!
- The computer allows you to mark questions for later review.
- You can also skip a question and go back to it at the end of the exam.
- You cannot mark key words in the question or right or wrong answers.
  - You may want to do this on the scratch paper that is available for this purpose.
- At the end of the exam, you can see a listing of your responses and a box showing the number of marked and incomplete questions.
  - You can review the marked and incomplete questions by clicking a button. You can also review the entire exam.
- When you are finished, you click the End Exam button.
- You should receive your results 1 to 2 weeks after the exam.

The ANCC GNP Exam Covers:
- General areas of scope of practice and ethics, health promotion and disease prevention, assessment, diagnosis, intervention, planning and education, and evaluation.
- Assessment includes history, physical examination, diagnostic studies/screening tests, and critical thinking/decision making.
- Diagnosis includes epidemiology, pathophysiology, and critical thinking/decision making.
- Planning and education includes teaching and critical thinking/decision making.
- Intervention includes pharmacologic, nonpharmacologic, and communication.
- Evaluation includes response to treatment plan and quality assurance.
- Health promotion/disease prevention includes primary and secondary prevention; family, ethnic, cultural, community, individual, developmental, and environmental factors; lifestyle/health behaviors; and health/wellness research.

- Scope of practice and ethics includes scope and standards of practice, ethical decision making and legal considerations, and client rights.

SAMPLE QUESTIONS

1. Staff members at a nursing home report that a resident regularly wanders into other residents' rooms, sometimes gets into bed with other residents, and often is found taking their belongings. The staff members ask the gerontological nurse practitioner to "do something" because the other residents' families are becoming angry. The nurse practitioner's most appropriate action would be to:
   a. Start the resident on a low dose of a benzodiazepine.
   b. Secure the doors and closets of the residents whose families are angry.
   c. Suggest that the resident's name and picture be put on the door to the resident's room.
   d. Have the resident undergo a Folstein Mini-Mental State Examination and dementia evaluation.

Comments: The correct answer is C. The question asks for the MOST appropriate action. Some of the other answers may also be appropriate, but c is the best. This question asks you to analyze the information and come up with an appropriate plan. You must choose the initial action that is the least invasive to the patient and other residents.

2. A nurse practitioner is asked to evaluate a protocol that requires routine urine screening of all older residents at a long-term care facility. The nurse practitioner should recommend that the protocol be:
   a. Discontinued because prevalence of asymptomatic bacteriuria in this population is very low.
   b. Discontinued because research studies have shown that routine screening of institutionalized older persons is not beneficial.
   c. Continued because current screening methods are highly sensitive and specific for significant disease.
   d. Continued because asymptomatic bacteriuria is an established risk factor for serious complications in institutionalized older persons.

Comments: The correct answer is B. This question asks you to apply facts. You must know that the elderly have a high incidence of asymptomatic bacteria but that screening and treatment of asymptomatic bacteriuria is not beneficial.

3. A 70-year-old client who has hypertension has been taking a beta-adrenergic blocking agent for 2 weeks. The client now is normotensive but complains of wheezing when walking fast. The nurse practitioner should:
   a. Add a beta-agonist to the regimen.
   b. Begin allergy testing.
   c. Advise the client to decrease the exercise intensity.
   d. Wean the client from the beta-adrenergic blocking agent.

Comments: The correct answer is D. In this question you must differentiate between options. This is a typical question about medications. The drug is identified by class. In other questions of this nature on the exam, drugs are also identified by specific name, such as digoxin (Lanoxin), so you must know the drug categories. The question is also typical in that it asks a safety question. You must know the adverse effects of the beta-adrenergic blockers. You also must know that it is necessary to wean patients from beta-blockers. And you must know that you don't add a drug to treat an adverse effect of the first drug. Using this knowledge, you choose the answer that removes the cause of the wheezing.

4. A 68-year-old client comes to the clinic with a complaint of acute low back pain for the past 2 days. The client attributes the pain to yard work he did over the weekend. The pain originates in

the left lower back and radiates into the left buttock. The client reports he is in good health with no previous back problems. The client has no known drug allergies and is not taking any medications. A focused examination is significant only for tender paravertebral muscles in the affected area and a positive straight left leg raise. The most appropriate initial intervention would be to:

a. Obtain lumbosacral spine x-rays to rule out underlying spinal pathology.
b. Recommend activity alterations to avoid back irritation and a nonprescription analgesic for pain relief.
c. Advise bed rest for 1 week and place the client on a nonsteroidal anti-inflammatory drug for pain relief.
d. Place the client on a narcotic analgesic for acute pain and schedule evaluation by an orthopedist.

Comments: The correct answer is b. This question asks you to differentiate between options. The information section in this question is longer than most questions on the exam and includes several statements that other questions assume. Remember you can assume anything not mentioned is normal. Note the focused exam is significant "ONLY for." (That means the rest of the exam is normal.) The stem asks for the MOST appropriate INITIAL intervention. Answers a and d are correct interventions, but they are not the INITIAL intervention for simple acute back pain. Answer c is incorrect, as bed rest is no longer recommended.

5. During a neurologic examination of a 65-year-old client, a negative Romberg's sign would indicate that:
a. Cerebellar function is adequate.
b. Cerebral function is adequate.
c. Brain stem function is disturbed.
d. Labyrinth function is disturbed.

Comments: Correct answer is a. This question asks you to recall a fact. This is a physical assessment question. Note you must read the answers carefully to get this question correct. The test expects you to know technical terms such as Romberg sign if it is commonly used. Do not expect esoteric signs to be on the test. In this case, a positive Romberg sign indicates pathology, so a negative Romberg would describe normal.

REFERENCES

Note: You will find many of these books, while old, are still available in print. Much of the clinical content is very basic and therefore still relevant today but would need to be updated with more recent journal or text materials.

The Process of Taking Exams

Gilbert, S. D. (1998). *How to do your best on tests*. New York: Harper Trophy.
Highfield, M. E., & Wong, J. (1992). *How to take multiple-choice tests*. Nursing 92, (October), 117–127.
Meyers, J. N. (2002). *The secrets of taking any test* (2nd ed.). New York: Learning Express, Inc.
Newman, E. (1996). *No more test anxiety: Effective steps for taking tests and achieving better grades*. New York: Learning Skillspubns.
Nugent, P. M., & Vitale, B. A. (1997). *Test success* (2nd ed.). Philadelphia: F. A. Davis.
Rozakis, L. (2002). *Test-taking strategies and study skills for the utterly confused*. New York: McGraw Hill.
Sides, M., & Korchek, N. *Nurse's guide to successful test taking* (2nd ed.). Philadelphia: J. B. Lippincott.

Books With GNP Review Questions

Kopac, C. A., & Millonig, V. L. (Eds.). (1996). *Gerontological nursing certification review guide for the generalist, clinical specialist, and nurse practitioner*. Potomac, MD: Health Leadership Associates.
Zerwekh, J. G., & Claborn, J. C. (1999). *Geriatric nurse practitioner: Certification review*. Philadelphia, PA: Saunders.

Other Resources:

- ANCC website Information—www.nursingworld.org/ancc
  /certify/review/index.htm—review courses
  /exams2.htm—for exam results
- ANA website—www.nursesbooks.org—catalog of ANA nursing scope and standards publications and other titles that may be listed on your test content outline, such as *Scope and Standards of Advanced Practice Registered Nursing*, ANA 1966, Pub. No. ADV-1.
- AANP website. Available at: www.aanp.org/certic.htm.
- National Conference of Gerontological Nurse Practitioners. Available at: http://www.ncgnp.org.
- National Guideline Clearinghouse. Available at: www.guideline.gov.

DIMENSIONS OF THE NP ROLE

HISTORY OF THE NP ROLE

The NP role began in 1965 at the University of Colorado, the brainchild of Henry K. Silver, MD, of the School of Medicine, and Loretta C. Ford, PhD, of the School of Nursing. Dr. Ford, who taught within the community health program at the School of Nursing, designed the original continuing education program for experienced community health nurses. They published extensively about their success in having experienced registered nurses with advanced training and skills additionally perform some of the clinical duties traditionally reserved for physicians. The Colorado program was established in the same year that the physician assistant role was being developed at Duke University. These early PNP programs were the prototype for all NP educational programs.

Early certificate-level NP programs were typically sixteen weeks in length. Many schools offered an NP certificate as part of a broader master's in Nursing curriculum. However, these CE programs were open to RNs with all types of preparation, including RNs with diploma and associate degrees that would not have been eligible for the MS programs. The first guidelines for PNP programs were published in a joint document from the American Nurses Association and the American Academy of Pediatrics in 1970. The National Board of PNP/A established an accreditation mechanism in 1973; the ANA quickly followed with moves to accredit these CE programs. Both organizations recognized the importance of achieving some standardization and control over quality.

The first certification exams for PNPs were offered by the American Nurses Association in the fall of 1976. Later, the American Nurses Credentialing Center (www.nursingworld.org/ancc) was established to write exams for nurses in all areas of practice.

The NP role gained momentum as a wide variety of programs were established in the late 1970s and early 1980s, fueled by the federal government's concern about the "shortage" of physicians and the realization that nurses were an underutilized resource in primary health care. This led to the Division of Nursing's funding of the first NP programs in Schools of Nursing. In addition, the Robert Wood Johnson Foundation fully funded "gold star" NP programs throughout the United States in 1980 and provided additional funding for "gold star" faculty to attend these programs. Most of these early programs were joint efforts of Schools of Medicine and Nursing.

The role of the GNP was developed through projects that emphasized the role of the GNP in nursing homes. The Mountain States Health Corporation project received funding from the W. K. Kellogg Foundation in 1976 to build a GNP program. The purpose was to improve the quality of care to elderly clients in long-term care facilities and other community settings. The impact of the gerontological nurse practitioners from this project was studied extensively, including patient care outcomes and career paths of the graduates. The Teaching Nursing Home Project funded by the Robert Wood Johnson Foundation emphasized improvement of care and utilization of GNPs in isolated healthcare institutions. As the GNP moved from the nursing home to other settings, the GNP model of practice became more varied. A newsletter from 1983 has job offerings for GNPs as a patient care coordinator, to establish a new program for 1100 geriatric community residents and to coordinate geriatric programs for a regional medical center.

Nurse practitioners have worked to have the nurse practice acts revised or replaced in all 50 states in order to recognize the diagnostic and treatment functions of the role. GNPs are prepared to provide a wide variety of services in a variety of clinical settings. GNPs can now be found in many settings: the nursing home, rehabilitation centers, primary care practices, clinics, Program for All-inclusive Care of the Elderly (PACE), Veteran's Administration Medical Centers, life care retirement communities, assisted-living facilities, adult day care centers, homecare, and hospitals.

Nurse practitioners rely heavily on their nursing education and background, integrating new assessment skills and diagnostic and treatment knowledge, to develop a totally new role. Their level of competence has brought growing acceptance of the NP role into the healthcare system.

CLINICAL PRACTICE OF GERONTOLOGICAL NURSE PRACTITIONERS

In 2003, the National Council of Gerontological Nurse Practitioners developed a position paper on GNP practice. In this paper they say that "Gerontological Nurse Practitioners (GNPs) are advanced practice nurses with specialized education in the diagnosis, treatment and management of acute and chronic conditions often found among older adults and generally associated with aging. Many such conditions lead to functional decline requiring therapeutic interventions to restore or maintain an optimal level of function or, when appropriate, palliative care. Such chronic or debilitating conditions are often complex and can occur in younger adults. The GNP has the clinical expertise to care for such aging persons.

"Practice sites of Gerontological Nurse Practitioners include traditional ambulatory care clinics, care management companies, acute and sub-acute hospitals, private homes, and all levels of long-term care. The GNP may treat adults of any age who have acute and chronic conditions. Other GNPs work in specialty areas with expanded scopes of practice that require specialized education and close collaboration with other healthcare providers.

"Gerontological Nurse Practitioners have been subjected to various age-related practice restrictions. Such restrictions are based upon the perception that practice scopes are defined by certification category rather than by education, ability, experience, and collaborative practice agreements. The National Council of State Boards of Nursing (1993) concluded that certification did not include a defined scope of practice. The Council stated, 'while different requirements for various areas of nursing may be acceptable for professional certification, inconsistency becomes problematic when attempts are made to apply professional certification requirements to regulatory systems.'

"NCGNP supports the position that the scope of practice of Gerontological Nurse Practitioners is concerned with the health problems of older adults that are generally associated with aging. Further, NCGNP supports the ANA (1996) position that 'the individual advanced practice registered nurse is responsible for identifying the scope of practice permitted by state and federal laws and regulations, the professional code of ethics, and professional practice standards.' Furthermore, the GNP's competence is circumscribed by his or her experience, education, knowledge, and abilities."

The National Council of Gerontological Nurse Practitioners' position paper includes the following as positions they have taken:

- Gerontological Nurse Practitioners (GNPs) are educated through nurse practitioner programs at the master's or post-master's level to meet the medical, bio-psycho-social, and functional needs of aging persons with acute and chronic illnesses through appropriate assessment, diagnostic, and management activities.
- GNPs have received advanced nursing education and training in the health problems of adults. All GNPs have received specialized education and training in the diagnosis, treatment, and management of acute and chronic conditions commonly found among older adults and generally associated with aging. The GNP may treat adults of any age who have acute and chronic conditions. The diversity of client groups served by GNPs is reflected in their varied practice settings and individualized scopes of practice.

- GNPs are recognized as advanced practice nurses in accordance with individual state rules and regulations concerning advanced practice nursing. Generally, GNPs are required to have specialty certification through a nationally recognized credentialing center.
- GNP scope of practice may be limited to a particular client group as delineated by the GNP's individualized scope of practice and/or collaborative practice agreements with other healthcare providers based on experience, education, knowledge, and abilities. See www.ncgnp.org.

IMPORTANT FACTORS INFLUENCING THE NP ROLE: LEGAL DIMENSIONS OF THE ROLE

LEGAL AUTHORITY FOR PRACTICE

State Nurse Practice Act—Rules and Regulations

- Authority for NP practice is found in state legislative statutes and in rules and regulations. The Nurse Practice Act of every state customarily authorizes the Boards of Nursing to establish statutory authority to define who may be called a nurse practitioner (title protection); what they may do (scope of practice); restrictions on their practice; the requirements an NP must meet in order to be credentialed within the state as an NP (educational, certification, etc.); and disciplinary grounds for infraction of regulations. (See http://www.ncsbn.org for listing of state nursing board requirements.) In many states, legislative acts may specifically require that an NP develop a collaborative agreement with a physician, describe what types of drugs might be prescribed, or define some form of oversight board for NP practice.
- Statutory law is implemented in regulatory language. The rules and regulations for each state may further define scope of practice and practice requirements and/or restrictions.
- Beginning in 1999, the National Council State Boards of Nursing (NCSBN) began implementation of an interstate compact for nursing practice to reduce state-to-state discrepancies in nursing requirements to practice. The Advanced Practice Registered Nurse (APRN) Compact addresses the need to promote consistent access to quality advanced practice nursing care within states and across state lines. The Uniform APRN Licensure/Authority to Practice Requirements, developed by NCSBN with APRN stakeholders in 2000, establishes the foundation for this APRN Compact. Similar to the existing Nurse Licensure Compact for recognition of RN and LPN licenses, the APRN Compact offers states the mechanism for mutually recognizing APRN licenses/authority to practice. A state must either be a member of the current nurse licensure compact for RN and LPN or choose to enter into both compacts simultaneously to be eligible for the APRN Compact. To determine which states participate, view the state compact map at www.ncsbn.org/nlc/index.asp.

NURSE PRACTITIONER PROFESSIONAL PRACTICE

Licensure

- "A process by which an agency of state government grants permission to individuals accountable for the practice of a profession to engage in the practice of that profession and prohibits all others from legally doing so." (DHEW, 1971)
- The purpose is to protect the public by ensuring a minimum level of professional competence. "This regulatory method is used when regulated activities are complex, require specialized knowledge, skill and independent decision-making. The licensure process includes the predetermination of qualifications necessary to perform a legally defined scope of practice safely and an evaluation of licensure applications to determine that the qualifications are met. Licensure provides that a specified scope of practice may only be performed legally by licensed individuals. Licensure provides title protection for those roles. It also provides authority to take disciplinary action should the licensee violate provision of the law or rules in order to assure that the public health, safety and welfare will be reasonably well protected." (NCSBN, http://www.ncsbn.org/regulation/nlc_licensure_aprn.asp, accessed 09/18/04)

Certification

- "A process by which a non-governmental agency or association certifies that an individual licensed to practice as a professional has met certain predetermined standards specified by that profession for specialty practice." (DHEW, 1971)
- The purpose is to assure the public that an individual has mastery of a body of knowledge and has acquired the skills necessary to function in a particular specialty. Some certifications are required for entry into practice (e.g., required for licensure within a state and thus have a regulatory function); some certifications denote professional competence and recognize excellence.

Accreditation

- "The process by which a voluntary, non-governmental agency or organization appraises and grants accreditation status to institutions and/or programs or services which meet predetermined structure, process and outcome criteria." (DHEW, 1971) The purpose is to assure that the organization has met specific standards.

Scope of practice

- Defines a specific legal scope determined by state statutes, boards of nursing, educational preparation, and common practice within a community. For example, ANPs are not legally authorized to care for children. The state might require an NP to have formal educational preparation in pediatrics. Broad variation exists from state to state.
- General scope of practice is specified in many published professional documents (e.g., *Scope and Standards of Advanced Practice Registered Nursing*, ANA, 1996). In addition, many organizations have completed role delineation studies that attempt to qualify the core behaviors that all APNs must possess, as well as the core knowledge and behaviors required of individuals in a particular specialty. For example, core knowledge for a PNP will be inherently different from that of a GNP. It is critical that these statements about specific scope and standards exist so that everyone—including nurses—will have access to materials to which they can refer when there are specific questions related to role. This is especially important when the traditional role of nurses is being changed or "advanced" at an uneven rate through changes in state law. As the nurse practitioner role has expanded into new practice settings, including hospice, hospitals, and home care, it is important that core knowledge as well as state law protecting NPs in these practice settings expand also, providing the legal authorization and title protection necessary for these practice settings.
- Prescriptive authority is recognized as within the scope of practice for nurse practitioners in all fifty states, though there is significant variability from state to state. This has created inherent difficulty in collecting data related to NP prescribing practices. A comprehensive update of legislative requirements and recent changes is published each by the *Nurse Practitioner Journal* in the January issue. Data collected by Nurse Practitioner Alternatives, Inc. since 1996 has documented stability within prescribing patterns by NPs. Data from 2004 documents that the majority of NPs possess their own Drug Enforcement Administration (DEA) number (72%), write between six and twenty-five prescriptions in an average clinical day (79%), recommend between one and twenty over-the-counter (OTC) preparations in an average clinical day (90%), and manage between 25% and 100% of their patient encounters independently (97%). (www.npedu.com)

Standards of practice

- Authoritative statements by which the quality of practice, service, or education can be judged (e.g., Scope and Standards of Advanced Practice Registered Nursing). (ANA, 1996)
- Professional standards focus on the minimum levels of acceptable performance as a way of providing consumers with a means of measuring the quality of care they receive. They may be written at the generic level to apply to all nurses (e.g., following universal precautions), as well as to define practice by each specialty.

- The presence of accepted standards of practice may be used to legally describe the standard of care that must be met by a provider. These standards may be precise protocols that must be followed or more recommendations for more general guidelines.
- *Healthy People 2010 Objectives* and WHO *"Health for All"* are, respectively, national and international policy statements that describe the objectives to be met to help all persons to obtain a level of health that will permit them to lead socially and economically productive lives. It is anticipated that, over time, these objectives will form the basis for international standards of practice.

CLIENT RIGHTS

Confidentiality
- The patient and family have a right to assume that information given to the healthcare provider will not be disclosed. This has several dimensions:
  - Verbal information—Healthcare providers shall not discuss any information given to them during the healthcare encounter with anyone not directly involved in providing this care without the patient's or family's permission.
  - Written information—Confidentiality of the healthcare encounter is protected under federal statute through Health Insurance Portability and Accountability Act of 1996 (HIPAA). The Administrative Simplification provisions of HIPAA require the Department of Health and Human Services to establish national standards for electronic healthcare transactions and national identifiers for providers, health plans, and employers. It also addresses the security and privacy of health data. Information may be accessed at http://www.cms.hhs.gov/hipaa/default.asp?
  - The individual's right to privacy is respected when requesting or responding to a request for a patient's medical record.
  - The statute requires that the provider discuss confidentiality issues with patients or parents in the case of a minor, establish consent, and clarify any questions about disclosure of information.
  - The provider is required to obtain a signed medical authorization and consent form to release medical records and information.
- Exceptions to guaranteed confidentiality occur when society determines that the need for information outweighs the principle of confidentiality. Examples might be when records are released to insurance companies or to attorneys involved in litigation; answering court orders, subpoenas, summonses; in meeting state requirements for mandatory reporting of diseases or conditions; cases of suspected child abuse; or if a patient reveals an intent to harm someone.

Informed consent
- The clinician has the duty to explain relevant information to the patient and family so that the family can make an appropriate decision. This information usually includes diagnosis, nature and purpose of proposed treatment or procedure, risks and benefits, prognosis, alternative methods of treatment and their risks and benefits, and even the remote possibility of serious harm.
- It must be documented in medical records that this information has been provided.

Advance directives
- When a patient is incapable of making decisions, a person's preferences may be expressed by way of a written living will or a healthcare durable power of attorney when he or she is still competent.
  - Living wills are written documents prepared in advance in case of terminal illness or non-reversible loss of consciousness.
    - Their provisions go into effect when:
      The individual has become incompetent
      When the patient is declared terminally ill
      No further interventions will alter the patient's course to a reasonable degree of medical certainty

Durable power of attorney for health care
- Individuals can identify in writing an agent to act on their behalf should they become mentally incapacitated. The decisions of the designated agent are:
  - Binding
  - Not limited to the circumstances of terminal illness
  - Flexible enough to carry out patient's wishes throughout the course of an illness
  - Often accompanied by a durable power of attorney over financial issues as well

Ethical decision making
- Moral concepts such as advocacy, accountability, loyalty, caring, compassion, and human dignity are the foundations of ethical behavior.
- The ethical behavior of nurses has been defined for professional nursing in an American Nurses Association policy statement. (ANA, 1988)
- Ethical behavior incorporates respect for the individual and his or her autonomy. Thus, no decision is truly ethical if the caregiver does not involve the patient in decision making to the full extent of the patient's capacity.
- Duty to help others (beneficence), avoidance of harmful behavior (nonmaleficence), and fairness are also foundational components of ethical behavior.

Quality assurance
- A system to evaluate and monitor the quality of patient care and the quality of facility management.
- Formal programs provide a framework for systematic, deliberate, and continuous evaluation and monitoring of individual clinical practice. Programs promote responsibility and accountability to deliver high-quality care, assist in the evaluation and improvement of patient care, and provide for an organized means of problem solving. Thus, a good program identifies educational needs, improves the documentation of care, and, overall, reduces the clinician's exposure to liability.
- Programs identify components of structure, process, and outcomes of care. They also look at organization effectiveness, efficiency, and client and provider interactions.
- These may be implemented through audits, utilization review, peer review, outcome studies, and measurements of patient satisfaction.

NURSE PRACTITIONER LEGAL AND FINANCIAL ISSUES
Liability
- Sources of legal risk
  - Patients, procedures
  - Quality of medical records
- Risk reduction or management
  - Activities or systems designed to recognize and intervene to reduce the risk of injury to patients and subsequent claims against healthcare providers.
  - Malpractice insurance does not protect a clinician from charges of practicing outside his or her legal scope of practice. It is universally recommended that all clinicians carry their own liability insurance coverage so they will have their own legal representation and attorney to advocate for them.
- Malpractice
  - Negligent professional acts of individuals engaged in professions requiring highly technical or professional skills
  - The plaintiff has the burden of proving four elements of malpractice:
    - Duty—The clinician has the duty to exercise reasonable care when undertaking and providing treatment to the patient when a patient–clinician relationship exists.
    - Breach of duty—The clinician violates the applicable standard of care in treating the patient's condition.

- Proximate cause—There is a causal relationship between the breach in the standard of care and the patient's injuries.
  - Damages—There are permanent and substantial damages to the patient as a result of the malpractice.
- National Practitioner Databank
  - The Health Care Quality Improvement Act of 1986 established a databank to scrutinize members of the healthcare profession and list those practitioners who have had a malpractice claim asserted against them.
  - Currently, very few NPs are listed in the National Practitioner Databank. There is very little history of successful litigation against NPs.

Reimbursement

- NPs are reimbursed as primary care providers in some form for their services under Medicare, Medicaid, Federal Employee Benefit Plan, Champus, Veterans and Military programs, and federally funded school-based clinics.
- Private insurance plans may elect to reimburse for NP services even if not mandated by state law. In some states, the insurance code may be interpreted rigidly to exclude reimbursement of NPs.
- Managed Care Organizations (MCOs) have frequently excluded NPs from being designated as primary care providers and allowing their own caseload. Thus, in many MCOs, the only employment arrangement left open to NPs is that of being a salaried employee. As a salaried employee, the NP contributions are often not visible and may be credited to their collaborating physicians, giving them a "ghost" provider status. Without a legitimate method to document services provided and revenue generated, NP job security is often at risk. A recent focus of legislative activity by many state NP organizations has been to enact state law that allows for NPs to be impaneled as primary care providers in both health maintenance organizations (HMOs) and preferred provider organizations (PPOs). These efforts have led to opposition from state medical organizations.
- There is considerable flux in state and national policy on what services and procedures NPs may bill for and whether they will be paid directly. Incorrect billing places the healthcare provider at risk of fraud and abuse charges whether they knowingly violate the law or are just ignorant of the regulations.
- NPs must be aware of specific regulations and policies for patient care services. Resources include Health Care Financing Agency bulletins, among others. See http://www.hcfa.gov.

Performance assessment

- The National Practitioner Data Bank (NPDB) and Health Integrity and Protection Data Bank (HIPDB) are maintained by the US Department of Health and Human Services (HHS), Health Resources and Services Administration (HRSA), Bureau of Health Professions (BHP), and Division of Practitioner Data Banks (DPDB). Developed as a result of the Health Care Quality and Improvement Act of 1986, the NPDB/HIPDB is a flagging system intended to facilitate a comprehensive review of healthcare practitioners' professional credentials. The information contained in the NPDB is intended to direct inquiry into a practitioner's licensure, professional society memberships, malpractice payment history, and record of clinical privileges, with a goal of improving the quality of health care. NPs may perform a self-query by visiting the site at http://www.npdb-hipdb.com/.
- Other programs monitoring and comparing health quality include the Health Plan Employer Data and Information Set (HEDIS®) developed by the National Committee on Quality Assurance (NCQA). HEDIS is a set of standardized performance measures designed to ensure that purchasers and consumers have the information they need to reliably compare the performance of managed healthcare plans. See http://www.ncqa.org/Programs/HEDIS/.

Current Trends

Some of the topics dominating NPs' discussions about their future

1. Fiscal issues
- Growing competition in job market for NPs as numbers of NPs have increased and NPs have begun to directly compete with physicians and physician assistants
- Reimbursement struggles with Medicare, private insurance
- Increasing costs for malpractice insurance. Many states have launched legislative initiatives in the area of medical tort reform in an attempt to hold down malpractice premiums.
- Beginning in May 2005, as a result of HIPAA, the Center for Medicare and Medicaid Services (CMS) will begin implementing a requirement that providers obtain a National Provider Identifier (NPI). All healthcare providers are eligible to be assigned NPIs. Information may be obtained at http://www.cms.hhs.gov/hipaa/hipaa2/default.asp.
- Growing concerns over reimbursement fraud and abuse issues as well as coding issues, both in the area of overbilling and underbilling, particularly for Medicare patients

2. NP education
- Recognition of need to ensure quality of NP education, faculty, and curriculum has led to efforts by the National Organization of Nurse Practitioner Faculties (NONPF) and the American Association of Colleges of Nursing (AACN) to promulgate core competency statements. These can be viewed at http://www.nonpf.org/finalaug2002.pdf.
- In addition, NONPF and AACN, along with numerous NP professional organizations, NP accrediting bodies, and educational organizations, have jointly promulgated criteria for evaluation of nurse practitioner programs. In combination with accreditation standards for graduate programs and for specialty areas, the criteria provide a basis for evaluating the quality of nurse practitioner programs. Documents may be viewed at http://www.nonpf.org/evalcriteria2002.pdf.
- As an alternative to research-focused doctoral degrees, the American Association of Colleges of Nursing, working with the National Organization of Nurse Practitioner Faculties (with input from other groups), has developed recommendations for a Practice Doctorate in Nursing that will be the degree associated with practice-focused doctoral nursing education. It is suggested that the practice doctorate in the future is to be the graduate degree for advanced nursing practice preparation, including but not limited to the four current APN roles: clinical nurse specialist, nurse anesthetist, nurse midwife, and nurse practitioner. A transition period would be planned to provide nurses with master's degrees who wish to obtain the practice doctoral degree, a mechanism to earn a practice doctorate in a relatively streamlined fashion with credit given for previous graduate study and practice experience. The transition mechanism would provide multiple points of entry, standardized validation of competencies, and be time limited. The draft also recommends that current APNs would not be required to obtain a DNP. (See http://www.aacn.nche.edu/.)

3. Practice environment
- Health disparities—There is growing recognition of disparities in the health services and outcomes of different populations in the United States. The National Center on Minority Health and Health Disparities (NCMHD) at the National Institutes of Health (NIH) is a government organization with a mission to promote minority health and to lead, coordinate, support, and assess the NIH effort to reduce and ultimately eliminate health disparities. See http://ncmhd.nih.gov/.
- Health literacy—It is now recognized that one of the largest contributors to health outcome is the ability of a patient and family to understand and act on health information. Both the Institute of Medicine (IOM) and the Agency for Health Care Research and Quality (AHRQ) have launched efforts to quantify and offer solutions to the problems that result from inadequate

health literacy. The IOM report may be viewed at http://www.iom.edu/report.asp?id=19723; the AHRQ study can be found at http://www.ahrq.gov/news/press/pr2004/litpr.htm.

- Patient Bill of Rights—In 2004, both the Senate and House passed different versions of a Patient Bill of Rights. These bills are an attempt to ensure that patients have access to their provider of choice and have access to an independent external appeals process to address health plan grievances. The bills have not yet been approved by a joint committee or been sent to the office of the president for signature. It is critical that NPs monitor legislation in this area to ensure that the rights of nonphysician providers are protected.

- There is increasing attention being paid to preparing registered nurses to gain disaster education so that they are prepared to assume emergency roles during a time of mass casualties from either natural disasters or terrorist attacks. Because some other countries have had more experience in dealing with terrorism, The International Nursing Coalition for Mass Casualty Education has been established and headquartered at Vanderbilt School of Nursing to help US nurses profit from their experience and to identify the educational competencies for registered nurses responding to mass casualty incidents. They desire to improve the ability of all nurses to respond safely and effectively to mass casualty incidents through identification of existing and emerging roles of nurses, ensuring appropriateness of education in mass casualty incidents, and helping to understand response frameworks and to ensure collaborative efforts. All NPs are expected to prepare themselves to play a larger role in delivery of care during a time of disaster. Information of the objectives and work that has been done toward a uniform curriculum in this area may be obtained through the Internet at www.incmce.org.

- Direct-to-consumer advertising—Patients frequently present to the office already having formed their diagnosis and wanting specific treatments. NPs are required to become knowledgeable about the newest products on the markets in order to appropriately counsel and treat patients.

- There is greater recognition of the use of complementary and alternative medicine by consumers. Research suggests that 40% to 50% of patients are currently using a form of complementary or alternative (CAM) therapy today, despite the fact that there is little research on which to base treatment regimens. NPs as providers need to learn about common CAM treatments and particularly about how some of the herbal products interact adversely with prescription drugs. The National Institutes of Health have established a center to begin research on these popular preparations. Until that time, it is suggested that providers need to move cautiously in prescribing these preparations for their patients. See http://www.nih.cam.gov.

- Since release of the Institute of Medicine's report To Err Is Human: Building a Safer Health System, http://www.iom.edu/report.asp?id=5575, there has been increased attention on changes all healthcare providers should make to decrease medical errors. In response, the Joint Commission on Accreditation of Healthcare Organizations (JCAHO), http://www.jcaho.org/, has issued a list of abbreviations that should not be used in health care, and the Institute for Safe Medication Practices (ISMP) has published a list of dangerous abbreviations related to medication use that it recommends should be explicitly prohibited (http://www.ismp.org/). The list of banned abbreviations includes many symbols traditionally used on patient charts and in writing prescriptions.

Professional Organizations

- Participation in professional organizations is important because nurse practitioners acting as a group can have more influence over our profession.
- State organizations: Every NP should belong to his or her state NP organization. State organizations work diligently to monitor and affect laws and regulations affecting NP practice. In addition, these associations provide a group of peers for discussion and continuing education.
- The American College of Nurse Practitioners (ACNP) is focused on advocacy and keeping NPs current on legislative, regulatory, and clinical practice issues that affect NPs in the rapidly changing healthcare arena. See www.nurse.org/acnp.

- The National Council of Gerontological Nurse Practitioners (NCGNP) is the professional organization that advocates for geriatric nurse practitioners who deliver health care in a variety of settings.
- The National Organization of Nurse Practitioner Faculties (NONPF) is an organization of nurse practitioner educators who are instrumental in setting standards for nurse practitioner education. NONPF has developed core competencies describing the domains of practice with critical behaviors that should be exhibited by all entry-level NPs. Originally written in 1995, the revised edition became available in 2000 to reflect the current NP practice. See www.nonpf.com.

CASE STUDIES

Case 1. Your 92-year-old female patient, who lives alone at home, has fallen several times in the past few months. She refuses to have physical therapy or to move to an assisted-living or nursing home. Her daughter, who has not talked to her for the past 10 years, wants you to sign a document stating that her mother is not competent so she can put her in a nursing home. The daughter also wants a copy of her mother's chart.
1. What are the legal issues involved?
2. Should you tell the daughter about the patient's condition or give her a copy of the chart?
3. Can you determine from the information given that the patient is not competent?

Case 2. An 82-year-old man is found to have lung cancer. This was an incidental finding on CXR for admission to assisted living. He has no symptoms. He is a widower with one son.
1. What healthcare documents would you ask the patient about?
2. What healthcare decisions would you look for on his durable power of attorney?
3. How would you decide how aggressively to manage this patient?
4. The patient becomes incompetent without writing down his wishes. You need to decide whether to put in a feeding tube. What question do you pose to the son?

Case 3. You just graduated from your nurse practitioner program.
1. What additional qualifications do you need in order to practice?

REFERENCES

American Nurses Association. (2000). Medicare and "Incident To" payment: Coverage of nursing services in hospital outpatient clinics and emergency departments. See http://www.ana.org/readroom/incident2/htm.

American Nurses Association. (1988). *Ethics in nursing: Position statements and guidelines.* Washington, DC: ANA Publication No. G-175.

American Nurses Association. (1996). *Scope and standards of advanced practice registered nursing.* Washington, DC: ANA Publication No. ADV-10.

American Nurses Credentialing Center. (2001). *ANCC certification.* Washington, DC: Author.

Baxter, M. L. (1999). Ethical issues. In J. T. Stone, J. F. Wyman, S. A. Salisbury (Eds.), *Clinical gerontological nursing* (2nd ed.). Philadelphia: W. B. Saunders.

Birren, J. E., & Schaie, K.W. (Eds.). (2001). *Handbook of the psychology of aging* (5th ed.). San Diego: Academic Press.

Buppert, C. (1999). *Nurse practitioners' business practice and legal guide.* Gaithersburg, MD: Aspen Publishers.

Burggraf, V. (1999). Advanced practice of gerontological nursing. In J. T. Stone, J. F. Wyman, S. A. Salisbury (Eds.), *Clinical gerontological nursing* (2nd ed.). Philadelphia: W. B. Saunders.

Ebersole, P. (1985). Geriatric nurse practitioners past and present. *Geriatric Nursing.* 6, 219–222.

Edmunds, M.W., & Mayhew, M.S. (2004). *Pharmacology for primary care providers* (2nd ed.). St. Louis: Mosby.

Federation of State Medical Boards of the United States. Non-physician duties and scope of practice position statement 210.003; July 1988.

Ford, L. C. (1992). Advanced nursing practice: Future of the nurse practitioner. In L. H. Aiken, C. M. Fagin (Eds.), *Charting nursing's future. Agenda for the 1990s*. Philadelphia: J. B. Lippincott.

The Institute of Medicine. (1999). To err is human: Building a safe healthcare system. Available at: http://www.iom.edu/report.asp?id=5575. Accessed November 28, 2004.

The Institute for the Futures. (2000). *Health & health care 2010: The forecast, the challenge*. San Francisco, CA: Jossey-Bass.

Kane, R. A., Kane, R. L., Arnold, S., Garrard, J., McDermont, S., & Keperele, L. (1988). Geriatric nurse practitioners as nursing home employees: Implementing the role. *The Gerontologist, 28*(4), 469–477.

McDougall, G. J., Roberts, B. (1993). A gerontologic nurse practitioner in every nursing home: A necessary expenditure. *Geriatric Nursing, 14*(4), 218–220.

Mullen, F., Plitzer, R. M., Lewis, C. T., et al. (1992). The National Practitioner Data Bank: Report from the First Year. *JAMA, 268*, 73–79.

Munden, J. (Ed.). (2001). *Nurse practitioner's legal reference*. Springhouse, PA: Springhouse Corporation.

National Council of State Boards of Nursing. (1993). Regulation of advanced nursing practice. National Council Position Paper, 1993. Chicago, IL: Author.

National Organization of Nurse Practitioner Faculties (NONPF). (2002). Nurse practitioner primary care competencies in specialty areas: Adult, family, gerontological, pediatric, and women's health. Washington, DC: Author.

Pearson, L. J. (2004). Annual update of how each state stands on legislative issues affecting advanced nursing practice. *The Nurse Practitioner, 29*(1), 26–51.

Radosevich, D. M., et al. (1990). Career paths of geriatric nurse practitioners employed in nursing homes. *Public Health Reports. 105*(1), 65–71.

Safreit, B. (Summer 1992). Health care dollars and regulatory sense: The role of advanced practice nursing. *Yale J Regulation, 9* (2), 417–488.

USDHHS, Division of Nursing. (2002). *Nurse practitioner primary care competencies in specialty areas: Adult, family, gerontological, pediatric, and women's health*. Washington, DC: US Department of Health and Human Services, Health Resources and Services Administration, Bureau of Health Professions.

US DHEW. *Report on licensure and related health personnel credentials*. Washington, DC: USDHEW Publication No. (HSM) 72–11.

US Office of Technology Assessment. (1986). Nurse practitioners, physician's assistants and certified nurse midwives: A policy analysis. Washington, DC: US Government Printing Office.

Walker, L., & Wetle, T. (1999). Ethical issues. In S. L. Molony, C. M. Waszynski, C. H. Lyder. *Gerontological nursing: An advanced practice approach*. Stamford, CN: Appleton & Lange.

HEALTH CARE ISSUES 3

GERIATRICS

- Most people use the age 65 to mark the beginning of geriatrics.
- Perhaps the most important public health concern of the early 21st century is the increasing numbers of individuals aged 65 and older.
- Not only will this number double in the next 20 years, but individuals who are not 65 years of age will, on average, live for another 20 years.
- Often geriatrics is divided into the young old (65 to 74), the old (75 to 84), and the oldest old (85 and above).
- Within those older than 65, the fastest growing subgroup is those over age 85.
- Variability between patients increases with age. This book presents many generalizations about the elderly. Just remember that every patient is unique.
- Cultural diversity continues to be an important factor in the assessment and management of the elderly.

Assessment

Nonspecific Presentation of Illness
- A crucial aspect of geriatrics is that the elderly often present with vague complaints or deterioration of functional independence as an early subtle sign of illness.
- This generally occurs in the absence of classical (typical) symptoms and signs of disease.
- When older adults become acutely ill, they most often present with:
  - Confusion, delirium, mental status changes: altered attention and orientation
  - Worsening dementia or delirium superimposed on dementia
  - Increased difficulty or taking longer to perform ADLs
  - Incontinence
  - Falls
  - Dizziness
  - Vague, generalized nonspecific pain
  - Decreased appetite, weight loss, failure to thrive
  - May not have high fever or increased WBC in presence of severe infection

Assessment of the Elderly
- **Functional status determines quality of life to an elderly patient.**
- Elderly define health in terms of independent function, not medical diagnosis.
- Elderly often have multiple chronic medical conditions that cannot be cured; therefore, care is focused on maintaining function while managing illness.
- An important difference from adult medicine is the need for systematic assessment of the complex and multisystem problems of the geriatric patient encompassing both medical and social needs.

- It is advisable to utilize appropriate standardized assessment instruments to measure factors relevant to patients' abilities.
- Assessment tools provide standardized data to follow trends and evaluate response to treatment.
- Cognitive and functional assessments are the keystone to geriatrics.
- Each GNP should have a set of assessment tools appropriate to his or her practice. See the book by Kane and Kane in the reference section.
- Components of a complete assessment of the elderly are:
  - Physiologic—normal changes of aging, medical diagnoses
  - Cognitive (mental status)—Folstein Mini-Mental State Exam (MMSE)
  - Functional—ADLs, IADLs, mobility, activities, get up and go test, Tinneti
  - Social—relationships, support systems
  - Psychological—anxiety, hope, depression, Geriatric Depression Scale
  - Nutritional in terms of appropriate weight and adequate intake of nutrients, nutritional assessment tool
  - Economic—ability to pay for medications and health insurance as well as basic needs food, housing, and utilities
  - Others—spiritual, physical environment, stressors, coping skills, values, quality of life

Cognitive Function

- Essential to differentiate between normal changes of cognitive function and dementia and delirium
- Many assessment tools have been developed
- MMSE is the most famous, used as a screening test but is not highly sensitive
- Other good dementia screening tools are the short portable mental status questionnaire and the clock drawing test
- Consider culture and education when interpreting score
- Cognitive function is divided into domains:
  - Attention—maintenance of alertness over time
  - Memory—ability to collect, store, and retrieve information
  - Orientation—memory of person, place, and time
  - Language—use and understand oral and written communication
  - Visuospatial abilities—perceive objects and spatial relationships
  - Psychomotor speed—rate of cognitive processing
  - Executive/problem solving—higher cognitive skills—judgment, insight, and abstract thinking, difficult to describe or assess
  - Intelligence—global levels of general cognitive functioning
- Memory is further divided into:
  - Working memory—ability to manipulate remembered items
  - Recent memory—memory of events with the last 24 hours, the first type of memory to go in dementia
  - Remote memory—memory of events that occurred in the distant past, often preserved late in dementia
  - Implicit and procedural memory—memory without awareness, memory to do a previously learned task such as dressing and eating

Functional Assessment

- Those activities of daily living necessary to survive in society
- They are usually divided into three categories:
  - Activities of daily living include bathing, dressing, eating, grooming, toileting, continence of bowel and bladder, and transferring

- Absolutely essential basic assessment of the elderly, as in nonspecific presentation of illness in the elderly
    - Many assessment tools; most famous is Katz
  - Instrumental activities of daily living include cooking, shopping, cleaning, money management, use of transportation, use of telephone, and medication administration; more complex tasks than the ADL
    - Common scale used is Lawton & Brody Instrumental Activities of Daily Living scale, OARS-IADL
  - Mobility includes walking, stairs, balance and transferring, the get up and go test is a common assessment tool; also Tinetti
- When using one of the functional assessment tools, judge:
  - Amount of human assistance required: independent, supervision, cuing/organization, hands-on help, dependent (total help)
  - Speed of performance
  - Degree of pain during performance, endurance
  - Quality of performance
  - Safety
- When relying on self-report, patients tend to overestimate ability while families and caregivers tend to underestimate
- Assistive devices help the patient prolong independence. These include hearing aids, glasses, respiratory equipment, and mobility aids, such as canes and walkers

Demographics/Epidemiology
- Population
  - The older population is large, growing fast, and becoming more diverse.
  - 13% of population is 65 or older; in 2020, 20% will be 65 or older
  - Includes 2% 85+; age 85+ growing fastest
  - Still largely white; other groups growing faster
  - More women than men: 59% at 65+; 71% at 85+
  - Nursing homes—5% reside in NH: 1% of ages 65 to 74; 20% of 85+
  - 33% are living alone
  - 10% live in poverty; higher among black and Hispanic
- Life expectancy
  - At birth, women 79.4 years; men 73.6
  - Women aged 65 can expect to live to 84; women aged 85 can expect to live to 92
  - Women live longer than men
  - Shorter expectancy among black and Hispanic
- Mortality
  - Leading causes of death

Heart disease	35%
Cancer	35%
Stroke	10%
COPD	6%
Pneumonia/influenza	7%

    Other: diabetes, Alzheimer disease, nephritis, accidents, septicemia
- Morbidity
  - Chronic conditions are prolonged illnesses that are generally never cured completely
  - In noninstitutionalized persons 70 years of age and older, 79% had at least 1 of the 7 chronic conditions common among the elderly:

Arthritis	63%
Hypertension	40%
Heart disease	25%
Respiratory illnesses	11%
Diabetes	11%
Stroke	9%
Cancer	4%

- Impairments commonly occur in older adults
  - Visual impairment
  - Hearing impairment
  - Decreased functional abilities
    3% over age 65 and 11% over age 75 report having some difficulty with at least one activity of daily living (ADL)
    7% over age 65 and 22% over age 75 report needing assistance with at least one instrumental activity of daily living (IADL)
    Approximately 15% are unable to walk one-quarter mile
  - There has been a decline in disability in the elderly in recent years

Health Insurance

Medicare
- The federal health insurance program for the elderly, disabled, and end-stage renal disease
- It is run by HCFA, Health Care Financing Administration, which can be found at www.hcfa.gov
- It covers 98% of elderly
- Two Medicare programs:
  - Part A Hospital Insurance
    Covers payments for inpatient hospital care, skilled nursing facility care, hospice care, home health services, and other health services and supplies
    Eligibility is automatic once work requirements are met
    The Hospice benefit may be selected instead of this benefit
  - Part B Supplementary Medical Insurance
    A voluntary plan; approximately 90% choose to enroll, monthly premium
    Covers physician services including office visits, clinical laboratory tests, durable medical equipment, flu vaccinations, drugs that cannot be self-administered, medical supplies, diagnostic tests, ambulance services, and some therapeutic services
    Pays the physician 80% of the allowable cost, as determined by Medicare
- Prescription coverage under Medicare is limited
  - Currently prescriptions cards are available to some; these cards provide discounts on medications
  - Medicare is mandated to provide prescription drug coverage, and plans are underway to develop guidelines for plans that wish to provide these services
- Medicare does not cover custodial care (assistance with ADLs and IADLs), nonskilled care in nursing homes, or assisted living facilities
- Many have a secondary insurance (Medi-gap), which is designed to pay the 20% of what Medicare does not pay
- About 15% of Medicare recipients are enrolled in HMOs

Medicaid is a state program for the poor
- It will fill in the gaps for certain qualifying elderly
- It covers payment for medications

Long-term care insurance
- Private insurance policy purchased in advance; depending on the policy, may reimburse for nursing home care, assisted living, or home health care

- Policies vary on the amount and time of reimbursement; a length of stay may be required before insurance becomes effective
- Currently covers less then 2% of all nursing home expenses and is unlikely to lead to substantial reduction in out-of-pocket expenses and decreased Medicaid use

Social Support
- Social isolation is a common problem in the elderly
  - Their friends and family die
  - They are often are living alone in their own home, unable to drive or use public transportation
  - People engage in fewer social activities as they age
  - Contact with family is the most common social activity
  - Women are more socially active than men
  - Disability limits social interaction
- High-quality interactions with others help individuals maintain or regain health.
- Types of supporting behaviors
- Instrumental support gives direct assistance and service.
  - Informational support uses advice, suggestions, and information in solving problem.
  - Emotional support comes when love, care, empathy, and trust are provided through a relationship
  - Appraisal support uses feedback and affirmation to help persons evaluate themselves
- Caregivers are important to the elderly
  - 35% of elderly have caregivers
  - 90% are unpaid family members, many are over 65 themselves (spouses, children, other relatives or friends)
  - Many elderly have unmet needs because of lack of adequate help; 44% of those needing help, lack enough assistance

Normal Changes of Aging
- What is normal becomes less uniform as patients age
- Many physiologic functions decline with aging. Within an individual, different systems will age more rapidly than others. Mental function is often the one most affected
- It is often difficult to discern what is normal aging, chronic disease, medication effect, or disuse
- Normal changes of aging usually mean less functional reserve: patient or specific organ system fails when stressed. Stress may be physical (infection) or psychological (death of spouse). Specific changes in each system will be discussed in the appropriate chapter
- Chronological age as a marker of functional capacity becomes less accurate as the patient ages. As patients age, their functional status becomes more important and can tell you more about the patient than their medical diagnoses. A patient with CHF can be functioning normally or unable to get out of bed. A 65-year-old with CHF may be less functional then a 90-year-old with CHF
- Geriatric patients are more heterogeneous as a group then younger patients, including response to same medications for the same illness in patients of the same age and sex

The Practice of Geriatrics

Communicating with the Demented Patient
- Get their attention—speak to them; if they don't respond, touch shoulder gently; position yourself so they can see you
- Assess hearing—do they react to what you say?
- Communicate nonverbally—smile, use friendly body language
- Keep it simple—one thought per sentence
- Repeat—in exact same words at first, then rephrase

- Give them time to respond—wait several seconds before asking another question
- Monitor their reaction—are they getting upset or confused?
- Continually adjust your approach
  - If they react quickly, you can speed up
  - If they cannot hear, see instructions below
  - If they get upset, slow down, relax, move back a little, wait until they have calmed down, and try something simpler

How to Obtain a History
- Compensate for the normal sensory changes of aging.
  - Make sure patient can see and hear you
  - Make sure the individual is wearing (clean) glasses and hearing aide (with working battery) if needed.
  - Eliminate background noise.
  - Ensure adequate lighting.
  - Use multiple sources of information: visual, auditory and sensory
- Establish relationship—treat with respect
  - Introduce yourself
  - Use formal address of Mr. or Mrs.
  - Do not condescend, patronize, or assume patient is demented because of age
  - Allow sufficient time with patient so encounter is not rushed
- Get information from patient/family/caregivers/and old records
- Patient is likely to have more than one chief complaint
- Even those with cognitive impairment can provide information about symptoms.
- Observe for symptoms as you ask about them.
  - Pain will be evidenced with a grimace, withdrawal, or aggressive behavior.
  - Give them water to see if they cough when they swallow.
  - Watch them walk, get out of chair
- Use open-ended questions to expand on current problems; geriatric patients may require more yes/no questions to get specific information.
- Repeat questions to confirm findings, ask questions so that they require different answers to validate that the patient understands the question.

The Physical Examination of the Elderly
- Establish the baseline (ask caregiver) and look for a change from baseline.
- Observe behavior—look for changes from baseline and watch for consistency.
- Facilitate exam by organizing evaluation so patient does not have to change position frequently.
- Focus on important, essential elements first in case patient becomes fatigued or agitated.
- Modify instructions—make things as simple as possible.
- Box 3-1 provides ideas for a senior-friendly setting.

Diagnostic Tests
- Does the proposed diagnostic test meet the "so what" test: Would the results change how you would treat the patient?
- Explore the risks versus benefits.
- Explore with the patient his/her willingness and ability to participate in diagnostic tests.
- Ask the older adults if they would consider additional treatment based on the findings of the test.

Management
- Explore with the patient and caregiver treatment options and the impact of each.
- Will the treatment improve quality of life and decrease suffering?

Box 3-1: Guidelines for Senior-Friendly Settings

*Keep the temperature between 70° and 80°F
*Use bright lights and avoid glare by having blinds or shades on windows
*Avoid any background noise (radios, etc.)
*Use higher-than-standard chairs for the waiting room and office rooms
*Have available a broad-based step stool with handrail for transfers to the exam table
*Have available exam tables that mechanically lift the patient from lying to sitting
*Raise the back on the exam table and provide support for sitting
*Have weight scale with bar for stability when getting on and off

- Will the treatment have an impact on outcomes, for example, increase length of life? Improve function? Decrease pain?
- Will the treatment be difficult or unpleasant to tolerate or recover from?
- What is the monetary cost of treatment or prescription? Can the patient pay for the treatment or service? Is there a source of financial assistance? Many pharmaceutical companies have programs for assistance with the cost of their medications. See www.NeedyMeds.com for listing of programs.

Pharmacology (See Table 3-1)

Start Low, Go Slow
- Polypharmacy is common.
  - 85% of those over 65 take medications
  - With multiple drug use, the drug interactions become very high.
  - These tend to be more frequent and serious in the elderly.
  - The effects of alcohol use must be considered.
  - Discontinue drugs as appropriate and evaluate at each visit.
- Drug toxicities are more common and more serious in the elderly.
  - Drug dosage guidelines are usually based on studies in younger people.
  - Recommended adult dosage guidelines are often too high for older patients.
  - Monitor blood levels when appropriate.
  - Behavioral side effects are more common in older people because the blood–brain barrier becomes less effective.
  - When there is an acute change in mental status, medication should always be considered as the cause.
  - The patient presents with fewer classic symptoms.
  - The adverse reaction may take longer to develop; can be months
  - It may be more pronounced once it occurs.
- Over-the-counter drugs can cause problems.
  - Medications considered safe in the adult cause adverse reactions in the elderly.
  - Patients take them because they think they are safe and cheap.
  - They forget to tell the provider they are taking them.
  - There has been an increase in use of herbal remedies and dietary supplements.
    These are not FDA regulated.
    Purity and quality of products may vary.
    Few controlled studies support safety and efficacy of supplements.
- Noncompliance is very common.

Table 3-1: Age-Related Changes That Impact Pharmacotherapy

Pharmaco-kinetics	Definition	Age Changes	Implications
Absorption	Receptor-coupled or diffusional uptake of a drug into the tissue	Increased GI pH Decreased GI motility Decreased absorptive surface area Decreased splanchnic blood flow Decreased first pass effect	Slower absorption and delayed onset Greater bioavailability of drugs with high hepatic extraction (first pass)
Distribution	Movement of the drug into the tissue or body compartment	Decreased total body fluid Increased body fat Decreased lean muscle mass Decreased albumin	Small older adults are more sensitive to usual doses Lipophilic drugs have increased half-life Hydrophilic drugs have increased peak concentrations Increased free drug Drug levels are difficult to interpret
Metabolism	Chemical change in a drug that causes it to be active or inactive	Decreased liver and kidney blood flow Decreased glomerular filtration rate Alteration in Phase I reactions and P450 system	Increased effect and toxicity of drugs metabolized by Phase I or P450 No change in drugs metabolized by conjugation
Excretion	Removal of a drug through the kidney, via bile, feces, the saliva, or the lungs	Decreased renal blood flow and filtration rate Decreased distal renal tubular secretory function Unchanged biliary excretion	Accumulation of drug eliminated unchanged Accumulation of metabolites Increased effect and toxicity of renally eliminated drugs

- Intentional
  - They can't afford the medication but don't tell you.
  - Because of cost, they medicate with borrowed, old medications.
  - Information about drugs from other sources, such as advertisements or friends and family, often confuse them.
  - They read the package insert and become scared.
- Unintentional
  - Drug regimen is overly complicated and confusing
  - Impaired mental status, normal age-associated forgetfulness
- Strategies to increase compliance:
  - Check ability to comply
    Patients should bring all medications, including OTCs, in original containers to every visit.
    Prescribe once-a-day medications whenever possible.
    Provide readable written instructions, including dose and time.
    Coordinate medication regimen with task such as meals.
    Medication boxes should be filled by appropriate individual or pharmacy.
    Reinforce regimens with responsible family members.

Theory

Theories of Aging
- Aging is a multifactorial process. Theories of aging include biological, sociological, psychological, and medical theories. These theories can be helpful to understand age-related changes and direct the care of older adults.
- Biological theories include:
  - Accumulation of oxidation damage by free radicals to DNA, RNA, proteins, and lipids
  - Regulation of aging by specific genes; the regenerative ability of cells is genetically determined
- Sociological theories include:
  - Disengagement theory suggests that, with age, there is a mutual beneficial process of reciprocal withdrawal between society and older adults.
  - Activity theory focuses on the belief that the way to age successfully is to keep active.
  - Continuity theory purports that the personality remains stable over time/age and helps direct behavior.
  - Subculture theory suggests that older adults have their own norms, expectations, beliefs and habits, that is, subculture.
  - Age stratification theory differentiates between those who age and the impact of age on society.
  - Person-environment fit theory considers the interrelationship between personal competence and the environment.
- Psychological theories include:
  - Human needs theories focus on the relationship between motivation and need.
  - Life-course and personality development theories identify personality types as predictive forces for successful/unsuccessful aging.

Developmental Theory
- All development is patterned, orderly, and predictable, with both a purpose and a direction.
- Development is continuous throughout life.
- Development may occur simultaneously in several areas, for example, physical and social, but the rate of change in each area varies.

- Development proceeds from the simple to the complex.
- The pace of development varies among individuals.
- Physical and mental stress during periods of critical developmental change, such as old age, may make a person particularly susceptible to outside stressors.

Erikson's Stages of Psychosocial Development (Erikson, 1963)
- This theory maintains that how well individuals accomplish developmental tasks will determine their success in accomplishing other tasks as they get older.
- Tasks to be mastered include:
  - Trust (failure causes mistrust)
  - Autonomy (failure leads to feelings of shame and doubt)
  - Initiative (failure leads to feelings of guilt)
  - Industry (failure leads to feelings of inferiority)
  - Identity (failure leads to role confusion)
  - Intimacy (failure leads to additional role confusion)
  - Generativity (failure leads to stagnation)
  - Ego identity (failure leads to despair)

Sadavoy Identified Critical Age-Related Stresses (Sadavoy, 1987)
- Interpersonal loss, loss of social support such as loss of spouse, family, friends
- Physical disability, loss of strength
- Loss of youthful appearance and beauty
- Change in social role, such as children caring for parent
- Forced reliance on caregivers
- Change in living arrangements, such as loss of house
- Confrontation with death

Stressors in the Elderly
- A common myth about the elderly is that they do not tolerate change.
- However, the elderly are faced with major life changes, especially losses of spouse and friends—that is, they often have to move, they lose their job, and the ability to do many activities declines, etc.
- These changes cause major stress in the elderly.
- Stress is the emotional and physical response to an increase in the environmental demands beyond the resources of an individual to cope with those demands.
- Stress theory is based on the General Adaptation Syndrome identified in 1974 by Selye, who described a continuum of stress. Small amounts of stress may add excitement and variety and increase the quality of life. Large amounts of stress may be overwhelming and lead to disease.
- The goal is to find the right balance of stress in life.
- Individuals often seem to have vulnerability in one system to stress (e.g., hypertension, ulcer, mental problems).
- Stress may be managed through various techniques or coping strategies:
  - Avoid unnecessary change during stressful times.
  - Manage time by keeping to predetermined goals and priorities.
  - Avoid stressful triggers when possible: people, activities, etc.
  - Create habits or routines to decrease stress.
  - Develop alternative activities or friendships that increase pleasure.
  - Physical exercise often decreases stress.
  - Participate in religious, motivational, or service projects that increase self-esteem or change focus to helping others,
  - Use biofeedback, tension-relaxation exercises, yoga, or imagery to control stress reactions.

Health Maintenance

Models and Theories Related to Health Care

Health Belief Model (Becker, 1972)
- Model to explain why healthy people do or do not take advantage of screening programs
- Involves variables, such as perceptions of susceptibility and seriousness of a disease, benefits of treatment, perceived barriers to change, and expectations of efficacy

Maslow's Hierarchy of Needs (Maslow, 1954)
- Suggests that some needs are more important than others and must be met before other needs can be considered. The hierarchy includes:
  - Survival needs: water, food, sleep
  - Safety and security: protection from hazards
  - Love and belonging: affection, intimacy, companionship
  - Self-esteem: sense of worth
  - Self-actualization: achieving potential

Trans-theoretical Model of Change (Prochashka and DiClemente, 1984)
- Six predictable stages of change:
  - Precontemplation
  - Contemplation
  - Preparation
  - Action
  - Maintenance
  - Termination

Self-efficacy or Social Cognitive Theory Model (Bandura, 1977)
- Self-efficacy is the perception of one's ability to perform a certain task at a certain level of accomplishment
- Outcome expectations are the beliefs that if the behavior is performed, there will be a specific outcome (e.g., if I exercise, I will get stronger)
- Behavior change and maintenance are a function of outcome expectations and efficacy expectations
- Verbal encouragement, actually performing the activity, seeing role models perform, and physiological feedback (sensations associated with the activity such as pain or fear) all influence self-efficacy and outcome expectations

Epidemiologic Principles

Etiology—defines the cause or the web of causation of a disease or problem
- Prevalence rates describe a group at a certain point in time and the number within a group that has a particular disease or problem. It is like a snapshot in time
- Incidence rates describe the rate of development of a disease in a group over a period of time. It describes the continuing occurrence of new cases of disease. This information is based on large-scale data collection from the Centers for Disease Control and Prevention.

Natural History of Disease—the course of disease development, expression, and progression. Whether based on microbiology principles of certain organisms or large scale research studies of causality, several stages appear to be universally descriptive:
- Stage of susceptibility
- Stage of presymptomatic disease
- Stage of clinical disease
- Stage of disability
- Goal is to intervene as early as possible to prevent disease or disability

Risk Factors

- Age, sex, social, cultural, familial, occupational, and lifestyle history represent potential sources of problems and diseases that may be difficult or impossible to alter.
- Risk reduction programs may be established to decrease the vulnerability of individuals to some problems by modifying some risks.

Communicable/Infectious Diseases—patterns in which organisms attack and invade vulnerable individuals

- Involves identification of causative agents
- Relies on microbiology principles in understanding life cycle of organism
- Focuses on intervention at vulnerable phases in course or disease or life cycle of organism to limit or eradicate disease

Epidemiologic Concepts

Host-Parasite Relations

- Pathogenicity
- Virulence

Reservoirs of Infection

- Cases
- Carriers

Mechanisms of Transmission of Infection

- Direct
- Indirect through vehicle, vector, or air

Concepts of Epidemic vs Endemic Infections

- Person-to-person transmission
- Generation time—time between receipt of infection and maximal communicability of that infection
- Herd immunity—resistance of a group to invasion and spread of an infectious agent

Control Measures

- Measures directed against the reservoir—isolation, quarantine
- Measures that interrupt the transmission of organisms—water purification, pasteurization of milk, inspection procedures
- Measures that reduce host susceptibility—immunization

Current Factors Supporting Greater Emphasis on Health Maintenance

- Increased emphasis on disease prevention and promotion of health as major causes of morbidity and mortality in general have shifted away from infectious etiologies.
- Changing demographics means more people living longer and with less disease and dysfunction
- Emphasis on containing costs means primary prevention preferred over secondary and secondary preferred over tertiary
- *Healthy People 2010* is the prevention agenda for the nation. They set national health objectives designed to identify the most significant preventable threats to health and to establish national goals to reduce the threats. The complete documents can be found at www.health.gov, then click on *Healthy People 2010*. *Healthy People* leading health indicators most relevant to geriatrics are:
  - Physical activity
  - Overweight and obesity
  - Tobacco use
  - Mental health
  - Injury and violence
  - Access to health care

Health Maintenance in the Elderly

- Goal is to preserve function and quality of life in the elderly, as well as reduction of morbidity and mortality
- Most research in this area has been done on much younger adults
- Because the research has not been done, there is insufficient data to make specific recommendation for the elderly
- Most organizations that recommend preventive measures use the cut off age of 65
- Screening is unlikely to be of benefit if the individual has less than a 10-year life expectancy
- Prevention and screening must be individualized in the elderly based on risk factors, potential for benefit, and on patient willingness to undergo treatment
- Emphasis should be on prevention of discomfort and maintaining quality of life
- Screening is less likely to be useful if patient:
  - Has consistently negative screening results in the past
  - Is frail
  - Is demented
  - Has limited remaining quality and quantity of life
  - Would not be a candidate for treatment
  - Is unable or unwilling to cooperate with the intervention

Levels of Prevention

Primary Prevention

- Emphasis is on reducing incidence of disease or problems by generalized health promotion and specific disease protection
- Important examples are exercise and nutrition
- Older adults can benefit from primary prevention, even at very old ages, as it may improve quality of life
- Cardiovascular disease (atherosclerotic cardiovascular and cerebrovascular disease), the most common cause of death, is amenable to primary prevention

Secondary Prevention

- Emphasis is on early detection of illness or problem while the outcome can be favorably altered
- Example, PSA tests, breast exams, smoking cessation programs, cholesterol screening
- Must explore with older adult the pros and cons of screening and determine willingness to have further evaluation and treatment of identified disease

Tertiary Prevention

- Emphasis is on treatment and rehabilitation of the illness or problem to return the patient to the highest level of functioning and to avoid or postpone complications.
- Example: poststroke or postmyocardial infarction rehabilitations programs
- Becomes very important in the elderly

Effective Health Promotion Interventions (See Table 3-2)

Exercise

- Exercise can be of benefit to almost every patient; research has included people in their 90s
- The main exception is patients with an unstable cardiac condition, such as angina or arrhythmia
- Caution is needed, particularly in patients with musculoskeletal disorders
- Recommendations are for 30 minutes of moderate physical activity of different types on most days of the week
- It is not necessary to achieve this goal to receive benefit from exercise
- Older adults should be encouraged to combine both aerobic exercise and resistive:
  - Walking, swimming, water walking, biking (stationary bike, recumbent bicycle)
  - Muscle strengthening

Table 3-2: Specific Health Behaviors Amenable to Intervention

Behavior	Strength of Evidence	Benefit	Age for Which Recommended	Recommendation
Exercise	Good evidence	Many, including cardiac disease, death	All ages; proven in men in their 90s	Individualize
Nutrition	Simple, focused intervention can be effective	Helps with many chronic conditions	No upper limit	Counseling re adequate diet
Calcium	Good evidence in high-risk patients	Reduces risk of osteoporosis	Postmenopausal women	1000–1500 mg/d; no recommendations for men
Cholesterol (cho)	Diet not proven to be sufficient to reduce cho level; normal cho levels proven to protect young to middle-aged men	Reduce hyperlipidemia-atherosclerotic cardiovascular disease	No support for screening and treatment over age 75	Cholesterol under 200, LDL depends on risk factors
Weight Loss	Well documented in adults up to age 65	Independent risk factor for atherosclerotic cardiovascular disease	Not studied in elderly	Maintain ideal body weight
Stop Smoking	Strongest recommendation, simple interventions can have 5%–10% quit rate	Cardiovascular, pulmonary, gastrointestinal diseases and malignancies	Quitting at any time improves pulmonary function and risk of MI and death	Ask about, encourage cessation at each visit
Alcohol	Cessation difficult to achieve in alcoholics	Puts elderly at risk for falls and confusion	No age limit to improved safety	Ask about, counsel to use in moderation
Drugs	Well documented	Polypharmacy has many risks or adverse reactions, drug interactions, a cause of death in the elderly	Never too late	Check medications at each visit, ask about OTC and herbal remedies. Use only medications that are medically necessary
Safety/Injury/ Abuse Prevention	Little data on effectiveness of prevention	Falls 6th leading cause of death	Different focus in the elderly	Home safety evaluation
Aspirin	Proved in middle-aged men; few studies in elderly	Primary and secondary prevention of cardiovascular and cerebrovascular disease	Recommended for over 40 or 50	Low dose 81–324 mg/d for cardiovascular health
Immunizations				
Influenza Pneumonia	Well documented 60% efficacy	Influenza *Streptococcus pneumoniae* infection	65+ 65+	Annually Once; may repeat in 5 years
Tetanus	Well proven	Tetanus	Indicated in the elderly	Every 10 years

- Stretching, including yoga, Tai chi
- Less strenuous activity is also beneficial, such as gardening or slow walking
- Health benefits include:
  - Reduced risk of chronic disease
  - Improved bone and muscle strength
  - Decreased risk of falling
  - Improved function
  - Improved quality of life
  - Improved bowel function
  - Decreased depression
  - Improved sleep
  - Improved overall sense of well-being

Nutrition
- Supply all essential body nutrients to maintain or regain health
- Maintain, gain, or lose weight if necessary for ideal body weight (IBW)—see Obesity in Endocrine Chapter 17
- Risk factors for malnutrition include drugs, chronic disease, depression, dental problems, decreased taste and smell, poverty, physical weakness, and isolation
- Adequate calcium intake—1000 mg to 1500 mg per day
- Adequate Vitamin D intake—800 IU per day
- Diet moderate in fat content to keep cholesterol within normal limits
- Adequate fluid intake—6 to 8 glasses of water per day
- Adequate fiber—grains, fruits, and vegetables
- Avoid excess sodium, most important in CHF, hypertension; elderly at risk for low sodium due to severe restriction of salt in their diet
- Frail elderly at risk for malnutrition low albumin levels

Smoking Cessation
- One of the most important preventive interventions
- Elderly can benefit from smoking cessation programs
- Usually safe to use nicotine replacement therapy or bupropion (Wellbutrin)

Safety-Injury Prevention
- Fall prevention with home safety evaluation
  - Bathrooms are the site of most falls
  - Throw rugs dangerous
  - Sufficient lighting both inside and outside the home
  - Safe and appropriate assistive devices
- Driving evaluations for safety
  - Driving essential for independence, patients reluctant to give up
  - Driving can be impaired due to dementia, impaired vision, slowed reflexes, musculoskeletal disorders, etc.
- Seat belts
- Smoke detectors
- Safety lock on firearms

Violence and Abuse (See section in Chapter 18)
- An estimated 1.5 to 2 million older adults in the United States are abused annually
- Anticipate problems in the care of older adults and help caregivers cope with these problems (e.g., urinary incontinence, short-term memory changes)
- Clinicians should ask about and watch for signs of physical abuse during encounters with clients.

- Patients will often admit to problems but only if they are asked
- Talk to caregivers about stress, coping, support systems, and respite care
- Know and utilize state laws in determining requirements to report suspected abuse

Alcohol (See section in Chapter 18)
- Depression is highly associated with alcohol abuse
- In older adults, signs and symptoms of alcohol abuse might include falls, changes in functional status and/or cognition, weight loss or malnutrition, abnormal lab values, and recent losses
- Older adults may have had a prior history of drinking, or this may be new in older age
- May begin or resume as part of grief reaction to loss
- Screening should be done by assuming there is regular alcohol use and asking the older adult not if they drink, but how much

Drugs
- See section of pharmacology in this chapter for a discussion of prescription and OTC drugs in the elderly
- Dependency is a common personality tendency that in its extreme form causes an individual to rely on other individuals or activities, such as eating food, drinking alcohol, having sex, gambling, or other components, to try to satisfy an emotional hunger
- Action begun voluntarily, which through repetition, becomes involuntary
- Dependency becomes an addiction when there is loss of control (compulsivity), continuation despite adverse consequences, and obsession or preoccupation with the activity

Estrogen
- For postmenopausal women to prevent osteoporosis
- See GYN Chapter 12 for discussion of risks versus benefits

Aspirin
- To prevent strokes and MIs
- Most effective in high-risk patients

Immunizations
- To obtain up-to-date standards for adult immunization practices, go to www.cdc.gov/nip/recs/rev-immz-stds.htm
- Many older adults remain without adequate immunization
- Influenza and pneumonia vaccines underutilized
- Tetanus a hidden risk
  - The largest age group acquiring tetanus infections is the elderly
  - Men often have not had a booster since they were in the military
  - Women may have never had full immunization series

Geriatric Screening Guidelines
See Table 3-3.

Health Care and Treatment Considerations
Cultural influences—If the healthcare provider becomes more sensitive to issues surrounding health care and the traditional health beliefs of the patient, more comprehensive health care can be provided
- **Family**—a group of adults and children who are usually related and whose adults participate in carrying out the essential functions of providing food, clothing, shelter, safety, and education of the children. The concept must be broadened beyond the traditional husband-wife-children pattern seen in the US The family initially teaches the belief patterns, religion, culture, and mores of a society
- **Ethnic**—the race, tribe, or nation with which a person or group identifies and which influence beliefs and behavior; the cultural background of an individual

- **Culture**—the learned beliefs and behaviors or socially inherited characteristics that are common among all members of a group and have both practical and symbolic components
- **Community**—a group of families often sharing the same race, tribe, or culture and who have beliefs or behavior not shared by others
- **Individual**—one member of a family, community, or cultural group
- **Environmental factors**—general circumstances, such as climate, altitude, and temperature, affect all people, while more specific items, such as air pollution, fluoride in the water, water contamination, crime, poverty, transportation, are examples of things that might be manipulated with a more positive or more negative effect on the population

Evidence-based Medicine

- In order to reduce the numbers of conflicting or varying recommendations for the diagnosis and treatment of common problems, the trend is to base decisions on evidence from randomized controlled research trials. Meta-analyses of these trials, together with individual trials, have gained acceptance as valid foundations on which care can be provided. Information about the status of research in these areas is growing through use of the computer.
- Outcome studies will replace tradition, intuition, and preference for how different clinical problems should be handled. NPs should have sufficient research skills to be able to critically evaluate and participate in outcome studies that will relate to their clinical practice.
- There is frequently no research that has been done on elderly patients; this severely limits evidence-based geriatric medicine. Elderly are different from younger adults and research done on younger adults must be interpreted with caution with reference to the elderly population. Age-related changes as well as more comorbid conditions may affect treatment outcomes in the elderly.

Clinical Guidelines

- Standards of practice are devised from research by experts in the field to guide and standardize practice across the nation. NPs should know how to analyze clinical guidelines to determine those that are written by objective scholars and are without organization, professional, or pharmaceutical bias. See the National Guideline Clearinghouse at www.guideline.gov
- Factors to consider in evaluating guidelines include source of guideline, appropriateness of methodology used to develop guideline, use of expert opinion/clinical experience in decision-making, public policy issue considerations, feasibility issues, use of peer review, congruence with other practice guidelines, timeliness, and funding source

Critical Thinking/Decision Making

- Critical thinking involves acquisition of knowledge with an attitude of deliberate inquiry. Part of critical thinking may be innate, but most people can learn to think critically
- Decision making is a higher level of critical thinking. It involves making decisions based on an understanding of the different options and the possible desirability of the outcomes of each option in the mind of the clinician and the patient
- Pattern recognition, similarity recognition, commonsense understanding, skilled know-how, sense of importance, and deliberative rationality are all important aspects that influence decision making

Communication—the written and oral transfer of information regarding the structure, process, and outcome of health care encounters. Health care providers are required to have good communication skills in interviewing and teaching patients, recording information and decisions, sharing or clarifying information with others involved in the patient's care. All communication is privileged and confidential and written documentation is subject to specific standards and audits
- Types of special communication
    - **Triage**—the prioritization and sorting of patients according to a preexisting standard; used in disaster and emergency settings

Table 3-3: Geriatric Screening Recommendations

Screening Procedure	Strength of Evidence	Screen for	Age for Which Recommended	Recommendations
Blood Pressure	Excellent, especially in elderly	Hypertension isolated systolic HTN	No age cutoff, important in the elderly	Every 1–2 years
Height and Weight	No data	Obesity	No age stated	Periodic
Clinical Breast Exam	Excellent	Breast cancer	Over age 40	Annually
Mammogram	Excellent	Breast cancer	Every year for ages 50–69; continue in willing/ appropriate patients	Continue every 1–3 years
Pap Smear	Excellent in adults	Cervical cancer	Adult	Can decrease to test every 2–3 years after ages 65–69, if 3 consecutive negative PAP smears unless immunocompromised
Rectal Exam /PSA	Good for rectal exam; PSA now discredited	Colorectal cancer; prostate cancer	Less likely to benefit elderly	Annual
Oral Cavity Exam	Good in high-risk patients	Cancer, gingivitis	No upper age limit	Yearly exam and counseling
Cholesterol Level	Less certain for elderly	Cardiovascular, cerebrovascular disease	Often no recommendation after 65, controversial	Every 5 years
Fecal Occult Blood	Good data	Colorectal cancer	No upper limit established	Annual

Sigmoidoscopy	Colorectal cancer	Significant benefit for adults, especially with risk factors; no data for elderly	No specific recommendations over 65; into healthy old age if healthy and willing	Every 5 years
TSH	Thyroid disorder	Some data	Elderly, esp women	Yearly
Glucose	Diabetes mellitus	Treatment shown to reduce complications	Those at increased risk	Every 3 years
Bone Density	Osteoporosis	Good data	Women aged 65 and older with increased risk for osteoporosis, or those on FDA-approved osteoporosis drug therapy; no recommendations for men	Every 2 years
Skin Exam	Skin cancer	No data	Older adults, no upper age limit	Periodic, depends on risk
Vision	Vision loss, glaucoma	Some evidence	Many recommend exam for patients 65 and older	Screen visual acuity of elderly with Snellen testing and refer persons at high risk for glaucoma to eye specialists
Hearing	Hearing loss	Some evidence	Over age 65	Assess hearing through physical exam and refer as needed
Urinalysis	Infection, cancer	Some evidence	High risk, such as DM, older patients	Periodically
EKG	Heart disease	Some evidence	Over ages 40–50	Periodically
Cognitive and Functional Assessment	Functional status, dementia	Insufficient evidence	Some recommend screening patients over ages 65 or 75	Periodic assessment
Depression	Depression	Some data	Some recommend in the elderly	Periodic assessment

- **Case management**

  Case management is a system of controlled oversight and authorization of services and benefits provided to clients

  The case manager is an advocate in the managed care environment for both consumers and providers, where managing can also mean balancing key issues of access, cost, and outcomes

- **Team management**

  The elderly have many interdisciplinary problems necessitating multiple-care providers

  The different specialties must communicate with each other to provide a unified plan of care

Interpersonal Relationships—NPs work closely with many other types of healthcare providers. The NP role boundaries are not always clear and may vary from state to state or even institution to institution. Some principles in establishing and maintaining relationships with others include:

- Flexibility
- Willingness to listen
- Respect for others views, beliefs, traditions
- Assertiveness in clarifying your own opinion, belief, traditions
- Tolerance
- Patience
- Ability to make change

CASE STUDIES

Case 1. You are asked to assess an 82-year-old man for admission to an assisted living facility.
1. What chronic conditions is he likely to have?
2. What impairments is he likely to have?
3. What kind of health insurance is he likely to have?
4. What cause is he most likely to die from?

Case 2. A 94-year-old nursing home patient with moderate dementia has had four falls in the past 2 days. She had not fallen for the past year.
1. What is this an example of?
2. How would you begin the evaluation of this problem?
3. What other aspects of the functional assessment would be important in this patient?

Case 3. You have a new patient in the nursing home, a 78-year-old woman with moderate dementia, impaired hearing, and impaired vision.
1. Your initial approach would be?
2. How would you alter the environment to improve communication?
3. How would you adjust your physical exam?

REFERENCES

Andersen, E., Rothenberg, B., & Zimmer, J. G. (1997). *Assessing the health status of older adults*. MD: Springer.

Bandura, A. (1986). *Social foundations of thought and action*. Englewood Cliffs, NY: Prentice-Hall.

Becker, M. (1972). The health believe model and personal health behavior. *Health Education Monographs, 2,* 326–327.

Brownson, R. C. (1998). *Applied epidemiology: Theory to practice*. London: Oxford University Press.

Caloras, D. (November 1999). The virtues of hospice. *Patient Care for the Nurse Practitioner,* 6–30.

Draye, M. A. (2000). Health promotion, health maintenance, and disease prevention. In P. V. Meredith, N. M. Horan (Eds.), *Adult primary care*. St. Louis: Harcourt Brace.

Edmunds, M. W., & Mayhew, M. S. (2004). *Pharmacology for primary care providers* (2nd ed.). St. Louis: Mosby.

Emanuel, E. (November 2000). A detailed examination of advance directives. *Patient Care for the Nurse Practitioner*, 31–51.

Erikson, E. (1963). *Childhood and society* (2nd ed.). NY: Norton.

Finkel, T., & Holbrook, N. J. (2000). Oxidants, oxidative stress and the biology of ageing. *Nature, 408*, 239–247.

Freedman, V. A., et al. (2002). Recent trends in disability and functioning among older adults in the United States. JAMA, 288, 3137–3146.

Friedman, M. (1998). *Family nursing: Research, theory and practice* (4th ed.). Stanford, CT: Appleton & Lange.

Goldberg, T. H., & Chavin, S. I. (1997). Preventive medicine and screening in older adults. *JAGS. 45*, 344–354.

Kane, R. A. (2001). Long term care and a good quality of life: Bringing them closer together. *Gerontologist, 41*(30), 293–304.

Kane, R. L., & Kane, R. A. (2000). *Assessing older persons*. Oxford University Press.

Kerlikowske, K., et al. (1999). Continuing screening mammography in women aged 70 to 79 years. JAMA, 282, 2156–2163.

Kramarow, E., et al. (1999). *Health and aging chartbook*. Hyattsville, MD: National Center for Health Statistics. Available online at: www.health.gov.

Lenburg, C. B., et al. (1995). *Promoting cultural competence in and through nursing education: A critical review and comprehensive plan for action*. Washington, DC: American Academy of Nursing.

Maslow, A. (1954). *Motivation and personality*. New York: Harper & Row.

Moon, M. (1996). What Medicare has meant to older Americans. *Health Care Fin Rev, 18*(2), 49–59.

Pender, N. (1996). *Health promotion in nursing practice* (3rd ed.). Norwalk, CT: Appleton & Lange.

Prochaska, J. O., & DiClemente, C. C. (1984). *The trans-theoretical approach: Crossing traditional boundaries of change*. Homewood, IL: Dow-Jones-Irwin.

Sadavoy, J., & Lesczc, M., (Eds.). (1987). *Treating the elderly with psychotherapy: The scope for change in later life*. Madison, CT: International Universities Press.

Selye, H. (1974). *Stress without distress*. PA: J. B. Lippincott.

Statistical Abstract of the United States. (1999). US Census Bureau. Available at: www.census.gov.

United States Department of Health and Human Services (USDHHS). (1996). *Healthy People 2000*. Washington, DC: US Public Health Service, 479–510.

United States Department of Health and Human Services (USDHHS). *Healthy People 2010*. Washington, DC: US Public Health Service.

United States Preventive Services Task Force (USPSTF). (2002). *Guide to clinical preventive services*. (3rd ed.). McLean, VA: International Medical Publishing.

Vladeck, B. C. (2001). Medicare: Can its benefits be sustained as cost of coverage grows? *Geriatrics, 56*(5), 50–53.

Websites for Geriatrics

Administration on Aging. Available at: www.aoa.gov.

AgeNet Eldercare Network. Available at: www.caregivers.com.

American Association of Homes and Services for the Aging. Available at: www.aahsa.org.

American Association of Retired Persons. Available at: www.aarp.org.

American Geriatrics Society. Available at: www.americangeriatrics.org.

American Health Care Association. Available at: www.ahca.org.

American Medical Directors Association. Available at: www.amda.com.

American Society of Consultant Pharmacists. Available at: www.ascp.com.

Gerontological Society of America. Available at: www.geron.org.

National Association of Area Agencies on Aging. Available at: www.n4a.org.

National Council on the Aging. Available at: www.ncoa.org.

National Guidelines Clearinghouse. Available at: www.guideline.gov.

NCOA Benefits Checkup. Available at: www.benefitscheckup.org.

Web Resources for Advance Directive

Aging with Dignity. Available at: www.agingwithdignity.org. advance directive

American Academy of Family Physicians. Available at: www.familydoctor.org/handouts/003.html.

Choice in Dying. Available at: www.choices.org.

Healthwatch. Available at: www.healthwatch.com.

Living Wills and Values History Project. Available at: www.euthanasia.org/vh.html.

The Medical Directive from JAMA. Available at: www.medicaldirective.org.

GERIATRIC MULTISYSTEM SYNDROMES

4

Nonspecific Presentation of Illness in the Elderly
- Geriatric patients usually have more than one chronic illness.
- Most presentations of illness in the elderly do not reflect the system causing the problem. The most common presentation of illness is delirium. Therefore, geriatric health care providers often evaluate older patients using a multisystem approach. This chapter will discuss some of the common geriatric multisystem syndromes.

DEMENTIA

Description
- Dementia: impairment of global intellectual and cognitive function characterized by memory loss, aphasia, agnosia, and apraxia with preservation of level of consciousness; difficulty with problem solving, organization, and abstract thinking
- Alzheimer disease (AD): gradual onset and progressive decline without focal neurological deficits
- Vascular dementia: dementing process caused by strokes characterized by step-wise decline
- Lewey body disease (LBD): dementia with visual hallucinations, parkinsonian-type movement disorder, and altered alertness
- Normal-pressure hydrocephalus (NPH): dementia with associated ataxic gait, urinary incontinence, and communicating hydrocephalus

Etiology
- Alzheimer disease
  - Mostly unknown
  - More neuritic plaques and neurofibrillary tangles are found on autopsy as compared with nondemented patients
  - 3 genes on different chromosomes have been identified in families with history of AD, although all cases may not be inherited
- Vascular dementia
  - Multiple lacunar infarcts
- NPH
  - Cause unknown
  - Diagnosis is made if symptoms improve with spinal fluid drainage

Incidence and Demographics
- Increased incidence with age over 85
- AD and related dementias affect 2 to 4 million Americans
- AD is the 7th leading cause of death in the elderly
- AD: 50%–60% of all dementias
- Vascular dementia: 10%–20% of all dementias

Risk Factors

- Age
- AD: Down syndrome, familial or inherited, apolipoprotein E
- Vascular dementia: hypertension, previous stroke, TIAs

Prevention and Screening
- Those over 65 should have cognitive and functional evaluation at least every 3 years.
- It is important that clinicians and families be aware of early symptoms to facilitate early assessment and recognition, and rule out age-related memory changes, unidentified conditions, or "reversible forms" of dementia.

Assessment
(See Table 4-1.)

History
- Detailed history of present illness, including time frame and progression, and any associated neurologic symptoms such as vision loss, aphasia, unilateral weakness
- Past medical history of hypertension, strokes, head trauma, psychiatric illness
- Psychiatric history of depression, anxiety, schizophrenia
- Social history: present living situation, marital status, occupation, education, alcohol, tobacco, illicit drug use
- Medications including over the counter, supplements, and home remedies
- Initial and periodic functional history and assessment
- Validate history with family member and/or caregiver, but also be aware of potential for self-serving motives; informants may exaggerate or deny symptoms
- Mental status test results are not diagnostic, serve as baseline for assessing trends in cognitive impairment
- Instruments include Folstein Mini-Mental State Examination, the Short Portable Mental Status Questionnaire, and Blessed Dementia Rating Scale
- Consider visual, sensory, language, physical disabilities, and education when administering mental status tests
- Functional and behavioral assessment. Instruments include Katz, Global Deterioration Scale (GDS), and Functional Assessment Staging (FAST)
- History of falls

Physical
- Complete with attention to focal neuro deficits
- Hearing and visual impairments
- Cardiac findings (murmurs, arrhythmias, heart enlargement)
- Evaluate for orthostatic hypotension
- Pulmonary findings
- Any evidence of infectious processes
- AD: no focal neurological findings
- Vascular: focal motor weakness or impaired sensation, reflex asymmetry, positive Babinski
- NPH: ataxia and incontinence

Diagnostic Studies
- CBC, chemistry profile, thyroid function tests, B_{12} level, folate level to rule out metabolic causes or unidentified conditions
- Computed tomography if
  - Early dementia of less than 2 years duration
  - NPH suspected, presence of ataxia and incontinence
  - Focal neurological findings
- Syphilis, HIV, and drug toxicity if indicated by history

Table 4-1: Stages of Alzheimer Disease

Stage	Characteristics	Interventions
Stage 1 Mild Dementia Functional Assessment Staging (FAST) (stage 2–4)	Short-term memory loss Impaired organizational, decision-making, and judgment skills Difficulty learning new skills and following directions Difficulty with driving, cooking, managing finances, and medications May get lost Decreased attention span Attempts to hide memory loss May exhibit anxiety, depression, agitation, or paranoia	Calm, structured environment with moderate stimulation in familiar surroundings Maintain a routine including meal and sleep patterns Clocks, calendars, and to-do lists Avoid distraction Simple one-step commands Repeat and rephrase Cholinesterase inhibitors Treat depression Advanced directive and long-term care planning Consider cholinesterase inhibitor
Stage 2 Moderate Dementia FAST (stage 5–6)	Problems recalling major current life events Increased problems following directions Word-finding difficulty Difficulty choosing appropriate clothing Verbal or physical agitation and aggression Delusions and hallucinations Wandering and pacing Purposeless and repetitive behavior Motor apraxia	Maintain safe independent function for as long as possible Plan for and determine when patient is no longer competent to make legal, financial, and medical decisions Avoid background noise Avoid arguing Try distraction Provide reassurance Avoid new or distressing social situations Consider cholinesterase inhibitor or NMDA antagonist
Stage 3 Severe Dementia FAST (stage 7)	Lose ability to communicate, become nonverbal Become chair bound or bedridden Totally dependent for care	Provide comfort care Consider long-term care placement Continue to speak to and touch patient, and maintain eye contact Consider NMDA antagonist

- Urinalysis if urinary tract infection suspected
- Arterial oxygen or pulse oximetry if hypoxemia is considered
- EEG is not useful
- Neuropsychological testing is recommended under certain circumstances
  - Abnormal mental status testing with normal function
  - Differentiate depression, stroke, or delirium in unusual presentations
  - Identify areas of preserved cognitive function to develop a care plan

Differential Diagnosis
- Delirium
- Other dementias: Lewey body disease, Pick disease, etc.
- Parkinson disease
- Depression and anxiety
- Hearing loss
- B_{12} and folate deficiency
- Trauma: consider subdural hematoma, history of falls may be forgotten if not witnessed
- Tumor
- Hypothyroidism
- Infectious process: chronic infection, AIDS, tertiary syphilis
- Cerebral vascular accident (CVA)
- Myocardial infarction
- Medications: polypharmacy, interactions
- Alcohol intoxication

Management
- Rule out or treat any conditions that may contribute to cognitive impairment.
- Discontinue all unnecessary medications, especially sedatives and hypnotics.
- Vascular dementia: nonpharmacologic and pharmacologic reduction of stroke risks (see management of TIA and stroke)
- Surgical shunting for NPH; approximately 50% improve; improvement may be immediate or take weeks and may be temporary

Nonpharmacologic Treatment
- Educate patient and family about the illness, treatment, community resources
- Assist with long-term planning, including financial, legal, and advanced directives
- Assess home and driving safety
- Behavior therapy identifies causes of problem behaviors and changes the environment to reduce the behavior
- Recreational, art, pet therapy, create pleasurable experiences for the patient
- Reminiscence therapy
- Maintain a simple daily routine for bathing, dressing, eating, toileting, and bedtime.
- Integrate cultural beliefs into the management of minority patients with dementia.

Pharmacologic Treatment
MILD TO MODERATE COGNITIVE SYMPTOMS
- Cholinesterase inhibitors
  - Donepezil (Aricept) 5–10 mg once a day
  - Rivastigmine (Exelon) 1.5–6 mg bid; increase gradually
  - Galantamine (Reminyl) 4–12 mg bid; increase gradually as tolerated
- Indicated for Alzheimer disease; may also be effective in patients with vascular dementia
- Modest clinical improvement in some patients with studies showing 2- to 3-point improvement in mental status testing
- Treats only symptoms, may improve agitated behaviors

- Does not prevent pathological progression of disease
- Not effective in severe end-stage disease
- Stop if side effects develop, usually nausea, vomiting
- Common adverse reactions: nausea, diarrhea, insomnia, vomiting, muscle cramps, fatigue, anorexia, agitation; Galantamine: bradycardia, syncope
- Moderate to severe cognitive symptoms
- NMDA antagonist
  - Memantine (Namenda) 5 mg qd to 10 mg PO bid; increase gradually as tolerated
- Adverse reactions: dizziness, headache, constipation, hypertension, pain, GI upset, somnolence, hallucination, dyspnea
- May be used in combination with cholinesterase inhibitors

PSYCHOSIS AND AGITATION
- Antipsychotics
  - Manage psychic disturbances such as paranoia, delusions, and hallucinations
  - Use lowest effective dose and attempt to wean periodically
  - Haloperidol (Haldol) 0.25–2 mg at bedtime or up to 3 times a day
    "Typical" phenothiazine high-potency antipsychotic medication with high risk for extrapyramidal side effects, tardive dyskinesia, and neuromalignant hypertensive syndrome, anticholinergic side effects, postural hypotension
  - Risperidone 0.25–0.5 mg at bedtime, up to 1–1.5 mg daily
  - Olanzapine 2.5–5 mg at bedtime
  - Quetiapine (Seroquel) 25 mg bid; up to 150 mg bid
    "Atypical" antipsychotics have lower risk for extrapyramidal side effects
    However, they have been associated with increased risk of hyper- or hypoglycemia and of stroke in the elderly, and their use is controversial
- Anxiolytics
  - Benzodiazepines may be used for treating anxiety or infrequent agitation but are not as effective as antipsychotics for severe symptoms
  - Lorazepam (Ativan) (prominent anxiety) 0.5–6 mg a day in divided doses as needed
  - High risk for increased confusion and ataxia with falls

DEPRESSION (see also Chapter 18)
- Paroxetine HCl (Paxil) 10–40 mg/day
- Sertraline HCl (Zoloft) 25–200 mg/day
- Escitalopram (Lexapro) 5–20 mg/day
- Nortriptyline HCl (Pamelor) 30–50 mg/day (also may improve insomnia and neuropathic pain)
- Mirtazapine (Remeron) 7.5–45 mg at bedtime (also good for may improve insomnia)
- Attempt to wean after 6 to12 months; patients may be less depressed as dementia progresses in that they are less aware of their circumstances

SLEEP DISTURBANCES
- Zolpidem (Ambien) 5–10 mg at bedtime
- Trazodone (Desyrel) 25–75 mg at bedtime

When to Consult, Refer, Hospitalize
- Neurology: unusual presentation
- Psychiatry: unable to differentiate from depression, intractable behaviors
- Social work for long-term planning
- Hospitalize if unable to manage at home for delirium, complications of comorbid or infectious conditions, or trauma with injury (CHF, COPD exacerbations, dehydration, pneumonia, hip fracture)
- Avoid hospitalization when possible

- Demented patients are likely to become more confused and delirious and fall when hospitalized.

Follow-up

Expected Course
- AD: slowly and steadily progressive downhill course leading to complications and death
- Vascular dementia: stepwise with new focal deficits and decline with each stroke; patient often declines at a faster rate as the dementia progresses
- NPH: poor outcomes if dementia severe or precedes ataxia

Complications
- Half will develop agitation as the disease progresses
- Less then half develop psychotic symptoms of delusions, hallucinations, and paranoia
- Incontinence and behaviors that cause family distress lead to institutionalization
- Depression is common; suicide is a risk when the patient is aware of their condition
- Complications related to comorbidity or complications due to immobility with severe end-stage dementia, such as pneumonia, decubiti, dehydration, and injury due to falls, and death
- NPH: 30% complications with shunting including subdural hematomas, stroke, seizures, and shunt malfunction

DELIRIUM

Description
- Acute disorder of attention with onset of hours to days, characterized by confusion, disorientation and fluctuation over the course of a day

Etiology
- Functional disorder of the brain caused by organic factors
- A derangement of cortical glucose metabolism or a cerebral metabolic insufficiency may be the underlying mechanism responsible for this global disturbance in attention and concentration
- Intracranial conditions such as head trauma, stroke, cancer, seizures
- Systemic disease
  - Infections: UTI, pneumonia
  - Cardiovascular: CHF, MI
- Fluid and electrolyte imbalance: dehydration, anemia, uremia, hypokalemia, hypoglycemia, hypoxia
- Exogenous toxic agent such as medications and poisons
- Withdrawal from alcohol and medications

Incidence and Demographics
- Highest incidence in hospitalized elderly
- Also common in patients with dementia in nursing home
- Delirium is a frequent presenting symptom of illness in the elderly
- 10% to 40% of patients over 65 have been found to have delirium on admission
- 25% to 60% will develop delirium during hospitalization with 10% to 65% mortality rate
- Delirium accounts for increased institutionalization, rehabilitation, home care and caregiver burden
- Medications contribute to 40% of delirium cases in the hospitalized elderly

Risk Factors
- Age, dementia, frailty, comorbidities, infections, dehydration, hypoxemia and hypercarbia, visual and hearing impairments, sleep deprivation
- Medications associated with increased incidence of delirium
  - Anticholinergics: oxybutynin, scopolamine, atropine, and antidiarrheals with atropine

- Antihistamines (histamine H_1 receptor blockers): loratadine and fexofenadine least likely to cause CNS disturbance
- Histamine H_2 receptor blockers: especially cimetidine
- Antidepressants: particularly amitriptyline and doxepin
- Antipsychotics: chlorpromazine, thioridazine, clozapine most likely to cause delirium, risperidone least likely
- Antiparkinson medications: especially anticholinergics (benztropine and trihexyphenidyl), and multiple medications in late stage disease
- Antiepileptics
- Antihypertensives including diuretics
- Benzodiazepines: particularly long-acting and any at high doses
- Narcotics: particularly meperidine and transdermal fentanyl
- Cyclobenzaprine (Flexeril)
- Metronidazole (Flagyl)
- Digoxin (anticholinergic effects)
- Trimethoprim-sulfamethoxazole

Prevention and Screening
- Eliminate unnecessary medications
- Maintain adequate hydration, nutrition, and oxygenation
- Monitor bowels, avoid constipation
- Correct visual and auditory deficits
- Continuity of care and environment

Assessment

History
- Detailed history of present illness, including cognition, time frame, and progression
- Comprehensive review of systems to identify underlying etiology
- Functional history and assessment
- Validate history with family member and/or caregiver
- Folstein Mini-Mental State Examination
- Geriatric Depression Scale

Physical
- Complete with attention to level of consciousness, focal neuro deficits
- Hearing and visual impairments
- Cardiac findings (murmurs, arrhythmias, heart enlargement)
- Pulmonary findings
- Any evidence of infectious processes
- Signs of trauma
- Evaluate for orthostatic hypotension, urinary retention, and fecal impaction

Diagnostic Studies
- Urinalysis if urinary tract infection is suspected
- CXR if pneumonia is suspected
- CBC, chemistry profile, thyroid function tests, B_{12} level, folate level to identify a reversible cause for cognitive impairment or etiology of delirium
- Other tests to consider
  - Computed tomography to identify infarcts, space occupying lesions
  - Syphilis, HIV, and drug toxicity if indicated by history
  - Arterial oxygen or pulse oximetry if hypoxemia is considered
  - EKG to identify cardiopulmonary cause

- EEG to rule out seizure
- Lumbar puncture for suspected encephalopathy or meningitis

Differential Diagnosis
- Dementia   • Depression

Management
- Identify and treat underlying cause

Nonpharmacologic Treatment
- Continuity of care
- Minimize environmental stimuli
- Provide eye glasses or hearing aides
- Clocks and calendars to maintain orientation
- Maintain hydration, nutrition, oxygenation
- Adequate bowel and bladder regimen
- Avoid physical restraints and any unnecessary IV lines and Foley catheters

Pharmacologic Treatment
- Treat agitation with
  - Haloperidol 0.5 mg PO or IM every 2–6 hours for agitation OR
  - Risperidone 0.25–2.5 mg once or twice a day
  - Olanzapine 2.5–5 mg each day
  - Quetiapine (Seroquel) 25 mg bid—300 mg in divided doses
  - Lorazepam 0.25–0.5 mg if sedation is desired to avoid extrapyramidal symptoms in Parkinson's patients or in alcohol or in sedative-hypnotic withdrawal
  - Monitor for extrapyramidal symptoms, prolonged QT interval, and neuroleptic malignant syndrome
- It may be necessary to treat the patient's agitation with an antipsychotic in order to be able to adequately examine the patient to determine cause of the delirium and to treat the cause
- Appropriate treatment of cause

How Long to Treat
- Discontinue the antipsychotic as soon as possible
- Depends upon etiology
- Continue nonpharmacologic therapy until baseline cognitive function returns

When to Consult, Refer, Hospitalize
- Consult physician for any primary care patient with suspected delirium
- Keep patient at home if patient has adequate supervision to ensure that the condition can be adequately treated and patient can be kept safe
- Delirious patients become more confused and agitated in the hospital setting
- Hospitalize when necessary to ensure patient safety, adequate hydration, and prescribed treatment

Follow-up

Expected Course
- Delirium generally resolves when etiology is adequately treated
- Depends on etiology

Complications
- Falls with injury
- Associated with increased morbidity and mortality
- If the delirium is not diagnosed and treated, death may result

DIZZINESS

Description
- Alterations in level of consciousness or functioning
- Generally with vague symptoms and typically occurring at inconvenient times
- Usually episodic
- Similar to fatigue/weakness in that it has many causes, often multifactorial, etiology often elusive
- Dizziness can be
  - Generalized unspecified dizziness: vague sensations of light-headedness, vague, unpleasant feeling in head, can be constant or episodic
  - Disequilibrium (unsteady, off balance): usually due to peripheral neuropathy
  - Syncope (loss of consciousness) and near-syncope: fainting, due to impaired cerebral blood flow, usually cardiovascular etiology
  - Fatigue: lethargy or excessive tiredness
  - Vertigo (sense of rotary motion): usually vestibular etiology See EENT Chapter 7
  - Drop attack (fall due to loss of muscle tone with no loss of consciousness): indicative of vertebral insufficiency
  - TIA (transient ischemic attack): brief episode of focal neurologic dysfunction that resolves completely without any residual deficit (see Chapter 15 Neurological Disorders)
  - Seizure: temporary and reversible behavioral alteration resulting from an excessive paroxysmal neuronal discharge in the brain. Often difficult to differentiate between other causes of dizziness (see Chapter 15 Neuro)
  - Orthostatic hypotension: drop of 20 or more in systolic blood pressure or drop of 10 or more in diastolic blood pressure; usually with increase in pulse

Etiology
See Table 4-2.

Table 4-2: Common Causes of Dizziness

Cause	Generalized	Disequilibrium	Syncope/Near Syncope
Multifactorial	Usually	Usually	Less likely
Combination Cardiac, Neuro, Age	Cause	Less likely	Major cause
Normal Changes of Aging		Many	Neuro
Sensory Deficit	Contribute	Important	Less likely
Cardiac	Usually not	No	Important, all causes
Orthostatic Hypotension	Important	Less likely	Important
Neuro	Many	PN, cerebellar, Parkinson's	TIA, migraines, other
Vestibular	Contributes	Important	Less likely
Metabolic	Many	Less likely	Hypoglycemia
Pulmonary	Yes	Less likely	Hypoxia, PE
Musculoskeletal	Cervical arthritis	Generalized arthritis	No
Psychological	Rare as main cause	Anxiety	Hyperventilation
Toxic	Yes	Yes	No
Medication	Many	Possible	Less likely (antiarrhythmics)

PN = peripheral neuropathy
PE = pulmonary emboli

- Multifactorial, most patients have more than one risk factor
- Combination cardiac and neurological and normal changes of aging
  - Orthostatic hypotension
  - Reflex reduction in cardiac output or systemic vascular resistance
  - Vasovagal
  - Postprandial
- Age-related cardiovascular, neurologic, especially autonomic, and neuroendocrine changes—see respective Chapters 9 and 17
- Sensory deficits (visual and hearing)
- Physical deconditioning
- Cardiac
  - Any cardiac condition with decreased cardiac output
  - Cardiovascular deconditioning
  - Acute MI
  - Arrhythmias, usually bradycardias
  - Valve disease—aortic stenosis
  - CHF
  - Cerebrovascular insufficiency
  - Carotid stenosis
- Neurologic
  - Normal changes of aging of the neurological system
  - Multiple neurosensory impairments
  - Vestibular (inner ear) disease
  - TIA
  - CVA
  - Cerebellar disease—from alcohol, other causes
  - Parkinson's disease
  - Peripheral neuropathy (PN)—from diabetes, alcohol use, B_{12} and folate deficiency, renal failure
  - Seizure
  - Brain tumor
  - Demyelinating disease such as multiple sclerosis
  - Vertebrobasilar migraine
- Metabolic
  - Electrolyte imbalance
  - Hypo/hyperglycemia
  - Kidney failure
  - Liver failure
  - Thyroid disease
  - Dehydration volume depletion
  - Acute anemia
  - Infection
- Pulmonary
  - Hypoxia
  - Pulmonary embolism
- Musculoskeletal
  - Cervical arthritis
  - Generalized arthritis
- Psychological
  - Depression
  - Anxiety
  - Panic attack
  - Hyperventilation
- Toxic
  - Alcohol—acute intoxication
- Medications that can cause dizziness
  - Cardiac
    Antihypertensives, especially beta blockers, calcium channel blockers, ACE inhibitors, vasodilators, adrenergic blocking agents; diuretics, antiarrhythmics, nitrates, digoxin

- Anxiolytics
  Benzodiazepines
- Antibiotics: aminoglycosides, erythromycin, ethambutol, griseofulvin, isoniazid, nitrofurantoin, polymyxin, rifampin, streptomycin, sulfonamides, trimethoprim, vancomycin
- Antihistamines
- Muscle relaxants
- Cold preparations
- Neuroleptic
  Phenothiazine
- Sedatives
- Antidiabetics Insulin or oral hypoglycemic agents
- Seizure medications
  Phenytoin (Dilantin)—ataxia
  Carbamazepine (Tegretol)
  Gabapentin (Neurontin)
- Antidepressants
- Opioids
- NSAIDs
- Polypharmacy especially dangerous

Incidence and Demographics
- One of the most common complaints in the elderly
- 30% of community-dwelling people age 72+ had complaint of dizziness in past 2 months

Risk Factors
- Risk of dizziness 68% in patients with 5 or more
  - Anxiety
  - Depressive symptoms
  - Past myocardial infarction
  - Use of more than 4 medications
  - Impaired balance
  - Postural hypotension
  - Impaired hearing

Prevention and Screening
- Review fall risks and prevention
- Eliminate all unnecessary medications, including OTC and herbal
- Manage medical illnesses closely
- Alcohol screening and counseling

Assessment
- Most important to determine if acute or chronic, or if condition is unstable

History
- Description
  - Have the patient describe the feeling without using the word "dizzy"
  - Interview family member or witness
- Course/Timing
  - Detailed history of event, frequency, when it occurs, prodromal symptoms
  - Length of loss of consciousness, seizure activity, fall hard or soft, any injuries including to tongue
  - Confusion or drowsiness after event
- What made it better/worse

- Precipitating factors
  - Rapid head movements
  - Change in position
- Associated symptoms
  - Diaphoresis
  - Blurred vision
  - Nausea
  - Hearing loss
  - Tinnitus
  - Associated cardiac or neurological symptoms: chest pain, palpitations, headache, diplopia, aphasia, unilateral motor weakness, paresthesia
  - Incontinence of bladder or bowel
  - Was event exertional
- How it interferes with their routine activities
  - Past medical history: cardiac, neurologic
  - Family history of heart disease, seizures
  - Medications

Physical
- Specific to etiology, look for
  - Cardiac abnormalities: orthostatic hypotension, arrhythmia, murmurs, cardiomegaly, bruits
  - Neurological abnormalities: focal deficits
  - Test vestibular function by rotational testing
  - Otologic evaluation
  - Evaluate vision and hearing
  - Respiratory exam

Diagnostic Studies

GENERAL
- CBC
- Metabolic panel, including fasting blood sugar
- Thyroid function test if suspect hypothyroidism

IF SUSPECT CARDIAC CAUSE
- Electrocardiography
- Echocardiography to rule out valvular disease
- Stress testing if exertional syncope to rule out ischemia
- Holter or event monitoring to rule out arrhythmia

IF SUSPECT NEUROLOGIC CAUSE
- Brain CT scan if mass lesion suspected
- Tilt table to evaluate autonomic dysfunction
- Electroencephalography if seizure history or seizures suspected
- Electronystagmography if vestibular origin is suspected
- Brain imaging if focal neuro signs
- Carotid or transcranial Doppler studies if bruits or rule out vertebrobasilar insufficiency

Differential Diagnosis
- Between the types of dizziness
- Between the causes of dizziness

Management
- Treat underlying cause

Nonpharmacologic Treatment
- Manage orthostatic hypotension
  - Change position slowly

- Exercise feet before standing
- Elastic stockings (put on before rising)
- Elevate head of bed
- Avoid activity in hot weather
- Exercise
- Fluid—ensure adequate intake
- Dietary interventions—adequate amount, good nutrition

Pharmacologic Treatment
- Discontinue unnecessary medications
- Use smallest doses of medications

How Long to Treat
- Usually lifelong

When to Consult, Refer, Hospitalize
- Hospitalize for unstable condition
- Refer to Cardiology for suspected cardiac cause
- Refer to Neurology for neurological cause, focal neuro signs
- Refer to Psychiatry if symptoms interfering with function and cannot be managed with first-line medications
- Refer older people that cannot be safely managed in their present living environment

Follow-up

Expected Course
- Depends on etiology

Complications
- Functional disability
- Falls, fractures, fear of falling
- Immobility
- Social isolation
- Nursing home placement
- Depression
- Death

DISEQUILIBRIUM

Description
- Imbalance, unsteadiness, "dizziness in the feet"

Etiology
- Vestibular: loss of vestibular function (see Vertigo Chapter 7)
  - Cause—ototoxic drugs, cerumen impaction, labyrinthitis, acoustic neuroma
- Proprioceptive and somatosensory
  - Symptoms numbness, weakness, bowel and bladder dysfunction
  - Cause—peripheral neuropathy secondary to alcohol, DM, renal failure
- Motor and cerebellar lesions
  - Symptoms—gait disturbances, ataxia
  - Cause—Parkinson's, cerebellum atrophy, tumors, infarcts, hydrocephalus
- Normal changes of aging
- Slowing of motor responses, weakness of support muscles, decreased proprioception

Incidence and Demographics
- Unknown

Risk Factors
- See Dizziness etiology

Prevention and Screening
- Treat risk factors

Assessment

History
- Occurs in standing position, with movement, or turning head

Physical
- Observe rising from chair and gait
- Neuro exam including cerebellar function and sensation (especially vibratory) in lower extremities

Differential Diagnosis
- See Dizziness etiology

Management

Nonpharmacologic Treatment
- Support with cane or walker
- Physical therapy with gait and balance training
- Tai Chi

Pharmacologic Treatment
- Depending on underlying etiology
- Manage diabetes, B_{12}, and folate deficiency

How Long to Treat
- Usually chronic, cannot be cured

When to Consult, Refer, Hospitalize
- Refer if etiology in doubt, treatment not effective, patient unable to function

Follow-up
- See Dizziness

SYNCOPE

Description
- Syncope: transient loss of consciousness and postural tone due to impaired cerebral circulation with spontaneous recovery
- Occurs from standing position, occasionally from seated position but not lying down
- Patient is neurologically baseline upon recovery
- Near-syncope: sensation of impending faint may be caused by all of causes of dizziness, especially psychogenic etiologies and hyperventilation

Etiology
- Unknown (37%)
- Vasovagal (20%)
- Cardiovascular (10%)
- Orthostatic hypotension (9%)
- Medications (7%)
- Vasovagal: due to impaired vasoconstriction resulting in hypotension with decrease cerebral perfusion
- Stimuli for vasovagal syncope include fear, emotions, pain, nausea, cough, defecation, micturition, swallowing, postprandial

Incidence and Demographics
- 30% of adults will experience at least one episode of syncope
- 3% of all emergency department visits and 1% to 6% of hospitalizations

- Associated with high morbidity and mortality, and falls
- Work-up can be expensive

Risk Factors
- Cardiac disease
- Diabetes
- COPD
- Polypharmacy: vasodilators, diuretics, adrenergic blocking agents
- Age-related cardiovascular, autonomic, and neuroendocrine changes
- Cardiovascular deconditioning

Prevention and Screening
- Adequate hydration
- Reduction of cardiac risk factors

Assessment

History
- Premonitory autonomic nervous system signs and symptoms preceding vasovagal syncope: sweating, pallor, nausea, palpitations, shortness of breath
- Associated cardiac symptoms before or after episode
- Any neurologic signs or symptoms: confusion, weakness, sensory disturbance, aphasia, aura

Differential Diagnosis
- See etiology of Dizziness

Management

Nonpharmacologic Treatment
- In cases of benign syncope (vasomotor) explain etiology to patient, advise to lie down when prodromal symptoms occur

When to Consult, Refer, Hospitalize
- Refer to cardiology for evaluation
- Hospitalize if hemodynamically unstable or new onset atrial fibrillation

Follow-up
- Patient with syncope from unknown cause should be followed closely

Complications
- Patients with syncope of unknown cause have a 30% increase in all cause mortality and in risk for MI
- Patients with syncope from vasovagal, orthostatic, or medication have no increased risk for death or MI

FATIGUE/WEAKNESS

Description
- Generalized fatigue and weakness, a vague complaint of lethargy or excessive tiredness
- Similar to dizziness in that it has many causes, often multifactorial, etiology often elusive
- Weakness of a particular part of the body should prompt investigation of CVA

Etiology

Physical
- Deconditioning
- Sleep disorder, insomnia, sleep apnea

- Diet
- Alcohol
- Sedentary lifestyle
- Drugs
- Obesity
- GU—cancer of bladder, uterus, and prostate, renal failure
- Hematopoietic—anemia, chronic leukemias, lymphoma, multiple myeloma
- Infection—acute or chronic
- Respiratory—COPD, asthma
- Cardiac disease—CAD, CHF
- Endocrine disorder—DM, thyroid, parathyroid, and Cushing's
- GI—pancreatic, colon carcinoma, chronic hepatitis, irritable bowel syndrome
- Neurological disease—neuromuscular, dementia, delirium, CVA
- Rheumatic disease—temporal arteritis, rheumatoid arthritis, polymyalgia rheumatic
- Other malignancies

Psychological
- Depression
- Stress
- Panic Disorder
- Anxiety

Incidence and Demographics
- Very common in the elderly

Risk Factors
- Chronic disease
- Medications

Prevention and Screening
- Specific to etiology

Assessment

History
- Overall, systemic, generalized lack of energy, fatigue, nonspecific malaise
- Trouble concentrating, lack of interest
- How is fatigue interfering with function
- History of weight change
- The family may report the patient is acting weak, has decreased activity, or is sleeping more

Physical
- Specific to the etiology
- Use functional assessment to look for impairments
- May have weight loss

Diagnostic Studies
- CBC
- Electrolytes, glucose, creatinine and BUN, calcium, ESR, liver function tests, thyroid function tests
- Urine for urinalysis and culture and sensitivity
- May need CXR and EKG and other diagnostic tests

Differential Diagnosis
- See Etiology

Management
- Treatment specific to etiology

Nonpharmacologic Treatment
- OT and PT to regain strength lost from deconditioning and to increase functional independence
- Energy conservation
- Plan day to complete necessary tasks
- Exercise to tolerance
- Diet counseling and supplements if appropriate to etiology

How Long to Treat
- As underlying etiology dictates

When to Consult, Refer, Hospitalize
- Appropriate consultant for underlying etiology
- Physical/Occupational therapy
- Dietitian
- Hospitalize if underlying etiology or acute exacerbation of etiology cannot be managed safely on an outpatient basis

Follow-up
Depends on etiology

GAIT DISORDERS

Description
- Instability when walking
- Impaired mobility
- Places patients at risk for falls, fractures

Etiology
- Multifactorial
- Normal changes of aging—a more stable, careful gait
- Sway while standing increases, postural support responses are slowed
- Greater reliance on proprioception
- Shorter, broader based stride, speed declines
- Arm swing decreases
- Sensory deficit
- Neurologic disorders
- Dementia
- Parkinson's flexed posture, diminished arm swing, festination, difficulty initiating movement, turns, impaired balance
- Normal pressure hydrocephalus—shuffling gait
- Cerebellar disease—lateral instability of trunk, widened stance, sensory ataxia, destabilized by eye closure
- Peripheral neuropathy
- Stroke—hemiparesis
- Frontal lobe gait apraxia—hesitation in starting, shuffling, difficulty picking up feet, turning, poor standing balance
- Myopathy
- Vestibular disfunction
- Musculoskeletal disorders
- Arthritis of lower extremities
- Myelopathy—compression of cervical cord
- Cervical spondylosis—chronic cord compression, spasticity, hyperreflexia in legs, dorsal column sign, urinary urgency, gait stiff legged

- Lumbar spondylosis
- Hip replacement surgery
- Foot disease
- Medications

Incidence and Demographics
- Unknown, leads to falls, which are very common

Risk Factors
- See Etiology

Prevention and Screening
- Depends on etiology

Assessment

History
- Time course
- Additional symptoms
- Medications
- Falls
- Does gait disorder interfere with ADLs?
- Physical
- Visual/sensory changes
- Neurologic
- Musculoskeletal
- Observe gait
- Get up and go test—stand up from a chair, walk 10 feet, turn around, come back and sit down
- Tinetti assessment tool

Diagnostic Studies
- Lab depends on history and physical
- Motor—CT scan or MRI rule out mass lesion, subdural hematoma, normal pressure hydrocephalus
- Balance—toxic and metabolic causes blood chemistries, B_{12}
- CT scan strokes
- Cervical spine films

Differential Diagnosis
- See Etiology

Management
- Specific to cause

Nonpharmacologic Treatment
- Physical therapy for assistive devices
- Home safety assessment for fall risk
- Proper footgear

When to Consult, Refer, Hospitalize
- Refer to neurology, physiatry, or orthopedics

Follow-up

Expected Course
- Depends on etiology

Complications
- Falls
- Fractures

FALLS

Description
- Person unintentionally comes to rest on lower level, not due to loss of consciousness or violent impact
- What did they hurt? Why did they fall?
- Falls are a marker for frailty and a predictor of death

Etiology
- Cause—multifactorial, remember nonspecific presentation of illness in the elderly
- Anything that causes dizziness, gait disorder, or fatigue
- Environmental hazards—need home evaluation
  - Handrails, rugs, lighting, footgear
  - Kitchen—overhead cabinets
  - Bathrooms, bedrooms, at night, rushing to bathroom, answer phone

Incidence and Demographics
- 30% of elderly living at home fall each year
- 5% result in serious soft tissue injury
- 5% result in fractures
- 50% of patient who fell will be alive in 1 year
- 50% of nursing home patients fall each year
- Accidents are the fifth leading cause of death
- Primary cause of accidental deaths in the elderly

Risk Factors
- Sensory: somatosensory, proprioception, and visual
- Vestibular: balance
- Musculoskeletal: strength, endurance
- Behavioral: attention, memory, fear of falling, depression
- Medications/drugs: sedatives, anxiolytics, especially benzodiazepines, diuretics, laxatives, alcohol
- Environment: home safety

Prevention and Screening
- Screen for risk factors
- Use one of many fall risk assessment tools, choice depends on setting—home, NH, hospital
- Exercise is the single most effective strategy for preventing falls

Assessment
- Complete history and physical
- History of previous falls
- Medications
- Circumstances of the fall: time of day, events, symptoms prior to fall, what happened after fall, loss of consciousness, could patient get up under own power or required assistance, how long on floor
- Patients perception of the cause of the fall: trip or slip, awareness
- Get up and go test—stand up from a chair, walk 10 feet, turn around, come back and sit down
- Tinetti assessment tool

Diagnostic Studies
- X-rays and other imaging as appropriate for injury or to diagnose underlying condition

Differential Diagnosis
See Etiology

Management
- Specific to etiology
- Physical conditioning, physical therapy, occupational therapy to include leg strength, flexibility, and balance
- Revise environment to eliminate hazards
- Vision improvement, lighting
- Assistive devices
- Tai Chi
- Aquatic therapy
- See osteoporosis management to decrease fracture risk
- Address behavioral issues, especially fear of falling, which may cause patients to be overly cautious and walk less, leading to deconditioning and more falls
- Personal response services to activate 911 when patient falls

Special Considerations
- Long periods down on floor before found are associated with increased morbidity, including hypothermia

When to Consult, Refer, Hospitalize
- Emergency department for serious injuries or life-threatening underlying condition
- Consult with appropriate specialty cardiac, neuro, ortho if suspect underlying condition

Follow-up
- Depends on etiology

Complications
- Fractures
- Painful soft tissue injuries
- Subdural hematoma
- Impaired mobility because of physical injury
- Fear of falling with decreased activity
- Social isolation
- Decreased independence

FRACTURES

Description
- A break in a bone
- Most common fractures in the elderly are hip, vertebral compression, and wrist (Colle's)

Etiology
- Falls
- Osteoporosis
- Tumor
- Osteomyelitis
- Osteomalacia

Incidence and Demographics
- Hip fractures are most frequent, followed by wrist fracture
- 50% hip fracture patients end up in nursing home
- Fewer than 30% regain prefracture level of physical functioning
- Hip—12% to 20% mortality associated with hip fracture repair
- White women over age 60 have a higher incidence of fracture than for men and other races due to osteoporosis

Risk Factors
- See Etiology

Prevention and Screening
- Maximize bone density during adolescence/young adulthood
- Treatment of osteoporosis/osteopenia

- Weight-bearing physical activity
- Adequate dietary intake of calcium
- Avoidance of smoking, excessive alcohol intake

Assessment
- Hip fracture—may occur with a fall or spontaneously due to osteoporosis
- Vertebral fractures may occur with sudden move such as sneezing, coughing, lifting, or stretching
- Colle's fracture of distal radius—occurs with fall with outstretched arm

History
- Pain is predominant symptom
- Pain worse with movement
- Swelling occurs rapidly, may be associated with bruising, variable degree of deformity

Physical
- Point tenderness over bone; muscle weakness/pain with movement; deformity
- Hip fracture: leg shortened, externally rotated; patient will not weight bear
- Vertebra: back pain, kyphosis
- Wrist: Colle's—exquisite tenderness to touch

Diagnostic Studies
- X-ray: most cost-effective; usually adequate for showing fracture; in elderly may take days for fracture to appear on x-ray
- Bone scan: useful for identifying occult/stress fracture
- CT: for evaluating degree of displacement, compression of fracture
- MRI: identifying lesions that may affect bone
- Laboratory studies not usually indicated

Differential Diagnosis
- Sprain
- Torn ligament
- Hematoma
- Tendinitis
- Tumor

Management

Nonpharmacologic Treatment
- Hip: surgery usually necessary
- Intertrochanteric—pin—associated with bleeding, instability, deformity
- Femoral neck—prosthesis—associated with avascular necrosis, infection
- Vertebra: pain management
- Wrist: cast

Pharmacologic Treatment
- Pain management—see section on pain

How Long to Treat
- Primary care treatment is immobilization and referral to orthopedic surgeon

Special Considerations
- If x-ray initially negative for fracture and pain does not begin to improve after 1 to 2 weeks, re-x-ray or consider bone scan to rule out occult fracture

Follow-up

Expected Course
- Fracture healing should occur in 6 to 12 weeks
- Persistent but gradually decreasing swelling and improving strength, may take another 4 to 6 weeks to resolve

Complications
- Persistent deformity, arthritis, compression neuropathy, fibrous union
- Failure to heal secondary to osteoporosis
- Functional decline, decreased ambulation
- Chronic pain, especially with vertebral fractures
- Loss of independence
- Increased health care utilization and institutionalization
- Death

SLEEP DISORDERS

Description
- Insomnia is a symptom, the most frequent complaint of the sleep disorders
  - Subjective problem of insufficient or nonrestorative sleep in spite of adequate opportunity to sleep
  - Short term—less than 3 weeks
  - Long term—at least 3 nights/week for more than 3 weeks
- Sleep apnea is a sleep-related breathing disorder, cessation of airflow at the nose and mouth for at least 10 seconds in repetitive episodes that disrupt sleep structure. Important sleep disorder in the elderly that is under diagnosed and undertreated

Etiology
- Insomnia
  - Short-term insomnia
    Acute stress
    Acute pain
    Environmental changes
    Drugs (decongestants)
    Stimulants, caffeine
    Withdrawal of sedatives, especially benzodiazepines
  - Long-term insomnia
    Psychiatric disorders
       Conditioned anxiety about being able to fall asleep
       Alcohol and substance abuse, caffeine, stimulants
       Depression (early morning awakening)
       Anxiety
       Grief
    Chronic pain
    Nocturia (often caused by diuretics)
    Medical disorders
       CHF
       Hyperthyroidism
       Rheumatologic diseases
       Dementia, Parkinson's
       COPD, asthma
       Esophageal reflux
       Restless leg syndrome
    Medication
- Sleep apnea
  - Central—failure to initiate breathing
  - Obstructive upper airway occlusion, usually accompanied by periods of snoring and restlessness

Incidence and Demographics
- Insomnia
  - 30% to 40% of all adults complain of insomnia
  - 10% to 15% have chronic and or severe insomnia
  - More prevalent with increasing age
  - The elderly consume 40% of all prescription sleep medications and 15% use them regularly
- Apnea
  - Unknown, underdiagnosed
  - More common in men than women

Risk Factors
- See Etiology

Prevention and Screening
- Public and patient education concerning the causes and risk factors associated with primary sleep disorders
- Regular bedtime routines
- Normalized daily routines and waking hours
- Physical exercise regime
- Stable interpersonal relations
- Family and social support systems

Assessment
History
- Ask sleep history
  - Timing—onset, duration
  - Time it takes to fall asleep
  - Frequency of awakenings
  - Difficulty going back to sleep after awakening
- What makes it better, worse
- Ask about symptoms during day/consequences of insomnia
  - Sleepy, lethargic during day
  - Poor performance in demanding situations
  - Difficulty concentrating
  - Fatigue
  - Irritability
- Patient to keep sleep diary
- Obtain history from the patient's bed partner to look for snoring, apnea, jerking, restlessness

Physical
- Specific to suspected etiology
- Physical exam should be tailored to the presenting symptomology, as primary insomnia is an illness of exclusion of other underlying medical conditions

Diagnostic Studies
- Depends on suspected etiology
- CBC, chemistry profile, electrolytes,
- Sleep study—polysomnography if suspect sleep apnea

Differential Diagnosis
- See Etiology

Management
- Specific to condition
- Treat short-term insomnia to avoid long-term insomnia

Nonpharmacologic Treatment
- Treat underlying cause
- Withdraw unnecessary medications
- Pain relief
- Sleep hygiene
  - Go to bed, wake up same time every day
  - Avoid long periods of wakefulness in bed
  - Do not use bed except for sleep (and sex)
  - Avoid napping
- Regular exercise (not too close to bedtime)
- Avoid alcohol, caffeine, smoking
- Stress management/relaxation therapy
- Herbal treatments, such as valerian root, camomile and melatonin, are unproven
- Provide individual with literature and community resources

Pharmacologic Treatment
See Table 4-3.
- Short term
  - Zolpidem (Ambien) 5–10 mg PO at night
  - Zaleplon (Sonata) 5–10 mg PO at night
  - Benzodiazepines short acting with caution
- Long term
  - Antihistamines
  - Antidepressants, sedating such as trazodone, mirtazapine (Remeron), paroxetine (Paxil) if patient also depressed
  - Discontinue gradually
  - Rebound insomnia may occur when medications discontinued
  - Be aware of potential for drug tolerance, dependence, and withdrawal with benzodiazepines
  - Do not prescribe for patients with a history of substance abuse or mental illness
  - Refer to a psychiatrist or other mental health specialist when symptoms are secondary to anxiety disorder or mood disorder not amenable to first-line treatment
- Sleep apnea
  - Refer to sleep specialist

How Long to Treat
- Patients should be followed weekly short term to monitor effectiveness of treatment, compliance, and potential abuse
- Once stable, monitor every 1 to 3 months

Special Considerations
- Habituation/tolerance is a major problem with benzodiazepam hypnotics
- The elderly are very vulnerable to the effects of sedative-hypnotics, especially confusion, delirium, sleep apnea, falls with fractures

Table 4-3: Insomnia Medications

Medication	Dose
Zaleplon (Sonata)	5–10 mg PO at night
Zolpidem (Ambien)	5–10 mg PO at night
Trazodone (Desyrel)	25–50 mg at night

When to Consult, Refer, Hospitalize
- When symptoms continue to occur for longer than 1 month, refer to a sleep disorder specialist, psychiatrist, or other qualified mental health practitioner
- Refer suspected sleep apnea to specialist

Follow-up
Expected Course
- Most patients have chronic lifelong insomnia that is best managed by nonpharmacologic treatment

Complications
- Insomnia can lead to chronic fatigue and decreased activity
- Sleep apnea can lead to sudden death

UNINTENTIONAL WEIGHT LOSS/FAILURE TO THRIVE

Description
- Weight loss in an elderly patient who is not trying to lose weight
- Weight loss exceeding 5% of baseline weight should trigger investigation
- Failure to thrive is defined as weight loss of greater than 5% of baseline, decreased appetite, poor nutrition, and inactivity

Etiology
- In the elderly, cause may be multifactorial
- Look for any treatable causes
- The cause is not found in about one-quarter of patients with weight loss
- If no diagnosis is made, follow over time, weeks to months for cause to be revealed
- Normal changes of aging
  - Decreased appetite, taste, smell
- Medical disease
  - Depression (cause in 30%)
  - Dementia—no longer recognize food (5%)
  - Cancer (cause in only 5%)
  - Hyperthyroidism
  - Infection
  - Any medical illness that causes fatigue/anorexia (COPD, CHF, CRF, etc.)
  - Neurological disease that causes dysphagia (stroke, Parkinson's)
  - Mouth problems causing poor dentition, unable or painful to chew, gingivitis
- Social and psychological factors
  - Poverty
  - Bereavement
  - Ability to get food
- Medications (cause in 3%)
  - That cause dry mouth, altered taste, anorexia, GI distress, nausea, vomiting, diarrhea, constipation, cognitive disturbance, increased metabolism
  - Include parasympathomimetics, anticholinergics, diuretics, digoxin, ACE inhibitors, psychotropics, antidepressants, anticonvulsants, antineoplastic, NSAIDs
- Prescribed diets (cause in 7%)
  - Cholesterol-lowering, low-salt, and diabetic diets may be unpalatable
  - Patients may take diet to extremes, for example, no fat, too low salt diets

Incidence and Demographics
- 20% to 65% of institutionalized patients are undernourished

- 5% to 10% of elderly outpatients are malnourished
- 20% to 35% of elderly outpatients have subclinical undernutrition

Risk Factors
- See Etiology

Prevention and Screening
- Weigh patients at routine visits
- Assess diet history
- Regular counseling regarding nutrition

Assessment
- Complete history and physical

History
- Search for depression
- Is food available and is patient able to prepare it?
- Are clothes loose fitting? Is there a change in clothing size or waistband size?

Physical
- Look for cancer; see following section
- Can the patient eat? Observe patient eating/drinking
- Serial weights
- General appearance: thin, cachectic, dehydrated, muscle wasting, disheveled, loose-fitting clothes

Diagnostic Studies
- CBC
- Metabolic panel—dehydration common
- Ca++—may be elevated in cancer
- Albumin/total protein, low in protein malnutrition
- Total cholesterol often low in total calorie undernutrition
- Thyroid function tests
- Urinalysis
- Stool hemoccult—cancer
- Chest x-ray
- PSA in men

Management

Nonpharmacologic Treatment
- Dietary supplements: easily eaten foods that are high calorie—ice cream, Ensure
- Flavor enhancement of food
- Assistance with preparing, eating
- Patient monitoring over time
- Consider multiple vitamin supplement

Pharmacologic Treatment
- Treat cause
- Drugs that may stimulate appetite
    - Progestin (Megace) indicated for AIDS at 800 mg/day; used in much lower doses in the elderly, dosage controversial, studies have not demonstrated decreased mortality with use
    - Methylphenidate (Ritalin)—not FDA indicated, but used in low dose in the elderly for depression and to stimulate appetite, starting dose 2.5 mg PO q AM, may increase to 5–10 mg daily
    - Mirtazapine (Remeron) antidepressant, has side effects of appetite stimulation, see Psych Chapter 18

Special Considerations
- Artificial nutrition and hydration via gastric tube is not needed if the patient has terminal disease

When to Consult, Refer, Hospitalize
- Nutrition consult recommended for most patients
- Consult if etiology is undetermined after workup
- Consult if patient continues to lose weight with intervention
- Hospitalize for severe dehydration

Follow-up
- Weekly weights may be useful in evaluating weight loss
- Monthly weights are useful to monitor for weight loss

Expected Course
- Depends on etiology
- Often not correctable
- Weight loss is a marker for a poor prognosis
- In many patients, weight loss means the patient is terminal

Complications
- General
  - Decreased quality and length of life
  - Impaired functional status
  - Delirium
  - Weakness/fatigue
  - Dehydration
  - Orthostatic hypotension
- Immune
  - Decreased response to infections and allergies
- Skin
  - Poor wound healing
  - Increased pressure ulcers
- Musculoskeletal
  - Decreased muscle mass and strength
  - Increased falls
  - Increased fractures

CANCER
- See relevant chapters for discussion of specific cancers

Normal Changes of Aging
- General decline in functional reserve of many organ systems
- Increase in comorbidities, disability, and geriatric syndromes (e.g., dementia, depression)
- Decline in renal function: glomerular filtration rate has a significant impact on the many chemotherapy drugs that are renally excreted
- Hepatic drug metabolism activity decreases (e.g., P450 system)—metabolism of some drugs affected

Age-Related Factors and Cancer Development
- Age-related accumulation of genetic damage
- Molecular changes: tissues may be more susceptible to environmental carcinogens
- DNA damage may lead to inactivation of tumor suppressor genes
- Damage more difficult to repair in older cells

- Biological behavior of tumors may change with aging
  - Breast and non–small cell lung cancer (NSCLC): generally more indolent
  - Acute myelogenous leukemia (AML), large-cell non-Hodgkin's lymphoma (NHL), celomic ovarian cancer: poorer prognosis

Presentation of Cancer

- Delayed diagnoses common; atypical presentations may be masked by aging changes or coexisting diseases
- Stage of cancer at presentation may vary with age
- Breast, colon, bladder cancers, melanoma often present at more advanced stages; NSCL cancer at earlier stage

Incidence and Demographics

COMMON CANCERS

- Increased incidence cancer and mortality in persons older than 65
- 50% of all cancers occur in 12% of population aged 65 and older
- Incidence of most common cancers over age 65: prostate (76.9%), breast (47.5%), lung (65.8%), non-Hodgkin's lymphoma (NHL) (51%), urinary/bladder (71.4%)
- Highest cancer mortality in US: lung, colon and rectum, breast, prostate
- Increased incidence in last 20 years of non-melanoma skin cancer, NHL, and malignant brain tumors

SPECIFIC CANCERS

- Prostate and colorectal cancer continue to increase after age 85
- Ovarian Cancer: fifth leading cause of death in women; 46% in women over 65; highest mortality of all GYN cancers
- 48% of breast and 46% ovarian cancer occur in older women
- Lung cancer incidence increases up to age 70

Prevention and Screening

- Benefits: increased prevalence of cancer; increased positive predictive value of screening tests
- Limitations: shorter life expectancy; magnitude of benefit may decrease with increasing age and comorbidity
- Consider life expectancy, quality of life (QOL), and individual factors
- Barriers: inadequate use of preventive services and limited access to care
  - Provider: inadequate knowledge; limited evidence based studies to demonstrated benefits and risks of screening those aged 75 plus; time factors; inadequate referrals for screening and specialized care
  - Patient: knowledge, transportation, economic limitations, and inadequate provider support for screening

Risk Factors

BREAST CANCER (BC)

- Age, prior history BC, family history, menarche before age 12, first birth after 35, menopause after 53, prior breast biopsies
- Exogenous estrogens, radiation exposure in childhood
- Lower risk of genetic transmission (1% in women aged 80 and older)
- Breast self-exam (BSE) monthly, clinical breast exam (CBE) yearly; mammogram every 1 to 2 years
- Controversial: screening intervals; screening over age 80

CERVICAL CANCER

- Increased risk in women who do not undergo regular pap tests
- Early age first intercourse, several sex partners

- Pap smear every 1 to 3 years

Ovarian Cancer
- Family history ovarian cancer, use of fertility drugs
- Nulliparous, late menopause
- Risk decreases with increasing parity, oral contraceptive use, breast-feeding
- CA 125, ultrasound useful in diagnosis
- Insufficient evidence to recommend routine screening

Lung Cancer
- Cigarette smoking: risk increases with quantity and duration of smoking
- Asbestos, radon, gas, environmental agents
- Insufficient evidence for routine screening

Prostate Cancer
- Age, family history, black race
- Only 9% thought to have genetic basis
- Digital rectal exam (DRE): poor detection anterior prostate cancer
- PSA: false positives due to BPH, prostatitis, finasteride, needle biopsy, procedures
- PSA + DRE: sensitivity 87.2%
- Screening controversial: many false-positives; high incidence indolent disease elderly

Colorectal Cancer
- Combination genetic and environmental factors likely
- DNA defects from inherited familial syndromes
- Hereditary nonpolyposis syndrome, chronic inflammatory bowel disease
- Annual fecal occult blood test (FOBT)
- Sigmoidoscopy age 50 and every 5 years
- Barium enema (BE) alternative screening test in low-risk persons
- If adenomas or polyps: colonoscopy and every 3 years thereafter
- Positive FOBT: colonoscopy

Non-melanoma Skin Cancer
- Older age, fair complexion, prior NMSC, cumulative sun exposure
- Screening controversial: insufficient evidence that routine skin examination decreases mortality

Assessment
- Comorbidity, functional status, mental status, depression, polypharmacy, nutritional status, social support, living situation
- Comorbidities: preexisting illnesses (hypertension, heart conditions, arthritis, frailty, other geriatric syndromes)
- Associated with increased risk of cancer-related complications and death
- Assess Activities of Daily Living (ADL), functional status (FS): ability to perform daily tasks
- Limitations in functional reserve and dependence in ADL may decrease tolerance of chemo-therapy

Frailty Criteria (1 or more)
- Age 85 or older at risk
- Limited functional reserve: dependence in one or more ADL
- Comorbidities: 3 or more
- Geriatric syndromes: dementia, depression, delirium, falls, osteoporosis, neglect

Management
- Decision making
  - Goals of treatment
    Preserve function and quality of life

Prevent morbidity

Delay pain in advanced disease

- Risk/benefit analysis

Benefits of treatment (prolong survival, QOL, palliation symptoms)

Risks/side effects (complications chemotherapy)

- Decision triad: consider tumor, treatment, and patient

Tumor: disease, stage

Treatment: effectiveness, tolerance

Patient: life expectancy, quality of life, function, comorbidity, access to care, preferences/values

Nonpharmacologic Treatment

- Surgery
  - Determination of surgical risk often difficult
  - Consider physiologic status, coexisting diseases
  - Similar mortality and morbidity to younger patients when no contraindications
  - Influenced by comorbidities, declines in function
  - Increased morbidity/mortality with advanced disease, emergency surgery
- Radiation
  - Adjunct to surgery/chemotherapy
  - May benefit older and frail persons as alternative to surgery/chemotherapy
  - Used for curative and palliative treatment
  - Symptoms palliation; organ and function preservation
  - Data regarding effectiveness and tolerance of radiation therapy in older person is limited
  - Available data suggest that older patients with good functional status tolerate radiotherapy as well as younger patients with comparable tumor responses and survival
  - Disadvantage long duration of therapy (6 to 7 weeks for curative therapy)

Pharmacologic/Other Considerations

- May need to adjust dose based on renal or hepatic function
- Frailty: risks of aggressive chemotherapy may outweigh benefits
- Supportive care may include modified chemotherapy or hormonal regimen for palliative treatment
- Malnourished may have low albumin: increased free drug concentration leads to toxicity
- Manage polypharmacy, comorbidities, social issues, malnutrition
- Complications
  - Myelotoxicity due to reduced hematologic reserve
  - Neutropenia may lead to infection-related death or hospitalization
  - Mucositis, cardiomyopathy, central and peripheral neuropathy
  - Chemotherapy and anemia-related fatigue may lead to functional dependence
  - Cognitive dysfunction

Special Considerations

- Many elderly undertreated due to fears of treatment-related toxicities
- Only one third of persons over 75 managed by multimodal therapy vs two-thirds younger patients
- Assess social, psychological, and economic concerns
- Assess social or family support and caregiver concerns
- Address potential barriers to treatment
- Older patients receive less aggressive therapy for similar cancers
- Reasons unclear, perhaps due to decreased expectations of the providers
- However, research has shown the elderly are often able to tolerate and to benefit from aggressive therapy

When to Consult, Refer, Hospitalize
- Refer patients to oncologist

Follow-up
- Lifelong monitoring for recurrences and metastases

Expected Course
- Depends on type of cancer

Complications
- Pain
- Death

PAIN

Description
- Noxious sensation that may or may not be associated with tissue damage, has emotion and cognitive associations, uncontrolled leads to loss of function and depression

Etiology
- Musculoskeletal: osteoarthritis, osteoporosis, muscle injury, chronic headache, back pain; can be due to bone metastasis
- Visceral pain: GI tract/soft tissue tumor involvement, chronic pelvic pain, interstitial cystitis, partial obstruction due to tumor
- Neuropathic pain: nerve compression due to tumor or other cause, diabetic neuropathy, postherpetic neuralgia
- Direct tumor involvement
- Pain related to cancer therapy (surgery, radiation, chemotherapy)

Incidence and Demographics
- 80% to 85% elderly will have a pain problem during their life
- 25% to 50% will experience significant pain, that impairs their functional status
- 45% to 80% of nursing home patients will have significant pain
- 74% elderly with metastatic disease experience pain

Assessment
- Challenging in presence of multiple sources of pains
- Complicated by communication difficulties, atypical illness presentations
- Pain in cognitively impaired especially difficult to assess
- Pain is a contributing factor to delirium and depression
- Evaluate distress from other symptoms, such as nausea
- Has the patient had an adequate evaluation into the direct cause of the pain?
- Nonverbal behavior can give clues to pain, such as grimace, restlessness
- Pain can be acute, chronic, or mixed
  - Acute: pallor, diaphoresis; anxiety, agitation
  - Chronic: subtle personality changes, changes in functional ability

History
- Believe your patient when they complain of pain; if in doubt, ask in different ways and look for consistency of answers
- Elderly may underreport symptoms (lowered expectations, fear of side effects)
- Have patient describe pain—throbbing, shooting, stabbing, aching, etc.
  - Musculoskeletal—aching
  - Visceral—cramping
  - Neuropathic—burning or tingling

- Past medical history, chronology of pain, and/or cancer
- Pain-related history (characteristics, responses to prior therapies)
- Multiple pain: assess each problem independently
- Use validated pain instruments (numerical rating scale [0–10])
- Consequences of pain on ADLs, function, sleep

Physical
- Careful musculoskeletal exam
- Detailed neurologic exam
- Functional assessment

Diagnostic Studies
- Specific to suspected etiology
- X-rays
- MRI

Management
- Usually requires multidisciplinary approach
- Continuity of care necessary
- Let the patient have as much control as possible over life
- Treat the specific cause of the pain
- Treat the complications of the pain, such as muscle spasm, depression, insomnia

Nonpharmacologic Treatment
- Emphasize nonpharmacologic treatment
- Adequate pain control before exercise or physical therapy
- Exercise, activity increases conditioning, endurance, flexibility, blood flow, strength
- Physical therapy: helpful in getting started on safe and effective exercise program
- Heat, ice: whichever patient prefers, alternate
- Vibration for muscle tension
- Massage: distraction, relax muscles, use carefully—DVTs, touch is therapeutic
- TENS: transcutaneous electrical nerve stimulation—low-voltage electrical stimulation—counterirritation, size of beeper, hook between brain and pain, tingles, fiddle with them, PT usually handles
- Acupuncture for established pain: neurostimulatory technique that treats pain by the insertion of small, solid needles into the skin at varying depths, typically penetrating the underlying musculature; acupressure also safe and effective, less scary
- Psychosocial interventions/coping strategies
- Relaxation
  - Relaxation exercises—tapes available in any bookstore
  - Requires cognitive ability, motivation
  - Progressive muscle relaxation, tense/relax
  - Biofeedback
- Distraction
  - Does not deny patient has pain, but helps get mind off pain
  - A social counterirritant—get involved with other people
  - Guided imagery—imagine yourself
- Manage daily routine
  - Regular daily schedule
  - Get out of bed
  - Get dressed, fixed up nice
  - Out of bedroom
  - Allow patient as much control over routine as feasible

Table 4-4: Choice of Pain Medication

	Musculoskeletal	Visceral	Neuropathic
Mild	Topical, acetaminophen NSAIDs	Acetaminophen	Topical, acetaminophen
Moderate	NSAIDs/mild opioid	Opioid	Adjuvant
Severe	Opioid, adjuvant	Opioid	Adjuvant/opioid

- Social involvement
  - Communication with family and friends
  - Avoid isolation
  - Maintain outside interests
- Treat the depression
  - With counseling and/or medications
  - Complex relationship between chronic pain and depression
  - Certain medications treat both depression and pain and can be very effective

Pharmacologic Treatment (See Table 4-4)
- Refer also to the American Geriatrics Society clinical practice guidelines—see references
- Principles
  - Expect to relieve the pain; pain can be successfully treated in the elderly
  - Monitor for and treat side effects of medications, which frequently limit medication usefulness
  - Regular dosing for chronic pain, not PRN
  - Monitor effectiveness, individualize regimen
  - Give PO if possible, then consider topical, transdermal, rectal, SQ, IM, pump
  - Treat aggressively to break cycle, get started on nonpharmacological management
  - Then decrease dosage, medications for maintenance
  - The main difference between treatment of chronic, nonmalignant pain, and cancer pain is the expected duration of treatment
  - Opioids are generally used earlier in cancer pain because of the limited life expectancy
  - Opioids cause dependence, do not use long term unless necessary
  - Recently providers are becoming less reluctant to use opioids in nonmalignant pain
  - Many patients still suffer needlessly because providers are reluctant to treat pain adequately
  - Adequate treatment of pain allows for quality of life, ability to function
  - Gradually increases dosages, increase dosing intervals, add medicines as disease progresses
- Topical
  - Rubs and liniments—use on intact skin
  - Counterirritant—camphor, capsicum, cloves, menthol, methyl salicylate, etc.
  - Antiseptics—chloroxylenol, eugenol, thymol
  - Local anesthetic—benzocaine, lidocaine
- Acetaminophen
  - Acetaminophen (Tylenol) 500 mg 2 tabs q 4 h (up to 4000 mg in 24 hours)
  - Also available in long-acting formulation for sleep
- NSAIDs
  - Prototype—Ibuprofen (Motrin) 200–800 mg PO bid–qid
  - Side effects—indigestion, GI bleed, CHF, renal failure, confusion
  - Use short term; may be used long term with caution
  - All NSAIDs are similar, but one may work better for a patient than another
  - COX-2 inhibitors—less incidence of GI side effects

- Opioids
  - Very effective for most types of pain
  - Underutilized due to fears of addiction
  - Addiction is not an issue in the dying
  - Physical dependence will necessitate increased doses
  - Start with mild opioid and change to stronger as needed
  - No upper limits to dose of narcotics needed to treat severe pain, acetaminophen and narcotic combination tablets limited by dose of acetaminophen, not to exceed 4000 mg in 24 hours
  - Give patient continuous long-acting opioid for chronic pain management
  - Provide a fast-acting rescue medication for "breakthrough" pain
  - Start with low dose, progress with caution
  - Monitor for side effects, which are common: sedation, drowsiness, CNS depression, respiratory depression, nausea, vomiting, constipation, urinary retention, hepatotoxicity
    Treat side effects at first sign
    Many treat preventatively for constipation at onset of opioid therapy
    Reduce dosage if possible
- Listed from weakest to strongest, with starting dose and comments
  - Codeine with acetaminophen (Tylenol #3) 30–60 mg PO q 3–4 h
  - Hydrocodone (Vicodin) 5–10 mg PO q 3–4 h
  - Oxycodone (Percocet) 5–10 mg PO q 3–4 h
  - Sustained release oxycodone (OxyContin) 10–20 mg PO q 12 h
  - Morphine sulfate (Roxanol, MSIR) 15–30 mg PO q 4–6 h used as rescue med
  - Sustained Release Morphine (MS Contin) 15–30 mg PO q 12 h
  - Transdermal fentanyl (Duragesic) 25 mcg/hr change patch q 3 days; good if patient has difficulty swallowing
  - Hydromorphone (Dilaudid) 1.5 mg PO q 3–4 h, generally used as last resort
- Adjuvant analgesic drugs
  - Tricyclic antidepressants—neuropathic pain, insomnia
    Amitriptyline (Elavil), Nortriptyline (Pamelor) 10–25 mg PO at night
    Side effects include anticholinergic, sedation, postural hypotension
  - Anticonvulsants—neuropathic pain
    Carbamazepine (Tegretol) 100–200 mg at night
      Side effects include dizziness, drowsiness, nausea, vomiting, bone marrow suppression
    Gabapentin (Neurontin) 100 mg PO qhs—600 mg tid—excellent for pain from many causes, titrate up slowly
      Side effects include somnolence, dizziness, ataxia, fatigue, nystagmus, visual disturbances
      Other medications
- Prednisone 2.5–5 mg PO qd—for inflammation
- Baclofen (Lioresal) 5 mg PO qd for muscle spasms, neuropathic pain

When to Consult, Refer, Hospitalize
- Complicated pain, pain with difficult psychosocial issues
- Team approach for pain management (palliative care team; anesthesia pain specialist)
- Hospitalize for uncontrolled pain syndromes (cancer-related, compression fracture, traumatic)
- Neurosurgeon for neuropathic pain unrelieved by management
- Palliative radiation and chemotherapy
- Hospice for pain management of terminally ill patients

Follow-up
- Monitor efficacy of pain regimen at regular intervals
- New pain or change in pattern: diagnostic workup, modify treatment plan
- Teach patient/family assessment tools for effective home management

Expected Course
- Most chronic pain is chronic progressive

Complications
- Impaired function
- Depression, anxiety
- Insomnia
- Cognitive impairment, delirium
- Unacceptable quality of life and suicide risk

DEATH AND DYING

Description
- Most elderly are more concerned about how they die than about death
- What is a "good death"—no one clear universally accepted definition
- Traditionally was a fight to the end against the disease, more popular with the medical provider than most patients; some patients still want "a good death"
- Patients more often define as including control, closure, and acceptance, usually at home

Etiology
- See Chapter 3 for causes of death in the elderly

Incidence and Demographics
- Many patients die prolonged and painful deaths
- Many receive unwanted, painful, and invasive care that impairs the quality of life in their last days with needless suffering and emotion distress
- Most deaths still occur in hospitals

Risk Factors—Important Factors at the End of Life
- Personal care
  - Freedom from pain and discomfort (respiratory distress, GI distress, and constipation)
  - Kept clean, free from odors
- Preparation for death
  - Financial affairs in order
  - Knowing what to expect
- Achieve a sense of completion
  - Having treatment preferences in writing and naming power of attorney
- Being treated as a person
  - Maintaining dignity
  - Maintaining sense of humor
  - Having someone who will listen
  - Trusting one's physician
  - Having a nurse with whom one feels comfortable

Assessment
- Disease/symptom status; prognosis
- Emotional/spiritual aspects
- Patient/family goals/preferences
- Family support/needs
- Therapeutic options (benefits/burdens)
- Available resources

History
- Symptoms near death that cause discomfort
- Pain—see pain management section, this chapter
- GI symptoms—nausea, abdominal pain, constipation
- Respiratory—shortness of breath
- Psychosocial—anxiety, fear, family wishes, and knowledge of what is happening

Physical
- As necessary

Diagnostic Studies
- Avoid unnecessary procedures to avoid discomfort

Management

Nonpharmacologic Treatment
- Hospice—reimbursed by Medicare; NP now able to act as attending healthcare provider
  - Criteria: estimated life span less than 6 months
  - Hospice involves the concepts of comfort and caring, and management of symptoms while allowing the patient to die with control and dignity
  - Multidisciplinary team including nurses, volunteers, chaplains, therapists, social workers, bereavement counselors, and clinicians
  - Spiritual component of care
  - Continues beyond death of the patient to provide bereavement support for family and friends
  - Patients are often referred much later than they could be, which causes unnecessary suffering
  - Support/education patient/family
  - Utilizes self-report measures to quantify distress; implementing treatment guidelines
  - Provides skilled nursing, medical care, and interventions
  - Realistic goals and therapies in context of ongoing interactions
  - Optimize quality of life and psychosocial, physical, spiritual needs
  - Team approach: easy access to caregivers; for example, nurse as manager
  - Assure dignity, attention to comfort measures, goals of dying person and family

Pharmacologic Treatment
- Symptom Management
  - Pain control—see section on pain management
  - Dyspnea is very frightening—oxygen, steroids, opioids
  - Excessive secretions—hyoscyamine SL, scopolamine patch
  - Delirium: neuroleptics to treat agitation—Haldol
  - Depression, anxiety—antidepressants, benzodiazepines (lorazepam)
  - Nausea—medication, see GI Chapter 10, prochlorperazine (Compazine) PO or per rectum
  - Restlessness—sedatives
  - Incontinence—Foley catheter for comfort
  - Fatigue, weakness—adequate rest periods
  - Comfort can be achieved in almost all patients
  - Treatment strategies are commonly underused or inadequate

Special Considerations
- Encourage communication
- Counsel family regarding bereavement
- Help family plan for death, make arrangements

When to Consult, Refer, Hospitalize
- Hospice
- Specialist for symptom management when not controlled

Follow-up
- Be available to family and patient
- Have emergency backup plan
- Follow up with family after death

Expected Course
- A good death

Complications
- Unnecessary suffering

CASE STUDIES

Case 1. An 82-year-old female comes to the clinic complaining of "nearly fainting" 3 times in the last month.
History: She states that several times in past month she has had episodes when she feels like she is going to faint. The spell lasts maybe a few minutes, then she slowly feels better. If she is at home, she eats something, then goes to lie down, which relieves it. She had a spell at church last Sunday, and her friends insisted she come to the clinic for an evaluation.
PMH: Type 2 diabetes, osteoarthritis, hypertension, hypothyroidism, rheumatic fever as a child.
Medications: glipizide (Glucotrol XL) 10 mg PO qd, hydrochlorothiazide 25 mg qd, metoprolol (Lopressor) 100 mg qd, Synthroid 125 mg qd, naproxen (Naprosyn) 250 mg bid
  1. What part of the physical exam is appropriate?
  2. Name as many possible causes and contributing factors as you can think of.
  3. What diagnostic tests would you order?

Case 2. An 87-year-old man comes to your office complaining of fatigue. The patient lives in assisted living, needs help with bathing and dressing, walks with difficulty with walker, becomes SOB walking 20 feet, and feels too tired to eat. Diagnoses include COPD, CHF, Parkinson's disease. He is on 10 medications.
Exam: 20-pound weight loss in past 6 months; abdomen reveals nontender mass in left lower abdomen
Lab: CBC shows mild microcytic hypochromic anemia; BUN and creatinine show renal insufficiency, stool has occult blood
  1. What is the most likely diagnosis?
     Tests show patient has advanced colon cancer with metastasis to bone. Patient refuses treatment for the problem and starts preparing to die. He complains that the pain in his low back will not let him sleep. You determine that he is competent to make his own decisions.
  2. What is your initial plan?
     Over the next month, the pain becomes severe and patient becomes bed-bound. Because of the Parkinson disease, he is having trouble handling his secretions. He is still able to take sips of PO liquids.
  3. What is your next plan?
  4. What issues are likely to be the most important to this patient?

Case 3. The daughter brings her 80-year-old female with moderate Alzheimer disease for a routine checkup. Her daughter reports the patient is more easily distracted, increasingly irritable, and less aware of her surroundings. Daughter is not sure how long this has been going on. She is on multiple medications for cardiac disease and Alzheimer disease.
  1. What part of the history would be most important?
  2. What would you look for on physical examination?
  3. What laboratory and diagnostic tests would you order?
  4. What is your differential diagnosis?

REFERENCES

Dementia

Alzheimer's and Related Disorders Association. Available at: www.alz.org.

Alzheimer's Disease Education and Referral Center. Available at: www.alzheimers.org.

Boustani, M., Peterson, B., Hanson, L., et al. (2003). Screening for dementia in primary care: A summary of the evidence for the U. S. Preventive Services Task Force. *Ann Intern Med, 138,* 927–937.

Cohen-Mansfield, J. (2001). Nonpharmacologic interventions for inappropriate behaviors in dementia. *Am J Geriatric Psychiatry, 9,* 361–381.

Doody, R., Stevens, J., Beck, C., et al. (2001). Practice parameter: Management of dementia (an evidence-based review). Report of the Quality Standards Subcommittee of the American Academy of Neurology. *Neurology, 56*(9), 1154–1166.

Forette, F., et al. (2002). The prevention of dementia with antihypertensive treatment. *Arch Intern Med, 162,* 2046–2052.

Knopman, D., DeKosky, S., Cummings, J., et al. (2001). Practice parameter: Diagnosis of dementia (an evidence-based review). Report of the Quality Standards Subcommittee of the American Academy of Neurology. *Neurology, 56*(9), 1143–1153.

Lyketsos, C. G., et al. (2002). Prevalence of neuropsychiatric symptoms in dementia and mild cognitive impairment. *JAMA, 288*(12), 1475–1483.

Medical Letter. (2002). Drugs that may cause psychiatric symptoms. *Med Lett, 4459*–4462.

Reisberg, B., Doody, R., Stoffler, A., et al. (2003). Memantine in moderate-to-severe Alzheimer's disease. *NEJM, 348,* 1333–1341.

Ross, G. W., & Bowen, J. D. (2002, May). The diagnosis and differential diagnosis of dementia. *Med Clin North Am, 86*(3), 455–476.

Trinh, N-H., et al. (2003, January 8). Efficacy of cholinesterase inhibitors in the treatment of neuropsychiatric symptoms and functional impairment in Alzheimer's disease: A meta analysis. *JAMA 289,* 210–216.

Delirium

American Psychiatric Association. (1999). Practice guideline for the treatment of patients with delirium. American Psychiatric Association. *Am J Psychiatry 156*(5 Suppl), 1-20.

Inouye, S. K. (2000). Assessment and management of delirium in hospitalized older patients. *Annals of Long-Term Care, 8*(12), 53–59.

Inouye, S. K., Bogardus, S. T., Charpentier, P. A., et al. (1999). A multicomponent intervention to prevent delirium in hospitalized older patients. *NEJM, 340*(9), 669–676.

Dizziness

Bath, A .P., et al. (2000). Experience from a multidisciplinary "dizzy" clinic. *Am J Otol, 21,* 92.

Garcia-Civera, R., et al. (2003). Selective use of diagnostic tests in patients with syncope of unknown cause. *J Am Coll Cardiol, 41,787*–790.

Kaufmann, H., et al. (2001). Why do we faint? *Muscle Nerve, 24,* 981.

Olshansky, B. (2000, April 1). Syncope: Step by step through the workup. *Consultant, 702*–709.

Soteriades, E. S., et al. (2002, September 19). Incidence and prognosis of syncope. *NEJM, 347,* 878–885.

Tinetti, M. E., Williams, C. S., & Gill, T. M. (2000). Dizziness among older adults: A possible geriatric syndrome. *Annals of Internal Medicine, 132*(5), 337–344.

Fatigue/Weakness

Hicks, J. E., et al. (1998, March 15). Persistent fatigue: A practical approach. *Patient Care.*

Gait Disorders/Falls

American Geriatrics Society, British Geriatrics Society, American Academy of Orthopaedic Surgeons Panel of Falls Prevention. (2001). Guideline for the prevention of falls in older persons. *J Am Geriatr Soc, 49,* 664–672.

Chang, J. T., et al. (2004, March 20). Interventions for the prevention of falls in older adults: Systematic review and met analysis of randomized clinical trials. *BMJ, 328,* 680–683.

Day, L., et al. (2002). Randomized factorial trial of falls prevention among older people living in their own homes. *BMJ, 325,* 128–131.

Gill et al. (2000). Environmental hazards and the risk of nonsyncopal falls in the homes of community living older persons. *Med Care, 38,* 1174–1183.

Jensen, J. et al. (2002). Fall and injury prevention in older people living in residential care facilities: A cluster randomized trial. *Ann Intern Med, 136* 733–741.

Mathias, S. N., et al. (1986). Balance in elderly patients: The "get up and go" test. *Arch Phys Med Rehabil, 67*, 387–389.

Stevens, et al. (2001). Preventing falls in older people: Outcome evaluation of a randomized controlled trial. *J Am Geriatr Soc, 49*, 1448–1455.

Tinetti, M. D. (1986, February). Performance oriented assessment of mobility problems in elderly patients. *J Am Geriatr Soc, 34*(2), 119–126.

Tinetti, M. E., (2003). Preventing falls in elderly persons. *NEJM, 348*, 42–9.

Sleep Disorders

Chervin, R.,D., & Guilleminault, C. (1996). Obstructive sleep apnea and related disorders. *Neurol Clin 14*, 583–609.

National Heart, Lung, and Blood Institute Working Group on Insomnia. (1999). Insomnia: Assessment and management in primary care. *Am Fam Physician, 59*, 3029–3038.

Umlauf, M., Chasens, E., & Weaver, T. (2003). Excessive sleepiness. In M. Mezey, T. Fulmer, I. Abraham, D. Zwicker (Eds.), *Geriatric nursing protocols for best practice* (2nd ed., pp. 47–65). New York: Springer Publishing Company, Inc..

Venugopal, M., & Susman, J. L. (June 2000). Insomnia in the elderly. *Consultant*, 1234–1247.

Weakness

Carmeli, E., et al. (2000). Muscle strength and mass of lower extremities in relation to functional abilities in elderly adults. *Gerontology, 46*, 249–257.

Verrill, D. E. (2002, July/August). Strength training for older adults. *Geriatric Times*, II.

Weight Loss/Failure to Thrive

Guigoz, Y., et al. (1996). Assessing the nutritional status of the elderly: The Mini nutritional assessment as part of the geriatric evaluation. *Nutr Rev, 54*, 559–565.

Huffman, G. B. (2002). Evaluating and treating unintentional weight loss in the elderly. *Am Fam Physician, 65*, 640–650.

Robertson, R. G., & Montagnini, M. (2004). Geriatric failure to thrive. *Am Fam Physician, 70*, 343–350.

Thomas, D. R., & Morley, J. E. (2000). Anorexia and weight loss in elderly outpatients. *Clinical Geriatrics*, (December Suppl.), 1–8.

Wilson, M.M.G., Vaswani, S., Liu, D., Morley, J. E., & Miller, D. K. (1998). Prevalence and Causes of undernutrition in medical outpatients. *The American Journal of Medicine, 104*, 56–63.

Cancer/Pain/End of Life

AGS Panel of Persistent Pain in Older Persons. (2002). The management of persistent pain in older persons. *J Am Geriatr Soc, 50*, S205–224.

American Academy of Pain Medicine. Available at: www.painmed.org.

American Cancer Society. Available at: www.cancer.org.

American Pain Foundation. Available at: www.painfoundation.org.

American Pain Society. Available at: www.ampainsoc.org.

American Society of Pain Management Nurses. Available at: www.aspmn.org.

Balducci, L., & Stanta, G. (2000). Cancer in the frail patient. *Hematology/Oncology*.

Balducci, L. (2000, March/April). Prevention and treatment of cancer in the elderly. *Oncology Issues*, 26–28.

Bernabei, R., et al. (1998). Management of pain in elderly patients with cancer. *JAMA, 279*(23), 1877–1882.

Brummel-Smith, K., et al. (2002, November). Outcomes of pain in frail older adults with dementia. *J Am Geriatr Soc, 50*(11), 1847–1851.

Byock, I. (1998). Hospice and palliative care: A parting of ways or a path to the future? *Journal of Palliative Medicine, 1*(2), 165–176.

Center to Advance Palliative Care. Available at: www.capc.org.

Dannemiller Memorial Education Foundation. Consumer and physician site. Available at: www.pain.com.

Extermann, M., & Aapro, M. (2000). Assessment of the older cancer patient. *Hematology/Oncology Clinics of North America, 14*(1), 63–77.

Field, M. J., & Cassel, C. K. (Eds.). (1997). Approaching death: Improving care at the end of life. (Report of the Institute of Medicine Task Force). Washington, DC: National Academy Press.

McDonald, M. (1999). Assessment and management of cancer pain in the cognitively impaired elderly. *Geriatric Nursing, 20*(5), 249–253.

Medical Letter. (2003). Drugs of choice for cancer. *Treatment Guidelines* (Vol. 1)(7).

Medical Letter. (2004). Drugs for pain. Treatment Guidelines, (Vol. 2)(23), 47–54.

National Cancer Institute—Cancer Net. Available at: http://cancernet.nci.nih.gov.

NIH National Cancer Institute. Available at: www.nci.nih.gov. Available by phone at: 1-800-4-cancer.

Quill, T. C. (2000, November 15). Initiating end of life discussions with seriously ill patients: Addressing the "elephant in the room." JAMA, 284, 2502–2507.

Walter, L. C., & Covinsky, K. E. (2001). Cancer screening in elderly patients: A framework for decision making. JAMA, 285, 2750–2756.

Wrede-Seaman, L. D. (2001). Treatment options to manage pain at the end of life. *American Journal of Hospice and Palliative Care, 18*(2), 89–101.

Zachariah, B., & Balducci, L. (2000). Radiation therapy of the older patient. *Hematology/Oncology Clinics of North America, 14*(1), 131–167.

INFECTIOUS DISEASE

5

GERIATRIC APPROACH

- The incidence of infectious diseases among the elderly in the United States has increased during recent years. This increase is the result of complex interactions between the aging immune system, unexpected pathogens, environmental factors, comorbidities, diagnostic challenges, and rapidly changing antibiotic tolerance and resistance.
- This chapter will discuss infections in general. It will also discuss HIV exposure, HIV, Lyme disease, West Nile disease, and SARS. Other specific infections will be discussed in their respective chapters. For example, urinary tract infections are discussed in the Renal Chapter 11.

The Immune System

FROM THE MYELOID STEM CELL
- Monocytes move into tissue and develop into macrophages; initiate immune response and start phagocytosis
- Granulocytes
  - Neutrophils are phagocytes in early inflammation.
  - Eosinophils mediate allergic reactions. They also are phagocytes and defense against parasites.
  - Basophils are found in the blood and become mast cells in the tissue. Both cause inflammatory response in allergic reactions. The mast cell is the most important activator of the inflammatory response.
    - Basophils produce histamine, bradykinin, serotonin, and heparin.
    - Mast cells produce leukotrienes and prostaglandins.

FROM THE LYMPHOID STEM CELL: These require an antigen to become activated.
- B cells produce immunoglobulins (antibodies) and mediate humoral immune response.
- T cells produce cytotoxic (killer), lymphokine-producing, helper, and suppressor cells to orchestrate cell-mediated immunity.

PLASMA PROTEIN SYSTEMS: Inactive proteins (proenzymes) when activated, initiate a cascade of reactions to produce potent mediators of the inflammatory response.
- Complement system
  - Consists of at least 10 proteins
  - Components participate in almost every inflammatory response
  - Activated by nonspecific particles such as:
    Antigen-antibody complexes (immune complexes)
    Products released from invading bacteria
- Kinin system
  - Bradykinin causes dilation of vessels, acts with prostaglandins to induce pain, increase vascular permeability
  - Important during the prolonged phase of inflammation

- Clotting system
  - Consists of intrinsic and extrinsic pathways
  - Activated by many of the substances released during inflammation

Normal Changes of Aging
- Immune system function declines with age.
- The thymus becomes extremely small (fewer B cells and T cells).
- T cell function and specific antibody responses decrease (decreased response to infection).
- Macrophages show a decreased ability to clear antigens and attack tumor cells.
- Decreased complement levels
- B cells produce antibodies that do not bind antigens well, causing suboptimal antibody response to vaccines and delayed hypersensitivity response (less response to a PPD test)
- Increase in autoantibodies

AGE-RELATED CHANGES IN OTHER BODY SYSTEMS: A few of the normal changes that predispose the elderly to infection. See each individual chapter for details.
- Renal
  - Impaired bladder emptying
  - Decreased ability of the kidneys to acidify urine
  - Benign prostatic hypertrophy
  - Menopause—urogenital atrophy
- Respiratory
  - Decreased cough reflex, oxygen uptake, and mucociliary function
  - Musculoskeletal stiffness leads to decreased depth of respiration
- Skin
  - Increased skin fragility and loss of subcutaneous tissue
- Other
  - Decreased hydrochloric acid in the stomach and small intestine
  - Decreased vascular supply to extremities
  - Impaired glucose metabolism

INFECTIONS

Description
- Most common/life-threatening infections in the elderly
  - Bacterial pneumonia and influenza: fifth leading cause of death in the elderly
  - Urinary tract infections: most common infection
  - Skin infections: cellulitis
  - Methicillin-resistant *Staphylococcus aureus* (MRSA)
  - Vancomycin-resistant *Enterococcus* (urinary tract and skin)
  - Sepsis
- Other important infections in the elderly
  - Herpes zoster
  - Infective endocarditis: increasingly seen in elderly due to degenerative valvular disorders and prosthetic valves
  - Prosthetic device infections: joints, pacemakers, vascular grafts, intraocular lens implants, etc.
  - Human immunodeficiency virus (rare, but increasing)

Etiology
- Emergence of more virulent strains (e.g., *E coli*, influenza)
- Reemergence of some infections (e.g., tuberculosis)
- Gram-negative bacilli more prevalent in elderly

- Vancomycin-resistant *Enterococcus* (primarily urinary tract and skin)
- Methicillin-resistant *S aureus* (treated with vancomycin, but there are reports of resistance)

Incidence and Demographics
- Account for 40% of all deaths in geriatric patients
- Pneumonia/influenza is the fifth leading cause of death in the elderly.
- Septicemia is the tenth leading cause of death in the elderly.

Risk Factors
- Normal changes of aging, decreased physiologic reserves, including immune system
- Decreased activity pattern, immobility
- Decreased fluid intake
- Malnourishment
- Invasive procedures
- Medications that are immunosuppressive agents, including steroids, chemotherapy
- Nursing home residence and hospital admissions can result in nosocomial infections and increased exposure to antibiotics.
- Comorbid conditions that predispose the elderly to infection
  - Diabetes mellitus
  - COPD
  - Malignancy: leukemia, multiple myeloma, or receiving chemotherapy
  - Bladder outlet obstruction
  - Condition causing decreased vascular supply to area

Prevention and Screening
- Avoid risk factors
- Three most important general measures:
  - Maintain activity pattern, avoid immobility
  - Maintain adequate fluid intake; can be very difficult, absolutely crucial intervention
  - Maintain nutritional intake. See section in Chapter 3.

Assessment
- As functional assessment is the key to diagnosis of infection in the elderly, standardized assessment tools are useful to detect changes from baseline and noting changes. See Chapter 3 for discussion of functional assessment of the elderly.

History
- Nonspecific presentation of illness in the elderly is the most common presentation of infection in the elderly.
  - Delirium or decrease in ADLs is the most frequent symptom.
  - Sudden onset of functional decline, falls, incontinence, fatigue, or anorexia
- Symptoms generally reflect the patient's weakest system, not the symptom that is infected
- Usual symptoms of the particular infection may be blunted or absent.

Physical
- Often no temperature; look for change from baseline, may be elevated and still within normal limits. If fever is present, consider bacterial infection.
- May not have leukocytosis due to decreased immune response; severe leukocytosis indicates poor prognosis.
- Tachycardia and dehydration seen frequently
- Absence of classic symptoms. For example, UTI may not produce dysuria, appendicitis may not have right lower quadrant pain, stiff neck may not be seen in meningitis.
- Since the 3 most common infections are urinary tract, respiratory, and skin, direct your search there first.

- Assess for risk factors for infections of other systems and search accordingly. For example, diabetics have a specific pattern of infection; see Endocrine Chapter 17 for details.

Diagnostic Studies
- Cultures of affected organ system before antibiotic, if possible
- WBC count and differential—leukocytosis may be blunted
- Urinalysis
- Blood cultures if patient appears septic—appears ill, tachycardia, fever
- Increased sedimentation rate may be seen in certain infections and inflammatory diseases but also may be elevated in healthy elderly.
- Low serum albumin may indicate undernutrition as a contributing factor.
- More specific studies may be required to identify source of infection (e.g., chest x-ray, CT scans, echocardiogram).

Differential Diagnosis
- Microorganisms not a pathogen in healthy adults
- Leukemia
- Multiple myeloma
- Drug reaction
- Viral or fungal infection

Management

Nonpharmacologic Treatment
- Focus on comfort care
- Frequent rest periods without prolonged immobility
- Maintain nutritional intake/supplements
- Encourage fluid intake, at least 1500 cc/day

Pharmacologic Treatment
- Review allergy history (drugs, type of reaction), recent antibiotic use
- Review other drugs patient takes to be aware of possible drug interactions.
- In general, use a single agent that will reach the infected area, has a narrow spectrum and low toxicity profile, and is least expensive.
- Choice of drug should be based on culture or Gram stain results when available.
- Severe illness may require empiric therapy. If so, consider a third-generation cephalosporin, since gram-negative infections are common.
- Avoid treating infections that are likely to be viral with antibiotics.
- Age, renal and liver function should be considered when determining dose
- Renal function monitoring and drug levels during therapy indicated for some antibiotics, especially aminoglycosides, to prevent toxicity
- Elderly may need longer course of antibiotic than younger adults
- Ensure patient/family understands instruction for administration and importance of completing course of medication
- Most antibiotics should be given on an empty stomach, 1 hour before or 2 hours after a meal.

How Long to Treat
- Must complete entire course of antibiotic; length of course depends on organism, severity, and location of infection
- Give specific length of treatment with antibiotic; elderly usually require a longer course of antibiotic

Special Considerations
- Chronic illnesses that reduce circulation, such as diabetes or CHF, may limit delivery of the antibiotic to the infected site.
- Antibiotics can be given orally, IM, and IV at home and in nursing homes, depending on support systems and severity of infection.
- Blunted fever and leukocytosis responses are indicators of poor prognosis.

When to Consult, Refer, Hospitalize
- Severe infection, sepsis
- Patient not taking adequate fluids
- Not responsive to antibiotic in 3 days

Follow-up

Expected Course
- Antibiotics take 2 to 3 days at least to have an effect.
- Elderly patients will take longer to recover from infections than adult patients, especially confusion and weakness

Complications
- Sepsis more likely, higher mortality in elderly
- Great risk of mortality
- Elderly more susceptible to adverse effects of antibiotics
  - Allergy
  - Drug toxicity (ototoxic and nephrotoxic in aminoglycosides)
  - Altered bacterial flora of the intestinal tract—*Clostridium difficile*
  - Frequent nausea, diarrhea
- Drug Resistance
  - Drug resistance causes infections that are harder to treat, last longer, and require hospitalization.
  - Future infections may also prove resistant to antibiotics.
  - More frequent infections with a narrowing range of therapeutic options
  - Development of resistant strains of bacteria that are then spread throughout the community
- Superinfection
  - New infection during antimicrobial treatment for the primary infection
  - Caused by altered bacterial flora of intestinal, genitourinary, and upper respiratory tracts
  - More likely to occur with broad-spectrum antibiotics or when course of treatment is prolonged
  - Example seen in elderly is C *difficile* diarrhea
- Low therapeutic response
  - No response in 3 days or deterioration in condition (dehydration, delirium) merits consultation, change in antibiotic, or hospitalization.

HIV Exposure

Description
- Exposure places patient at risk for HIV infection and therefore requires consideration for post-exposure prophylaxis (PEP)
- Defined as a percutaneous injury, contact of mucous membrane or nonintact skin, or contact with intact skin when the duration of contact is prolonged (e.g., several minutes or more) or involves an extensive area, with blood tissue, or other body fluids

Etiology
- Fluids with known risk of HIV transmission: blood, bloody fluids, semen, and vaginal fluids
- Fluids with suspected risk of HIV transmission: pleural fluid, cerebrospinal fluid, peritoneal fluid, synovial fluid, and pericardial fluid
- Materials with doubtful risk of HIV transmission: feces, vomitus, urine, saliva, sweat, tears (unless bloody)

Incidence and Demographics
- Factors that may increase risk for HIV transmission after an exposure include (1) a device visibly contaminated with the patient's blood, (2) a procedure that involved a needle placed directly into a vein or artery, or (3) a deep injury.

- Risk of HIV transmission after a percutaneous exposure to HIV-infected blood is approximately 0.3%, mucous membrane exposure is 0.09%, skin exposure less

Risk Factors
- Contact with blood or other body fluids from patients with HIV

Prevention and Screening
- Universal or Standard Precautions
- Wear gloves when possible contact with blood or bodily fluids
- Use of "personal protective equipment" (masks, goggles, gowns) when engaging in procedures that involve blood or bodily fluids
- Prevention of needle injuries; use of puncture-proof containers, using "safety" needles, refrain from recovering or post-use manipulation of needles

Assessment

History
- Evaluate exposure: type of fluid, type of exposure (needle gauge, depth of needlestick, visible blood, mucous membrane) and duration of exposure
- Evaluate exposure source person: prior HIV testing results, CD4 levels, history of possible HIV exposures, and risk for HIV (IV drug use, sexual contact, acute HIV syndrome)
- If source person is HIV positive, document current HIV RNA levels, CD4 levels, and current or previous antiretroviral treatment

Physical
- Assess site or wound, anxiety level of patient

Diagnostic Studies
- Source person: If HIV serologic status is unknown, request HIV antibody after incident, pretest counseling, and consent form.
- If consent cannot be obtained, follow local and state laws.
- If source person is HIV seronegative, no testing of patient is needed
- Exposed patient: HIV antibody testing offered for baseline evaluation with consent
- Maintaining confidentiality of test results and documentation is critical.

Management

Nonpharmacologic Treatment
- Immediately following exposure:
  - Skin: wash thoroughly with soap and water
  - Eyes: rinse thoroughly with sterile saline, eye irrigate, clean-water flush
  - Mouth, nose: clean-water rinse/flush
  - Depending on type of fluid, source risk, and type of exposure; consider and discuss risks and benefits of postexposure prophylaxis
  - Counsel exposed patient to follow measures to prevent secondary transmission, especially the first 6 to 12 weeks: sexual abstinence or use of condoms, refrain from donating blood, plasma, organs, tissue, or semen
  - Serology for HIV antibody (baseline) with consent, hepatitis B serology for immune status
  - Serological testing on "source" for hepatitis C, hepatitis B antigen, and HIV

Pharmacological Treatment
- Tetanus vaccine (if not vaccinated within the last 5 years)
- Hepatitis B vaccine (if not already vaccinated in the past)
- Hepatitis B immune globulin (if source antigen positive or high risk for hepatitis B and patient not immune)
- After evaluation/assessment of HIV infection risk, determination made regarding need for post-exposure prophylaxis

- Data supports zidovudine (ZDV), spell out efficacy for postexposure prophylaxis

How Long to Treat
- Postexposure prophylaxis should be administered for 4 weeks if patient can tolerate

When to Consult, Refer, Hospitalize
- All potentially exposed patients should have a consult with infectious disease specialist who should determine treatment

Follow-up
- Advise exposed patient to seek medical evaluation for any acute illness occurring during the follow-up period. Illness characterized by fever, rash, myalgia, fatigue, malaise, or lymphadenopathy may indicate acute HIV infection.
- For patients exposed to HIV+ source or high risk: HIV antibody testing at 6 weeks, 12 weeks, and 6 months

Expected Course
- Patient to finish 4-week medication regimen

Complications
- HIV seroconversion
- Side effects from antiretroviral therapy, such as nausea/vomiting, nephrolithiasis, hemolytic anemia, hyperglycemia, or patient unable to finish medication

HIV and AIDS

Description

HIV
- Infection with human retrovirus, human immunodeficiency virus (HIV)
- Invades body and enters any susceptible cell; circulating CD4 lymphocytes, macrophages, and monocytes, destroying the immune system

AIDS
- HIV-positive person with opportunistic infections OR
- HIV-positive person with CD4 cells counts <200/mL or a CD4 percent <14%

Etiology
- Viral transmission: HIV usually transmitted through sexual intercourse (homosexual/ heterosexual), IV drug use, transfusions of blood or blood products, needle stick or mucous membrane exposures to person, injections with unsterilized, used needles such as acupuncture, tattooing, or medical injection
- Seroconversion: takes an average of 3 weeks from transmission. Using standard serologic tests, more than 95% of patients seroconvert within 5.8 months following HIV transmission
- Median time from infection with HIV to AIDS is 10 years
- Stages of HIV infection include: viral transmission, primary HIV infection (acute retroviral syndrome), seroconversion, asymptomatic chronic infection, symptomatic HIV infection, AIDS, advanced HIV infection

Incidence and Demographics
- Initially seen in elderly from blood transfusions for coronary artery bypass or other surgery (given 1978–1985)
- Being seen with increasing frequency in the elderly from prior sexual activity
- Currently 20% of HIV cases are in the elderly; part of this is because people with AIDS have been living longer
- Reported in elderly women without other risk factors who are caregivers to children and grand-children infected with AIDS, presumably transmitted through breaks in skin of hands
- 11% of new AIDS cases occur in patients over age 50

Risk Factors
- Blood transfusion outside of the US or in US during the period from 1977–1985
- Unprotected sex
- Exposure of person to infected blood and body fluids through breaks in skin or mucous membranes

Prevention and Screening
- HIV antibody testing of plasma, organ, and tissue donors
- HIV education programs

Assessment

PRIMARY HIV INFECTION: ("acute HIV infection")
- Experienced by an estimated 80% to 90% of HIV-infected patients
- Typical symptoms include: fever (96%), adenopathy (74%), pharyngitis (70%), rash (erythematous maculopapular) (70%), myalgias or arthralgias (54%), diarrhea (32%), headache (32%), nausea and vomiting (27%), hepatosplenomegaly (14%), and thrush (12%)

ASYMPTOMATIC INFECTION
- Patient clinically asymptomatic, generally has no physical findings except in some cases "persistent generalized lymphadenopathy"

EARLY SYMPTOMATIC HIV INFECTION: (AIDS-Related Complex, "ARC" or "Stage B")
- Clinical conditions that are more common and more severe in the presence of HIV infection but are not AIDS-indicator conditions. Examples: thrush, oral hairy leukoplakia, peripheral neuropathy, cervical dysplasia, constitutional symptoms (fever, weight loss), recurrent herpes zoster, idiopathic thrombocytopenic purpura, and listeriosis.

AIDS: CDC DEFINITIONS
- HIV+ persons with CD4 cell counts <200 mm or a CD4 percent <14%
- With opportunistic infection such as *Pneumocystis carinii* (now *P jiroveci*) (PCP), esophageal candidiasis, cryptococcal meningitis, or tuberculosis

History
- Unprotected sex

Physical
- Vital signs: fever may be present
- Weight loss, lymphadenopathy, hepatosplenomegaly
- Complete physical to look for opportunistic infections
- Neurological: signs of dementia or neuropathy

Diagnostic Studies
- CBC for lymphopenia/neutropenia, thrombocytopenia, anemia
- Comprehensive metabolic panel: evaluate renal and hepatic function

Criteria for HIV Infection
- Persons with repeatedly (2 or more) reactive screening tests (ELISA) + specific antibodies identified by a supplemental test (e.g., Western blot)
- Other specific methods of diagnosis of HIV-1 include virus isolation, antigen detection, and detection of HIV genetic material

Differential Diagnosis
- Cancer
- Endocrine diseases
- Dementia
- Enterocolitis
- Tuberculosis

Management
- All 50 states, Washington, DC, and US territories require reporting of AIDS cases to local health authorities

- Refer to specialist for evaluation and management
- Treatment is similar to that of adults
- Frequent interactions between HIV drugs and other drugs the patient is taking
- Adverse reactions to medications tend to occur more frequently and be more serious

Follow-up

Expected Course
- Average progression of disease without treatment is approximately 10 to 12 years from seroconversion to death in young adults
- Elderly experience a more rapid downhill course, perhaps due to impaired T-cell replacement
- Viral burden and the CD4 count highly predictive of prognosis; time to AIDS and death decreases with a decline of CD4 cells and higher viral burden

Complications
- Many complications occur as the immune system becomes depleted: neuropathy, chronic diarrhea, wasting syndrome, lymphoma, cancers, opportunistic infections, dementia, death

Influenza

Description
- Acute viral illness that occurs in epidemics usually in the fall and winter

Etiology
- Caused by an orthomyxovirus that appears in antigenic types A and B
- Frequent mutations produce new strains each flu season

Incidence and Demographics
- Very common
- Frequently leads to pneumonia in the elderly, contributing to the fifth leading cause of death in the elderly

Risk Factors
- Nursing home residents
- Residing with children

Prevention and Screening
- Influenza vaccine provides immunity to 85% of those inoculated
- Protection begins about 2 weeks after vaccination and lasts a few months
- Influenza virus mutation means that flu vaccine is reconstituted every year and that people need a flu shot every year to be protected.
- Those who should be vaccinated include patients over age 50 and health care workers.
- Amantadine or rimantadine given shortly after exposure to influenza A
- Oseltamivir and zanamivir after exposure in influenza A or B

Assessment

History
- Acute onset
- Malaise
- Headache
- Nausea
- Muscle aching
- Nasal stuffiness

Physical
- Fever, chills
- Mild pharyngeal injection
- Conjunctival redness

Diagnostic Studies
- CBC: leukopenia is common
- Nasal or throat swab for identifying the influenza antigen

Differential Diagnosis

- Colds
- Bronchitis
- Pneumonia
- Other acute febrile illnesses

Management

Nonpharmacological Treatment

- Rest
- Encourage fluids

Pharmacological Treatment

- Analgesics
- Cough syrup
- Antivirals must be started within 2 days of onset of symptoms to be effective.
- Amantadine (Symmetrel) 100 mg qd or bid or rimantadine (Flumadine) 100 mg PO bid x 7 days for influenza A
- Oseltamivir (Tamiflu) 75 mg PO bid or zanamivir (Relenza) 2 inhalations bid x 5 days for influenza A or B

Follow-up

Expected Course

- Usual duration is 1 to 7 days
- Often a longer and more severe course in the elderly

Complications

- Pneumonia
- Death

Lyme Disease

Description

- Bacterial infection that often begins with a rash (erythema migrans), then headaches, arthritis; severe neurologic complications may occur in up to 20% of patients; most do not have permanent sequelae

Etiology

- Caused by the spirochete *Borrelia burgdorferi*
- Transmitted to humans by ixodid tick (deer tick); not transmitted by larger dog tick
- Size of tick is 2 to 9 mm
- Painless bite; ticks usually drop off unnoticed in 2 to 4 days; must be imbedded more than 24 hours to transmit disease
- No person-to-person transmission
- Incubation period from bite to appearance of erythema migrans is 3 to 31 days; usually 7 to 14 days

Incidence and Demographics

- Accuracy of diagnosis remains a problem
- Probably overreported and overtreated
- Majority of cases reported in 3 distinct geographic areas: the majority of cases occur in Northeast from Massachusetts to Maryland, a lower frequency is reported in the upper Midwest (Minnesota and Wisconsin), and less commonly on the West Coast (Northern California)
- Incidence is increasing
- Occurs during tick season, spring through the first frost

Risk Factors

- Age: middle-aged gardeners, people of all ages who are outdoors

Table 5-1: Stages of Lyme Disease

Stage 1: Early Localized Disease	Flu-like symptoms of fever, chills, myalgia, arthralgia, headache 50%–90% of patients develop a distinctive rash termed erythema migrans within about 1 week of tick bite; begins as red macule or papule, expands rapidly over several days to annular, erythematous patch with central clearing, ≥5 cm and may be as large as 30 cm. Resolves in 3–4 weeks without treatment. Usually in area of tick bite, but may occur anywhere
Stage 2: Early Disseminated Disease	Begins roughly 3–5 weeks after initial infection, as spirochete spreads. Wide variety of symptoms, most notably persistent fatigue. Migratory arthralgia common. Cranial nerve palsies (especially facial nerve) common. Meningitis, conjunctivitis may occur; carditis with heart block rare. Most common manifestation is multiple erythema migrans, usually smaller than initial lesion
Stage 3: Late Disease	Months to years after initial infection, characterized by recurrent pauciarticular arthritis, usually affecting large joints (knees). Central and peripheral nervous system affected may develop subacute encephalopathy, distal paresthesias. Memory, mood, sleep problems may be noted. Cardiac involvement

- Live in endemic region
- Exposed skin: short pants and sleeves, no use of repellents

Prevention and Screening (See Table 5-1)
- Long pants, long sleeves when working outdoors; tuck shirts into pants; wear insect repellents
- Walk in middle of path, inspect skin and scalp after spending day outside
- When a patient in an endemic area presents with a flu-like illness in the summer, consider Lyme disease.
- Prophylactic antibiotics are not recommended following tick bites.

Assessment
History
- Most unable to identify tick bite

Physical
- Without reliable history of tick bite and presence of characteristic rash, PE may demonstrate findings consistent with above listed symptoms but may lead to a variety of other diagnoses

Diagnostic Studies
- Antibodies to *B burgdorferi* can be detected by ELISA several weeks after the bite; however, false-positive rate is fairly high and false-negatives are also reported.
- Western blot analysis is more specific after the first few weeks of the infection.
- Positive ELISA and negative Western blot indicate no Lyme disease
- If joint tap done, joint fluid will have 500 to 110,000 cells/mm³; cells are primarily neutrophils

Differential Diagnosis
FOR ERYTHEMA MIGRANS
- Tinea corporis
- Erythema multiforme
- Granuloma annulare
- Nummular eczema

- Rheumatoid Arthritis
- Septic Arthritis
- Systemic Lupus Erythematosus
- Postinfectious Arthritis
- Fibromyalgia

Management

Nonpharmacologic Treatment
- Supportive: fluids, keep skin lubricated
- Remove tick using firm tension and fine tweezers; be sure head is completely removed; clean site

Pharmacologic Treatment
- Early Lyme disease
  - Doxycycline 100 mg PO q 12 h for 10 days
  - Amoxicillin 500 mg q 8 h
  - Cefuroxime 500 mg q 12 h

Follow-up

Expected Course
- Erythema migrans usually resolves within several days of initiating treatment.
- Treatment of erythema migrans almost always prevents progression of disease
- Most respond promptly to treatment; complete resolution of symptoms in 4 weeks
- Retesting of Lyme titer not indicated as will remain elevated for months to years
- Long-term outcome unclear; depends on promptness and adequacy of treatment

Complications
- Subacute encephalopathy: memory loss, mood changes and sleep disturbances; distal sensory paresthesias, radicular pain
- Chronic arthritis or synovitis
- Myocardiopathies (rare)

West Nile Virus

Description
- Viral infection causing febrile illness, rash, arthritis, myalgias, weakness, lymphadenopathy, and meningoencephalitis

Etiology
- Arbovirus of family Flaviviridae spread by mosquitoes and birds
- Humans and horses are affected by contact with either
- Infection spread through blood transfusions, organ transplantation, and intrauterine transmission

Incidence and Demographics
- Reported in Asia, Africa, Europe, and US (first in 1999)
- In 2003, over 3500 cases of WNV in US with ~60% having mild disease and ~30% severe disease; 66 deaths occurred
- Incubation period 5 to15 days
- 20% of infected people develop mild illness lasting 3 to 6 days
- 1/150 develop severe neurological disease, encephalitis more than meningitis
- Mortality 5% with most deaths in older adults

Risk Factors
- Outdoor workers
- Blood transfusion and organ transplant recipients
- Elderly

Prevention and Screening
- Avoidance of mosquito bites: wear protective clothing, use insect repellent containing DEET, drain standing water
- Control of vectors by public health spraying against mosquitoes
- Use of gloves when disposing of dead birds
- Report dead birds to local health department
- Blood donations screened for WNV using nucleic acid-amplification test

Assessment
History
- Determine exposure to mosquitoes
- History of blood transfusion or organ transplantation

Physical
- Nondescript fever with maculopapular or morbilliform rash on neck, trunk, arms, and legs
- Arthritis, myalgias, generalized weakness, and lymphadenopathy
- Meningitis: fever, headache, and nuchal rigidity
- Encephalitis: fever, headache, and altered mental status ranging form confusion to coma with or without additional signs of brain dysfunction (paresis, flaccid paralysis, ataxia, sensory deficits, optic neuritis, seizures, and abnormal reflexes)

Diagnostic Studies
- CSF with IgM antibody for WNV is confirmative. CSF with pleocytosis (increased number of lymphocytes)
- WNV antibody in serum is presumptive of recent infection in patients with acute CNS infection. A more than 4-fold increase in antibody titers 2 to 4 weeks apart is confirmative.
- Pleocytosis increased number of lymphocytes in CSF

Differential Diagnosis
- California encephalitis
- Eastern equine encephalitis
- Western equine encephalitis
- Powassan encephalitis
- St. Louis encephalitis
- Colorado tick fever
- Dengue fever

Management
Nonpharmacologic Treatment
- Supportive care
- Monitor for complications

Pharmacologic Treatment
- Appropriate treatment of complications

How Long to Treat
- Continue supportive care until improvement

Special Considerations
- CDC website for West Nile virus: http://www.cdc.gov/ncidod/dvbid/westnile/background.htm

When to Consult, Refer, Hospitalize
- West Nile virus encephalitis cases should be reported to the local state health department.
- Patients with deteriorating mental status should be referred to a physician for hospitalization.

Follow-up
- Majority have very minor illness and recovery without complications

Complications
- Central nervous system abnormalities
- Death

Severe Acute Respiratory Syndrome (SARS)

Description
- Severe febrile viral lower respiratory tract illness

Etiology
- Caused by SARS-associated coronavirus (SARS-CoV)

Incidence and Demographics
- First reported in Asia in February 2003
- Spread to North America, South America, Europe
- According to CDC: 8089 cases of SARS and 774 deaths worldwide
- In US, 8 people with lab evidence of SARS; all had traveled to SARS areas
- Incubation period 2–10 days with median of 4–6 days
- Spread by close (within 3 feet) respiratory droplet transmission or fomites

Risk Factors
- Recent travel to mainland China, Hong Kong, or Taiwan
- Close contact with persons ill with SARS
- Occupations at high risk: health care workers, laboratory technicians
- Cluster of atypical pneumonia without other diagnosis

Prevention and Screening
- Avoid travel to high-risk areas
- Isolation of persons with possible SARS infection

Assessment

History
- History of exposure to SARS patient or SARS location

Physical
- Fever more than 100.4°F, headache, body aches, mild respiratory symptoms; headache and myalgia may precede fever
- 10% to 20% have diarrhea
- After 2 to 7 days, dry cough develops with dyspnea and pneumonia

Diagnostic Studies
- No specific clinical or lab test available
- Obtain CBC with differential (70% to 90% with lymphopenia), blood cultures
- Chest x-ray and/or chest CT scan: chest CT may show infiltrate before CXR. Obtain CT if + epidemiological link to known SARS case and negative CXR 6 days after symptoms develop. Repeat CXR on day 9 of illness.
- Pulse oximetry
- Sputum for Gram stain and culture
- Viral respiratory testing for Influenza A and B and RSV
  - Lab tests available through state health department: RT-PCR for SARS-CoV on blood, stool, and respiratory secretions; serology for SARS-CoV antibodies and viral culture for SARS-CoV. A signed consent should be obtained. Due to the possibility of false-positive results, lab studies should be obtained only on patients meeting certain criteria. See CDC website for information. www.cdc.gov/ncido/sars/index.htm

Differential Diagnosis

- Influenza
- RSV
- Mycoplasma
- Bacterial pneumonia
- Viral pneumonia

Management

Nonpharmacologic Treatment

- Supportive care

Pharmacologic Treatment

- No specific treatment for SARS
- Appropriate treatment for complications

Special Considerations

- Persons with possible SARS must be quarantined in the home for 10 days or until fever resolved and free from respiratory symptoms

When to Consult, Refer, Hospitalize

- Hospitalize any patients with worsening illness
- Consult with state health department and/or CDC for lab testing and management of possible SARS cases

Follow-up

Expected Course

- Mild cases resolve without complication

Complications

- 10% fatality rate overall with more than 50% older than 60 years

ILLNESSES OF UNKNOWN ORIGIN
Infections Caused by Bioweapons

Description

- Biological agents that have the potential for use as a bioweapon are characterized as Category A agents. These agents can be easily disseminated or transmitted from person to person, cause high mortality with potential for major public health impact, and require prompt action. Numerous viruses, several bacteria, and toxins may be used as weapons, but those that are known to have been weaponized, have effective dispersal methods, and are environmentally stable include anthrax, botulism, plague, smallpox, tularemia, and viral hemorrhagic fevers (Ebola, Marburg, Lassa, dengue, yellow fever and others).

Etiology

- Naturally occurring organisms that have been altered to increase lethality

Incidence and Demographics

- Smallpox no longer is found in wild form. All other potential bioagents occur naturally. Inhalation anthrax is rare, though dermatologic infection is still found fairly often in farm workers. Large scale outbreaks of botulism have never occurred.

Risk Factors

- Any population can be at risk, though bioweapons attacks are more likely to occur in densely populated, urban areas or at large, crowded events such as football stadiums.

Prevention and Screening

- Primary care providers must maintain an elevated level of suspicion.

Table 5-2: Potential Bioweapons (BW) Agents

Biological Agent	Transmission/Incubation	Clinical Presentation	Diagnosis	Management
Anthrax (*Bacillus anthracis*); Gram-positive, spore-forming aerobic rod that causes cutaneous or pulmonary infection. Cutaneous anthrax does not have BW potential poison.	Inhalation of aerosolized spores. Person-to-person transmission does not occur. 1–7 day incubation.	Biphasic, with initial prodrome of nonspecific febrile flu-like illness. May be followed by brief period of improvement, then rapid onset of high fever, severe respiratory distress. Shock, death within 24–36 hours.	Chest x-ray–mediastinal widening. Gram-positive bacilli on unspun peripheral blood smear	Ciprofloxacin or doxycycline; standard contact precautions. Prophylaxis should be offered with the same agents. A vaccine is available, but supply is limited.
Botulism—caused by neurotoxin produced by *Clostridium botulinum*, spore-forming, obligate-anaerobe found in soil. Botulinum toxin is the most lethal known natural poison.	Toxin can be aerosolized; sources of entry include wounds, GI tract, respiratory. It can also be dispensed in food. There is no person-to-person transmission. 12–36 hour incubation period.	Symmetric cranial neuropathies (e.g., drooping eyelids, weakened jaw clench, difficulty swallowing, speaking), blurred vision or diplopia, symmetric descending weakness in a proximal to distal pattern, respiratory dysfunction	Routine laboratory tests usually unremarkable. Definitive diagnostic testing for botulism available only at the CDC. Diagnosis is primarily clinical.	Supportive care, including ventilator support. Passive immunization with equine antitoxin.
Plague (*Yersinia pestis*), nonmotile bacillus	Bubonic: transmitted by bites from infected fleas, most common type. Pneumonic: inhalation of respiratory droplets from a human or animal with respiratory plague, may be aerosolized. Secondary cases would occur from contact with infected individuals. A BW attack most likely to produce pneumonic plague. 2–4 day incubation.	Bubonic: Enlarged, painful, regional lymph nodes (buboes), fever, chills and prostration with bubonic plague. Pneumonic: fever, weakness, and rapidly developing pneumonia with shortness of breath, chest pain, cough, and sometimes bloody or watery sputum	Clinical diagnosis important as treatment must be begun in ≤24 hours. Large numbers of patients with severe pneumonia particularly if accompanied by hemoptysis must trigger prompt presumptive treatment and isolation. Prophylaxis of close contacts.	Streptomycin, gentamicin, tetracycline, or chloramphenicol begun within 24 hours greatly improves prognosis. Isolation and supportive care necessary. Prophylactic therapy begun within 7 days is very effective in preventing infection. No vaccine is available.

| **Smallpox**—caused by a DNA virus in the orthopox-virus family. | Person-to-person transmission; spread by inhalation of air droplets or aerosols. Small-pox virus is specific for humans; animal infection does not occur. Weapon-ized smallpox can be spread by aerosol or by bombs or missiles. Secondary infection would occur from direct person-to-person spread, via both droplet and infected fomites (clothing, bedding) | High fever, malaise, severe aching pains, prostration. Later, a papular rash develops over the face and spreads to the extrem-ities, soon becomes vesicular and, later, pustular. Rash is most dense on face. 12–14 day incubation. | Patients are most contagious from time of onset of rash until scabs form. Initial diagnosis must occur at a military facility. After confirmation of community disease, subsequent diag-noses made on basis of clinical presentation | No known effective antiviral agents. Treatment is supportive. All potentially infected indi-viduals should be hospitalized in their homes. In event of widespread outbreak, specific hospitals would be designated for treatment of smallpox patients. Widespread vaccination would be indicated; smallpox vaccine is effective only if administered within 4 days of exposure. Vaccine is available, though supply is government controlled. |
| **Tularemia** (*Francisella tularensis*). Gram-negative coccobacillus. Type A most virulent and likely to be weap-ized. Very small amount (10–50) organ-isms can produce disease. | Naturally occurring in temp-erate areas of North America, Europe, and Asia. Weaponized tularemia can be delivered via aerosol, with infection occurring secondary to inhalation, skin or mucus membrane contact, or GI exposure from contaminated soil, water, food, or animals. Person-to-person trans-mission is not known to occur. | Presentation dependent on route of administration. Inhalation most likely. Symptoms include abrupt onset of fever with progression to pneumonia and respiratory disease, hilar lympha-denopathy, and pleuritis. Inhalation can also cause sepsis without respiratory symptoms; this syndrome has a high fatality ratio. 1–4 day incubation dependent on virulence of strain, site, and size of inoculum. | No means of rapid testing is widely available. Diagnosis is initially clinical. *F tularensis* may be identified by culture done in biological safety level (BSL) 3 labs. | Streptomycin IM or gentamicin IV for infection. Ciprofloxacin or doxycycline at usual doses recommended for mass casualties or postexposure. Vaccine is not widely available and immunity is incomplete. |

continued

Table 5-2: *Continued*

Biological Agent	Transmission/Incubation	Clinical Presentation	Diagnosis	Management
Viral Hemorrhagic Fevers (VHF)—refer to a group of illnesses that are caused by several distinct RNA viruses (Arenaviridae, Bunyaviridae, Filoviridae, Flaviviridae) and include Ebola hemorrhagic fever, Marburg virus, Lassa fever, hantavirus pulmonary syndrome (HPS)	Incubation dependent on virus. Humans are not the natural reservoir of these viruses and are infected when they come into contact with secretions of infected hosts. However, with some viruses, after the accidental transmission from the host, humans can transmit the virus to one another. Naturally occurring human cases occur sporadically.	Specific signs and symptoms vary by the type of VHF; initial signs and symptoms include marked fever, fatigue, dizziness, muscle aches, loss of strength, and exhaustion. Patients often show signs of bleeding under the skin, in internal organs, or from body orifices like the mouth, eyes, or ears. Full-blown VHF evolves to shock and generalized bleeding from the mucous membranes.	High index of suspicion, detailed travel history important. Lab findings supportive of infection vary; typically leucopenia, thrombocytopenia occur. Immunoglobulin (Ig) M antibody by enzyme linked immunosorbent assays (ELISA) during the acute illness. Diagnosis by viral cultivation requires 3–10 days and can only be done at BSL 4 labs (CDC, military facilities).	There is no cure or established drug treatment for VHFs, though Ribavirin has been tried with Lassa fever. Therapy is supportive and barrier isolation techniques should be initiated. No vaccines are available.

- NPs must be aware of modes of transmission, incubation periods, and communicable periods of these diseases. Excellent source of information is the CDC Emergency Preparedness & Response website: http://www.bt.cdc.gov/index.asp.
- Rapid isolation of patient and contacts

Assessment

History
- Symptoms for most agents may initially mimic those of common viral illnesses and include fever, fatigue, malaise, muscle aches, headache, cough, vomiting, diarrhea, rashes.
- For most agents, symptoms will quickly increase in intensity and severity.
- First indication of unannounced biologic attack will likely be an unusual increase in number of persons seeking care.

Physical
- Ill-appearing patient, often out of proportion to degree of illness prevalent in the community

Diagnostic Studies
- Blood cultures, CBC, electrolytes
- Other studies dictated by clinical picture

Differential Diagnosis
- Common wild virus agents (Fifth's disease, coxsackie, Varicella)
- Other potential biological agents

Management

Nonpharmacologic Treatment
- Rapidly notify public health authorities
- Psychological and mental health problems brought on by the event will require significant expertise.

Pharmacologic Treatment
- See Table 5-2.
- Empiric therapy may be indicated if large numbers of individuals present with a nonspecific febrile illness in a limited time frame and location under credible threat of attack. Empiric therapy is ciprofloxacin or doxycycline PO or IV at routine recommended doses.

Special Considerations
- Appropriate management of postexposure prophylaxis and its complications will be critical in containing spread of infection.

Follow-up

Complications
- Dependent on agent
- Most potential agents have high lethality, 30% to 100%.

CASE STUDIES

Case 1. A 96-year-old woman resides in a nursing home. She usually gets up, dresses herself, and walks to breakfast in the dining room, but today the nursing assistant reports she won't get out of bed. She is agitated, trying to hit the staff, and crying out incoherently; she was incontinent of urine overnight.
PMH: moderate dementia, osteoporosis, type 2 DM, CHF

Medications: metformin (Glucophage) 500 mg PO bid, furosemide (Lasix) 20 mg PO qd, lisinopril (Zestril) 10 mg PO qd, digoxin (Lanoxin) 0.125 mg PO qod, alendronate (Fosamax) 70 mg PO q week, donepezil (Aricept) 5 mg PO qd

1. What other history or review of systems would be needed?
2. What components of the physical exam would you perform?
3. What is your differential diagnosis?
4. What diagnostic tests are needed?

Case 2. A 68-year-old woman complains of diarrhea. It is soft to liquid and profuse. There is no nausea or vomiting. The patient was recently in the hospital for a cholecystectomy and had Foley catheter during hospital stay. She was started on trimethoprim-sulfamethoxazole. The culture came back with resistant to TMP-SMZ, so she was switched to Cipro. While on Cipro, she developed a pneumonia, so the Cipro was switched to Biaxin.

1. What other history or review of system would be needed?
2. What components of the physical exam would you perform?
3. What is your differential diagnosis?
4. What diagnostic tests are needed?
5. What treatment should be instituted pending diagnosis?

Case 3. A 74-year-old female, living independently, presents with many vague complaints including fatigue, weight loss, intermittent diarrhea, painful rash on trunk, numbness and tingling of toes, and white coating in mouth. Patient's social history consists of 45 years of an unhappy marriage to a distant husband, who died of a mysterious illness in 1995 at age 80.
PE: weight 108, down from 126 in past year, temporal wasting
Rash vesicles on erythematous base in dermatome pattern on right side of trunk
Decreased reflexes to LE
White exudate that sticks to tongue in mouth, malodorous
Normal abdominal and rectal exam

1. What is your differential diagnosis?
2. What diagnostic tests are needed?
3. What treatment would you initiate?

REFERENCES

Bartlett, J. G. (2002). Antibiotic-associated diarrhea. *NEJM, 346*, 334–339.

Bartlett, J. G., & Gallant, J. E. (2000). *2000–2001 Medical Management of HIV Infection.* Maryland: John Hopkins University, Department of Infectious Diseases.

Benenson, A. S. (2001). *Control of Communicable Diseases Manual* (18th ed.). Washington, DC: American Public Health Association.

Cassell, G. H., & Mekalanos, J. (2001). Development of antimicrobial agents in the era of new and reemerging infectious diseases and increasing antibiotic resistance. *JAMA, 285*, 601–605.

Center for Disease Control and Prevention. Available at: www.cdc.gov.

Centers for Disease Control, Emergency Preparedness and Response. Available at: http://www.bt.cdc.gov/agent/index.asp. (Accessed 09/28/04).

Gilbert, D. N., et al. (2004). *Sanford Guide to Antimicrobial Therapy.* Vienna, VA: Antimicrobial Therapy, Inc. Available at: www.sanfordguide.com.

Gradon, J. D. (2004). HIV Infection in the older population. *Clinical Geriatrics 12*(6), 37–45.

Kaplan, J. E., et al. (2002). Guidelines for prevention opportunistic infections among HIV infected persons—

2002. Recommendations of the US Public Health Service and the Infectious Diseases Society of America. *MMWR Recom Rep, 51*(RR-8), 1.

Mandell, G. L., Bennett, J. E., & Dolin, R. (2000). *Mandell, Douglas & Bennett's principles and practices of infectious diseases*. Philadelphia: Churchill Livingstone.

Mouton, C. P., Pierce, B., & Espino, D. (2001). Common infections in older adults. *Am Fam Physician, 63*, 257–268.

Monnet, D. L., et al. (2004, August). Antimicrobial drug use and methicillin resistant *Staphylococcus aureus*, Aberdeen, 1996–2000. *Emerging Infectious Diseases*. Journal available at: www.cdc.gov.

Wormser, G. P., et al. (2003, May 6). Duration of antibiotic therapy for early Lyme disease: A randomized, double blind, placebo controlled trial. *Ann Intern Med, 138*, 697–704.

DERMATOLOGY

6

GENERAL INFORMATION

Skin layers include: (See Table 6-1)
- **Epidermis** (visible) made up of stratum corneum (protector of underlying tissues), stratum lucidum, stratum granulosum, stratum spinosum, and stratum germinativum (producer of new skin, anchors epidermis to dermis)
- **Dermis** made up of connective tissue, gives skin strength and flexibility (contains blood and lymphatic vessels, sweat and sebaceous glands; composed of fibroblasts that are responsible for formation of collagen)
- **Subcutaneous layer** made up of adipose and connective tissue, major blood and lymphatic vessels, and nerves; appendages of skin include hair, nails

GENERAL DERMATOLOGIC SIGNS TO BE ASSESSED AND DOCUMENTED
- **Morphology** of lesions (macule, papule, nodule, vesicle, pustule, purpura, patch, plaque, tumor, bulla, abscess, ecchymosis, wheal, cyst, comedo, telangiectasia)
- **Secondary** lesions (sequential lesions that have evolved from other skin conditions) such as scar, erosion, ulcer, fissure, scale crust
- **Distribution** of lesions (generalized or localized, central or peripheral, symmetric or asymmetric, predilection for certain body areas such as extensor or flexor surfaces and intertriginous areas, sun-exposed or pressure areas/bony prominences)
- **Arrangement** of lesions (discrete, confluent, scattered, linear, zosteriform, polycyclic, grouped, patchy, arcuate, reticular, scarlatiniform)
- **Shape** or **configuration** of the primary lesion (annular, oval, nummular, iris, pedunculated, verrucous, umbilicated, gyrate or serpiginous)

Table 6-1: Morphologic Definitions for Primary Skin Lesions

Term	Definition and Example	Size
Macule	Flat, nonpalpable colored spot (freckle)	Up to 5 mm
Papule	Solid elevated circumscribed lesion (acne)	Up to 5 mm
Nodule	Solid, elevated, circumscribed lesion (erythema nodosum)	0.5–1.2 cm
Vesicle	Fluid-filled, elevated, circumscribed lesions (herpes simplex)	Up to 5 mm
Cyst	Encapsulated, fluid-filled mass (epidermoid cyst)	Variable
Bulla	Fluid-filled, elevated, circumscribed lesion (second-degree burn, severe poison ivy)	Larger than 5 mm
Pustule	Pus-filled, elevated, circumscribed lesion (acne)	Up to 5 mm
Wheal	Circumscribed, reddening with transient elevation (mosquito bite, hives, urticaria)	0.5–10 cm diameter
Tumor	Solid, elevated mass	Larger than 1 cm

- **Color** of lesions (erythematous, violaceous, hypomelanotic, depigmented, flesh colored, hyper-melanotic, variegated)
- **Borders** or **margins** of lesions (well demarcated or ill defined)
- **Palpable** qualities (soft, firm, mobile, fixed, hard, fluctuant, tender, hot/warm/cool, smooth, rough, indurated)
- **Measure** dimensions (diameter, width, length, elevation, depression)
- **Descriptive** terms (lichenified, atrophied, sclerosed, pigmented, friable, hyperkeratotic, weeping, crusted, mobile or nonmobile, hypertrophic/keloidal, excoriations)
- **Associated symptoms** involving the hair, nails and mucous membranes, lymphadenopathy or hepatosplenomegaly, ophthalmologic, and/or neurologic

GERIATRIC APPROACH

Normal Changes of Aging (See Table 6-2)
- **Epidermis:** thinner, connection to dermis less adhesive and more easily traumatized, more susceptible to blisters and skin tears, less of a barrier; keratinocytes have lower proliferation rate, which leads to slower wound healing; fewer functioning melanocytes leads to less protection from ultraviolet light; decreased number of Langerhans' cells means less immune defenses
- **Dermis:** about 20% thinner, skin feels thin and looks transparent; reduced capillary network leads to atrophy of skin; reduced size and number of fibroblasts
- **Subcutaneous layer:** thinner, less protection from trauma and cold
- **Hair:** graying, thinning, and loss
- **Nails:** rate of growth slows; thin and brittle or thick and dystrophic
- **Sebaceous glands:** may be hypertrophy, function diminishes leading to dry skin
- **Wound healing:** The normal changes of aging listed above all contribute to delayed healing and weaker scars after healing; the presence of multiple medical problems add to this compromised healing process.

Clinical Implications

Assessment

History
- Most important part of the evaluation
- Dermatologic complaints can indicate dermatological or systemic disorder.
- Dermatologic disorders can have profound impact on self-image; psychological assessment needs to be included

Physical
- Physical exam best performed in well-lit room with a handheld light for illumination and shadowing, Wood's lamp for fluorescing certain types of lesions, a magnifying lens, glass slides for diascopy and skin scrapings, KOH solution, 5% acetic acid for acetowhitening, mineral oil for suspected scabies, Giemsa or Wright stains, and a regular and dark-field microscope.
- Appearance of patient and vital signs (comfortable, agitated, toxic) with referral to an ER considered for a toxic patient
- Rule out skin cancer with any suspicious lesion.

Management

Nonpharmacologic Treatment
- Care of underlying age-related xerosis often important for improvement and control of many signs and symptoms
- Consider external/functional factors when looking for cause (e.g., incontinence, poor self-care/hygiene abilities, repeated motor activities)
- Know what the patient's or family's goal of care is: cure or comfort?

Table 6-2: Age-Specific Dermatologic Changes

Skin Condition	Pearl	Description	Risk Factors	Treatment
Photo-aging	Cause of 90% of undesirable skin changes of elderly	Wrinkling, yellowing, mottled pigmentation, atrophy, easy bruising	Changes in skin as a direct result of repeated sun exposure superimposed on normal aging of the skin	Protection from further damage still needed, and both clothing and use of sunscreen SPF 15 recommended with any sun exposure
Xerosis	Almost universal	Dry, scaly, often pruritic skin Common on legs, back, and arms	Worse during winter in heated building with low humidity	Decrease use of soaps and hot water. Use skin emollient regularly. If inflamed or pruritic, use low dose topical steroid (e.g., 1%–2.5% hydrocortisone ointment)
Pruritus	Due to decreased inflammatory response, underlying skin disease can be difficult to detect.	Localized or generalized itching that may interrupt sleep and cause scratching that excoriates skin	Xerosis often primary cause. Systemic diseases (e.g., renal failure, liver disease, cancer, thyrotoxicosis, and DM may cause pruritus). Need to rule out drug reaction	Treat underlying cause. Use topical emollients, antipruritic agents, and oral antihistamines with caution secondary to sedative effects.
Skin Tags	Benign	Found especially around neck and flexural areas; pink to brown color	Frequently found in obese patients	Removed with scissors or light electrodesiccation if irritated or cosmetically desired
Cherry Angiomas	Common	Typically 1–4 m dome shaped, red	More numerous, larger with age	Removal not necessary
Spider Veins	Common	Dilated, star-shaped blue veins on feet and legs	Increased number in older women	Treatment with sclerotherapy by consultant if desired

Table 6-3: Common Topical Steroids Ranked by Potency (Group 1 Most Potent)

Group	Example
Group 1	Betamethasone dipropionate ointment 0.05% (Diprolene)
Group 2	Desoximetasone ointment 0.25% (Topicort)
	Fluocinonide cream, gel, 0.05% (Lidex)
Group 3	Betamethasone valerate ointment 0.05% (Valisone)
	Triamcinolone acetonide ointment, 0.5% (Aristocort, Kenalog)
Group 4	Flurandrenolide ointment 0.05% (Cordran)
	Fluocinolone acetonide cream 0.2% (Synalar-HP)
Group 5	Desonide ointment 0.05% (Tridesilon)
	Fluocinolone acetonide cream 0.025% (Synalar)
	Hydrocortisone valerate cream 0.2% (Westcort)
Group 6	Betamethasone valerate cream 0.2% (Celestone)
	Hydrocortisone 1% (Hytone)
	Methylprednisolone cream 0.25% (Medrol)

Pharmacologic Treatment (See Table 6-3)
- Steroid medications play a big role in treatment of many skin conditions.
  - Use lowest dosage steroid possible, starting with strength below usual standard adult dosage.
  - Do not use fluorinated steroids on the face as it causes thinning of the tissue.

COMMON SKIN PROBLEMS
Allergy
Contact Dermatitis

Description
- An eczematous cutaneous eruption that results from one of two different processes—either irritant or allergen

Etiology
- Irritant contact dermatitis due to direct contact with an irritant that has a toxic effect on the skin (e.g., from detergent); damages one of the components of the water-protein-lipid matrix of the outer layer of the skin
- Allergic contact dermatitis results from a delayed hypersensitivity reaction to a contact allergen; cell-mediated hypersensitivity response with two phases
  - An initial exposure to the allergen sensitizes the skin and produces proliferation of T lymphocytes.
  - An elicitation phase, which causes the antigen-specific T lymphocytes present in the skin to combine with the allergen to produce an inflammatory response
- Most common recognized allergens: Rhus plants (poison ivy, sumac, and oak); also nickel, rubber chemicals, chemicals used in personal products such as cosmetics, shampoos, drugs

Incidence and Demographics
- Less common in blacks
- Common in elders in incontinence diapers

Risk Factors
- Exposure to irritant, including ammonia of incontinent urine—very common in infants/children
- Includes metal, plant, chemical, or food substance, topical antibiotics, preservatives, anesthetics, etc.
- When older individuals have multiple use of topical medications may trigger reaction

Prevention and Screening
- Avoidance of known irritants/allergens

Assessment
- Due to elder's decreased inflammatory response of skin, dermatitis may be mild.

History
- Pruritic rash in unnatural pattern on exposed skin
- Known exposure to irritant or allergen
- May include systemic symptoms of toxicity if extensive involvement

Physical
- Morphology: erythematous papules, vesicles, or bullae on inflamed background
- Location/distribution: exposed skin surfaces in unnatural pattern mimicking possible irritant
- Particular irritant or allergen may be obvious by location of symptoms
- Metal allergy: most common offender is nickel in jewelry and clothing
  - Distribution: neck, wrists, waist, strap line
  - Generally mild and chronic with scaling, pigmentation changes, and pruritus
- Plant dermatitis:
  - Distribution and arrangement: often linear pattern
  - Most commonly caused by poison ivy, oak, or sumac
  - Secondary signs: weeping, scaling, edema, crusting, and excoriations

Diagnostic Studies
- Clinical diagnosis, patch testing may be warranted for severe or recurrent episodes with unclear etiology

Differential Diagnosis
- Atopic dermatitis
- Insect bites

Management

Nonpharmacologic Treatment
- Removal of offending irritant or allergen
- Wash potentially contacted clothing
- Bathe in tepid water with soap to wash allergen/irritant off skin
- Cool compresses with astringent, Domeboro solution, or colloidal oatmeal suspension to treat pruritus (Aveeno)

Pharmacologic Treatment
- Oral antihistamines (diphenhydramine or hydroxyzine) for pruritus; use with caution due to sedation, dizziness, confusion
- Topical steroids bid; use lowest potency especially for less severe lesions and lesions covering large surface area
- Systemic steroids for severe or extensive involvement
- Oral antibiotics for impetiginized lesions

How Long to Treat
- Length of treatment determined by extent of involvement and response

When to Consult, Refer, Hospitalize
- Consultation/referral to allergist for unresponsive cases
- Hospitalization should be considered for toxic patient or unstable patients.

Follow-up
- Course is usually dictated by irritant or allergen and extent of involvement.
- Metal allergies tend to be low-level and chronic with possible lichenification and hyperpigmentation.

Complications
- Toxicity and impetiginization
- Oral antihistamines may cause excessive drowsiness or confusion in the elderly.

Eczematous Conditions
Nummular Eczema

Description
- Chronic, pruritic, inflammatory dermatitis in coin-shaped plaques of 4 to 5 cm

Incidence and Demographics
- More common in older males and in young adults
- Patients often have an atopic background

Risk Factors
- Atopic history
- Male sex
- Xerosis

Assessment

History
- Coin-shaped rash usually on anterior aspects of lower legs but may also appear on trunk, hands, and fingers
- Pruritus often intense
- More common in winter and fall months

Physical
- Morphology: round or coin-shaped plaques composed of grouped papules, vesicles on erythematous base, well-demarcated borders; may be more pronounced than centers
- Distribution: legs, trunk, hands, and fingers
- Secondary signs: exudative, crusting, scales, excoriations, and lichenification
- Frequently colonized with *S aureus*

Diagnostic Studies
- Cultures to rule out bacterial infection

Differential Diagnosis
- Contact dermatitis
- Dermatophytosis (fungal infections)
- Psoriasis

Management
- Emollients
- Low-dose topical steroids

Special Considerations
- Black skin may be more prone to postinflammatory hyperpigmentation.

Follow-up
- Chronic recurrent condition

Complications
- Bacterial superinfection
- Postinflammatory hyperpigmentation

Seborrheic Dermatitis

Description
- Chronic, recurrent, and sometimes pruritic inflammatory disease of skin where sebaceous glands are most active (face, scalp, body folds)

Etiology
- Unknown with questionable role of *Pityrosporum ovale*

Incidence and Demographics
- Very common chronic problem
- 20% of elderly
- Males more than females

Risk Factors
- Family history
- HIV infection
- Zinc or niacin deficiency
- Parkinson's disease

Assessment

History
- Gradual onset of greasy, scaly rash on face and scalp (often referred to as dandruff by patient)
- Possibly associated with slight pruritus

Physical
- Morphology: lesions are yellowish-red, greasy, moist, sharply marginated, 5 to 20 mm scaling macules and papules
- Distribution: scalp, eyebrow, eyelids, nasolabial folds, cheek, behind ears, intertriginous areas
- Secondary signs: possible inflammatory base, sticky crusting (more common on ears), fissures (more common at ear attachments to scalp)

Diagnostic Studies
- Diagnosis is usually made clinically

Differential Diagnosis
- Psoriasis
- Rosacea
- Impetigo
- Pemphigus (bullous autoimmune disease)
- Dermatophytosis (fungal infection)
- Lupus erythematosus

Management

Nonpharmacologic Treatment
- Avoiding cold creams and moisturizers
- Removal of scaling of eyelashes with baby shampoo

Pharmacologic Treatment
- Frequent shampooing with selenium sulfide (Selsun or Exsel), tar (Polytar, T-Gel, or Tegrin), or zinc (Head and Shoulders) shampoos
- Salicylic acid may be helpful in removing crusts
- Hydrocortisone lotion for stubborn areas and/or Nizoral (ketoconazole) cream
- Treatment of face includes sulfur-based soap
- Topical steroids (1% hydrocortisone lotion with sulfur) low potency; avoid fluorinated/potent corticosteroids

How Long to Treat
- Chronic condition requires initial therapy until symptoms resolve followed by maintenance therapy of ketoconazole shampoo, lotions, and/or topical steroids every day.

Special Considerations
- Most severe form is generalized and develops into erythroderma.

When to Consult, Refer, Hospitalize
- Consult or refer for unresponsive cases

Follow-up

Expected Course

- Chronic condition requiring initial treatment phase and then maintenance therapy
- Visits every 1 to 2 months during maintenance phase to monitor disorder and for signs of skin atrophy

Complications

- Bacterial superinfection
- Skin atrophy from chronic topical steroids

Psoriasis

Description

- Chronic, scaling papules and plaques in characteristic distribution on knees, elbows, and scalp

Etiology

- Alteration in cell kinetics of keratinocytes with shortening of cell turnover rate resulting in increased production of epidermal cells

Incidence and Demographics

- Affects about 1% to 2% of population
- Onset and persistence in latter decades not uncommon
- Rare in West Africans, Japanese, Eskimos, and very rare in North and South American Indians
- Family history common

Risk Factors

- Trauma
- Infections (streptococcal) can lead to guttate psoriasis
- Stress can lead to exacerbations
- Genetic predisposition

Prevention and Screening

- Stress management

Assessment

History

- Skin lesions usually with insidious onset but may be acute
- Pruritus may or may not be present
- May be associated with acute systemic illness with fever and malaise
- About 7% may be associated with arthralgias/arthritis, usually distal phalanges

Physical

- Morphology—silvery-white scaling papules and plaques; usually attached at only one point
- Drops of blood may form where scale peels off
- Distribution usually symmetrical, involves scalp, extensor surfaces, and areas subject to trauma
- May involve pitting of nails
- Köbner phenomenon: injury or irritation of normal skin induces lesions
- Variations: guttate psoriasis (lesions 3–10 mm in diameter)
  - Pustular psoriasis
  - Psoriatic arthritis

Diagnostic Studies

- Serum antistreptolysin titer and/or throat culture in evaluating guttate psoriasis
- KOH to rule out fungal infection
- HIV screen

Differential Diagnosis
- Seborrheic dermatitis
- Atopic dermatitis
- Drug eruptions
- Lichen simplex chronicus
- Fungal infections
- Candidiasis
- Reiter's syndrome

Management

Nonpharmacologic Treatment
- Avoid rubbing or scratching lesions

Pharmacologic Treatment
- Topical high to highest potency steroids
  - Start with 2–3 weeks of bid use
  - Then use in pulse fashion bid x 2 days once a week
- Interlesional steroids
- Avoid oral steroids, which can cause rebound flares
- Calcipotriene ointment 0.005% (vitamin D analog) 1 to 2 x day
- Tazarotene gel (topical retinoid) topical 1 to 2 x day
- Tar preparations such as Fototar cream
- Scalp treatment: tar shampoo, 6% salicylic acid gel, steroid solution
- For generalized disease: UUVB light exposure
- Systemic therapy: oral retinoids, methotrexate, cyclosporine

When to Consult, Refer, Hospitalize
- All patients should be referred to a dermatologist for confirmation of diagnosis and assistance in developing plan of care.

INFECTIONS
Fungal (Dermatophyte) Infections
Tinea

Description
- Superficial fungal infection of nonliving, keratinized portions of skin, including stratum corneum (epidermomycosis), nails (onychomycosis), and hair (trichomycosis)
- Infections are named by the body part involved
  - Tinea corporis: body
  - Tinea manuum: hand
  - Tinea pedis: feet
  - Tinea cruris: groin
  - Tinea capitis: scalp (trichomycosis)
  - Tinea barbae: beard (trichomycosis)
  - Onychomycosis (tinea unguium): nails
  - Tinea versicolor: named by its multicolored appearance; usually seen on torso and neck

Etiology
- Caused by several dermatophytes with regional predominance
- In the United States there are 3 common dermatophytes: *Microsporum, Trichophyton,* and *Epidermophyton*
- Can be spread by direct contact with an active lesion of an animal, another human, or fomites, such as clothing, linens, or gym mats or rarely from the soil

Incidence and Demographics
- Very common in elderly, particularly on feet, nails, and groin

- Affects all ages, races, genders; adult blacks believed to have lower incidence
- More common in tropical climates, warmer months in temperate climates
- More common in immunocompromised, including when secondary to prolonged use of topical steroids, with greater risk of intractable infection
- Systemic corticosteroids decrease host resistance to fungal infection
- More common in peripheral nerve disease: reduced blood flow to periphery

Risk Factors
- Heat and humidity
- Obesity: creates body warmth and perspiration, thus recreating the hot, humid conditions that can encourage fungal growth
- Exposure to fungal infections of animals and humans with whom the person has close physical contact (pets, household members, other nursing home residents)
- Exposure to fomites in hot humid environments
- Mechanical pressure from shoe: predisposes susceptible individuals to onychomycosis

Prevention and Screening
- Climate control as appropriate: air-conditioning; loose, cotton clothing
- Management of obesity
- Air drying or using electric hair dryer to completely dry intertriginous areas prior to dressing
- Completely dry shoes between wearing
- Frequently changing shoes, white cotton socks during day; wearing sandals
- Do not share combs, brushes, and hair ornaments
- Avoid occlusive ornaments: acrylic nails, synthetic jewelry, belts, shoes

Assessment

History
- Known exposure to others with tinea or high-risk population
- Mild to moderately pruritic localized "rash" or isolated lesion

Physical
- Presentation differs based on location of lesion
- Scaling erythematous plaque ranging from less than 1 cm up to 20 cm
- Varying shapes: round, arciform, or polycyclic
- With or without pustules/vesicles
- Usually has elevated, sharp border with central clearing; annular configuration ("ringworm")
- Color is erythematous or hyperpigmented

TINEA CRURIS ("jock itch")
- Similar but usually arciform or polycyclic and is duller red in coloring
- Often coexists with tinea pedis; infection transferred from feet to groin by hands
- Maceration common in intertriginous areas

TINEA PEDIS ("athlete's foot")
- Erythema
- Diffuse desquamation with superficial white scales and possible bulla formation
- Hyperkeratosis of soles
- Painful fissuring/cracking along lateral borders of the soles and toe webs
- Usually bilateral foot involvement
- Maceration seen in intertriginous areas between toes
- Moccasin type is caused by *T rubrum*
- More common in atopic individuals

TINEA MANUUM
- May be unilateral (50%) or bilateral (50%)
- Frequently coexists with tinea pedis or tinea cruris

TINEA VERSICOLOR
- Superficial *Pityrosporum orbiculare*
- Yeast that colonizes all human skin
- Clinically significant only in some individuals
- Distribution on trunk and neck
- Hypo- or hyperpigmented nummular macules
- Discrete, scattered, or confluent patches
- Usually asymptomatic but may be mildly pruritic

TINEA CAPITIS AND TINEA BARBAE (Trichomycosis)
- Involve dermatophyte invasion of the hair follicle by *Trichophyton* dermatophytes
- Inflammation of the hair follicle
- Painful, boggy suppurative nodules with crusting/scabs
- Alopecia

TINEA UNGUIUM (Onychomycosis)
- Nails become white, brown, yellow, or black
- Nails thicken and surface becomes roughened
- Nails eventually separate from the nail bed

Diagnostic Studies
- Wood's lamp
  - Tinea capitis fluoresces green
  - Tinea versicolor fluoresces faint yellow-green scales
  - Tinea cruris does not fluoresce, but Wood's lamp exam can identify erythrasma, a bacterial infection that fluoresces coral-red.
- KOH mount—skin scrapings placed on a slide in 10% to 30% KOH solution with a cover slip; can be viewed under a microscope after warming for 30 to 60 seconds; will demonstrate mycelia and hyphae
  - Tinea capitis appears as spores invading hair follicles
  - Tinea cruris appears as mycelia with septate hyphae and scattered buds
  - Tinea versicolor appears as long hyphae and few buds ("spaghetti and meatballs")
- Fungal cultures can identify a fungus but usually take weeks to grow.
  - Indicated only when an infection is resistant to treatment

Differential Diagnosis: based on location of lesions

TINEA PEDIS
- Impetigo
- Psoriasis
- Erythrasma
- Candidiasis
- Contact dermatitis
- Dyshidrotic eczema

TINEA MANUUM
- Atopic dermatitis
- Contact dermatitis
- Psoriasis
- Lichen simplex chronicus
- In situ squamous cell carcinoma
- Pityriasis rubra pilari

TINEA CRURIS
- Erythrasma
- Inverse pattern psoriasis
- Candidiasis

TINEA CORPORIS
- Atopic dermatitis
- Seborrheic dermatitis

- Contact dermatitis
- Annular erythema
- Psoriasis
- Erythema migrans
- Pityriasis rosea

TINEA CAPITIS
- Seborrheic dermatitis
- Psoriasis
- Atopic dermatitis
- Alopecia areata
- Lichen simplex chronicus
- Chronic SLE
- Impetigo
- Ecthyma
- Crusted scabies

TINEA BARBAE
- Beard folliculitis
- Acne vulgaris
- Acne rosacea
- Furunculosis

TINEA TRICHOMYCOSIS
- Paronychia
- Herpetic whitlow
- Eczematous dermatitis
- Allergic contact dermatitis
- Lichen planus
- Pseudomonal nail infection (black-green coloring)
- Reiter's syndrome
- Traumatic
- Injury to the nail

Management

Nonpharmacologic Treatment
- Managing and treating predisposing conditions
  - Obesity
  - Diabetes
  - Immunosuppression
- Advise patient of need to avoid tight or occlusive clothing or ornaments
- Change shoes and socks during the day and/or wear sandals
- Completely drying intertriginous areas after bathing

Pharmacologic Treatment
- Tinea corporis, manuum, pedis, cruris: use cream or lotion
- Tinea capitis and barbae (trichomycosis): use solution
- Topical antifungal preparations: Apply to affected area including a 2-cm peripheral border and rub in bid
  - Clotrimazole 1% cream, solution, lotion
  - Econazole 1% cream or lotion
  - Ketoconazole 2% cream, shampoo
  - Miconazole 2% cream
  - Oxiconazole 1% cream
  - Sulconazole 1% cream
  - Naftifine 1% cream or gel
  - Tolnaftate 1% cream
  - Terbinafine (Lamisil) 1% cream
- Onychomycosis (tinea unguium) nails:
  - Ciclopirox (Penlac) 1% bid
  - Naftifine gel 1% bid
- Tinea versicolor
  - Selenium sulfide lotion apply from neck to waist qd, leave on 5–15 min, qd x 7 days
  - Ketoconazole shampoo for weekly maintenance
- Oral antifungal medications: synthetic antifungal agents are effective but should be reserved for severe or extensive cases: for example, griseofulvin, ketoconazole

How Long to Treat
- Resolution is slow, treatment length depends on location; all take several weeks
  - Tinea capitis and tinea barbae: 8 to 16 weeks
  - Tinea corporis, tinea manuum, cruris: 4 to 6 weeks
  - Tinea pedis: 4 to 12 weeks
  - Tinea versicolor: 4 to 6 weeks, with frequent relapses
  - Onychomycosis: 8 to 12 months

Special Considerations
- Side effects from systemic antifungal agents include hepatotoxicity, lowering of serum testosterone. Evaluate LFTs prior to starting oral agents, then every 4 to 6 weeks

When to Consult, Refer, Hospitalize
- Consultation and/or referral appropriate for extensive involvement or unresponsive infections.
- Consider hospitalization for immunosuppressed patients with extensive disease.

Follow-up
- Every 4 weeks for reevaluation and LFTs

Candidiasis

Description
- Yeastlike fungus that proliferates and causes infections on moist cutaneous and mucosal sites in susceptible individuals when local immunity is disturbed

Etiology
- *Candida* species (*Candida albicans* most common, *C glabrata*, *C tropicalis*) that are normal inhabitants of mucosal surfaces and intestinal tract of healthy individuals

Incidence and Demographics
- Frequently seen in elderly, especially in diabetics, and in those debilitated
- Both sexes equally and all races can be affected

Risk Factors
- Predisposing factors that alter local immunity
- Immunocompromised states, HIV
- Chronic debilitation; inability to perform personal hygiene
- Chemotherapy
- Diabetes or polyendocrinopathy
- Systemic broad-spectrum antibiotic therapy
- Moisture from repeated immersion in water or urine
- Obesity with redundant skin folds
- Occlusive clothing that traps moisture (adult diapers, incontinence pads, rubber boots)
- Hyperhidrosis (excessive sweating)
- Corticosteroid use

Prevention and Screening
- Management of underlying predisposing factors such as obesity, DM, etc.
- Avoid occlusive clothing, repetitive moisture exposure
- Frequent toileting of incontinent elderly
- Limitation of corticosteroid use

Assessment

History
- Pruritic and or burning sensation and "rash" in characteristic locations, such as intertriginous areas, anogenital region, and redundant skin folds (often under pendulous breasts, in the axillae, or redundant folds of an obese abdomen)

- Painful or sensitive white "stuck on" lesions of the oral mucosa with decreased taste and odynophagia ("thrush")
- Corners of mouth thickened with slight erythema (perlèche or angular cheilitis)
- White, curdlike vaginal discharge usually associated with pruritus, external dysuria, and dyspareunia (vulvovaginitis)
- Painful fissuring of foreskin in uncircumcised males with dysuria and dyspareunia (balanoposthitis)
- Painful, inflamed nail folds, discolored nails, and a creamy discharge (paronychial candidiasis)
- Painful, congested ear canal with moist exudate (otitis externa)

Physical
- Bright red, smooth macules
- Maceration is typical of all intertriginous infections
- Scaling elevated border
- "Satellite" lesions: similar macules outside main lesion
- Oral and vaginal candidiasis; white, stuck-on but removable plaques on inflamed mucosa
- Balanoposthitis: flattened pustules, edema, erosions, fissuring on erythematous surface
- Candida otitis externa: edematous ear canal with macerated appearance and moist white scaly exudate

Diagnostic Studies
- 5% KOH preparation under microscope demonstrates buds and pseudohyphae in clusters
- Cultures may be done to identify specific species, but this is usually not done because it takes 1 to 2 weeks for results

Differential Diagnosis

ORAL CANDIDIASIS
- Hairy leukoplakia
- Pernicious anemia
- Geographic tongue
- Bite irritation

GENITAL CANDIDIASIS
- Bacterial vaginosis
- Lichen planus
- Scabies
- Condyloma acuminatum
- Erythrasma
- Inverse pattern psoriasis

INTERTRIGINOUS AREAS
- Eczema
- Atopic dermatitis
- Contact dermatitis
- Dermatophytosis

PARONYCHIAL CANDIDIASIS
- Herpetic whitlow
- S. aureus paronychia

Management

Nonpharmacologic Treatment
- Management of underlying predisposing factors such as obesity, DM, etc.
- Air exposure to affected areas such as diaper region in incontinent elderly
- Careful drying of intertriginous areas and redundant skin folds
- Wearing cotton undergarments and avoiding tight, synthetic clothing
- If incontinent, change diapers frequently

Pharmacologic Treatment
- Oral: nystatin oral suspension 500,000 units, swish in mouth and swallow 3–5 x per day, Clotrimazole 10 mg troches 3–5 x per day, systemic ketoconazole 200 mg qd to bid, fluconazole 100 mg qd to bid, itraconazole 100 mg qd, amphotericin B 3/mg/kg/day for resistant cases in immunocompromised hosts

- Intertriginous and anogenital infections: Castellani paint x 1
- Topical antifungal: imidazole topical creams, sol., powder bid, clotrimazole 1% cream, miconazole 2% cream, ketoconazole 2% cream, econazole (Spectazole) 1% cream, terconazole (Terazol) 0.4 or 0.8% cream, terbinafine (Lamisil) 1% cream or solution bid, tolnaftate (Tinactin) 1% cream, solution, powder bid
- Oral antifungal treatment may be necessary in extensive or recurrent infections or when host immunity is suppressed.
- Oral fluconazole (Diflucan 150 mg) x 1 has been successful in treatment of vaginal candidiasis

How Long to Treat
- Oral candidiasis: 10 to 14 days
- Intertriginous and anogenital candidiasis: 1 to several weeks depending on extent of the infection and the immune status of the host
- Paronychial candidiasis: 2 to 4 weeks

Special Considerations
- Immunosuppressed patients are subject to extensive and recurrent infections and may require a daily maintenance dose to limit recurrences

When to Refer, Consult, Hospitalize
- Immunosuppressed patients with extensive or severe candidiasis, particularly oral/esophageal candidiasis, may require hospitalization or home IV infusion therapy of amphotericin B and nutrition supplementation.

Follow-up

Expected Course
- Resolution can be expected in patients without immunosuppression but other predisposing factors such as obesity and poorly controlled diabetes mellitus may make recurrences common. Patients should be seen in follow-up in 2 to 4 weeks and PRN to evaluate progress.

Complications
- Bacterial superinfection of excoriated lesions
- Weight loss secondary to odynophagia with esophagitis

Bacterial Infections of Skin
Cellulitis

Description
- Acute infection of the dermis and subcutaneous tissues

Etiology
- S aureus
- Streptococcus pyogenes (Group A beta-hemolytic)
- Streptococcus agalactiae (Group B)
- Gram-negative bacilli, anaerobes such as:
  - Escherichia coli
  - Pseudomonas aeruginosa
  - Clostridium spp.

Incidence and Demographics
- Common in older adults

Risk Factors
- Elders with chronic diseases and age-related factors that delay wound healing
- Breaks in skin from trauma (lacerations, abrasions, excoriation, pressure ulcers, skin tears)
- Underlying dermatosis, stasis ulcers with dermatitis

- Diabetes mellitus
- Hematologic malignancies
- Chronic lymphedema (postmastectomy or coronary artery grafting)
- Immunocompromised
- Previous episodes of cellulitis

Prevention and Screening
- Avoid scratching; maintain short, clean nails
- Educate diabetic patient to examine feet daily for any breaks in skin, lubricate to prevent cracking of skin

Assessment

History
- May be unaware of original break in skin
- Possible history of fungal infection or dermatitis of the affected area
- Possible fever, malaise, anorexia, pain that is increased with weight bearing or dependency
- Possible occlusive symptoms if cellulitis involves the face (erysipelas)

Physical
- Puncture wound, fissure, pressure ulcer, skin tear, or laceration may be visible
- Decreased age-related immune response may lessen clinical sign of infection
- Erythematous plaque that is edematous, hot and tender with sharply defined, irregular border
- Vesicles, bullae, abscesses may be seen within the plaque
- Lymphangitis—surrounding erythematous streaking
- Regional lymphadenopathy
- Systemic toxic signs may be present, especially if involved area large, patient immuno-compromised
- Necrotizing fasciitis, deep infection of subcutaneous tissue appears as a large erythematous plaque with a central area of necrosis; beta-hemolytic *Streptococci* usually invading organism; staph may or may not be involved

Diagnostic Studies
- Cultures are usually not warranted and result in false-negatives in about 75% of cases
- WBCs and sedimentation rate are indicated if the patient appears toxic

Differential Diagnosis
- Deep vein thrombosis or thrombophlebitis
- Early contact dermatitis
- Giant urticaria
- Fixed drug eruption
- Erythema migrans
- Early herpes zoster

Management

Nonpharmacologic Treatment
- Rest, elevate involved extremity (bedrest with up to bathroom only if leg is involved)
- Application of hot, moist compresses x 20 to 30 minutes qid (closely monitored secondary to increased risk of burn)

Pharmacologic Treatment
- Antibiotic
  - Dicloxacillin 250–500 mg qid x 5–10 days
  - Cephalexin 250–500 mg
  - Clindamycin 150–300 mg q 6 h
- MRSA (community acquired)
  - Clindamycin 300 mg oral q 6 h
  - Trimethoprim-sulfamethoxazole 1 oral q 12 h

- Fluoroquinolone (levofloxacin 500 qd, moxifloxacin 400 mg orally qd, or gatifloxacin 400 mg qd)
- NSAIDs PRN analgesia, fever, decreased inflammation (risk of gastritis, UGI bleed)

How Long to Treat
- 5 to 10 days depending on the extent of involvement

Special Considerations
- Immunocompromised patients and patients with synthetic heart valves: greater risk of toxicity, may warrant hospitalization
- Medical management of predisposing conditions such as diabetes, IV drug use, malignancies, or chronic lymphedema will augment treatment.
- Immunocompromised patients as well as patients on dialysis may be more prone to develop infections from drug resistant bacteria.

When to Consult, Refer, Hospitalize
- Consult with infectious disease specialist if the patient is not responding.
- A toxic patient may require transfer to a hospital.
- Hospitalization and surgery may be necessary to debride the necrotic tissue and prevent further tissue damage.
- Facial cellulitis (erysipelas) may require hospitalization to prevent spread of infection to brain and to monitor for and manage obstructive symptoms if they occur.

Follow-up

Expected Course
- Clinical response to treatment may be difficult to assess if initial site also has age-related changes.
- Erythematous plaque should be outlined with an indelible pen on initial assessment; patient should return daily to monitor progression or regression of the involved area.
- Incremental improvement should be noted and documented and resolution expected in 5 to 10 days depending on the initial level of involvement, patient's compliance with therapeutic regimen of elevation, antibiotics, and hot, moist compresses.

Complications
- Toxicity or septicemia
- Meningitis or respiratory distress secondary to occlusion from head and neck cellulitis
- Diabetic patients have the potential to require amputation due to severe cellulitis.

Abscess, Furuncle, and Carbuncle

Description
- Abscess is a circumscribed collection of purulent exudate associated with tissue destruction and inflammation, may arise from any organ or structure
- Furuncle is an infection deep in a hair follicle, usually caused by S. aureus folliculitis
- Furunculosis refers to several discrete furuncles.
- Carbuncle is deeper infection, involves subcutaneous tissue, arising in several contiguous hair follicles, interconnected by sinus tracts; may have several pustular openings onto skin; may be associated with systemic symptoms of fever and malaise

Etiology
- Usually S aureus, rarely other bacteria

Incidence and Demographics
- Often seen in elderly with chronic illness (e.g., DM, obesity)
- Sex: Male more than female

Risk Factors
- Chronic staph carrier state (nares, axillae, anogenital, intestine)
- Diabetes
- Obesity
- Poor hygiene, inability to perform hygiene
- Metabolic abnormalities (chronic granulomatosis, high serum IgE)

Prevention and Screening
- Education about good hygiene, improving the status of underlying predisposing factors, such as diabetes and obesity

Assessment

History
- Painful, hot lesion developing over days
- Sometimes accompanied by systemic symptoms of fever and malaise
- Predisposing factors or history of prior abscesses, furuncles, or carbuncles

Physical
- Abscess: initially tender nodule that develops over days to collect purulent exudate, becomes inflamed
- Central fluctuance found in a fully developed or "ripe" abscess
- Furuncle: firm, tender nodule with a central necrotic plug, fluctuant below plug, usually with a pustule over the plug
- Carbuncle: several adjacent, coalescing furuncles with multiple, loculated abscesses, draining pustules, and necrotic plugs

Diagnostic Studies
- Laboratory studies usually not indicated
- Gram staining usually demonstrates gram-positive cocci with multiple polymorphonuclear neutrophils (PMNs).
- Culture and sensitivity may be done to confirm S aureus or identify methicillin resistant S aureus or other bacteria that may be resistant to treatment.
- Blood cultures are indicated if the patient remains febrile or appears toxic.

Differential Diagnosis
- Ruptured epidermal or pilar cyst
- Hydradenitis suppurativa
- Necrotizing HSV

Management

Nonpharmacologic Treatment
- Warm, moist compresses or sitz baths x 10 minutes q 2–3 h

Pharmacologic Treatment
- Topical antibiotics are usually not effective in treating acute abscess, furuncle, or carbuncle
- Mupirocin ointment (Bactroban) tid to nares is helpful in eliminating chronic S. aureus carrier state
- Systemic antibiotics:
  - Dicloxacillin 250–500 mg qid
  - Cephalexin (Keflex) 250–500 mg qid
  - Amoxicillin and clavulanic acid (Augmentin) 250–500 mg
  - Erythromycin-EES 400 mg tid
  - Clarithromycin (Biaxin) 250–500 mg bid
  - Trimethoprim-sulfamethizole DS (Bactrim or Septra) bid
  - Ciprofloxacin (Cipro) 500 mg bid
  - Vancomycin IV for severe infections

Surgical Treatment
- Incision and drainage usually required to effectively treat
- Breaking through the interior walls allows drainage of the exudate
- Sterile packing is often necessary to allow the incision to continue to drain.

How Long to Treat
- 7 to 10 days

Special Considerations
- Diabetic patients may have delayed wound healing

When to Consult, Refer, Hospitalize
- Referral to general surgery is indicated for extensive abscess involvement.

Follow-up
- Initially daily to monitor response to therapy and to remove packing from surgical site

Complications
- Rarely endocarditis from manipulation of abscess
- Rare cavernous sinus thrombosis from manipulation of abscess near nasolabial folds

Viral Skin Infections
Herpes Zoster

Description
- "Shingles": acute, painful, unilateral, cutaneous infection in dermatomal distribution

Etiology
- Varicella-zoster virus (VZV)
- Usually contracted in childhood as chickenpox
- Lies dormant in a nerve ganglion
- Reactivation of virus causes eruption along course of the nerve
- Cause of reactivation unclear

Incidence and Demographics
- Occurs most often in persons over age 50; less than 10% of cases occur under age 20
- In those over 80 years, more than 10 cases per 1000

Risk Factors
- Found in patients without immunosuppression, but severity of disease is increased if immuno-compromised, such as decreased immunity of aged
- Advanced age

Prevention and Screening
- Most of adult population in US today is positive for anti-VZV antibodies
- Varicella vaccine now included in routine childhood immunization schedule may prevent development of herpes zoster in later life
- Varicella vaccine later in life when anti-VZV antibodies are declining may be effective in preventing development of herpes zoster

Assessment

History
- Frequently pain (piercing, stabbing, boring), paresthesia (tingling, burning, itching), and allodynia (heightened sensitivity to mild stimuli) preceding eruption by 3 to 5 days along neuronal pathway
- Generalized malaise, fever and headache in about 5%

Physical
- Initially grouped vesicles along a unilateral dermatomal pathway followed by bullae within 2 days (more than one contiguous dermatome may be involved but noncontiguous dermatome involvement is rare)
- By day 4 become pustules, followed by crusting in 7 to 10 days
- Lesions occur on erythematous, edematous cutaneous base

Diagnostic Studies
- Tzanck smear, serum VZV antibodies, viral culture
- EKG to rule out cardiac etiology, x-ray to rule out pleural or abdominal etiology, ultrasound to rule out cholelithiasis/nephrolithiasis

Differential Diagnosis

PRODROMAL STAGE
- Migraine
- Cardiac or pleuritic pain
- Acute abdomen
- Disc disease

VESICULAR-CRUSTING STAGE
- Herpes simplex
- Plant dermatitis
- Erysipelas
- Bullous impetigo
- Necrotizing fasciitis

Management

Nonpharmacologic Treatment
- Moist dressings (water, normal saline, or Burrow's solution) or colloidal oatmeal suspension (Aveeno) may decrease pain

Pharmacologic Treatment
- Acyclovir (Zovirax) 800 mg 5 x d
- Valacyclovir (Valtrex) 1000 mg tid
- Famciclovir (Famvir) 500 mg tid
- IV acyclovir 10 mg/kg tid
- IV foscarnet for acyclovir-resistant strains
- Pain management with non-narcotic and narcotic pain medications or NSAIDs
- Gabapentin (start at 100 mg qd) or nortriptyline (start at 10 mg qhs) may be used to manage chronic pain of postherpetic neuralgia
- Capsaicin ointment (0.025%–0.075%) tid–qid may be tried for postherpetic neuralgia

How Long to Treat
- 7 to 10 days

Special Considerations
- May become disseminated in immunocompromised patients; if so, requires hospitalization or in-home IV therapy
- Monitor hydration and renal function of frail elderly on antiviral medication.

When to Consult, Refer, Hospitalize
- Disseminated disease
- Ophthalmology consult if fifth cranial nerve affected

Follow-up

Expected Course
- Initial course generally resolved in 2 to 3 weeks

Complications
- Postherpetic neuralgia: may be long term, need chronic pain management; elderly at greater risk

with 20% to 50% affected; severity of acute phase does not predict the risk or severity of post-infection neuralgia
- Local hemorrhage, gangrene or super-infection
- Systemic meningoencephalitis, cerebral vascular syndrome, cranial nerve syndromes (ophthalmic, trigeminal, facial, and auditory), peripheral motor weakness

Parasitic Infestations
Scabies

Description
- Infestation by mite, spread by direct contact leading to generalized pruritus, which is a hyper-sensitivity reaction to the scabies

Etiology
- *Sarcoptes scabiei* that thrive and multiply only on human skin; spread by human-to-human contact; mites may live up to 2 days on clothing and bed linens
- Sensitization to *S scabiei* must occur prior to developing generalized pruritus associated with infestation. In initial infestation, sensitization takes about 10 days. Subsequent infestations advance to pruritic stage much more quickly.

Incidence and Demographics
- Common in the elderly and infirm in residential facilities
- Epidemics occur in cycles

Risk Factors
- Exposure to others with scabies
- Institutional living particularly in those with neurologic disorders and dementia
- Crusted scabies
- Immunocompromised status

Prevention and Screening
- Education about the mode of transmission

Assessment
History
- Often history of family members or close contacts with similar symptoms
- Severe generalized pruritus, sparing head and neck
- Pruritus and scratching often interfere with sleep

Physical
- Scattered vesicles, burrows, or nodules with excoriations
- Common distribution: axillae, anogenital region, wrists, hands, waist, and flexor surfaces of elbows
- May develop generalized erythroderma
- May also develop lichen simplex chronicus
- In atopic individuals, an eczematous dermatitis is common
- Postinflammatory hyperpigmentation may occur
- Secondary infections to denuded sites are common
- Crusted vesicles or burrows results after infestation of several months

Diagnostic Studies
- Serum eosinophilia
- By placing a drop of mineral oil over a burrow and scraping the burrow with a blade, mites and their eggs or fecal droppings can be collected and placed on a slide with mineral oil and a cover slip. This can then be examined under the microscope.

Differential Diagnosis

- Drug eruption dermatitis
- Atopic or contact dermatitis
- Pityriasis rosea
- Herpetiform dermatitis
- Pediculosis dermatitis
- Insect bites
- Delusions of parasitosis
- Metabolic pruritus

Management

Nonpharmacologic Treatment

- Not effective alone
- Wash bedding and clothing after application of medication

Pharmacologic Treatment

- Management of pruritus relies on pharmacologic eradication of mites and their eggs and pharmacologic treatment of pruritus.
- Permethrin 5% cream overnight (8–14 hours) x 1
- A tapered course of systemic steroids starting at 70–80 mg qd and tapering by 5 mg qd is often necessary to treat wide spread pruritus
- Topical steroids bid to severely pruritic areas
- Systemic antihistamines, such as diphenhydramine 25–50 mg q 4–6 hours for treatment of pruritus

How Long to Treat

- One-time treatment with lindane or permethrin may be effective but a repeat treatment in 14 days is often necessary to eliminate infestation
- Systemic steroids are generally tapered over 10 to 14 days
- Systemic antihistamines are used PRN

Special Considerations

- In the elderly, lesions may appear as excoriations on the back

When to Consult, Refer, Hospitalize

- When resolution is not achieved with above regimen

Follow-up

Expected Course

- Mites may be eradicated with 1 or possibly 2 treatments with the above medications, but the generalized pruritus may persist for several weeks since it is a hypersensitivity reaction to the mite.
- Patients should be brought back for follow up in 1 to 2 weeks and then at weekly intervals if there is extensive dermatitis.

Complications

- Secondary bacterial infection, abscesses and/or cellulitis are possible complications as a result of the associated scratching.

Miscellaneous
Acne Rosacea

Description

- Chronic acneform inflammation of central area of face
- Does not involve any comedones, which are the classic lesion of acne vulgaris

Etiology

- Cutaneous vascular disorder of increased reaction of capillaries to heat-"flushing"

Table 6-4: Skin Phototype Based on Sun Sensitivity

Skin Type	Sunburn and Tanning History
I	Always burns easily; rarely tans
II	Always burns easily; tans minimally
III	Burns moderately; tans gradually and uniformly to a light brown color
IV	Burns minimally; always tans well to moderate brown color
V	Rarely burns; tans profusely to dark brown color
VI	Rarely burns; deeply pigmented black color

Incidence and Demographics
- Frequently seen in elderly
- Commonly found in fair-skinned, middle-aged to elderly people
- Severe form with rhinophyma is seen almost exclusively in men over 40

Risk Factors
- Found more commonly in individuals with fair skin (skin phototype I, II, and III) (See Table 6-4) due to increased sensitivity to sun exposure
- Positive family history of rosacea is a risk factor
- Excessive ETOH consumption is associated with flares

Prevention and Screening
- Education about the risks of excess consumption of ETOH and hot drinks

Assessment (See Table 6-4)

History
- History of abnormal flushing of the central portion of the face after drinking hot or alcoholic beverages or eating spicy foods

Physical
- 2 mm to 3 mm papular and pustular discrete and clustered lesions on the central portion of the face on any erythematous base
- Dilatation of superficial capillaries causing flushing, eventually leads to telangiectasia
- Ocular symptoms may be associated and include blepharitis, conjunctivitis
- Chronic symptoms can lead to lymphatic changes causing cellulitis
- Irreversible hypertrophy of the nose, rhinophyma, is a result of chronic inflammation and is seen almost exclusively in men over 40

Diagnostic Studies
- Based on clinical presentation; culture or biopsy is not necessary

Differential Diagnosis
- Acne vulgaris
- Butterfly rash of SL
- Folliculitis
- Pustular tinea

Management

Nonpharmacologic Treatment
- Avoid triggers that cause facial flushing such as hot beverages, ETOH, highly spicy foods, exposure to sun and wind, emotional stress, certain medications such as niacin

Pharmacologic Treatment
- Topical metronidazole 0.75%, erythromycin 2%, or clindamycin topical gel bid
- Doxycycline 100 mg bid
- Erythromycin 250 mg tid or bid

How Long to Treat
- Length of treatment: long term, initially bid or tid, taper to qd maintenance dosing

Special Considerations
- ASA may be given to lessen the flushing associated with niacin cholesterol therapy

When to Consult, Refer, Hospitalize
- If suboptimal response with above regimen, refer to dermatology

Follow-up

Expected Course
- Response usually seen in 3 weeks, maximum response from one regimen usually seen by 9 weeks

Complications
- Rhinophyma as described above

Burns

Description
- Damage to the epidermis, dermis, and/or subcutaneous tissue

Etiology
- Exposure to intense heat of fire or steam or to chemicals or electricity

Incidence and Demographics
- Approximately 1.25 million burn injuries annually in US
- Flame burns most common in adults
- Scald burns more common in early dementia
- Unsupervised demented elderly at home or at nursing home

Risk Factors
- Unsupervised elders with dementia and/or progressive debilitating diseases
- Exposure to scalding liquids (steam), chemicals. or electricity at home or nursing facility

Prevention and Screening
- Fire safety and safe handling of hot liquids, chemicals. and electricity education in the community; caretakers to review home for risk factors
- Lower thermostat of water heater
- Educate patients and families regarding safe use of heating pads
- Practice evacuation drills in community settings, homes, and nursing facilities

Assessment

History
- Exposure to fire, chemicals, scalding liquids. or electricity
- Intense pain and site of exposure (third-degree burns are usually painless)

Physical
- Burns classified by extent and depth of tissue involvement, patient age, and associated illness or injury
- Patient's age and health status is critical; even a minor burn in an elderly patient may be fatal
- Extent of involvement can be measured by using the "rule of nines" (see Table 6-5)
- Another estimate of extent of involvement is to equate the patient's palm size as 1% of total body size
- Depth of injury described as first-, second-, or third-degree burns
  - First-degree burns: superficial burns involve the epidermis only; redness and blanching erythema (demonstrating capillary refill) of affected area with no initial blistering
  - Second-degree burns: partial-thickness burns involve entire epidermis and variable portions of the dermis; red, moist and edematous skin with small or large bullae

Table 6-5: Rule of Nines

Body Part Affected	Percentage
Anterior head and neck	4.5%
Posterior head and neck	4.5%
Torso and abdomen	18%
Back	18%
Anterior arms	4.5% each
Posterior arms	4.5% each
Genitalia	1%
Anterior legs	9% each
Posterior legs	9% each

- Third-degree burns: full-thickness burn involving entire dermis and subcutaneous tissue; pale, white, tan, or charred wound that may appear dry and depressed below surrounding skin. Skin may feel tight and leathery.

Diagnostic Studies
- Immediate clinical triage is essential to allow patients to be treated in most appropriate setting.

Management
- Office management
  - First-degree burns (e.g., sunburn)
  - Superficial second-degree burns of up to approximately 5% to 6% total body surface area (TBSA) that do not affect areas of function or cosmetic appearance
  - Selected, deeper second-degree burns if not on lower extremities, hands, face, genitals, or areas of function or cosmetic importance; probably do not cover more than 1% to 2% TBSA
  - Patient or family must be reliable and the home situation functional
  - Emergency stabilization of serious burn patients

Nonpharmacologic Treatment
- Burns involving eye should be irrigated with water, saline, or lactated Ringer's solution
- Wound should be cleaned and debrided using plain soap and water, Betadine diluted with water, or saline solution. Any dead skin should be removed.
- Elevate involved extremities

Pharmacologic Treatment
- Topical silver sulfadiazine (Silvadene) in a half-inch layer over entire surface, covered with nonabsorbent gauze (Kerlix or Telfa) and wrapped in at least a 3-inch-thick nonadhesive wrap
- Analgesia with narcotics
- Tetanus prophylaxis
- Antibiotic coverage for superinfection

How Long to Treat
- Dressing changes bid
- Until resolution with frequent reevaluation

Special Considerations
- Elderly or debilitated patients are at higher risk for hemodynamic compromise.

When to Consult, Refer, and Hospitalize
- Refer patients with the following burn characteristics to a burn center:
  - Deep second-degree or third-degree burns
  - Burns of greater than 10% TBSA in patients less than 10 years and more than 50 years

- Burns of greater than 20% TBSA in all other patients
- Burns of the face, hands, and feet, over a joint or of the perineum, or burns that are circumferential
- Burns resulting from elder abuse
- Inhalation injury
- Electrical burns
- Chemical burns
- Suspected toxic epidermal necrolysis syndrome

Follow-up

Expected Course
- Depends on the extent and location of the burn

Complications
- Hemodynamic compromise
- Multi-organ failure
- Sepsis
- Scarring
- Post-traumatic stress
- Increased photosensitivity of healed skin

TUMORS
Seborrheic Keratosis

Description
- Hereditary benign epithelial tumors that appear in adulthood
- Normal changes with age

Etiology
- Probable autosomal dominant inheritance
- Results from proliferation of keratinocytes, melanocytes, and plugged follicles

Incidence and Demographics
- Often seen in elderly secondary to photoaging
- Slightly more common and with more extensive involvement in males

Risk Factors
- Family history

Assessment

History
- Gradual onset of asymptomatic skin lesions appearing after the age of 30
- Rarely mild pruritus
- Painful if secondarily infected

Physical
- Initially 1 mm to 3 mm scattered and discrete, lightly tan colored round or oval macules appearing on the face, trunk, and upper extremities
- Slowly develops into a very slightly raised papule or plaque that has usually darkened in color to brown, gray, or black
- This lesion has a stuck on appearance with a warty surface and multiple plugged follicles or "horny cysts," which are very typical of seborrheic keratosis.

Diagnostic Studies
- Usually not indicated
- Biopsy should be done if diagnosis is unclear; rule out carcinoma or melanoma

Differential Diagnosis

- Solar lentigo
- Actinic keratosis
- Basal cell carcinoma
- Squamous cell carcinoma
- Malignant melanoma
- Verruca vulgaris

Management

Nonpharmacologic Treatment

- Electrocautery, cryosurgery, and curettage if a problem

Special Considerations

- Patients with a history of actinic keratosis or skin cancer should have lesions biopsied by an experienced clinician with attention to excising with a margin around the borders to rule out malignant lesions.

When to Consult, Refer, Hospitalize

- To dermatology for excision and biopsy if primary care clinician is not experienced with excision procedures or to oncology for malignant lesions

Follow-up

Expected Course

- Lesions are considered benign and may continue to develop throughout a lifetime; may recur after removal or destruction with cryosurgery

Complications

- Secondary infection

Actinic/Solar Keratosis

Description

- Discrete, dry, scaly lesions occurring on prolonged or recurrently sun-exposed skin of susceptible adults, often precursor to squamous cell carcinoma (SCC)

Etiology

- Recurrent or prolonged sun exposure of SPT I, II, and III skin

Incidence and Demographics

- Common in elders secondary to photoaging of skin
- Males more commonly than females
- Appears in middle adulthood, earlier in Australia and the Southwestern US

Risk Factors

- SPT I, II, or III type skin
- Prolonged or recurrent unprotected sun exposure
- Outdoors work or frequent outdoor sports

Prevention and Screening

- Education about the risks of unprotected sun exposure
- Use of sun block and protective clothing during periods of exposure

Assessment

History

- Gradual onset of light tan, brown, or red dry, roughened lesions on sun-exposed skin
- Minimal sensation but may be mildly tender
- May bleed if irritated

Physical

- Single or multiple discrete adherent hyperkeratotic scaly lesions

- Approximately 1 cm in size and round or oval
- Color ranges from light tan to brown with or without reddish tinge

Diagnostic Studies
- Biopsy demonstrates atypical keratinocytes

Differential Diagnosis
- Discoid lupus erythematosus
- Seborrheic keratosis

Management

Nonpharmacologic Treatment
- Cryotherapy
- Excision

Pharmacologic Treatment
- Topical 5% 5-fluorouracil cream bid until resolved

How Long to Treat
- Several days to weeks

Special Considerations
- Identifying at risk patients is essential

When to Consult, Refer, Hospitalize
- For excision of large or extensive lesions or for management if primary care clinician is unfamiliar with excision and management protocols

Follow-up

Expected Course
- Treatment is effective in eradicating lesions but vigilant follow-up is warranted to monitor for new lesions.

Complications
- Squamous cell carcinoma in untreated lesions

Basal Cell Carcinoma (BCC)

Description
- Most commonly seen skin cancer
- Requires a hair follicle to develop
- Slow growing
- Rarely metastasizes
- Can become invasive if located on the face, in the ear canal, or in the posterior auricular sulcus

Etiology
- Excess sun exposure, particularly in fair-skinned individuals
- Result of proliferating atypical basal cells with various amounts of stroma

Incidence and Demographics
- Accounts for 75% of 1 million cases of skin cancer diagnosed annually in US
- Basal cell skin cancer is the most common cancer in the US today
- Age: 95% between 40 and 79 years
- Male more than female
- Fair skin with poor tanning ability (SPT I or II)
- Dark skin rarely affected

Risk Factors
- Excess sun exposure
- Fair skin with poor tanning ability (SPT I or II)
- Prior treatment with x-ray for facial acne

Prevention and Screening
- Primary prevention involves avoiding sun exposure and sun protection
- Secondary prevention involves screening for skin lesions with premalignant or malignant characteristics during routine health exams, referral for lesions of concern
- Tertiary prevention involves removal of precancerous lesions such as suspicious moles and actinic keratoses, usually done by dermatologist or surgeon

Assessment
History
- Patients may or may not be aware of suspicious lesions.

Physical
- 85% occur on head and neck, and one-fourth of lesions occur on nose
- "Pearly"-appearing firm, round or oval papules or nodules on sun-exposed skin (80% on the face and neck)
- "Ulcer" or "sore" with a rolled border ("rodent bite ulcer")
- Crusting may be present
- Pink or red, pigmented lesions may be brown, blue, or black
- Central umbilication possible

Diagnostic Studies
- Clinical diagnosis of suspicious lesions on sun-exposed skin
- Biopsy demonstrating atypical basal cells

Differential Diagnosis
- Molluscum contagiosum
- Solar lentigo
- Actinic keratosis
- Squamous cell carcinoma
- Malignant melanoma
- Verruca vulgaris

Management
- Excision, cryosurgery, or electrosurgery
- Mohs' surgery—microscopically controlled surgery for lesions in the danger zones of nasolabial folds, around eyes, in ear canal, and posterior auricular sulcus
- Radiation therapy is alternative in areas of possible cosmetic disfigurement

Special Considerations
- Refer to dermatologist for biopsy and excision of lesions or lesions of cosmetic disfigurement

Follow-up
Expected Course
- Resolution with above therapies is the norm but at-risk patients should be followed to monitor for new lesions.

Complications
- Cosmetic disfigurement

Squamous Cell Carcinoma (SCC)

Description
- Second most common type of cutaneous carcinoma
- Malignant tumor of epithelial keratinocytes; develops on skin and mucous membranes
- Bowen's disease is form of SCC arising de novo on any area of skin

Etiology
- Skin exposure to exogenous carcinogens
- Sunlight, arsenic ingestion, tobacco, ionizing radiation, HPV

Incidence and Demographics
- Higher incidence in Sunbelt
- Age—older than 55
- Male more than female
- More common than basal cell carcinoma in black individuals; occurring at sites of scars or chronic inflammation rather than sun-exposed areas

Risk Factors
- Fair skin with poor tanning ability (SPT I or II)
- Sun exposure—outdoor workers and sportsman
- Arsenic ingestion
- Tobacco use
- Radiation exposure
- Solar keratosis

Prevention and Screening
- Education about the risks of unprotected sun exposure, tobacco, and arsenic ingestion and radiation exposure
- Use of sun block

Assessment
History
- Suspicious lesion developing over months to years
- Most often on sun-exposed skin (face, lips, hands, neck, and forearms)

Physical
- Indurated papule, nodule, or plaque
- Thick adherent, keratotic scale
- Honey-colored exudate extruded from periphery
- May be eroded, crusted, ulcerated, hard, erythematous, isolated, or multiple lesions

Diagnostic Studies
- Biopsy demonstrating atypical squamous cells

Differential Diagnosis
- Nummular eczema
- Psoriasis
- Paget disease
- Basal cell carcinoma

Management
- Surgery or radiation depending on the size, shape, and location of the tumor

When to Consult, Refer, Hospitalize
- Refer to dermatology for microscopically controlled surgery

Follow-up
- Remission achieved in 90% of cases

Malignant Melanoma

Description
- Least common but most lethal of all cutaneous carcinomas
- Classification by type:
  - Superficial spreading melanoma (SSM)—starts fourth to fifth decade; commonly on upper back and legs; haphazard combination of many colors (especially red, brown, black); size about 2.5 cm diameter, irregular surface
  - Nodular melanoma (NM)—occurs in fifth or sixth decade; raised growth; brown, red, black with variety of shapes; frequent crusting and bleeding

- Lentigo maligna melanoma (LMM)—starts sixth or seventh decade; brown/black color; may stay flat; irregular borders; starts as nonmelanoma with slow progression; better prognosis
- Acral-lentiginous melanoma (ALM)—seen on palms, soles, terminal phalanges, mucous membranes; brown/black, usually flat; often slow growing; most in blacks and Asians; elevated lesions very aggressive

Etiology
- Proliferating malignant melanocytes

Incidence and Demographics
- Incidence rates rising dramatically over past 4 decades with estimated lifetime risk of 1 in 90 Americans
- There is greater incidence and greater death among the elderly
- Men more than 50 years old account for nearly half of all deaths from MM
- 5% of all cutaneous carcinomas in US
- More common in Sunbelt
- Associated with excessive sun exposure

Risk Factors
- Family history
- Excessive sun exposure
- Severe sunburn, particularly at an early age
- Outdoor occupations
- Fair skin

Prevention and Screening
- Education about the risks of unprotected sun exposure and genetic predisposition

Assessment

History
- Asymptomatic skin lesion for month

Physical
- Macules, papules, or nodules
- Colors ranging from pink to brown, blue, or black
- Boarders most often irregular
- Size may vary from a few millimeters to centimeters
- The 5 cardinal signs of malignant melanoma are:
  - **A** Asymmetry
  - **B** Border is irregular and often scalloped
  - **C** Color is mottled with haphazard display of brown, black, gray, and/or pink
  - **D** Diameter is large—greater than 6.0 mm
  - **E** Elevation is almost always present with subtle or obvious surface distortion, best assessed by side-lighting of the lesion

Diagnostic Studies
- Biopsy including margins and depth of invasion assessment
- Lymph node biopsy is often also indicated

Differential Diagnosis
- Benign nevi   • Pigmented basal cell carcinoma

Management
- Aggressive surgical management by excision with margins intact
- Chemotherapy for patients with high-risk melanomas

Special Considerations
- Refer for excision and chemotherapy as indicated

Follow-up
- Prognosis—death due to melanoma is preventable with early diagnosis
- Periodic and regular interval exams for high-risk patients
- Self or family member exam every month
- Dermatology follow-up every 6 months for suspicious lesions
- Depth of invasion or tumor thickness is the single most important prognostic factor (Breslow's depth)

PRESSURE ULCERS

Description
- Areas of local tissue trauma caused by unrelieved pressure to tissues that are compressed between a bony prominence and external surface
- A sign of local tissue necrosis and death

Etiology
- Mechanical injury to skin, underlying tissues; primarily caused by pressure and shear
- Increased pressure gradient over bony prominences where there is less available compressible tissue, leads to more pressure ulcers at these points
- Unrelieved pressure over time occludes blood and lymphatic circulation causing tissues to be deprived of oxygen, nutrients, and waste removal, leading to tissue breakdown and eventual death

Incidence and Demographics
- Highest incidence noted in both acute and long-term facilities and private homes where mobility of person and their capability to perform self-care has been altered
- Orthopedic surgery and spinal cord injury have higher risk than other institutionalized patients
- Terminally ill elderly at high risk

Risk Factors
- Use validated risk assessment tool, such as Braden Scale or Norton Scale, to determine level of risk and to have data base to start prevention and/or treatment plan
- Risk factors include:
  - Decreased mobility, activity, sensory perception/alertness, pain
  - Extrinsic factors of increased moisture (incontinence/perspiration/leakage), friction, shear
  - Intrinsic factors of increased age, decreased nutrition, and arteriolar pressure

Prevention and Screening
- Any patient at risk should have thorough skin inspection regularly
- Start program of care that would address risk factors identified
- Diligent skin cleansing of waste, regular moisturizing, and skin barrier ointments for incontinence/leakage, etc.
- Nutritional guidance and support
- If immobility present, needs proper pressure-relief devices for bed and chair and proper and frequent repositioning of patient
- Provide adequate pain management to facilitate ease of movement and change of position
- Provide/arrange for education for caregivers and patient

Assessment
History
- Recent or gradual change in health, mobility, continence; injury, trauma, surgery; self-care abilities
  - Postoperative surgery, especially orthopedic

- Recent or worsening of paralyzing or spastic neurological illness; for example, CVA, spinal cord injury, Parkinson disease
- Injury or illness causing pain and secondary immobility or restlessness

Physical
- Pressure ulcers and surrounding tissues should be examined, measured, and staged regularly. Acute and long-term healthcare facilities mandated to perform assessments weekly
- Ulcer bed should be described in terms of types of tissue present (e.g., granulation, necrotic, epithelial)
- Photograph if possible
- Evidence of frank wound infection to be monitored
- Stages
  - I: nonblanchable erythema of intact skin; in individuals with darker skin, discoloration of the skin, warmth, edema, induration, or hardness may also be indicators
  - II: partial-thickness skin loss involving epidermis, dermis, or both; the ulcer is superficial and presents as an abrasion, blister, or shallow crater
  - III: full-thickness skin loss involving damage to or necrosis of subcutaneous tissue that may extend down to, but not through, underlying fascia; presents as a deep crater with or without undermining
  - IV: full-thickness skin loss with extensive destruction, tissue necrosis, or damage to muscle, bone, or supporting structures
- If eschar present, ulcer cannot be accurately staged until eschar removed
- Sequential monitoring of ulcer should be documented on a flow record; researched tools available (e.g., Pressure Sore Status Tool, Sussman Wound Healing Tool)

Diagnostic Studies
- Clinical diagnosis based on precipitating factors
- Serum albumin level useful in diagnosing undernutrition

Differential Diagnosis
- Arterial/diabetic ulcer
- Venous ulcer
- Malignancy
- Rheumatoid disease
- Pyoderma gangrenosum

Management

Nonpharmacologic Treatment
- Basics: (1) nutritional assessment and support, (2) management of tissue loads, (3) ulcer care
- Nutrition: as compatible with patient's wishes, supplement diet as needed to provide at least RDA of vitamins and minerals, and minimum of 30–35 calories/kg/day and 1.25–1.5 g protein/kg/day
- Tissue load management: proper positioning, frequent repositioning, adequate pressure relief devices in chair and bed to facilitate healing and comfort
- Ulcer care
  - Cleansing—adequate, nontraumatic with noncytotoxic cleanser at safe irrigation pressure (4–15 psi)
  - Debridement—remove devitalized tissue when appropriate, choosing method of debridement based on condition and goals (sharp, mechanical, enzymatic, autolytic)
  - Dressings—moist wound healing shown to be most physiologically ideal (e.g., hydrocolloid, hydrogel dressings); protect periulcer area from maceration with skin barrier; control excess exudate from ulcer without drying out ulcer bed

Pharmacological Treatment
- For wound infection or surrounding cellulitis, or evidence of early osteomyelitis, use antibiotic appropriate for treatment of probable *S aureus*, gram-negative rods (swab cultures not used to diagnose infection as pressure ulcers are usually colonized)

- Use analgesics to control pain around the clock and/or prn before care

How Long to Treat
- Until ulcer healed or if terminally ill, until death, evaluating treatment plan about every 2 weeks for progress (if healing is goal) and adjust plan as needed

Special Considerations
- Approach to care and goal of treatment must be based on whether elder's wishes are for cure or for comfort

When to Consult, Refer, Hospitalize
- Physical therapy for adjunctive treatments (e.g., electrotherapy, electrical stimulation)
- Plastic surgeon if surgical repair may be appropriate
- Wound care center if treatment plan is failing
- In advancing cellulitis or osteomyelitis not appropriate for out patient treatment, consider hospitalization

Follow-up

Expected Course
- If elder can maintain adequate nutrition, cooperate with care, and avoid serious concurrent illnesses, healing is expected
- Slow or poor healing may be secondary to chronic physical and cognitive illnesses

Complications
- Wound infection/cellulitis
- Osteomyelitis
- Loss of extremity
- Necrotizing fasciitis
- Septicemia—death

VENOUS STASIS DERMATITIS AND ULCERS

Description
- Distal lower extremity may have dry or wet dermatitis and/or open ulcerations as a result of venous disease

Etiology
- Sustained venous hypertension of lower extremities
- Valvular incompetence in venous system of lower extremities
- Leakage of fibrinogen from vascular system into dermis leads to decrease in oxygen and nutrients
- Trapping of WBCs in microcirculation secondary to altered inflammatory mechanisms

Incidence and Demographics
- Estimated 500,000 to 700,000 patients in US
- About 40% have ulcer first occur at age 65 and older
- More than 50% have ulcer last more than 1 year
- About 70% have recurrence of ulcers

Risk Factors
- Obesity
- Lower extremity edema
- History of thrombophlebitis
- Multiple pregnancies
- Positive family history
- Trauma
- Advancing age
- Previous venous ulcer

Prevention and Screening
- Control of edema with elevation and compression
- Avoidance of trauma to lower extremities
- Monitor for skin color and consistency changes in gaiter area of leg (area around and proximal to ankle)
- Good moisturizing of lower legs

Assessment

History
- Past lower extremity phlebitis, injury, surgery, ulcer, edema
- Family history

Physical
- Location: lower leg, usually proximal to medial or lateral malleolus
- Skin: hyperpigmented, eczematous dermatitis, lipodermatosclerosis, often edema, palpable pulses, varicose veins
- Ulcer bed: shallow, irregular shape; beefy red and/or fibrinous necrosis; often moderate to heavy exudate
- Pain: usually mild, relieved with elevation

Diagnostic Studies
- Often diagnosis of clinical determination
- Rule out arterial insufficiency with Ankle Brachial Index (ABI); (not appropriate in diabetic; toe pressure studies may be helpful)
- Rule out deep-vein thrombosis (DVT) with ultrasound

Differential Diagnosis
- Arterial ulcer
- Diabetic ulcer
- Pressure ulcer
- Vasculitis
- Pyoderma gangrenosum
- Malignancy
- Osteomyelitis

Management

Nonpharmacologic Treatment
- Dermatitis: emollients, compression and elevation for edema
- Ulcers
  - Irrigate and/or mild whirlpool with noncytotoxic agent at safe irrigation pressure of 4 to 15 psi
  - Select appropriate dressing that fits wound(s) and provides basis for moist wound healing (e.g., hydrocolloid or foam dressing if drainage minimal, alginate if excess drainage, hydrogel if wound dry)
  - Compression is cornerstone to success: use medium to high (if ABI $\oplus$ 0.8) compression if tolerated (e.g., special-order knee high stockings, Unna's or Duke Boot, multilayered compression wrap, pneumatic compression device)

Pharmacologic Treatment
- Use topical mild steroids and antifungals as needed
- Oral pentoxifylline (Trental) or cilostazol (Pletal) may improve blood flow and improve function and reduce symptoms, particularly if claudication is present
- Systemic antibiotics if surrounding cellulitis; short-term use only of topical antibiotics (excess use can lead to secondary reactive dermatitis)

How Long to Treat
- Continue until healed, altering approach as ulcer and surrounding skin changes
- If not improving in 6 to 12 weeks, consider biopsy at edge

When to Consult, Refer, Hospitalize
- To vascular surgeon if considering evaluation of superficial venous system for possible corrective surgery
- To physical therapy if increased joint mobility and increased ambulation is needed
- To hospital for extensive cellulitis at level beyond appropriate for out patient treatment
- To wound care center for treatment failure more than 3 months if skin biopsy negative, or if considering advanced treatment (e.g., skin substitutes, growth factors)

Special Considerations
- Concurrent arterial disease makes treatment more complex and can impact healing

Follow-up

Expected Course
- Prolonged healing time of ulcers and recurrences are common.
- Compression therapy needed continuously even if skin healed
- Progression of venous disease and secondary skin changes expected with age

Complications
- Cellulitis
- Woody fibrosis and nonpitting edema with secondary ankle restriction
- Lifestyle change with negative aspects of prolonged treatment, change in mobility, change in body image, and powerlessness over healing

CASE STUDIES

Case 1. An 86-year-old female resident of a long-term care facility for 2 years secondary to late-stage dementia has fallen and suffered a right hip fracture. She was sent to the hospital for internal fixation and returned to the nursing home 2 days postop and now has 3 x 3 cm bulla on posterior right heel. Prior to fall, she was underweight, needed assistance to ambulate, and had poor short-term memory and poor safety insight. Meds include MVI with minerals, Peri Colace, and Lovenox injection.
1. What was probable cause of right heel bulla?
2. What were her risk factors for pressure ulcers pre- and post-op?
3. How could this heel ulcer have been prevented?
4. What are basics for treatment?
5. What are possible complications of this pressure ulcer?

Case 2. A 75-year-old blond white male, previous construction worker, complains of a raised lump on the back of his neck, which is often irritated by his shirt collar, and his wife has noticed that it seems to be getting larger in color over the past few months. He has no other significant medical history. Medications: Ecotrin, Lipitor, lisinopril
1. How common are skin cancers?
2. How does this patient follow the demographics and risk factors for skin cancer?
3. Does location of lesion help in assessment?
4. What diagnostic test is necessary?
5. What is appropriate treatment for lesions, and what is expected outcome?

Case 3. Your 95-year-old nursing home patient has dementia and is no longer ambulatory. She must be fed, and she is incontinent of urine. She is obese and has diabetes mellitus, polymyalgia rheumatica, and gastroesophageal reflux. Her medications are Avandia

4 mg PO qd, prednisone 3 mg PO qd, Tylenol prn, Prilosec 20 me PO bid. The nursing assistant noticed red skin on her abdomen and in perineal area when cleaning her today. You find bright red smooth macules with maceration and satellite lesions under her breasts, in skin folds on abdomen, and in perineal area.

1. What is your most likely diagnosis?
2. What risk factors does she have?
3. What nonpharmacologic treatment would you order?
4. What pharmacologic treatment would you order?
5. How long would it take for this to work?

REFERENCES

Balin, A. K. (2002). Seborrheic keratoses. Emedicine.com. Available at: http://222.emedicine.com/DERM/topic397.htm.

Berger, T. G. (2005). Skin, hair and nails. In L. M. Tierney, et al. *Current medical diagnosis and treatment* (44th ed.). New York: Lange Medical Books/McGraw Hill.

Blount, B.W. (2002). Rosacea: A common, yet commonly overlooked, condition. *American Family Physician*, 66 (3), 435–440.

Crawford, F., et al. (2000). Topical treatment for fungal infections of the skin and nails of the foot. Cochrane Database. *Syst Rev CD001434*.

Edmunds, M. W., & Mayhew, M. S. (2004). *Pharmacology for the primary care provider* (2nd ed.). St. Louis, MO: Mosby.

Fitzpatrick, T. B., Johnson, R. A., Wolff, K.,& Suurmond, D. (2000). *Color atlas & synopsis of clinical dermatology* (4th ed.). New York: McGraw-Hill.

Gnann, J. W., Jr. (2002). Clinical practice: Herpes zoster. *New England Journal of Medicine*, 347(4), 340–346.

Goldstein, B. G., et al. (2001). Diagnosis and management of malignant melanoma. *Am Fam Physician*, 63, 1359.

Goroll, A. H., & Mulley, A. G. (2000). *Primary care medicine* (4th ed.). Philadelphia: Lippincott, Williams & Wilkins.

Griffith, H. W., & Dambro, M. R. (2000). *The 5 minute clinical consult*. Malvern, PA: Lea & Febiger.

Habif, T. P., et al. (2004). *Clinical dermatology: A color guide to diagnosis and therapy*. St Louis, Mo: Mosby.

Hall, J. C. (2000). *Sauer's manual of skin diseases* (8th ed.). Philadelphia: Lippincott, Williams & Wilkins.

Jerant, A. F., et al. (2000). Early detection and treatment of skin cancer. *Am Fam Physician*, 62, 357.

Kaplan, D. L. (2001). Dermclinic: Cutaneous conundrums, dermatologic disguises. *Consultant*, 41(4), 571–579, 523–525, 529–530.

Marghoob, A. A. (2002). Dermatologic look-alikes: Skin cancer concerns. *Clinical Advisor*, 5(4), 121–122, 127.

Meredith, P. V., & Horan, N. M. (2000). *Adult primary care*. Philadelphia: WB Saunders.

Nicol, N. H. (2000). Managing atopic dermatitis in children and adults. *Nurse Practitioner*, 25(4), 58–81.

Rees, M. T. (2002). Managing atopic eczema. *Primary Health Care*, 12(8), 27–32.

Stankus, S. J., et al. (2000). Management of herpes zoster (shingles) and postherpetic neuralgia. *American Family Physician*, 61, 2437.

Tierney, L. M., McPhee, S. J., & Papadakis, A. (2005). *Current medical diagnosis and treatment* (44th ed.). NJ: Appleton & Lange.

Witman, P. M. (2001). Concise review for clinicians: Topical therapies for localized psoriasis. *Mayo Clinic Proceedings*, 76(9), 943–949.

EYE, EAR, NOSE, AND THROAT DISORDERS

7

EYE DISORDERS
GERIATRIC APPROACH

Normal Changes of Aging
- Tear production diminishes, predisposing to dry eyes
- *Arcus senilis:* age-related gray-white ring around limbus; no clinical significance
- Lens denser, less elastic, decreased accommodation. Results in *presbyopia* (far-sightedness). The dull lens may lead to **glare**
- Corneal sensitivity to touch decreases with age, may lead to corneal damage
- Pupil size diminishes; reacts more slowly to light, dilates more slowly in the dark
- Liquefaction of vitreous humor leads to **"floaters"**
- Retina may become duller
- **Retinal cell loss** affects color discrimination
- Loss of neurons in the visual pathways beyond the retina

Clinical Essentials

History
- Any visual changes since last visit; evaluate difficulty driving (night or daytime), changes in reading habits
- Date of last complete ophthalmologist exam
- Glasses or contact lenses
- Medications (ocular, systemic, OTC, herbal); consider ocular effects of systemic medicines (e.g., steroids, anticholinergics, antiarrhythmics)

Physical
- Test of visual acuity is keystone of exam. Assess vision using the Snellen chart, Rosenbaum pocket screen, or other standardized measurement of visual acuity
- Funduscopic exam should be attempted. If lens opacities prevent visualization, the patient should be evaluated for possible cataracts

Assessment
- Many eye disorders present in a similar fashion
- Determine effects of low vision on patient and family members
- The eyes offer a unique opportunity to visualize arteries directly. The *arteriosclerosis* visible in the retinal blood vessels mirrors the arteriosclerosis elsewhere in the body. See Cardiovascular Chapter 9 for details. This is due to changes in arteriole wall leading to loss of transparency

Treatment
- Refer immediately any sudden painless loss of vision. Most eye problems require ophthalmology referral
- Monitor for effects of topical treatments on eye

Table 7-1: Indicators of Vision-Threatening Disorders

Symptoms	Signs
• Blurred vision that does NOT clear with blinking • Sudden loss or decreased vision • Halos around sources of lights • Flashing lights • Sudden floating spots or sensation of "cobwebs" across field of vision • Photophobia • Periocular headache • Ocular pain	• Ciliary flush • Corneal damage (opacities, trauma) • Abnormal pupils • Increased intraocular pressure • Appearance of RBCs or WBCs in anterior chamber • Proptosis (forward displacement of the eye globe within the orbit of the eye) • Severe green-yellow d/c, erythema, chemosis, and lid edema • Acute onset limited ocular movement • Facial cellulitis

- Local—irritation, inflammation, hypersensitivity
- Systemic effects of drug as when given PO
- Because of potential for severe damage if given in the setting of undiagnosed herpes infections, **steroid preparations should only be prescribed by a physician.**
- Contact lenses may be damaged by ophthalmologic preparations: Instruct patient not to administer eye drops when wearing contacts.
- Have patient demonstrate the proper administration of eye drops.

THE ACUTE EYE

See Tables 7-1 and 7-2.

COMMON NONURGENT PROBLEMS

- **Dry eyes:** generalized redness, dry cornea due to decreased tear production, inadequate blink, poor lid closure, medications, environmental factors, develops slowly; sensation of dry, burning, foreign body. Use artificial tears
- **Subconjunctival hemorrhage:** bright red area due to blood beneath the conjunctiva; asymptomatic, sudden onset; no precipitating event usually identified; may be associated with trauma, cough, Valsalva, HTN, anticoagulant; rule out hyphema; completely benign, reassure patient; resolves spontaneously over 2 to 3 weeks
- **Foreign body:**(FB) dust, dirt lying on the epithelium of the cornea; sudden sharp pain, photophobia, urge to rub eyes; complete exam, refer to ophthalmology unless superficial and resolves within 24 hours. Irrigate eye with NS for 10 minutes or more. Evert eyelid to remove FB with moistened sterile Q-tip only if FB superficial. DO NOT PATCH. Recheck in 24 hours
- **Ectropion:** eyelid turns out away from the eyeball due to decreased tone in orbicular oculi muscles that close the eyelid and cause dry eye; treat with artificial tears, surgery
- **Entropion:** eyelid turns in to eyeball due to muscle spasm of the orbicular oculi; causes chronic irritation from rubbing the eyeball with each blink; artificial tears and surgical treatment
- **Xanthelasma:** asymptomatic, benign growths, slightly raised, well-circumscribed yellowish plaques along the nasal aspect of the eyelids; occur in diabetics and those with hypercholesterolemia. These can be surgically removed for cosmetic reasons
- **Blepharitis:** obstruction and inflammation of the sebum and sweat glands on the lid margins; symptoms: burning and itching of eyes; treat with warm compresses, scrub lids with baby shampoo and water 1:1 with cotton-tipped swab and ophthalmic antibiotics as needed

Table 7-2: Conditions of the Eye Requiring Emergency/Urgent Referral

Disease	Etiology	Risk Factors	History	Physical	Management/Comments
Keratitis	Inflammation of cornea	Irritation or infection, dry eye	Acute pain, visual loss, photophobia, foreign-body sensation	Red eye, ciliary flush	Refer immediately to ophthalmologist
Uveitis	Inflammation of the uveal tract: iris, ciliary body, and choroids	Caused by immune system, infection, or systemic disease	With or without pain, blurred vision, photophobia	May be inflamed injected, small pupils, cloudy cornea	Refer immediately to ophthalmologist
Corneal Abrasion	Superficial injury of the corneal epithelium	Often due to dry eye, trauma	Pain photophobia foreign body sensation	Generalized redness	Refer to ophthalmologist, urgency depends on severity
Acute Angle Glaucoma	Anterior chamber drainage is blocked	Anatomically narrow anterior chamber	Sudden severe pain in or around eye, photophobia	Acute red, hard tender eye; IOP 40–80 mm Hg	**Emergency** bedrest until ophthalmologic consult, may lead to blindness
Retinal Tear/ Detachment	Separation of the sensory retina from the pig-ment epithelium	Age Diabetes Myopia (nearsightedness) Cataract surgery Ocular injury	Tear: new onset light flashes, new floaters, shadows Detachment: "curtain coming down over my eye"	Tear: crescent-shaped, red or orange in color Detachment: gray, cloud-like, hanging in vitreous	**Emergency referral** position so gravity aids in reposition of retina during transport
Retinal Artery Occlusion	Blockage of the arterial supply to the retina	Carotid artery athero-sclerosis Diseased cardiac valves	Sudden onset of painless loss of vision in one eye	Pale swollen retina, "cherry red" spot at fovea	**Emergency** treatment to prevent blindness
Retinal Venous Occlusion	Obstruction of central retinal vein or its branches	Hypertension Diabetes Glaucoma	Sudden painless decrease in vision, complete or partial	Swollen disk, tortuous veins, retinal hemorrhage	Immediate referral, results in visual loss

- **Pingueculae:** yellowed areas of thickened conjunctiva near the corneal limbus in the eyelid fissure; may be due to sunlight exposure; bilateral, more nasally than temporally, present in a majority of elderly
- **Chalazion:** obstructed and inflamed meibomian gland on inner aspect of eyelid, caused by infection or debris; localized, firm nodule on inner aspect of eyelid, subacute onset, pain and tenderness; treat with warm compresses and ophthalmic antibiotic as needed
- **Hordeolum** (also called **stye**): infection of the glands that lubricate lashes and outer eyelid, similar to chalazion, except on outer aspect of eyelid; treat as chalazion, may need systemic antibiotics
- **Pterygium:** a triangular growth of conjunctival tissue growing from inner canthus toward pupil that vascularizes and invades cornea; may be due to sunlight exposure and genetic factors; may obstruct vision as reaches center of cornea; refer for surgery; may recur
- **Conjunctivitis:** commonly called "pink eye," is dilation of the blood vessels of bulbar and palpebral layers of conjunctiva; vision may be slightly blurry but clears with blink; may be viral or bacterial (see Table 7-3)

IMPAIRED VISION

Description
- Many eye conditions lead to low vision or blindness in the elderly
  - Consequences of low vision
  - Low vision is a frequent cause of limited independence and ability to maintain ADLs
  - Patients with central or severe peripheral vision loss will not be able to drive

Management
- There are many visual aids including special computers, high-intensity light and special lenses, books on tape
- Encourage sun glasses, night lights, high contrast in design of facilities for the aged (e.g., dark frames and light walls)
- Refer patient to organization such as Lighthouse for the Blind
- Include family, other supports in planning
- Http://www.familyvillage.wisc.edu/lib_blnd.htm provides a list of resources for those with low vision or blindness

Glaucoma

Description
- Disorders causing vision loss from increased intraocular pressure (IOP) that exerts progressive damage on the optic nerve
- Irreversible damage to the optic nerve can occur if IOP is not lowered
- There are three types of glaucoma:
  - Angle-closure (ACG), also called narrow-angle glaucoma or acute-angle closure
  - Open-angle (OAG), also called chronic glaucoma
  - Secondary glaucoma (SG)

Etiology
- ACG—anatomically narrow anterior chamber is suddenly blocked, resulting in an abrupt increase in IOP
- OAG—less dramatic increase in IOP related to resistance to outflow of aqueous humor
- SG—obstruction of outflow tracts caused by complications of other diseases (diabetes and hypertension)

Table 7-3: Conjunctivitis

Condition	History	Physical	Nonpharmacologic Treatment	Pharmacologic Treatment
Conjunctivitis	Subacute, no photophobia, feels gritty	Conjunctiva injected, no ciliary flush	Cool compresses for comfort, warm compresses to remove crusts	Erythromycin, Bacitracin, ciprofloxacin; only ophthalmologist should prescribe steroids
Allergic Conjunctivitis	Intermittent with seasons Feels itchy, gritty: other allergic signs and symptoms	Generalized redness, cobblestone edema of palpebral conjunctiva Discharge thir, watery, stringy	Cool compress useful in decreasing itching	Topical vasoconstrictors or antihistamines add local NSAID and mast cell stabilizer if needed
Viral	May have URI May begin unilaterally, spread to other eye Feels gritty	Generalized redness If herpetic, may see cold sores Discharge mucoid	Compresses for comfort	Some give topical antibiotic for bacterial prophylaxis
Bacterial	May begin unilaterally, spread to other eye Feels gritty, burning	If severe, may have palpable periauricular nodes Generalized redness Discharge mucopurulent, crusting on lids/lashes	Compresses for comfort Hand washing Contact precautions	Topical antibiotic with coverage for S. pneumoniae, H. influenzae or S. aureus Gram-negative coverage may be needed

FB = Foreign body. URI = Upper Respiratory Infection

Table 7-4: Comparison of ACG and OAG

ACG	OAG
IOP 40–80 mm Hg	IOP up to 22 mm Hg
Acute onset	Insidious onset
Severe pain	No early symptoms
Profound visual loss	Progressive loss of peripheral vision
Hard, red eye, ciliary flush, steamy cornea, dilated pupil	Optic nerve head pale, with increased cup to disc ratio

Incidence and Demographics
- Affects 2.5 millions Americans, with 80,000 diagnosed as legally blind
- About 10% of all cases of blindness in US are related to glaucoma
- OAG is most common, comprising about 90% of cases. OAG occurs about 6 times more often among African Americans, in whom it is the leading cause of blindness
- ACG accounts for less than 10% of glaucoma cases. Angle-closure glaucoma is more common among Asian Americans

Risk Factors
- Family history
- Age

ACG
- Hyperopia (far-sightedness) due to shape of eyeball, with narrowed angle
- Use of anticholinergic (atropine-like) drugs
- Anatomic small eye with shallow anterior chamber
- Pathology of the eye: cysts of the iris or ciliary bodies, cataracts, intraocular tumor

OAG
- Diabetics and those taking topical, oral, or inhaled steroids

Prevention and Screening
- Annual screening, including visual fields and IOP measurement

Assessment
History and Physical
See Table 7-4.

Diagnostic Studies
- IOP measurement
- Peripheral visual field testing

Differential Diagnosis
- See Table 7-2 under The Acute Eye

Management
Nonpharmacologic Treatment

ACG
- Bed rest pending surgery
- Laser iridotomy is curative

Pharmacologic Treatment
- OAG—medical management in OAG aimed at decreasing aqueous production and increasing aqueous outflow (see Table 7-5)

Table 7-5: Pharmacologic Management of OAG

Medication Class	Examples	Mechanism of Action	Local Effects	Systemic Effects
Beta Blocker	Timolol	Suppress aqueous production	Transient discomfort, tearing, blurred vision	Side effects of beta blockers: CHF, asthma, bradycardia, etc.
Parasympathetic	Pilocarpine	Increase aqueous outflow	Constricted pupil	Diarrhea, sweating, bronchospasm
Adrenergic	Epinephrine	Decreases inflow and increases outflow	Allergic lid reaction and eye irritation	Increased heart rate, palpitations
Prostaglandin Agonist	Latanoprost (Xalatan)	Increases outflow	Eye pigment change Local irritation	Rare
Carbonic Anhydrase Inhibitors	Trusopt, Dorzolamide	Suppresses aqueous production	Conjunctivitis	Side effects of sulfonamides

When to Consult, Refer, Hospitalize
- ACG, immediate referral to an ophthalmologist
- OAG, less urgent referral to ophthalmologist
- Secondary glaucoma, refer to ophthalmologist

Follow-up

Expected Course
- Damage caused by uncontrolled glaucoma is permanent
- ACG surgery curative, stops vision loss
- OAG not cured, controlled by lifelong administration of medications

Complications
- Loss of visual fields and visual acuity
- Damage to optic nerve, leading to blindness if left untreated
- Corneal damage: chronic edema, fibrosis, vascularization or cataracts
- Atrophy of iris, multiple synechiae (iris adhesions to cornea)
- Malignant glaucoma, central retinal vein occlusion

Diabetic Retinopathy

Description
- Retinal changes related to prolonged high blood glucose in diabetes; frequently leads to blindness

Etiology
- Nonproliferative diabetic retinopathy-dilated vessels steal circulation from retinal surface; aneurysms form, leak, and bleed with macular edema and vision loss
- Proliferative "wet"—fragile new vessels form to repair circulation; their support tissue may cause retinal detachment; they may grow into and bleed into vitreous

Incidence and Demographics
- Third leading cause of blindness

Prevention and Screening
- Good control of blood sugars may delay onset and minimize severity
- Regular ophthalmology exam for diabetics at least yearly

Assessment

History
- "Floaters," spots, cloudy vision related to vitreous hemorrhage; "curtain over the eye" if retinal detachment

Physical
- In nonproliferative, small red spots with sharp edges around the optic nerve and macula. Retinal hemorrhages, hard and soft exudates, and areas of dilated capillaries are later seen; macular edema indicates prompt action is needed to preserve vision
- In proliferative, neovascularization may be seen or visualization may be obscured due to vitreous hemorrhage

Diagnostic Studies
- Glucose, hemoglobin A_{1C}

Differential Diagnosis
- Hypertensive retinopathy
- Retinal detachment
- Glaucoma
- Macular degeneration

Management
- Optimal blood sugar control
- Refer to ophthalmology

Follow-up

Complications
- Progressive visual loss leading to blindness

Macular Degeneration

Description
- Age-related macular degeneration (AMD): a progressive deterioration of central vision that may be classified as atrophic (dry) when it is related to ischemia or exudative (wet) when it is related to increased vessel permeability and leakage. Both conditions lead to a loss of central vision

Etiology
- Disturbance of retinal pigment epithelium, which supports and nourishes the sensory retina; cause unknown
- Wet AMD: neovascularization with hemorrhage or exudation of fluid between retinal pigment epithelium and sensory retina, death of photoreceptor cells, with a loss of central vision
- Dry AMD: Atrophy of retinal pigment epithelium and photoreceptor cells; associated with presence of drusen, but exact relationship is unclear

Incidence and Demographics
- Leading cause of blindness in the elderly
- "Wet" AMD comprises 10% of cases and 90% of blindness

Risk Factors
- Smoking
- Cardiovascular disease
- Family history

Prevention and Screening
- Amsler grid used to screen at annual vision checkup

Assessment

History
- Loss of central vision (may be sudden)
- Alteration of vision with straight lines appearing blurry, wavy, or with missing segments (e.g., grid lines, power or telephone wires), patchy or blurry vision, distorted central visual field

Physical
- Decreased visual acuity and visual fields, central vision loss
- Amsler grid is seen with wavy or broken lines or open areas
- "Wet" AMD, neovascularization, retinal pigment change, exudation of fluid, and hemorrhage
- "Dry" AMD, drusen and macular pigmentary changes

Differential Diagnoses
- Diabetic retinopathy
- Hypertensive retinopathy

Management
- Nonexudative—no known treatment
- Exudative—Encourage patients to use Amsler grid to check for changes in vision; if sudden change is noted, refer to ophthalmologist for laser photocoagulation

Follow-up

Expected Course
- Nonexudative—progressive and usually bilateral, with preservation of peripheral fields and ability to navigate for ADLs

- Exudative—further visual loss may be prevented in about half of those treated, however only one-fifth retain the benefit at 5 years post-treatment

Complications
- Blindness

Cataracts

Description
- Opacities of the lens, reducing visual acuity

Etiology
- Protein changes in the lens causing opacity and scattering of light

Incidence and Demographics
- Virtually universal, increasing with aging, females more than males
- Cataract surgery is the most frequently performed surgical procedure in those over age 65
- Occur in 92% of persons over 75 years

Risk Factors
- Aging
- Cigarette smoking
- Poor nutrition
- Corticosteroid use
- Atopic dermatitis
- Exposure to UV light (sunny climates)
- Trauma
- Diabetes

Prevention and Screening
- Use sunglasses with UV protection

Assessment

History
- Progressive decrease in visual acuity without pain. Loss may be complete, central, or peripheral
- "Second sight," temporary improvement in presbyopia as development of central lens opacities alters refractive power of lens and induces myopia
- Glare from bright lights, related to scattering of light by opacified lens

Physical
- Opacity is a black silhouette against the red reflex, irregular, gray/brown, looks like a rock
- More complete cataracts can be seen progressively as whitish-blue clouding through the pupil

Diagnostic Studies
- None

Differential Diagnosis
- Corneal scar
- Macular degeneration
- Retinal tear

Management

Nonpharmacologic Treatment
- Referral for surgical correction is made when vision loss is severe enough to significantly impact function and when surgeon feels that vision can be sufficiently corrected (more than 20/30)

Follow-up

Expected Course
- 85% to 95% of patients have excellent post-op vision

Complications
- Incomplete correction with residual decrease in visual acuity
- Retinal detachment, glaucoma, hemorrhage, infection post-op
- Blindness

EAR DISORDERS

Normal Changes of Aging
- Presbycusis is the hearing loss of old age caused by a combination of the normal changes of aging
- Vestibular function is also affected by the changes of aging

EXTERNAL EAR
- Number and activity of cerumen and apocrine glands decrease, leading to increased dryness of cerumen. Men have more hair in the canal resulting in decreased movement of cerumen
- The walls of canal thin and becomes drier. This dryness may be a factor in the itching commonly seen in elderly patient
- The tympanic membrane (TM) becomes thicker and wider, which may impede sound wave transmission
- Blockage of transmission through ear canal causes *conductive hearing loss*

MIDDLE EAR
- The joints of ossicular chain are affected with calcification and other degenerative changes; however, studies have not demonstrated that these changes cause any related decrease in hearing

INNER EAR
- Degeneration of organ of Corti and basal end of cochlea destroys sensory cells results in *sensory presbycusis*, with loss of ability to hear high-frequency tones
- Decreased sensory neurons with a functional organ of Corti is associated with loss of speech discrimination: One can hear but cannot understand speech. This is the picture of *neural presbycusis*
- Degenerative changes in CNS may also contribute to presbycusis
- Debris collecting in ampullae of semicircular canal move with head motion, causing neural stimulation and episodes of intense *vertigo*, the sensation of spinning. This can be either the feeling that patient is spinning in place or that things are spinning around patient

Clinical Implications

History
- Obtain confirming information from family regarding extent of problem
- Assess for depression caused by social isolation of deafness

Physical
- External ear should be examined for any skin lesions
- Painful gouty tophi, lesions exuding chalky monosodium urate deposits, may be seen on the pinna, as well as nodules of rheumatoid arthritis

Assessment
- Ear pain (*otalgia*) should be carefully evaluated and etiology sought. Pain may be referred from temporomandibular joint pain related to poorly fitting dentures or bruxism (teeth grinding)
- Tumors of the head and neck may also cause referred ear pain

Treatment
- *A perforated eardrum is a contraindication to any use of otic drops*
- Provide clearly written instructions for any medication administration; have patient demonstrate the correct use of drops
- When drops are used, the affected ear should be kept facing up (head tilted or patient lying down) for 2 minutes after instilling the medication, or a cotton plug should be inserted
- Ophthalmic drops are sometimes used in the ear; however, otic drops are **never** used in the eye

HEARING LOSS

Description
- Diminished hearing due to either mechanical obstruction of sound transmission, neurological impairment, or both
- Presbycusis is a high-frequency hearing loss and is considered a nonpathologic normal function of aging
- There are two types of hearing loss—conductive and sensorineural
- Sensorineural is further divided into
  - Sensory degeneration of the organ of Corti
  - Neural degeneration of the higher auditory pathways

Etiology
- Conductive hearing loss involves outer or middle ear abnormalities that interfere with the conduction of sound waves. It is caused by a physical obstruction of the normal conduction of sound as in occlusion of external canal by wax, infection, or foreign object, perforated TM, bony growth, or tumor interfering with ossicles in middle ear
- Sensorineural involves the inner ear. This is the usual cause of presbycusis. It is loss of transmission of sound for processing due to damage of inner ear (cochlear apparatus) and of cranial nerve VIII. Causes include:
  - Exposure to loud noises
  - Ototoxic medications
    - Antibiotics: streptomycin, gentamicin, vancomycin, aminoglycosides
    - Diuretics: ethacrynic acid and furosemide
    - Miscellaneous: salicylates, cisplatin (and other antineoplastic agents)
  - Cranial nerve VIII dysfunction
  - Neurologic disorders, such as MS, syphilis, Ménière's disease

Incidence and Demographics
- Third most common major chronic disability in those older than 65 years
- 75% of those in nursing homes have significant loss of hearing
- 33% of those aged 65 to 75 have hearing loss, and 50% of those above 75 have hearing loss
- Men more than women
- Elderly people of lower economic status have poorer hearing than those of higher economic status

Risk Factors
- Family and occupational history, chronic otitis media, physical trauma
- Worsened by other disease states: diabetes mellitus, chronic lung disease, hypothyroidism, hypertension, cerebrovascular disorders, alcohol abuse
  - Contributory cardiovascular disorder such as stroke or vasculitis

Prevention and Screening
- Routine screening after age 65 (US Preventive Task Force); specific time frame not mentioned but at least an annual exam seems prudent
- Avoidance of flying or diving (changes in barometric pressure) when ill with upper respiratory infection
- There is no specific prevention for the age-related changes leading to presbycusis

Assessment

History
- Does patient hear better in one place than another (e.g., hears fine in quiet exam room but has trouble on a busy street or a room with television on)?
- Do family and social contacts think patient has problems with hearing?

- Any episodes of dizziness or vertigo?
- Patient with hearing loss may appear to be confused and demented

Physical
- Treat any conditions of the ear canal before testing hearing.
- The whispered voice test for hearing impairment is a good screening device.
  - Stand at arm's length behind a seated patient, whisper a combination of numbers and letters, ask patient to repeat; test each ear while covering the other
- Office screening AudioScope will test over four frequencies at three intensity levels with accuracy for screening of 75% to 80% (see Table 7-6)

Diagnostic Studies
- Studies ordered by ENT/audiology for new onset hearing loss

Differential Diagnoses
- See Etiology

Management
- Treat cause if possible

Nonpharmacologic Treatment
- Many patients will benefit from a hearing aid.
- Be sure to consider the patient's personal and cultural attitudes toward hearing loss. These will determine the successful use of hearing aids more than fit of the hearing aid or improvement of hearing
- Reassure patient and family that decrease in hearing does not mean decrease in cognitive function
- While some conductive and sensorineural loss may be treated, for many hearing loss is a permanent thing and must be accommodated
- Contrary to myth, sensorineural hearing loss CAN be corrected with hearing aids
- Assist patient in realistic expectations re: aids-hearing will not be perfect in difficult situations such as increased background noise, areas with poor acoustics, poor visualization of speaker
- Patient and family should be educated in speech reading: communication strategies to improve patient's comprehension of spoken language. These include facing patient when speaking, speaking clearly and distinctly, slightly louder without shouting; lessen background noise; not turning away and speaking while back is turned

Pharmacologic Treatment
- Only about 5% of hearing loss (conductive) can be treated medically
- Discontinue ototoxic drugs if possible; if not, modification of dosing schedule may decrease ototoxicity. Patients with decreased renal function are more at risk

How Long to Treat
- Depends on etiology
- For most, hearing loss is a way of life; hearing aids may greatly improve quality of life, but presbycusis and many sensorineural losses cannot be reversed

Special Considerations
- Resource for patient with hearing loss and families: http://www.hearingexchange.com

When to Consult, Refer, Hospitalize
- All patients with newly diagnosed or acute onset hearing loss should be referred to ENT
- Refer to an audiologist when hearing loss becomes a problem to the patient
- Refer patient as needed for aural rehabilitation: speech reading, and auditory assistive devices such as amplified doorbells and telephones, low-frequency ringers, telephone devices for the deaf (display a written message on LED display or printer)
- Refer to social services

Table 7-6: Characteristics of Types of Hearing Loss

Type of Loss	History	Pattern of Loss	Exam
Conductive	Unilateral loss low tones Can produce 60–70 dB deficit May experience tinnitus Gradual or acute decrease in hearing dependent on etiology	Good understanding (discrimination) of speech, loss of volume (i.e., can understand when volume is loud enough)	AC < BC; Weber lateralizes to affected ear May visualize cerumen or FB in ear canal; may see fluid level behind TM; TM may be stiff to insufflation, retracted or bulging
Sensorineural	Slow onset, generally bilateral; loss of high frequency and pitch; may experience tinnitus or vertigo	Loss of both tone and discrimination. Can hear but cannot understand. Volume is sufficient but consonant sounds are lost. Increased discrimination loss may indicate a central processing problem Sudden loss: look for acoustic neuroma	No abnormalities seen. AC ≥ BC; Weber lateralizes to better ear
Mixed	Bilateral sensorineural, with unilateral conductive component; may have tinnitus or vertigo; may have slow onset with acute loss	Loss for both volume and discrimination	Weber & Rinne non-conclusive; physical findings otherwise as under conductive

AC = Air conduction, BC = Bone conduction

Follow-up

Expected Course
- Presbycusis and sensorineural loss may not be reversed; progression may be slowed or halted

Complications
- Decreased function, depression, and social isolation

OTHER EAR PROBLEMS
Cerumen Impaction

Description
- Obstruction of ear canal by hardened wax

Etiology
- Cerumen is naturally occurring lubricant of ear canal; with aging, cerumen becomes drier and accumulates, obstructing canal

Incidence and Demographics
- Extremely common in elderly
- Most common cause of correctable hearing loss in elderly

Risk Factors
- Age
- Improper cleaning methods
- Hearing aide

Prevention and Screening
- Instruct patients in appropriate cleaning techniques (see management)
- Assess on annual exam and with any new decreased hearing

Assessment
- Assess TM patency to determine treatment
- If TM is not visible, look for pain and risk factors for damaged TM

History
- Recent onset of fullness, itching, tinnitus, pressure, hearing loss
- May present with acute onset pain if Q-tip broke off and became lodged in canal, swelling and putting pressure on sensitive canal or TM
- Significant pain indicates possible damage to TM
- History of perforation of TM
- Often bilateral

Physical
- Otoscopy shows TM partially or completely obscured by dark brown cerumen in canal
- Scratch marks along canal may be present if patients have used Q-tip to clean or to remove obstruction on their own

Diagnostic Studies
- None indicated

Differential Diagnosis
- Foreign body in canal
- Tumor
- Otitis externa

Management

Nonpharmacologic Treatment
- Presence of perforated TM is contraindication to ear drops or irrigation
- Soften ear wax with 1 to 2 drops of baby or mineral oil daily for 5 days; if not successful, then

- Irrigate ear with solution of hydrogen peroxide and warm water 10:1; avoid excess pressure, aim toward anterior wall of canal
- Patient education
  - Attempts to "clean" ear canal and remove wax using Q-tip, washcloth, bobby pin, or other item may force wax medially and cause impaction or perforation of TM
  - Cleaning of ear with alcohol and water can exacerbate ear canal problems

Pharmacologic Treatment
- OTC preparations, such as Cerumenex, may be used to soften wax
- If no contraindications exist, antibiotic drops, such as Cortisporin otic drops, 1 to 2 drops qid for several days, may be used after irrigation if ear canal is abraded

How Long to Treat
- Excess, dry cerumen is usually an ongoing problem; use mineral oil on weekly or monthly basis to prevent buildup

When to Consult, Refer, Hospitalize
- Referral to otolaryngology if affected ear is only ear with intact hearing, if there is suspected perforation of the TM, or if coexisting problems of ear are present, such as severe infection, unexplained hearing loss, or hearing loss that did not clear with treatment of the impaction

Follow-up
- Patients with hearing aids should have their ears monitored for buildup of wax and have their ears cleaned regularly

Expected Course
- Acute problem is generally resolved by irrigation
- Prophylactic mineral oil may ↓ recurrence

Complications
- Perforation of TM
- Infection
- Trauma to ear canal with bleeding
- Severe pain, fever, and chills, mastoid tenderness, cellulitis, malaise, facial nerve palsy may indicate necrotizing malignant otitis externa and should be considered an emergency and urgently referred

Tinnitus

Description
- Perception of abnormal external or internal sounds
- Two types of tinnitus
- Subjective tinnitus, which only patient hears
- Objective tinnitus, where the examiner is able to detect the sounds as well

Etiology

SUBJECTIVE
- Cerumen obstruction
- Hearing loss
- Perforation of TM
- Serious otitis media
- Ménière's disease
  - ASA
  - NSAIDs
  - Antineoplastic drugs
- Otosclerosis
- Depression
- Caffeine
- Alcohol
- Medications

- Aminoglycosides
- Tricyclic antidepressants
- Loop diuretics
- Oral contraceptives
- Neurologic disorders
  - Multiple sclerosis
  - Meningitis
  - Acoustic neuroma, may be unilateral

OBJECTIVE
- Vascular disorders (pulsatile quality, may be subjective), may be unilateral
  - Arteriovenous malformation
  - Aneurysm
  - Carotid occlusive disease
- Cardiovascular conditions causing increased flow (again, may be objective and pulsatile in rhythm)
  - Anemia
  - Hyperthyroidism
  - Atherosclerosis
  - Transmitted cardiac murmurs

Incidence and Demographics
- 25% of the elderly have tinnitus, severe in 1 of 6 and disabling in 1 of 30
- More prevalent among women than men

Risk Factors
- See Etiology

Prevention and Screening
- Avoidance of toxic medications
- Protection from noise exposure

Assessment

History
- Note onset of tinnitus, intensity, pattern. Note exacerbating and relieving factors (Is it worse in quiet room, unnoticed in noisy one?) and effect on function (Does it interfere with concentration or sleep?); progression of symptoms
- May be described as high-pitched, low-pitched, clicking, buzzing, hissing, roaring
- Assess for history of anemia, thyroid disorders, diabetes, cardiovascular disorder, trauma, neurologic disorder

Physical
- Assess for hearing loss, and if present, pattern and changes and association with tinnitus
- Assess for cerumen obstructing canal and fluid or mass behind the TM
- Focused head, neck, and CV evaluation; usually no abnormalities are found
- Assess for bruits over precordium, neck, and temporal bone
- Assess neurologically for any focal abnormalities; cranial nerve testing and cerebellar functioning are key

Diagnostic Studies
- Work-up for cardiovascular/tumor causes includes CT or MRI as needed to define pathology
- Lab studies to rule out etiology as indicated

Differential Diagnosis
- See Etiology

Management

Nonpharmacologic Treatment
- Hearing aids may help resolve tinnitus by increasing normal sounds
- Audiologist will determine sound frequency of tinnitus and evaluate patient for effectiveness of hearing aids or masking devices in relief of patient symptoms
- A white noise generator at bedside may enable patient to sleep
- Biofeedback has been useful in some cases

Pharmacologic Treatment
- There is no clear pharmacologic treatment for tinnitus
- Oral antidepressants have been most successful in relieving symptoms
- *Ginkgo biloba* has also been used

How Long to Treat
- Depends on etiology

When to Consult, Refer, Hospitalize
- Unilateral and/or pulsatile tinnitus should be promptly referred to rule out vascular or tumor cause
- New onset tinnitus should be referred for evaluation if it is not promptly resolved by medication adjustment (e.g., ASA excess) or clearing of cerumen impaction

Follow-up

Expected Course
- Approximately 75% of patients with tinnitus can be helped with nonpharmacologic measures
- Tinnitus due to bilateral sensorineural hearing loss may worsen over time
- Tinnitus due to aminoglycosides and antineoplastic agents may be partially reversible
- Tinnitus due to ASA and loop diuretics is reversible when drug stopped

Complications
- In severe cases, functional disruption, with inability to carry out activities of daily living due to interrupted concentration and impaired sleep
- Vascular disaster (stroke) if atherosclerotic or aneurysmal etiology is not identified
- Progressive acoustic neuroma, causing deafness, disequilibrium, visual loss, chronic headache

Vertigo
(*See also Chapter 4, Dizziness*)

Description
- Sensation of movement (frequently rotary) by either environment around patient or of patient within environment. May present as an exaggerated sense of motion in reaction to normal bodily movement: "rolling" unsteady sensation in response to walking
- Vertigo is the distinctive symptom of vestibular disease
- Distinguish from other forms of dizziness, see Chapter 4, Geriatric Multisystem Syndromes
- Two types: peripheral and central

Etiology

PERIPHERAL: ARISING FROM THE EAR, CHANGES IN THE VESTIBULAR OR LABYRINTHINE SYSTEM
- Benign positional vertigo: believed to be caused by free-floating debris in the semicircular canals. As patient reclines or changes position, debris settles and signals are sent to brainstem, stimulating sensation of vertigo and nausea
- Labyrinthitis: infection of inner ear, most likely viral, often follows an upper respiratory infection
- Ménière's disease: exact etiology is unknown; it is believed that swelling of endolymphatic system of inner ear is the cause; tears in membrane separating endolymph and perilymph allow mixing and distention, causing vertigo

CENTRAL: CNS DISTURBANCE
- Brain stem vascular disease: vertebrobasilar insufficiency TIA, may be caused by hypertension, atherosclerosis, embolic events
- Multiple sclerosis: demyelinization of nerve cells
- Acoustic neuroma: slow growing tumor arising from audio-vestibular nerve, compresses VIII cranial nerve with resultant hearing loss and tinnitus; vertigo is a late symptom

Incidence and Demographics
- Benign positional vertigo most common in those over 60
- Labyrinthitis affects any age, usually after upper respiratory infection
- Ménière's occurs between ages 40 and 70

Risk Factors
- Age
- Upper respiratory infection

Assessment
- Peripheral vertigo generally has sudden onset, is fatigable, with hearing loss, nausea, and vomiting
- Central vertigo generally has gradual onset and is progressive, becomes disabling, not fatigable; exception is TIAs

History
- In elderly, vertigo/dizziness may have a combination of etiologies. Obtain clearest history possible with detailed description. Be careful not to lead patient by using words like "vertigo" or "dizziness"

Physical
- Complete neurologic exam with attention to cranial nerves
- Nystagmus is indicative of vertigo, but may be central or peripheral
- Otologic exam
- Assess gait and balance
  - Romberg test: patient stands with feet together and eyes open then closed; inability to maintain balance is failed test
  - Hallpike maneuver: lie patient flat with head to one side, sit patient up quickly, repeat with other ear down; reproduction of symptoms and nystagmus are positive for positional vertigo

Diagnostic Studies
- MRI if central lesion suspected
- Audiogram to evaluate sustained hearing loss
- Depending suspected etiology: CBC, chemistry panel, lipids, thyroid function studies, or ESR
- Unilateral hearing loss requires evaluation to r/o acoustic neuroma

Differential Diagnosis
- Otitis media
- Otitis externa
- Other causes of dizziness (see Chapter 4)
- Cerebellar disease
- Cerumen impaction

Management

Nonpharmacologic Treatment
- Rest in quiet, darkened room
- Safety precautions: change positions slowly; cane or walker during episodes
- Bland diet with small portions, fluids if nausea and vomiting present
- See Table 7-7 for specifics

Table 7-7: Peripheral Vertigo

Disorder	History	Physical	Nonpharmacologic Treatment	Pharmacologic Treatment	Refer
Benign Positional Vertigo	Severe vertigo seconds after changing head position. Lasts seconds to minutes	Controlled head movements recreate symptoms; + nystagmus	Habituating exercises: vestibular rehab Self-limiting	Short course of vestibular suppressant (e.g., Meclizine 6.25–25 mg q 4–6 h prn)	If associated with auditory findings
Ménière's Disease	Sudden episodes of vertigo, associated with tinnitus and diminished hearing, lasting minutes to hours; asymptomatic between	May be non-specific; + nystagmus during acute episode May be progressive	Salt and fluid restriction Avoid caffeine Surgical intervention if episodes are incapacitating	Meclizine acutely Diuretic: HCTZ 12.5–25 mg qd or Triamterene 50 mg/day Monitor electrolytes	To ENT for unilateral hearing-loss evaluation
Labyrinthitis	Disabling vertigo; may experience hearing loss Lasts hours to days	Symptoms URI; sensorineural hearing loss, nystagmus first 24–48 h	Usually resolves in several days Support symptomatically		If any suspicion of hearing loss

Pharmacologic Treatment
- See Table 7-7.
- Antihistamines can cause drowsiness, confusion, and anticholinergic symptoms of dry mouth, constipation, and urinary retention and/or precipitate acute narrow-angle glaucoma
- Stop drugs when symptoms resolved; do not use prophylactically or as maintenance

How Long to Treat
- Taper and stop when symptoms resolve, generally within 1 to 2 weeks

When to Consult, Refer, Hospitalize
- Hospitalize for dehydration and inability to take oral rehydration, secondary to severe nausea and vomiting
- Neurology referral if there are focal neuro deficits, severe headaches, transient neurological events, seizures, or other suggestions of central nervous system problems
- ENT for any patient with vertigo and unilateral auditory symptoms to r/o acoustic neuroma

Follow-up

Expected Course
- Peripheral generally lasts several days to weeks; may reoccur

Complications
- Hearing loss
- Falls with injury
- Dehydration with associated nausea and vomiting

NOSE

Normal Changes of Aging
- Nose becomes longer and narrower, with a sagging tip, due to influence of gravity and changes in support structures
- Cartilage of nose softens and thins and skin becomes more loose
- Nasal dryness is caused by decreased mucus production due to atrophy of mucus-producing cells. The mucus membrane thins and there is less submucosal tissue
- Thinned blood vessel walls leads to increased risk of epistaxis
- Changes in vasomotor secretory fibers may result in rhinorrhea when patient is exposed to some foods or cold air
- Olfaction, the sense of smell, comprises 85% of "taste." Neural degeneration causes a decrease in smell and fine taste, which may result in lack of interest in eating, and poor nutrition, smoking, and exposure to environmental pollutants may also decrease sense of smell

Clinical Implications

History
- Acute onset of anosmia (loss of sense of smell) suggests tumor and requires investigation
- Ask about self-treatment of nasal symptoms and use of other medications that may cause dryness or rhinorrhea

Physical
- Pale, dry mucosa

Assessment
- Rhinitis, sinusitis, epistaxis, allergies, and nasal fractures are as common an occurrence in the elderly as in younger adults

Management
- The anticholinergic effects of some antihistamines can cause syncope, vertigo, excessive sedation, hypotension, incoordination, constipation, and urinary retention in the patient with BPH, as well as thickening secretions and making the airway more difficult to clear

- Sympathomimetics, such as decongestants, stimulate the cardiovascular system and can cause tachycardias, hypertension, confusion, agitation, and urinary retention
- Septal hematomas should be promptly evaluated by ENT and treated to prevent necrosis
- Nasal saline safe and often provides comfort for rhinitis

RHINITIS

Description
- An inflammation of the mucous membranes of the nose, usually accompanied by increased production of clear secretions (rhinorrhea); produces tissue inflammation of the nasal mucosa

Etiology
- *Allergic rhinitis* is an IgE-mediated hypersensitivity reaction
- *Seasonal* allergic rhinitis is related to inhaled seasonal pollen allergens (tree, grass, hay fever)
- *Perennial* allergic rhinitis is caused by always available allergens of dust mites, pets dander, cockroaches, molds, and indoor pollutants
- *Viral rhinitis (common cold)* is most commonly due to rhinovirus, as well as coronavirus, influenza, parainfluenza, and adenoviruses viruses
- *Vasomotor rhinitis* etiologies are not well understood; thought to be an autonomic response that results in vascular dilatation of the nasal submucosal vessels. Influencing or triggering factors include temperature or humidity change, odors, selected drugs, emotional response, and body positions, such as lying down
- *Atrophic rhinitis* uncommon, sometimes seen post nasal surgery; characterized by loss of cilia and abnormal patency of nasal passage, with formation of thick dry odorous crusts
- *Rebound rhinitis* is caused by overuse of nasal decongestants (e.g., oxymetazoline HCl [Afrin]) with rebound vasodilatation of the mucous membranes and nasal congestion after continuous use (see Table 7-8)

Prevention and Screening
- Frequent hand washing to reduce risk of infection; avoid close contact, particularly with con-fused elders who are unable to cover their mouth and nose when sneezing or coughing
- Avoidance of known allergens and use of environmental control measures indoors, such as frequent vacuuming with particulate filters, air cleaners (HEPA filters), mattress and pillow encasements, removal of carpeting, air conditioner, keep indoor humidity at least 50%, mop tile, dust furniture, etc.

Management
Nonpharmacologic Treatment
- General measures: hydration, humidification, intranasal irrigations with saline solutions

Pharmacologic Treatment
- Antihistamines for allergies
- Inhaled nasal corticosteroids are first-line option to reduce edema
- Many formulations: fluticasone propionate (Flonase), triamcinolone acetonide (Nasacort)
  - Aqueous preparations may be more comfortable, cause less irritation. Nasal inhalants may dry mucous membranes and cause irritation and bleeding
  - Oral: nonsedating: loratadine (Claritin), fexofenadine (Allegra)
  - Oral: less sedating: cetirizine (Zyrtec)
  - Topical: azelastine HCl 0.1% (Astelin)
- Decongestants
  - Oral for congestion: generally avoided in this age group due to side effects, such as tachycardia; in healthy older patient, give pseudoephedrine (Sudafed) 15–30 mg q 6 h with caution

Table 7-8: Differentiating Rhinitis Presentations

	Allergic Rhinitis	Viral Rhinitis (Cold)	Vasomotor Rhinitis	Atrophic Rhinitis
Onset	Any age	Anytime	Adulthood	Geriatric
Common Primary Symptoms	Nasal congestion, sneezing, itchy nose, clear drainage	Congestion, obstruction, nasal crusting, cloudy white to yellow drainage	Abrupt onset congestion and pronounced watery postnasal drip, sneezing	Nasal congestion, thick postnasal drip, repeated clearing of throat, bad smell in nose
Associated Symptoms	Cough, sore throat, itching and puffy eyes	Cough, sore throat, malaise, headache, fever >100°F (37.8°C)	Watery eyes	None
Physical Exam Findings	Nasal mucosa pale and boggy, violaceous Enlarged turbinates, Clear watery d/c	Edema and hyperemia of mucous membranes Throat erythema Postnasal drainage Cervical lymph nodes tender, enlargement	Turbinates pale and edematous No other findings	Nasal mucosa dry, nonedematous Airway patent No other findings
Diagnostic studies (if indicated): Hansel or Wright nasal smears	Positive for eosinophils	Positive for neutrophils Consider CBC, throat culture if suspect strep, advanced infection or complications	Normal smears	Not indicated

- Intranasal decongestants for short-term use only with monitoring not to exceed 3–5 days (e.g., oxymetazoline [Afrin], phenylephrine HCl [Neo-Synephrine])
- Specific recommendations
  - Allergic rhinitis: oral antihistamines, intranasal steroids
  - Viral rhinitis: acetaminophen or NSAIDs for pain or fever, decongestants (avoid antihistamines as may over dry and reduce ability to clear secretions)
  - Vasomotor rhinitis: saline solution nasal spray, some relief with intranasal anticholinergic (e.g., ipratropium [Atrovent])
  - Atrophic rhinitis: guaifenesin to liquefy mucus, or intranasal saline solution spray

How Long to Treat
- Viral rhinitis: treatment for symptom relief only
- Allergic rhinitis: treated prn for symptom relief, long-term treatment with intranasal corticosteroids
- Vasomotor rhinitis symptomatic treatment prn

Special Considerations
- Monitor closely for adverse affects from medications and drug interactions with antihypertensives, antidepressants, other cardiac drugs
- Use OTC decongestants with caution in patients with diabetes, HTN, or glaucoma
- Patient education: DO NOT combine these medications with herbal treatments, as some contain the same ingredients (e.g., Ephedra) that can cause side effects or overdosage if used concomitantly

When to Consult, Refer, Hospitalize
- Referral to an allergist to consider allergen immunotherapy for allergic rhinitis that is not easily managed by medications or avoidance of known allergens
- Referral to ENT for those with symptoms unmanageable with above described treatments, if complications, or if nasal polyps or other growths are seen or suspected

Follow-up

Expected Course
- Viral rhinitis usually resolves within 7 to 10 days.
- Allergic, vasomotor, or atrophic rhinitis are ongoing problems managed, not cured

Complications
- Worsening of related pulmonary conditions (e.g., COPD, asthma)
- Development and spread of bacterial infection: acute sinusitis, bronchitis, pneumonia

SINUSITIS

Description
- Inflammation and infection of the maxillary, frontal, ethmoid, or sphenoid sinuses due to viral, bacterial, or fungal agents or allergic reaction. Risk for sinusitis is increased by sinus structure in some patients
- Categorized as acute, recurrent, subacute, or chronic
- *Acute sinusitis* is an infection lasting 3 to 4 weeks
- *Recurrent sinusitis* if there are more than 3 acute episodes/year
- *Subacute sinusitis* is resolved in less than 3 months
- *Chronic sinusitis* is prolonged inflammation more than 3 months duration. There may be irreversible damage to mucosa

Etiology
- Three major common factors:
  - Drainage of the sinus is blocked

- Mucus secretions accumulate, providing media for bacterial infection
- Change in quality of sinus secretions
- The most common bacterial pathogens in acute sinusitis are *Streptococcus pneumoniae*, *Haemophilus influenza*, *S. aureus*, *Enterobacteriaceae*, and *Moraxella catarrhalis*
- Other infectious causes include viral (rhinovirus, coronavirus, adenovirus) and fungal (Aspergillus), especially in the immunocompromised
- Commonly caused by allergic rhinitis

Incidence and Demographics
- Common among the elderly
- Sinusitis frequently exacerbates asthma

Risk Factors
- Decreased immune system in the elderly, especially in patients with concurrent illness
- Rhinitis
- Nasal polyps or other obstruction
- Dental infections (roots extend to max. sinus)
- URIs

Prevention and Screening
- Appropriate treatment of allergies and infections
- Correction of mechanical obstruction such as polyps, septal deviation
- Avoidance of adverse environmental factors, such as known allergens, cigarette smoke, and other polluting agents

Assessment

History
- Acute and chronic sinusitis typically present with a history of precipitants such as allergic or nonallergic rhinitis, or an upper respiratory infection that has persisted beyond 5 to 7 days
- Classic presenting symptoms include nasal congestion, yellow/green rhinorrhea, postnasal drainage, facial or dental pain or pressure, headache, altered sense of smell, cough that is worse at night, sinus pressure when bending over
- Other associated symptoms of fever, malaise, fatigue, sore throat, halitosis, and nausea, increased snoring may be present
- Complaints of orbital pain or vision disturbances are indicators of a more serious problem

Physical
- Complete HEENT and pulmonary exam:
  - Face/sinuses: tenderness overlying the involved sinuses
  - Ears: middle ear abnormalities and eustachian tube dysfunction
  - Nose: erythema of the mucosa and purulent drainage
  - Mouth: purulent postnasal drainage on posterior pharyngeal area
  - Chest: potential for wheezing, congestion associated with asthma or URI

Diagnostic Studies
- CT scans are used to confirm the diagnosis and identify obstruction and need for surgical intervention in recurrent sinusitis. Cost of CT is similar to standard sinus films
- MRI is most useful for assessing the presence of fungal sinusitis and tumors and differentiating between inflammatory disease vs. malignant tumors
- Recurrent or chronic sinusitis may warrant culture

Differential Diagnosis
- URI
- Allergic rhinitis
- Nasal polyps
- Nasal septum deviation
- Nasopharyngeal tumor

Management
Nonpharmacologic Treatment
- Comfort measures to decrease inflammation and promote drainage: adequate rest, adequate hydration, analgesics as needed, warm facial packs, steamy showers, using saline nasal sprays, and sleeping with the head of bed elevated, increased humidity in home

Pharmacologic Treatment
- Antibiotics used for 14 days
  - Amoxicillin or amoxicillin-clavulanate should be used first line; trimethoprim/sulfamethoxazole DS bid; first-generation macrolide for patients with penicillin allergy
  - Second-line agent—amoxicillin/clavulanic acid 250 mg tid for 14 days; second-generation cephalosporin. Failure to respond to first line antibiotics within 5 to 7 days warrants switching to a new antibiotic, such as cefuroxime, clarithromycin, or a fluoroquinolone
- Nasal corticosteroids for those with underlying rhinitis or associated bronchial hyperresponsiveness
- Oral corticosteroids short-term, for those with significant anatomic obstruction, invasive nasal polyposis, or who have demonstrated marked mucosal edema radiographically
- Decongestants topically to help with drainage of sinuses

How Long to Treat
- Recommendations are not consistent; however, a 14-day course of oral antibiotics is typical for acute sinusitis
- Chronic sinusitis relapses may be treated for an extended period

When to Consult, Refer, Hospitalize
- Serious complications requiring urgent referral and treatment: external facial swelling, erythema, cellulitis over an involved sinus, vision changes such as diplopia, difficulty moving eyes (EOMs), proptosis (forward displacement of eye), and any abnormal neurologic signs
- Refer to ENT or allergist for treatment failure, chronic or complicated sinusitis management

Follow-up
Expected Course
- Improvement of symptoms within 72 hours and resolution of sinusitis within 10 days

Complications
- Asthma, bronchitis, bronchiectasis, or pneumonia
- Facial or orbital cellulitis
- Ophthalmoplegia and visual loss
- Osteomyelitis of facial bones
- Meningitis
- Subdural empyema
- Intracranial complications

EPISTAXIS

Description
- Hemorrhage from the nostrils, nasopharynx, or nasal cavity
- A symptom of an underlying problem or disease, not a disease of its own

Etiology
- Localized irritation secondary to rhinitis of all types, sinusitis
- Excessive drying of the membranes by low humidity or nasal oxygen
- Trauma, such as nose picking, forceful blowing of nose, or nasal fracture may precipitate bleed
- Tumor

- Arteriovenous malformation (AVM)
- Hypertension a rare cause (bleed may be worsened by but not caused by HTN)
- Use of NSAIDs or aspirin (even cardio-protective baby aspirin)
- Coagulation disorders or medications, such as warfarin

Incidence and Demographics
- Common among the elderly

Risk Factors
- Age-related mucosal and vessel wall changes

Prevention and Screening
- Adequate moisturizing of the mucous membranes: humidifier, saline nasal spray
- Keep nails short and away from the nose
- Apply petroleum jelly (Vaseline) or K-Y jelly to nares routinely for lubrication
- Humidify oxygen

Assessment

History
- Patients may present with actively bleeding nose or may consult for episodes that were resolved with self-care
- Determine
  - Bleeding unilateral (which nostril) or bilateral
  - Precipitating events
  - Past history of epistaxis
  - Associated symptoms URI, nausea and vomiting (swallowed blood), other signs/symptoms of systemic bleeding (coffee-ground emesis, hemoptysis, melena) (see Table 7-9)

Physical
- Inspect for site of bleed: note localized or diffuse mucosal irritation, bleeding from one or two nostrils, duration of bleeding

Diagnostic Studies
- Only recurrent or severe cases warrant extensive evaluation
- If significant blood loss is suspected, obtain an hemoglobin and hematocrit
- If bleeding disorders are suspected, then obtain a CBC, PT, and PTT

Table 7-9: Characteristics of Nasal Bleeding Sites

	Anterior Epistaxis	Posterior Epistaxis
Presentation	Typically unilateral, one nostril	Unilateral or bilateral
Timing	Lasts between a few to 30 min, in isolation or recurrently	Intermittent
Source of Bleed	90% are venous from Kiesselbach's plexus	Typically arterial from posterior nasopharynx
Miscellaneous Facts	Usually less severe, easier to treat	May have nausea or coffee-ground emesis
	Direct pressure frequently stops bleeding	Frequently requires nasal packing
		More common in the elderly

Differential Diagnosis
- See Etiology

Management

Nonpharmacologic Treatment
- For simple nosebleed
  - Application of direct pinching-type pressure just below the bridge of the nose for 10 to 15 minutes will stop the bleeding
  - Keep the patient in an upright position and leaning forward, drain blood into bowl and not swallowed
  - Apply ice packs over the bridge of the nose
  - See Prevention

Pharmacologic Treatment
- For anterior hemostasis, vasoconstrictors: oxymetazoline (Afrin) .05% with topical anesthetic agents (tetracaine and lidocaine) are used
- Silver nitrate stick cautery is very painful; give local anesthetic
- If packing is necessary, antibiotics may be given prophylactically to prevent sinus infection
- Correct any coagulopathies, iatrogenic or otherwise, so clot can form
- Acute treatment with antihypertensives if associated with an acute HTN crisis

How Long to Treat
- Treatment is episodic for the actual bleeding incident
- Ongoing monitoring and treatment indicated for the associated underlying disorders

When to Consult, Refer, Hospitalize
- Immediate referral to an ER or ENT for severe bleeding or bleeding unresponsive to first-line treatment
- Recurrent epistaxis is cause for referral to a specialist
- Patient requiring posterior packing may be admitted to hospital for respiratory monitoring

Follow-up
- Retained anterior gauze packing is frequent foreign body in the elderly. Monitor carefully

Expected Course
- Excellent prognosis for isolated, idiopathic epistaxis
- In other cases, variable outcome depending on underlying cause

Complications
- Sinusitis
- Nasal obstruction
- Abscess from excessive trauma during packing of nose
- Septal perforation from cauterization therapy
- Vasovagal episode during packing
- Anemia from blood loss during recurrent or severe epistaxis

MOUTH
GERIATRIC APPROACH

Normal Changes of Aging
- Some atrophy of oral epithelial tissue, remains functional and intact with a slight decrease in salivary production
- Periodontal changes: increase in dental plaque and gingival recession and bleeding
- In larynx, muscle atrophy, decreased vibratory mass, decreased support by fibrous tissue, and squamous metaplasia are seen

- Bowing of the vocal cords (due to decreased elasticity and decreased muscle mass) combine with decreased pulmonary volume and expiratory effort to produce a high, quivery voice

History
- Problems eating, food taste
- Lumps or sores in the mouth or on the lips
- Dentist visit, dentures or partials, fit
- Tobacco, alcohol use
- Medications

Physical
- Note fit of dentures
- Have patient remove dentures or partials, and using a flashlight and tongue depressor, examine thoroughly all surfaces
- Lesions in back and under side of tongue are easily missed: look carefully
- Palpate for any masses
- If any plaques are noted, see if they are fixed or if they can be scraped off
- Note the tongue, large lesions, and those persisting more than 2 weeks should be referred for biopsy
- Assess for gingivitis (inflammation of gums), which leads to periodontal disease and loss of teeth.

Assessment
- Decreased salivary function and decreased taste combine to put the patient at risk for decreased oral intake. Carefully assess patient's nutritional status and hydration status
- Patients with a history of heavy tobacco and alcohol use are at higher risk for malignant oral lesions and should be carefully evaluated for any ulcer that is atypical in appearance and/or does not heal in 2 weeks

Management
- Good nutritional support and hydration are key to resolution and prevention of oral lesions. Poor dentition may have led to poor nutrition and should be referred for dental correction
- Patients should be encouraged in good dental hygiene: brushing with soft brush including gum surfaces, flossing, and use of a fluoride dentifrice and/or rinse
- Patient should see dentist every 6 months to 1 year

COMMON MOUTH PROBLEMS
- Aphthous ulcers (canker sores) are common, benign, and generally resolve spontaneously
- Denture sores appear where dentures rub
  - Ill-fitting dentures are common due to weight loss.
  - Infected denture sores that do not heal by taking dentures out of the mouth overnight should be treated by dentist
- Oral candidiasis can manifest in several ways, including:
  - Thrush: leukoplakic plaques easily removed with an erythematous base beneath
  - Hyperplastic candidiasis: confluent leukoplakic plaques that cannot be removed
  - Atrophic candidiasis: erythematous mucosal lesions, often found beneath dentures
  - Risk factors for oral candidiasis include diabetes, medications such as antibiotics, corticosteroids, antineoplastics, other immunosuppressants. Precipitating cause of infection should be sought and treated
  - Topical treatment such as nystatin oral suspension (100,000 U/mL) 5 mL qid (swish for 5 minutes and swallow) should be given for 10 to 14 days
- Angular cheilitis: leukoplakic fissures formed in the redundant skin of the lip commissures, usually resolves with treatment with mild topical steroid

- Ulcers that do not completely heal within 2 to 3 weeks of treatment or that present with no clear etiology should be referred for ENT evaluation. The most common site of malignancies of the head and neck is the oral cavity. Extrinsic risk factors include tobacco and alcohol use. **Oral cancer should always be included in the differential diagnosis**
- Gingivitis is the inflammation of gums with swelling, receding, easily bleeding gums, and cold sensitivity. Periodontal disease is inflammation and destruction of supportive structure of tooth, causing loosening then loss of teeth
    - More common and extensive among those who have not had recent dental care, especially underserved populations such as African American, refugees, and Hispanics
    - Those with gingival hyperplasia (seen as a side effect of calcium channel blockers, phenytoin, and cyclosporine) are more prone to this disorder
    - Gingivitis and periodontitis are managed by the dentist and oral surgeon and should be referred
- Xerostomia: sensation of dry mouth related to decreased saliva production due to
    - Sjögren syndrome (autoimmune exocrinopathy)
    - Dehydration
    - Other oral conditions, such as infection, salivary gland obstruction (sialolith, a stone), trauma, and neoplasms may result in decreased salivary output
    - Stress (sympathetic nervous system effect)
    - Mouth breathing (nasal obstruction)
    - Medications, such as anticholinergics, antidepressants, antihistaminics, anxiolytics, diuretics, antidepressants, and antiparkinsonian agents
    - Oncologic treatment: radiation therapy and cytotoxic chemotherapy
    - Management
        - Modify medication regimen: substitute medications that are less anticholinergic, decrease dosages, or split dosages throughout the day
        - Stimulate salivation by sugarless mints and gums
        - Moisturizing gels and rinses, artificial saliva
        - Institute good oral hygiene
        - Lubricants can be used to prevent painful lip cracking
        - Pilocarpine 5 mg tid and at night may be tried
- Decreased taste: alteration in perceptions of flavor of food or drink due to
    - Xerostomia
    - Anticholinergic medications
    - In healthy older individuals, there is no decrease in taste/smell
    - Medical illnesses such as chronic renal failure, diabetes mellitus
- Places patient at risk for anorexia, malnutrition, and dehydration

CASE STUDIES

Case 1. An 83-year-old female nursing home patient is observed to have crusting on both eyelashes in the mornings.

HPI: Patient diagnosed with Alzheimer disease is a resident in a long-term care (LTC) facility. You are told that there have been several cases of conjunctivitis in the facility in the past week. The patient is nonverbal but has been observed rubbing her eyes in the past few days.

PMH: Resident has been in LTC for several years. Her personal care is provided by nurse aides, and she is in general good health otherwise. She is under treatment for seborrheic dermatitis. She has no food or drug allergies.

Medication: Hydrocortisone 1% crème sparingly to affected facial area daily; multivitamin daily.

1. Which are the most likely differential diagnoses for the presenting problem?
2. Review the risk factors for the possible diagnoses.
3. What further history would you obtain?
4. What key findings would you look for in the physical exam?

Exam: Eyelids are found to be inflamed with broken and misdirected lashes. Scaling of lids noted. Conjunctiva are mildly injected. Golden crusting is noted along lid edges; drainage is reported to be worse in the morning, staying clear through the day.

5. What treatment plan would you develop, based on these findings?
6. What follow-up would you recommend?
7. Under what circumstances would you make a referral?

Case 2. An 82-year-old man comes to the clinic accompanied by his wife. He has not been back for his routine visits for 8 months. He has no complaints and says no to every question you ask. Wife states he is driving her nuts; she thinks he is getting senile or going crazy because he has lost interest in socializing and has stopped watching TV. Chart shows patient was a construction worker. He smoked and drank heavily for many years before quitting about 15 years ago. His medical diagnoses are hypertension, osteoarthritis, and COPD; medications are atenolol (Tenormin) 50 mg PO qd, enalapril (Vasotec) 5 mg PO qd, theophylline sustained release (Theo-Dur) 100 mg PO bid, and aspirin as needed for arthritis pain.

1. What part of this history suggests hearing loss?
2. What risk factors for hearing loss does he have?

Exam: The patient can hear sound but cannot understand many of the words.

3. What kind of hearing loss does this suggest?
4. Would a referral for a hearing aid be appropriate for this kind of hearing loss?

Case 3. A 65-year-old female presents with complaint of "a cold." She states symptoms have been present for 6 days, include a "runny nose, cough, and she just feels miserable," They have gotten worse in the past 2 days. She gives history of "allergies to pollen." She takes no regular medications but has been taking ibuprofen and pseudoephedrine to control symptoms.

Exam: Patient appears mildly ill but not in distress; temperature 100.2 oral; pulse 100, respiration 20, mouth breathing, but no acute respiratory distress. Ears: canals clear, TMs bilaterally dull and retracted, nasal mucosa swollen, red, with green discharge. Palpable enlarged lymph nodes tender to palpation; chest is clear, heart normal.

1. What further history would you like?
2. What else is included in your physical exam?
3. What is your diagnosis?
4. What would you do for the patient on this visit?

REFERENCES

American Academy for Allergy, Asthma, and Immunology: *The Allergy Report*. Available at: http://www.aaaai.org/ar/working_vol2/009.asp. Accessed 10/10/2004.

American Academy of Audiology. Available at: www.audiology.org.

American Academy of Ophthalmology. Available at: www.aao.org.

American Glaucoma Society. Available at: www.glaucomaweb.org.

Browning, G. (2002). Wax in the ear. *Clinical Evidence*, 7, 490.

Evans, J. R. (2002). Antioxidant vitamin and mineral supplements for age-related macular degeneration. *Cochrane Database Syst Rev*, CD000254.

Gates, G. A., et al. (2003). Screening for handicapping hearing loss in the elderly. *J Family Practice, 52,* 56.

Goolsby, M. J. (2000) The red eye: Differential diagnosis and management. *The American Journal for Nurse Practitioners, 4*(6), 7–19.

Gottlieb, J. L. (2002). Age-related macular degeneration. *JAMA, 288,* 2233–2236.

Guitton, M. J., Wang, J., and Puel, J. L. (2004). New pharmacological strategies to restore hearing and treat tinnitus. *Acta Otolaryngoly, 124*(4), 411–415.

Hanley, K., et al. (2001). A systematic review of vertigo in primary care. *British J General Practice, 51,* 666.

Healthy Hearing. Available at: www.healthyhearing.com. Information on hearing aids.

Hearing Aid Help. Available at: www.hearingaidhelp.com. Information on hearing aids.

Kaliner, M. A. (2002). H1 Antihistamines in the elderly. *Clinical Allergy Immunology, 17,* 465.

Leske, M. C., et al. (2003). Factors for glaucoma progression and the effect of treatment: The early manifest glaucoma trial. *Archives Ophthalmology, 121,* 48.

Macular Degeneration Foundation International. Available at: www.maculardegeneration.org.

Macular Degeneration Partnership. Available at: www.macd.net.

NIH National Eye Institute. Available at: www.nei.nih.gov.

Pirozzo, S., et al. (2003, October 25). Whispered voice test for screening for hearing impairment in adults and children: Systematic review. *British Medical Journal, 327,* 967–970.

Shields, S. R. (2000). Managing eye disease in primary care. Part 1. How to screen for occult disease. *Postgraduate Medicine, 108,* 69.

Shields, S. R. (2000). Managing eye disease in primary care. Part 2. How to recognize and treat common eye problems. *Postgraduate Medicine, 108,* 83.

Shields, S. R. (2000). Managing eye disease in primary care. *Postgraduate Medicine, 108,* 99.

RESPIRATORY DISORDERS

8

GERIATRIC APPROACH

Normal Changes of Aging

CAPACITY

- Total lung capacity (TLC) (volume of gas in the lungs after a maximal inspiration) remains unchanged
  - Decreased elastic recoil makes it easier to expand the lungs
  - Chest wall is stiffer with aging, limiting the amount the lungs expand (a normal musculo-skeletal change of aging)
- Residual volume (RV) (volume of air remaining in the respiratory system when subjects have expired as much air as possible) increases with aging
  - Vital capacity (VC) is the difference between the maximal lung capacity (TLC) and the residual volume (RV). This is the air that is being moved in and out of the lungs
  - Since the RV increases while the TLC stays the same, the VC (amount of air being moved in and out) decreases
- Functional residual capacity (FRC) (the lung volume at the end of normal quiet respiration) increases slightly with age

FLOW RATE (See Table 8-1)

- Peak expiratory flow (PEF) rate decreases
- The initial PEF rate (maximal flow) decreases slightly, this is FEV_1
  - The rate is determined by recoil of lung and chest wall and the speed with which the respiratory muscles generate positive pleural pressure
  - The initial maximal flow decreases slightly
  - Forced expiratory volume (FEV_1) decreases at the rate of about 30 mls per year
- The FEV_{25-75} decreases significantly (see below)
  - Major reductions in maximal expiratory flow occur at lower lung volumes
  - The maximal flow throughout the remainder of the VC after FEV_1 is determined by the intrinsic properties of the lung: elastic recoil pressure, the cross sectional area of the airways, and airway compliance
  - Much of the decrease is caused by lung elastic recoil with aging
- Healthy black elderly have a 10% decrease in FEV_1
- Respiratory drive is reduced due to hypoxia, elevated PCO_2 levels, and resistance changes
- Increase airway reactivity

Clinical Implications

History

- Frequent nonspecific presentation of respiratory problems as confusion, decreased ADLs, and falls
- Obtain complete smoking history of patient and spouse

Table 8-1: Definitions of Pulmonary Function Tests

Test	Definition
Spirometry	
FVC	Forced vital capacity—volume of gas that can be forcefully expelled from the lungs after max. inspiration
FEV_1	Forced expiratory volume in 1 second—volume of gas expelled in the first second of the FVC
FEF_{25-75}	Forced expiratory flow from 25% to 75% of the FVC—maximal midexpiratory airflow rate
PEFR	Peak expiratory flow rate—maximal airflow rate achieved in the FVC maneuver
MVV	Maximum voluntary ventilation—maximum volume of gas that can be breathed in 1 minute (measured in 15 seconds and multiplied by 4)
Lung Volumes	
TLC	Total lung capacity—volume of gas in the lungs after a maximal inspiration
RV	Residual volume—volume of gas remaining in the lungs after maximal expiration
ERV	Expiratory reserve volume—volume of gas representing the difference between functional residual capacity and residual volume
FRC	Functional residual capacity—volume of gas into the lungs at the end of a normal tidal expiration
SVC	Slowed vital capacity—volume of gas that can be slowly exhaled after maximal inspiration

Adapted from: Tierney, L. M., et al. (2004). *Current medical diagnosis & treatment*. New York: McGraw Hill. p. 269.

- Is cough productive or nonproductive? Note color, amount, consistency of sputum
- Exercise tolerance/activity level; how far can they walk before getting short of breath?

Physical
- Elderly patients may have difficulty following instructions when asked to take a deep breath; subtle findings may be missed
- If patient is unable to sit up, roll patient onto side, auscultate the higher side then roll patient onto opposite side and auscultate other side
- Respiratory and cardiac problems closely related, evaluate both systems
- Spirometry for lung status in acute illness
- Chest x-rays are frequently necessary for accurate diagnosis
- Pulse oximetry for resting and exercise oxygenation

Assessment
- Elderly patients tend to present with confusion when their PO_2 is decreased for any reason
- Majority of respiratory infections are viral, but risk of secondary bacterial infection great
- Exacerbations in COPD (chronic obstructive pulmonary disease) symptoms are usually due to infection
- Elderly often have baseline low peak flow rates; however, monitoring may useful

Treatment
- Respiratory medications have increased adverse reactions in the elderly
- Dizziness causes falls
- May not tolerate oral decongestants due to tachycardia or agitation and nervousness
- When using metered dose inhalers (MDIs) instruct in proper use and use spacer and have them give return demonstration; many elderly have difficulty manipulating inhalers
- Nebulizers instead of inhalers for bronchodilators and steroids may be more effective
- Need to remain well hydrated, but watch fluid overload

- Influenza vaccination annually
- Pneumovax vaccination every 10 years

ASTHMA

Description
- Chronic inflammatory disorder of the airways in which there is episodic and reversible symptoms of airway narrowing and obstruction

Etiology
- Caused by allergic and nonallergic triggers
  - Allergic triggers: seasonal or environmental allergens—pollens, feathers. pet dander, dust mite and cockroach excrements, molds, food additives, preservatives, such as sulfites
  - Nonallergic triggers: smoke, fumes, dyes, air pollutants
- Respiratory/cardiac diseases or infections, such as chronic heart failure, bronchitis, and viral respiratory infection
- Drug induced—ASA, NSAIDs, topical and systemic beta-blockers

Incidence and Demographics
- Prevalence is similar to adults
- Usually develops in younger people, but onset in the elderly is not unusual
- Deaths 3 times greater among blacks and Hispanics than among whites

Risk Factors
- Family history asthma or allergies
- Nasal polyps
- Eczema/atopic dermatitis

Prevention and Screening
- Use of air filters and air conditioners
- Treat upper respiratory infections when present

Assessment
History
- Classic symptoms—episodic acute onset of wheezing (absent in severe exacerbations), chest tightness, dyspnea, chronic dry or nonproductive cough. Symptoms worse at night, with exercise, exposure to cold temperatures, patient's triggers
- Confusion, slight shortness of breath, decreased exercise tolerance
- Severity of symptoms (see Table 8-2 Classification and Treatment of Asthma)
- Frequency of episodes, previous treatment
- Smoking history

Physical (See Table 8-2)
- General: diaphoresis, use of accessory muscles to breathe, tachycardia, tachypnea
- Lungs: decreased breath sounds, wheezing, prolonged expiration, hyperresonance
- Look for signs of chronic heart failure or dehydration
- If allergic, may see nasal discharge, sinus tenderness, mucosal edema and erythema, postnasal drainage
- Severe exacerbation: cyanosis, barely audible to absent breath sounds, pulsus paradoxus (>20 mm Hg fall in blood pressure during inspiration)

Diagnostic Studies
- Routine monitoring of pulmonary function is essential with peak flow meter
  - Peak flow meter measures peak expiratory flow (PEF).
  - Used for monitoring lung status, not to confirm diagnosis

Table 8-2: Classification and Treatment of Asthma

Step	Symptoms	Nighttime Symptoms	Lung Function	Treatment
Step 4 Severe Persistent	Continual symptoms Limited physical activity Frequent exacerbations	Frequent	FEV_1 or PEF ≤60% predicted PEF variability >30%	Corticosteroid inhaled high dose AND β$_2$-agonist inhaled long acting AND, if needed: Corticosteroid PO long term, 2 mg/kg/d, not to exceed 60 mg/day (make repeat attempts to reduce systemic steroids and maintain control with high-dose inhaled steroids)
Step 3 Moderate Persistent	Daily symptoms Daily use of inhaled short acting β$_2$-agonist Exacerbations affect activity Exacerbations ≥ 2 times a week; may last days	>1 time a week	FEV_1 or PEF >60% to <80% predicted PEF variability >30%	Corticosteroid inhaled low-to-medium dose AND one of the three following: β$_2$-agonist inhaled long acting Leukotriene modifier Theophylline OR Corticosteroids inhaled medium dose
Step 2 Mild Persistent	Symptoms >2 times a week but <1 time a day Exacerbations may affect activity	>2 times a month	FEV_1 or PEF > 80% predicted PEF variability 20%–30%	Corticosteroid inhaled low dose OR Cromolyn leukotriene modifier, nedocromil OR Theophylline sustained release to serum concentration of 5–15 mcg/ml
Step 1 Mild Intermittent	Symptoms <2 times a week Asymptomatic and normal PEF between exacerbations Exacerbations brief (from a few hours to a few days); intensity may vary	<2 times a month	FEV_1 or PEF >80% predicted PEF variability <20%	No daily medication needed

*The presence of one of the features of severity is sufficient to place a patient in that category. An individual should be assigned to the most severe grade in which any feature occurs. The characteristics noted in the figure are general and may average because asthma is highly variable.
Adapted from: *National Asthma Education and Prevention Program Expert Panel Report: Guidelines for the diagnosis and management of asthma—Update on Selected Topics 2002, NIH Publication No. 02-5075.*

- Values vary with height, age, gender; with the very old patients are greatly decreased
- Values less than 200 L/min may indicate severe airflow obstruction
- 80% to 100% of patient's "personal best"—good control, maintain treatment
- 50% to less than 80%—acute exacerbation, adjust treatment
- Less than 50%—severe asthma exacerbation, emergency treatment
- Pulmonary function tests (PFT)/spirometry—reveal obstructive dysfunction
  - See Table 8-1 Definitions of Pulmonary Function Tests
  - Used to diagnose obstructive and restrictive airway disease
  - Airflow obstruction indicated by reduced FEV_1/FVC ratio (<75%).
  - Partial reversibility—improvement in FVC or FEV_1 of at least 15% or improvement in FEF of at least 25%, after bronchodilator treatment differentiates asthma from COPD
- Arterial blood gases (ABG)—normal to mild hypoxia and respiratory alkalosis less likely due to higher PCO_2 level
- Complete blood count (CBC)—slight increase of white blood cells during acute attack
- Chest x-ray—hyperinflation in uncomplicated episodes
- Sputum exam—if allergic, see mucus casts, eosinophils and elongated rhomboid crystals

Differential Diagnosis
- Chronic obstructive pulmonary disease (COPD)
- Chronic heart failure (CHF)
- Pulmonary embolism
- Bronchogenic carcinoma
- Foreign body aspiration
- Acute infections: bronchitis/pneumonia, tuberculosis, mycoplasma
- Vocal cord dysfunction/upper airway obstruction
- Gastroesophageal reflux disease (GERD)
- Anxiety

Management
- National Heart, Lung and Blood Institute of the National Institutes of Health have developed general guidelines for the treatment of asthma in adults (Table 8-2)

Nonpharmacologic Treatment
- Identify and avoid factors that trigger asthma
- Avoid cigarette smoke
- Promote adequate hydration to provide adequate bronchial toilet
- Yoga may be effective in adjunctive treatment of asthma; studies show improvement in mechanical aspects of breathing as well as reduction in stress.

Pharmacologic Treatment
- Management of acute exacerbations

SEVERE EXACERBATION
- Beta-agonist nebulization or 2–4 puffs q 20 min for total of 3 treatments
- Send to ER

MODERATE EXACERBATION
- Beta-agonist nebulization or 2–4 puffs q 2–4 h
- Course of systemic corticosteroids may be needed

MILD EXACERBATION
- Beta-agonist 2–4 puffs q 3–4 h
- Double dose for 7–10 days for patients on inhaled steroids

- Short-acting beta-agonist—onset of action 1–10 minutes
  - Relax the smooth muscle of the airway
  - May be less effective in elderly asthmatics with COPD
  - Albuterol (Proventil, Ventolin)—90 mcg/inhalations, 1–2 inhalations/nebulized 0.083% solution q 4–6 h prn
  - Levalbuterol (Xopenex) (single-isomer albuterol) 0.63 mg via nebulizer tid
  - Metaproterenol (Alupent)—0.65 mg/inhalations, 2 inhalations/nebulized 0.4% solution q 4–6 h prn
- Anticholinergics—onset of action 15 minutes
  - Inhibits vagal reflex with resulting bronchial smooth muscle relaxation
  - Good choice for elderly asthmatics with COPD, due to activity on larger airways
  - Ipratropium bromide (Atrovent)—18 mcg/puff, 2 puffs or nebulized 0.02% solution qid
- Systemic Corticosteroids—onset of action 12–36 hours
  - Need to carefully monitor use (e.g., coexisting diabetes, risk of steroid induced hyperglycemia, greater risk of steroid related psychosis in elderly, risk of increased osteoporosis)
  - Prednisone (Liquid Pred, Deltasone)—5–60 mg/day in divided doses bid, tid, or qid
  - Prednisolone (Delta-Cortef, Prelone)—5–60 mg/day in divided doses

LONG-TERM MANAGEMENT
- Stepwise approach
  - Gain control quickly
  - Gradual stepwise reduction in treatment if possible
  - If control not maintained, stepwise increase in medication
- Inhaled corticosteroids—onset of action 2 to 3 days
  - Good choice to avoid systemic corticosteroid use (e.g., large dosing range with reduced systemic effect)
  - Beclomethasone dipropionate (Beclovent, Vanceril, Vancenase)—42 mcg/puff 2 puffs or 84 mcg/puff 1–2 puffs bid–qid, not to exceed 840 mcg daily
  - (Flovent)—44 mcg/spray, 110 mcg/spray, 220 mcg/spray, 2–4 puffs bid–qid, should not exceed 660 mcg daily
  - Triamcinolone acetate (Azmacort)—100 mcg/puff, 2 puffs tid–qid
- Long-acting beta$_2$ agonists
  - Salmeterol (Serevent)—aerosol 25 mcg/spray, 2 puffs q 12 h
  - Formoterol (Foradil)—12 mcg dry powder via inhaler q 12 h
  - Caution: not for treatment of acute attacks; use with caution in patients with cardiovascular disease
  - Well tolerated in the elderly generally
- Methylxanthines
  - Theophylline—(Theo-Dur, Slo-bid)—Individualize dose: 16 mg/kg/24/h or 400 mg/24/h, whichever is less in divided doses at 6–8 h intervals
  - Dose to therapeutic range of 10–20; most elderly have fewer side effects on lower end of range; dose must be individualized
  - Adverse reactions: arrhythmias, nausea, restlessness
  - Watch for drug interactions with other medications commonly used (e.g., Digoxin, Coumadin, macrolides, quinolones, beta blockers, and corticosteroids)
  - Theophylline products are not interchangeable; absorption varies with brands
  - Theophylline should be used with caution, if other medications not effective, in the elderly due to the potential for adverse reactions and drug interactions
- Mast cell stabilizers
  - Cromolyn sodium (Intal)—inhalation 20 mg; 2 sprays 800 mcg/spray qid

- Leukotriene receptor antagonists
  - Zafirlukast (Accolade)—10 mg bid
  - Zileuton (Zyflo)—600 mg qid
  - Montelukast (Singulair)—10 mg daily

How Long to Treat
- Dependent on the severity of the attacks
- Goal of treatment is to gain control as quickly as possible and decrease treatment gradually to the least amount of medication needed to maintain control.

When to Consult, Refer, Hospitalize
- Severe asthma exacerbation or severe persistent asthma, requiring Step 3–4 Care
- Patient not meeting goals of treatment after 3 to 6 months of therapy
- Other conditions complicating asthma (infections, GERD, COPD)
- Additional diagnostic testing is indicated
- Continuous use of oral corticosteroid therapy or high-dose inhaled corticosteroids

Follow-up

Expected Course
- Patients should monitor peak flow rates regularly
- For acute exacerbations, follow up in 24 hours then in 3 to 5 days. Follow up weekly until symptoms are controlled and peak flow is consistently 80% of predicted, and then monthly
- Once stabilized follow up every 2 to 3 months
- Monitor theophylline levels 2 weeks after initiation of therapy, then every 4 months
- Use of quick relief medications more than 2 times a week in intermittent asthma (daily or increasing use in persistent asthma) may indicate the need to initiate (increase) long-term therapy.

Complications
- Exhaustion, dehydration, cor pulmonale, airway infection, tussive syncope
- Change in mental status, frequent falls, and exacerbation of other existing illnesses
- Pneumothorax, hypercapnia, hypoxic respiratory failure, and death

CHRONIC OBSTRUCTIVE PULMONARY DISEASE (COPD)

Description
- Limitation of expiratory airflow caused by destruction of airway tissue caused by emphysema, chronic bronchitis, or chronic asthma
- The obstruction is progressive and unresponsive to bronchodilators.
- Emphysema—dyspnea from abnormal remodeling of air spaces within the terminal bronchioles
- Bronchitis produces a productive cough most days of the month for at least 3 months over 2-year period.
- Asthma produces permanent remodeling of the basement membrane resulting from chronic inflammation.
- Most patients have characteristics of both emphysema and chronic bronchitis.

Etiology
- Smoking 80%

Incidence and Demographics
- Seventh ranking chronic condition
- Fourth leading cause of death in US (1997)
- Mortality rates continue to increase
- Affects patients older than age 50

Risk Factors
- Smokers
- Secondhand smoke
- Persons in occupations involving high concentrations of dust and fumes are also at high risk—coal miners, metal molders, grain handlers, farmers, asbestos exposure
- Air pollution
- Allergies
- Genetic predisposition
- Male gender

Prevention and Screening
- Smoking cessation
- Reduction in secondhand smoke exposure
- Treatment and control of upper respiratory illnesses and allergies

Assessment

History
- Presenting symptoms usually dyspnea with cough
- Duration and characteristics of cough
- Smoking history of patient and family members
- Exercise/activity tolerance, dyspnea on exertion or at rest
- Work history—disability
- Chills/fever, weight gain/loss, edema, fatigue, angina
- Sleep habits—number of pillows used
- Respiratory illness history—asthma, bronchitis, sinusitis, allergies
- Other existing illnesses—cardiovascular diseases

Physical
- General—weight loss, tachycardia, tachypnea
- Respiratory—pursed-lip breathing, use accessory respiratory muscles with breathing, increased AP diameter of chest, decreased breath sounds with prolonged expiratory phase, poor diaphragm mobility

Diagnostic Studies
- Chest radiographs—in emphysema, hyperinflation, subpleural blebs, parenchymal bullae, flattened diaphragm; in chronic bronchitis ("dirty lungs") nonspecific peribronchial and perivascular markings at bases
- Pulmonary function tests (PFT)—typically airflow obstruction of 70 or more diffusion capacity—determine air trapping and hypercapnia
- ECG—may show sinus tachycardia; abnormalities typical of cor pulmonale in advanced disease with pulmonary hypertension; supraventricular arrhythmia, ventricular irritability, right ventricular hypertrophy
- Arterial blood gases (ABGs)—should be done for baseline, hypoxemia in advanced chronic bronchitis; compensated respiratory acidosis with chronic respiratory failure in chronic bronchitis

Differential Diagnosis
- Asthma
- Bronchiectasis
- Interstitial fibrosis
- Bronchopulmonary mycosis
- Cor pulmonale
- CHF
- Cardiomyopathy

Management
- See Table 8-3 Step Therapy for COPD

Table 8-3: Step Therapy for COPD

Step	Symptoms	Therapy
1	Mild, variable	• Selective ß$_2$-agonist inhaler PRN
2	Mild to moderate, continuing	• Ipratropium inhaler on regular basis PLUS • Selective ß$_2$-agonist PRN or on regular basis
3	If Step 2 not satisfactory or mild to moderate increase	• Add sustained-release theophylline for nocturnal bronchospasm
4	If control suboptimal	• Consider course of oral steroids. If improvement, wean to low daily or alternate-day dose (e.g., 7.5 mg) • If no improvement, stop abruptly • If steroid appears to help, consider use of aerosol MDI, particularly if patient has evidence of bronchial hyperactivity
5	For severe exacerbation	• Increase ß$_2$-agonist dosage • Increase ipratropium dosage • And add an antibiotic, if indicated

Modified from, American Thoracic Society. (1995). Standards for the diagnosis and care of the patient with chronic obstructive pulmonary disease. *American Journal of Respiratory and Critical Care Medicine, 152.*

- Refer to American Thoracic Society Guidelines

Nonpharmacologic Treatment
- Smoking cessation
- Encourage well-balanced diet to maintain ideal body weight
- Monitored exercise program
- Avoid exposure to colds and influenza
- Avoid respiratory irritants: secondhand smoke, dust, and other air pollutants
- Increase fluids and humidification
- Breathing exercises; effective cough techniques
- Avoid outdoor activities when air pollutant concentrations are high

Pharmacologic Treatment
- Based on severity and etiology of COPD

ANTICHOLINERGICS
- First-line drugs
- Ipratropium bromide (Atrovent)—0.65 mg/inh, 2 inh q 6 h, max 12 inh or 500 mcg via neb q 6–8 h
- Tiotropium (Spiriva) 18 mcg 1 cap via inh qd
- Side effects mild—dry mouth, cough, nervousness, dizziness, GI upset

BRONCHODILATORS—BETA$_2$-AGONIST
- Second-line drugs
  SHORT ACTING
  - Albuterol (Proventil, Ventolin)—90 mcg/inh, 2 inh q 4–6 h OR neb 0.083% 2.5 mg 3–4 x day
  - Side effects—tremor, nervousness, headache, dizziness, hypokalemia, insomnia, tachycardia
  LONG ACTING
  - Formoterol (Foradil) 12 mcg dry powder via inhaler bid
  - Salmeterol (Serevent Diskus) 50 mcg dry powder via inhaler bid
  - Side effects—hypertension, nasal congestion, headache, dizziness

- Third-line drugs
- Theophylline—(Theo-24, Uniphyl)—individualize dose: 16 mg/kg/24 h or 400 mg/24 h, whichever is less, in divided doses at 1–2 x day
- Side effects—GI upset, headache, CNS stimulation, arrhythmias, seizures
- Theophylline has a narrow therapeutic window, close monitoring with serum levels necessary

CORTICOSTEROIDS—INHALED/ORAL
- Most effective for acute exacerbations
- Approximately 10% of stable COPD patients respond to oral steroids
- Beclomethasone dipropionate (Beclovent, Vanceril, Vancenase)—42 mcg/puff 2 puffs or 84 mcg/puff 1–2 puffs 3–4 x day
- Triamcinolone (Azmacort)—100 mcg/puff 2–4 puffs bid–qid
- Prednisone (Liquid Pred, Deltasone)—1 mg, 2.5 mg, 5 mg, 10 mg, 20 mg, 50-mg tabs, or 5 mg/5 ml oral solution, 5–60 mg/day in divided doses bid, tid, or qid
- Prednisolone (Delta-Cortef, Prelone)—5-mg tabs, 15 mg/ml and 50 mg/ml oral syrup, 5–60 mg/day in divided doses

OXYGEN
- The only drug documented to alter the natural history of COPD
- Medicare coverage for patients with resting hypoxemia:
  - PaO_2 less than or equal to 55 while awake
  - During sleep (nocturnal O_2 only): PaO_2 less than or equal to 55 OR decrease in PaO_2 more than 10, OR more an 5 decrease with associated symptoms of hypoxemia
  - During exercise (use during exercise only): PaO_2 less than or equal to 55 AND evidence that O_2 improves the hypoxemia
- 1–3 L/min via nasal cannula 15 h/day

How Long to Treat
- Chronic condition requiring ongoing therapeutic treatments and monitoring

Special Considerations
- Acute exacerbation of COPD—characterized by an increase in baseline symptoms: increased dyspnea, cough, increased sputum production
- Bacterial infection usual underlying cause—responds well to broad spectrum antibiotics (see Pharmacologic Treatment for CAP), increase of maintenance MDIs, treat based on severity of symptoms
- Other possible comorbidities should be investigated—chronic heart failure, pulmonary embolus, TB, pneumothorax

When to Consult, Refer, Hospitalize
- Signs and symptoms of respiratory failure
- Severe exacerbations
- Symptoms of cor pulmonale
- Progression of disease
- Poor response to therapy

Follow-up

Expected Course
- Exacerbation should resolve within 7 to 10 days, if persists, obtain CBC, chest x-ray, PFTs
- Degree of pulmonary dysfunction at initial visit is most important predictor of survival
- Poor prognosis especially for severe disease and emphysematous form—median survival approximately 4 years

Complications
- Acute exacerbation of COPD, pneumonia, pulmonary thromboembolism, spontaneous pneumothorax, acute bronchitis, pulmonary hypertension, cor pulmonale, chronic respiratory failure, left ventricular heart failure, death

COMMUNITY-ACQUIRED PNEUMONIA

Description
- An acute pulmonary infection that begins outside the hospital and is associated with symptoms of infection, parenchymal infiltrate on chest radiograph, and bronchial breath sounds or rales on auscultation
- Community-acquired pneumonia may also begin within 48 hours of hospital admission in a patient who has resided less than 14 days in a long-term care facility before symptom onset.

Etiology
- Bacterial more common than viral
- Most common is *S pneumoniae*
- Less common—*Haemophilus influenzae, Moraxella catarrhalis, Mycoplasma pneumoniae, Chlamydia pneumonia, S aureus, Neisseria meningitidis, Klebsiella pneumoniae,* legionella, gram-negative bacilli
- Many have multiple organisms
- Viral: influenza, adenovirus, parainfluenza, respiratory syncytial virus

Incidence and Demographics
- Common, 2 to 3 million cases each year
- Sixth leading cause of death

Risk Factors
- 65 years of age or older
- Nursing home residents
- Alcoholism
- Altered mental status—decreased gag and cough reflex
- Smoking
- Sedating drugs
- Influenza
- Poor dental hygiene
- Neurological deficits, aspiration secondary to stroke, Parkinson's, etc.
- Feeding tubes

Prevention and Screening
- Influenza vaccine
- Polyvalent pneumococcal vaccine
- Good nutritional screening

Assessment
- Assess preexisting conditions that influence ability to care for patient at home
  - Hemodynamic instability
  - Acute hypoxemia
  - Chronic oxygen dependency
  - Ability to take oral medication
- Assess severity
  - Characteristics that confer increased risk include advanced age, alcoholism, comorbid diseases, altered mental status, respiratory rate 30 or more, hypotension, and elevated BUN or sodium
  - Use PORT (Pneumonia Patient Outcomes Research Team) score, see Fine, M.F., et al.

- Assess overall health and suitability for home care
  - Frail physical condition
  - Social or psychiatric problems compromising home care
  - Unstable living situation

History
- Confusion or nonspecific presentation of illness may be the only symptoms
- Classic presentation: fever, chills, sweats, rigors AND
- Cough (productive or nonproductive), dyspnea
- Fatigue, myalgias, chest discomfort, headache, failure to thrive
- Anorexia, abdominal pain may or may not be present or intermittent

Physical
- Patient may only appear mildly ill, mental confusion
- Hypothermia, fever, or normal temperature
- Tachypnea over 30, very reliable indicator of pneumonia in the elderly, tachycardia
- Abnormal breath sounds and rales present. "A to E" changes on auscultation
- Percussion dullness if effusion present

Diagnostic Studies
- Chest x-ray
- CBC
- BUN, glucose, electrolytes, liver function
- Gram's stain and culture of sputum
- TB testing if atypical or at high risk

Differential Diagnosis
- Upper respiratory tract infections
- Reactive airway disease
- CHF
- Bronchiolitis
- Malignancy
- Myocardial infarction
- TB
- Pulmonary embolism
- Pulmonary vasculitis
- Atelectasis

Management
- Patient must be hospitalized if unable to take adequate PO fluids
- Refer to practice guidelines—Infectious Disease Society of America—see reference

Nonpharmacologic Treatment
- Rest
- Increase fluids
- Humidification
- Smoking cessation

Pharmacologic Treatment (See Table 8-4)
- Treat Gram's stain results if available
- Treat culture results when available

ANTIMICROBIALS
- Macrolides
  - Erythromycin 250–1000 mg q 6 h
  - Clarithromycin (Biaxin) 500 PO q 12 h x 14 d
  - Azithromycin (Zithromax) 500 me PO x 1 day, then 250 PO qd x 4 d
- Doxycycline—100 mg PO q 12 h
- Fluoroquinolone
  - Levo Floxin (Levaquin) 500 mg PO qd
  - Gatifloxacin (Tequin) 400 mg PO qd

Table 8-4: Initial Empiric Therapy of Community-Acquired Pneumonia

Patient Variable Outpatient	Treatment Options
Previously healthy	
No recent antibiotic therapy	Macrolide (erythromycin, azithromycin, clarithromycin) OR doxycycline
Recent antibiotic therapy (within 3 months)	Respiratory fluoroquinolone (moxifloxacin, gatifloxacin, levofloxacin, or gemifloxacin) OR Advanced macrolide (azithromycin or clarithromycin) PLUS High-dose amoxicillin (1 g PO tid) OR Advanced macrolide PLUS high-dose amoxicillin-clavulanate (2 g PO bid)
Comorbidities: COPD, diabetes, renal, failure, CHF, malignancy	
No recent antibiotic therapy (within 3 months	Advanced macrolide OR respiratory fluoroquinolone (as outlined above)
Recent antibiotic therapy (within 3 months)	Respiratory fluoroquinolone OR Advanced macrolide PLUS Beta-lactam: high-dose amoxicillin, high-dose amoxicillin-clavulanate, cefpodoxime, cefprozil or cefuroxime (as outlined above)
Suspected aspiration with infection	Amoxicillin-clavulanate (as outlined above) OR clindamycin
Influenza with bacterial superinfection	Beta-lactam OR respiratory fluoroquinolone (as outlined above)

- Moxifloxacin (Avelox) 400 mg qd
- Gemifloxacin mesylate not yet available
- Beta-lactams
  - Cefpodoxime (Vantin) 200 q 12 h
  - Cefprozil (Cefzil) 500 q 12 h
  - Cefuroxime (Ceftin) 250–500 q 12 h

ANTITUSSIVES
- Generally, cough should not be suppressed and antitussives should not be used
- However, in patients with severe chest discomfort and persistent cough, may consider use of non-narcotic or low-dose narcotic antitussive for night use only

How Long to Treat
- Treat bacterial infections until patient is afebrile or asymptomatic for 72 hours
- Treat for 7 to 14 days, except when using azithromycin

When to Consult, Refer, Hospitalize
- Refer to physician moderate to severe pneumonias
- Hospitalize patients with comorbid conditions, altered mental status, tachycardia, tachypnea, systolic blood pressure less than 90 mm HG, and temperature is elevated or subnormal, institutional acquired

Follow-up
- After discharge should be followed weekly until clear chest x-ray and asymptomatic

Expected Course
* Dependent upon pathogen, patient response, complications

Complications
* Heart failure, renal failure, pulmonary embolism, bacteremia, acute myocardial infection, death

PRIMARY LUNG MALIGNANCIES

Description
* Bronchogenic carcinomas include two classes:
  * Non-small cell lung carcinoma (NSCLC), which includes squamous cell carcinoma, adenocarcinoma, and large cell carcinoma
  * Small cell lung carcinoma (SCLC) also known as oat cell carcinoma

Etiology
* Cigarette smoking
* Secondhand smoke
* Ionizing radiation (radon gas, therapeutic radiation)
* Asbestos exposure (most common occupational cause), synergistic action with smoking
* Heavy metals (nickel, chromium), industrial carcinogens

Incidence and Demographics
* Lung cancer is the leading cause of cancer death for both men and women
* Smoking causes 85% to 90% of lung cancer
* 25% of cancer-related deaths in women, more than breast cancer 32% in men
* Most cases present between ages 50 and 70
* Non-small cell lung carcinoma—80% of lung cancers, small cell carcinomas, 20%
* High mortality and low 5-year survival rates due to inability to diagnose at early stage

Risk Factors
* See Etiology

Prevention and Screening
* DO NOT SMOKE
* Annual chest x-rays and cytology as preventive screening have not had significant impact on survival
* Low-dose helical computed tomography (LDCT) is being evaluated for screening current or former heavy smokers

Assessment

History
* Initial symptoms: cough associated with smoking that persists for greater than 1 month after cessation of smoking, change in characteristics of cough
* Later symptoms: chest pain—often made worse by deep breathing; hoarseness; weight loss and loss of appetite; dyspnea; fever without a known reason; recurring infections such as bronchitis, pneumonia; new onset of wheezing
* Symptoms of metastasis: bone pain, weakness or numbness of the arms or legs, dizziness, jaundice, skin tumors, lymphadenopathy, obstruction of trachea and esophagus
* Hemoptysis most frequently associated with lung cancer but can be from other causes ranging from minor erosions to severe necrosis of mucosa due to inflammation, pulmonary infarct, or gastrointestinal bleeding. Other noncancer causes include TB, coagulopathies, infection, and pulmonary edema. Investigation as outlined below would be similar.

Physical
* Findings vary on exam, may have none to fairly benign findings

- General: weight loss, hoarse voice
- Lung dyspnea, hemoptysis, wheezing, stridor, decreased breath sounds with effusion
- Pneumonia

Diagnostic Studies
- Chest radiographs—most important initial diagnostic test in predicting whether a bronchogenic carcinoma is potential cause of chronic cough
- Histologic confirmation is essential, cytology via bronchoscopy

Differential Diagnosis
- Asthma
- CHF
- Tuberculosis
- COPD
- Pulmonary embolism

Management

Nonpharmacologic Treatment
- Surgical resection
- Radiation therapy
- Palliative therapy includes general care of the patient with particular attention to pain control, maintenance of adequate nutrition, and psychological support; consider hospice referral

Pharmacologic Treatment
- Multiple anticancer chemotherapeutic agents are used to treat lung cancer
- For a more complete listing of specific agents, refer to American Cancer Society at www.cancer.org.

How Long to Treat
- Duration of treatment depends on type and stage of cancer.

When to Consult, Refer, Hospitalize
- Any patient with suspect lung malignancy should be referred to a pulmonologist and oncologist for evaluation and treatment.
- Hospitalization for frank hemoptysis

Follow-up

Expected Course
- Overall 5-year survival rate 10%–15%
- 5-year survival rate after curative resection of squamous cell carcinoma is 35% to 40%
- 25% for adenocarcinoma and large cell carcinoma
- Patients with small cell carcinoma rarely survive for 5 years after diagnosis

Complications
- Superior vena cava syndrome, phrenic nerve palsy, recurrent laryngeal nerve palsy, death
- Weight loss is a significant adverse indicator of prognosis, associated nausea, vomiting, and anorexia can increase this problem

TUBERCULOSIS

Description
- Chronic infectious acid-fast bacillus disease most frequently of the lungs
- In 15%, the bacilli cause disease in other regions, such as the skin, kidneys, bones, or reproductive and urinary systems
- Requires immediate respiratory isolation and reporting to public health
- See Table 8-5 Classification of Tuberculosis

Etiology
- Inhalation of aerosolized droplets containing *Mycobacterium tuberculosis* (M *tuberculosis*) causes infection.

Table 8-5: Classification of Tuberculosis

Classification	Status	PPD
0	No TB exposure—not infected	Negative
1	TB exposure—no evidence of infection	Negative
2	TB infection—no disease	Positive
3	TB clinically active	Positive
4	TB not clinically active	Positive
5	TB suspect	Pending result

Adapted from: American Thoracic Society. (1990). Diagnostic standards and classification of tuberculosis.
American Review Respiratory Disease, 142, 725–735.

- The bacteria are ingested by macrophages and will either die or grow, depending on the effectiveness of the immune system of the patient.
- If the immune system is effective, the bacteria will be walled off in a granuloma.
- The bacteria remain dormant in the granuloma until the patient's immune system weakens.
- This can be from old age, chronic disease, steroids, etc.
- Most tuberculosis in elderly patients is from reactivation of dormant bacteria

Incidence and Demographics
- Causes more deaths worldwide than any other infectious disease
- Approximately 15 million people in the US are infected with M. *tuberculosis*
- Persons 65 or older comprise 25% of all active TB cases
- 75% of active TB is in the lungs of elderly
- TB of the spine is most common form of extrapulmonary TB in elderly
- Minorities affected disproportionately by TB

Risk Factors
- Diabetes mellitus
- HIV infection
- Malignancy
- Chronic renal failure
- Poor nutrition
- Immunosuppressive drugs
- Close contacts of people with newly diagnosed infectious TB
- People with positive TB skin tests
- Abnormal chest x-rays compatible with inactive TB

Prevention and Screening
- Identifying and treating infected individuals early
- INH prevents the disease in most people in close contact with infected people or who are infected but who do not have active TB.
- Preventive therapy indicated for patients in the following groups with positive tuberculin skin test results:
  - Close contacts of newly diagnosed patients with infectious TB
  - Converters: people whose skin test results have recently converted from negative to positive
  - Patients with preexisting medical conditions, such as HIV infection, diabetes mellitus, end-stage renal disease, chronic malabsorption syndromes, and hematologic malignancies
  - Patients on corticosteroid therapy; immunosuppressive therapy
  - Patients with x-ray changes without previous adequate therapy

Assessment

History
- Elderly with TB infection may have no symptoms
- Elderly with TB disease may have any, all, or none of the following symptoms: chronic productive cough, fatigue/malaise, weight loss, anorexia, fever, hemoptysis, night sweats, pleuritic chest pain, changes in functional capacity

Physical
- Appear chronically ill, weight loss
- Chest exam: normal or reveal apical rales, increased tactile fremitus on palpation; percussion dull

Diagnostic Studies
- Tuberculin skin tests: Mantoux (PPD)—standard test, establishes exposure to TB—0.1 mL given intradermal on volar surface of forearm, reaction read in 48 to 72 hours (see Table 8-6 PPD Interpretation)
- Elderly require "boosting" for accurate results. The PPD should be done twice, with second test applied within 2 weeks of the first.
- Chest x-ray—high incidence of atypical chest x-ray presentation—middle, lower lobes and pleura; primary TB frequently middle and lower lobes as well as hilar and mediastinal lymph nodes.
- Sputum smear—suggestive of, does not confirm diagnosis of TB
- Sputum cultures—definitive diagnosis of TB
- CBC with differential and platelets
- Bronchoscopy with bronchial washings and biopsy

Differential Diagnosis
- COPD
- Pneumonia
- Carcinoma
- Pleurisy
- Histoplasmosis
- Silicosis

Management
- Follow national treatment guidelines, protocols, and latest findings from CDC

Nonpharmacologic Treatment
- Isolation for new cases of confirmed tuberculosis

Table 8-6: PPD Interpretation

Reaction Size	Patient Characteristics
≥5 mm	<ul><li>HIV infection or persons at risk for HIV infection</li><li>X-rays suggestive of previous healed TB infection</li><li>Close contacts of people with active TB</li></ul>
≥10 mm	<ul><li>Immigrants from Asia, Africa, Latin America</li><li>Residents of long-term care facilities—nursing homes, correctional institutes, or mental institutions</li><li>Medically underserved and low-income populations</li><li>Recent converters</li><li>Preexisting medical conditions : ≥10% below ideal body weight, diabetes mellitus, gastrectomy, jejunoileal bypass, silicosis, chronic renal failure, immunosuppressive therapy, cancer</li></ul>
≥15 mm	<ul><li>All persons</li></ul>

Information from: American Thoracic Society(1990). Diagnostic standards and classification of tuberculosis. *American Review Respiratory Disease, 142*, 725–735.

Pharmacologic Treatment
- Most common medications: isoniazid (INH), rifampin, pyrazinamide, ethambutol, streptomycin
- Geriatric TB generally responds well to INH and rifampin
- Most geriatric cases are reactivation of disease, thus less likely to have multiple-drug resistance
- Treatment changes often with changing patterns of resistance

Treatment of Exposure to TB
- Patients who are infected with M. *tuberculosis*, even if they do not have symptoms, harbor the bacteria
- Recent converters should receive chemoprophylaxis
- Isoniazid prophylaxis 300 mg per day for 6 to 12 months is recommended
- This will reduce the incidence of reactivated tuberculosis
- The major risk with INH treatment is liver toxicity

How Long to Treat Person Exposed to TB
- Duration of treatment depends on medications used
- Generally, patients are treated for 6 to 12 months

When to Consult, Refer, Hospitalize
- All suspected or confirmed cases of tuberculosis should be reported to the local and state health departments.
- Refer all patients to specialist for treatment.
- Hospitalize patients if incapable of self-care or if patient is likely to expose new susceptible individuals

Follow-up

Expected Course
- 90% cure rate with proper treatment; relapse rate less than 5% with current treatments
- Sputum exams should be monthly
- Monitor liver function test due to high risk of liver toxicity; at baseline and monthly while on medication Hepatic toxicity high with INH in geriatric patients

Complications
- Treatment failure most often due to noncompliance.
- The death rate for untreated TB patients is between 40% and 60%.
- Most deaths result from overlooked disease.

PULMONARY EMBOLISM (PE)

Description
- An obstruction of a pulmonary artery caused by a blood clot (or fat, air, bone) that has traveled to the area through the circulatory system

Etiology
- Deep venous thrombosis (DVT) causes 90%; blood clot initially develops in deep venous circulation. The vessels at highest risk are the popliteal and iliofemoral.
- Other sites of origin of blood clot: right atrium (due to atrial fibrillation), right ventricle, renal, pelvic, hepatic, subclavian and jugular veins
- Fat emboli sources: hip fractures and repairs, long bone fractures, pelvic fractures

Incidence and Demographics
- Primary cause of death in 100,000 people annually
- Contributing cause of death in additional 100,000 annually; many found only on autopsy
- Misdiagnosis in about 30% of cases, commonly in elderly due to high incidence of pulmonary and cardiovascular conditions

Risk Factors
- Venous stasis
- Estrogen use
- Immobility
- Surgery
- Injury to vessel wall
- Femoral vein catheters
- Altered clotting states

Prevention and Screening
- Prophylactic anticoagulation
- Mobility
- Anti-embolism devices: TED hose, alternating compression hose, and mattresses

Assessment

History
- Most common complaints: shortness of breath, chest pain with possible pleuritic component, anxiety, leg pain or swelling, hemoptysis and syncope
- Can also see a variety of symptoms such as confusion, fever, wheezing, congestion, changes in mentation, unexplained palpitations, transient shortness of breath

Physical
- Classic presentation of dyspnea, chest pain, and hemoptysis
- Most PE will present with DVT although symptoms maybe subtle: calf tenderness, edema, increased leg temperature
- Other common findings: arrhythmias, tachycardia, chronic heart failure, pleural friction rub, fever, and cyanosis

Diagnostic Studies
- Chest x-ray contributes to but not diagnostic, see atelectasis, effusion, elevated hemidiaphragm, infiltrate
- EKG may show signs of right side heart failure if significant PE exists
- ABGs will show signs of hypoxia, possible lower CO_2 levels,
- Lung scan—most diagnostic, noninvasive testing, will show degree of probability of embolus based on amount of perfusion defect
- Pulmonary angiography—most diagnostic test will show constant intraluminal filling defect and sharp cutting off of flow. Low incidence of false-negatives results. This is gold standard test. Invasive test with use of contrast material therefore higher risk of complications
- Venous duplex or Doppler studies—most common and quickest way to diagnosis DVT, non-invasive, may be used to monitor calf embolus if suspect risk of popliteal or femoral vein involvement. NOT used to diagnosis PE

Differential Diagnosis
- COPD
- Right-sided heart failure
- CHF
- Pulmonary hypertension
- Rib fractures
- Pneumothorax
- CAD
- Cardiac arrhythmias
- Heart valve disease

Management

Nonpharmacologic Treatment
- Education in regard to outpatient anticoagulation: foods and medications to avoid, bleeding risks, monitoring of therapeutic levels. See CV Chapter 9
- Exercise, antiembolism stockings if DVT involved

Pharmacologic Treatment
- Streptokinase—inpatient
- Heparin—inpatient
- Warfarin (Coumadin)
  - Generally started in hospital, will continue in outpatient setting
  - Requires 3 to 5 days to achieve therapeutic range
  - Monitored by prothrombin time (PT) and international normalizing rate (INR)
  - Goal of therapy is usually a INR of 2 to 3

How Long to Treat
- Time length varies, generally minimum of 3 to 6 months post event

Special Considerations
- Risk of falls in elderly resulting in possibly serious bleeding when on anticoagulation therapy
- Warfarin and heparin have many drug interactions.
- Coexisting diseases also affect action of heparin and warfarin.

When to Consult, Refer, and Hospitalize
- Refer to physician for hospitalization for initial treatment.
- Reoccurrence or extension of embolus with therapy
- Inability to control clotting times
- Pulmonary consult with any pulmonary embolus event with at least one outpatient follow-up
- Reaction to anticoagulant

Follow-up
- Initially should be seen within 10 days of discharge
- INRs should be monitored weekly until stable within therapeutic range
- Reevaluation of DVT with Doppler studies should be considered based on extent and location
- Length of therapy depends on severity of disease, risk of reoccurrence, and prior history.
- Multiple events should prompt consideration of placement of filter in vena cava.

Complications
- Acute respiratory failure
- Death

CASE STUDIES

Case 1. A 70-year-old male comes to clinic with productive cough and shortness of breath. Denies fever or upper respiratory symptoms. Patient is a retired construction worker with history of asthma.

HPI: Medications include asthma medications: Alupent prn, Serevent 2 puffs bid, triamcinolone (Azmacort) 2 puffs bid, and Claritin PM allergies.

    1. What additional history would you like?

Physical Exam: Vital signs stable. No acute respiratory distress, lungs without wheezes or rales (crackles), breath sounds are decreased bilaterally with prolonged expiration. Heart rate regular. Peak flow rate 300 and his baseline is 350.

    2. What is your assessment?
    3. What do you think is happening?
    4. What is your initial plan?

Case 2. A 75-year-old female presents with complaints of productive cough, fever, chills, chest discomfort and chest congestion; has had fatigue and headache for 3 days.

PMH: Bronchitis. Medications: Robitussin DM and Tylenol extra-strength for headache. Allergic to penicillin.

1. What additional history would you ask?

Exam: Patient appears ill; temp 100.8, tachypnea with exertion, skin warm to touch; ENT exam normal; chest splinting with fremitus and rales (crackles) in right lower lobe.

2. What diagnostic tests will you order?
3. What are the most likely diagnoses?
4. Based on your current impression, what treatment will you order?

Case 3. A 67-year-old male complains of shortness of breath, both at rest and on exertion. He is unable to perform normal activities without becoming "winded." Notes occasional cough.
PMH: Hypertension. Former smoker—1 and $^1/_2$ packs per day for 40 years. Medications: OTC cough medicine, enalapril (Vasotec) 5 mg every day for hypertension

1. What additional history would you ask?

Exam: Vital signs: B/P 152/90; no tachypnea; ENT: normal findings; chest: increased AP diameter, hyperresonance on percussion, decreased expansion on respiration, no abnormal breath sounds; extremities: no edema, no nail clubbing

2. What diagnostic tests would you order?
3. What is your differential diagnosis?
4. What would you do for this patient on this visit?

REFERENCES

American College of Chest Physicians Consensus Statement. (1998). Managing cough as a defense mechanism and as a symptom. *Chest, 114* (2; Suppl. 2).

American Lung Association. Available at: www.lungusa.org.

American Thoracic Society. (1990). Diagnostic standards and classification of tuberculosis. *American Review Respiratory Disease, 142,* 725–735.

American Thoracic Society. (1997). Standards for the diagnosis and care of patients with chronic obstructive pulmonary disease. *American Journal Respiratory Critical Care Medicine, 152,* 577–5120.

Bach, P. B., et al. (2003). Screening for lung cancer: The guidelines. *Chest, 123* (Suppl. 1), 83S.

Bach, P. B., et al. (2001). Management of acute exacerbations of chronic obstructive pulmonary disease: A summary and appraisal of published evidence. *Ann Intern Med, 134,* 600.

Barnes, P. J. (2000). Chronic obstructive pulmonary disease. *NEJM, 343,* 269.

Bartlett, J. G., et al. (2000). Practice guidelines for the management of community-acquired pneumonia in adults. *Clinical Infectious Diseases, 31,* 347–382.

Bilello, K. S., et al. (2002). Epidemiology, etiology, and prevention of lung cancer. *Clinical Chest Medicine, 23, 1.*

Busse, W. W., et al. (2001). Asthma. *NEJM, 344,* 350.

Drugs for asthma. (1999 January 15). *Med Letter, 41,*1044, 5–10.

Gilbert, D. (2004). *Sanford guide to antimicrobial therapy.* Hyde Park, VT: Antimicrobial Therapy, Inc.

Mandell, L. A., et al. (2003). Update of practice guidelines for the management of community-acquired pneumonia in immunocompetent adults. *Clin Infect Dis, 37,* 1405–1433.

National Asthma Education Program. (1997). Expert Panel Report 2: Guidelines for the diagnosis and management of asthma. NIH Publication No. 97-4051. Washington, DC: US Government Printing Office.

National Asthma Education and Prevention Program. (2002). Expert Panel Report: Guidelines for the diagnosis and management of asthma update on selected topics. NIH Publication No. 02-5075, Washington, DC: US Department of Health and Human Services. Available at: www.nhlbi.nih.gov/guidelines/asthma/index.htm.

National Cancer Institute. National Cancer Institute Cancer Net. (1999). Non-small Cell Lung Cancer (PDQ) Treatment—Health Professionals. Available at: at cancernet.nci.nih.gov/index.html.

National Institute of Allergy and Infectious Disease. (July 1999). Tuberculosis fact sheet. National Institutes of Health. Available at: http://www.niaid.nih.gov/factsheets/tb.htm.

Pauwels, R. A., et al., for GOLD Scientific Committee: Global strategy for the diagnosis, management, and prevention of chronic obstructive pulmonary disease: National Heart, Lung, and Blood Institute and World Health Organization Global Initiative for Chronic Obstructive Lung Disease (GOLD) executive summary. *Respir Care*, 46, 798–825, 2001. Available at: www.goldcopd.com.

Small, P. M., et al. (2001). Management of tuberculosis in the United States. *NEJM, 345*, 189.

CARDIOVASCULAR DISORDERS

GERIATRIC APPROACH

Normal Changes of Aging
- Normal changes of aging of the cardiovascular system are difficult to separate from changes due to atherosclerosis or lifestyle.

Vascular structure
- The large elastic arteries increase in wall thickness, become dilated, decrease in elastin, and increase in collagen, which cause the arteries to be stiffer and less elastic.
- The average systolic BP increases slightly, probably due to decreased elasticity. Diastolic BP is low, stops rising around midlife, and then decreases slightly.

Cardiovascular function at rest
- Heart rate decreases slightly, as does the respiratory variation in heart rate.
- Right side of the heart takes longer to fill: preload (amount of blood going into the heart)
  - Time between aortic valve closure and mitral valve opening becomes prolonged
  - Peak rate at which the LV fills with blood in early diastole is decreased
  - Reduced filling rate may be due to decreased muscle speed of contraction of heart muscle
- Afterload (the force against which the ventricle must contract to eject blood, or the arterial pressure, resistance)
  - Stroke volume determined by level of myocardial contractility, vascular afterload, compliance of the arteries
  - Age-related arterial stiffness increases afterload resistance against which heart works to push out the blood
  - Cardiac pump and myocardial contractile function is decreased, causing a decreased ability to compensate for increased afterload
- In conclusion, overall resting cardiac output not affected as the heart adapts to decreased elasticity of the arteries

Cardiovascular response to stress
- Slower response to change in position
- There is an age-related decrease in cardiac output during exercise. This is because the heart does not increase its rate as much as when younger due to the slowed cardiac refilling in the diastolic interval.
- The stroke volume does not decline with age.
- Beta-adrenergic stimulation—myocardial and vascular responses to beta-adrenergic stimulation decline with age

Clinical Implications

History
- Remember nonspecific presentation of illness in the elderly; many cardiovascular conditions present with vague symptoms in the elderly

Physical
- Supine and standing blood pressure to detect postural hypotension
- "White coat" hypertension—excessive variability in BP in presence of person taking BP; if suspected, obtain series of BPs taken outside of office setting

Assessment
- Incidence of coronary atherosclerosis increases with age, but disease is not universal aspect of aging
- Problems related to myocardial infarction are one of the four leading causes of malpractice lawsuits. In order to reduce legal liability in a patient with chest pain, the clinician must accurately answer two questions: (1) Does the patient have a significant problem? (2) Can the patient go home today?

Treatment
Clinical practice should adhere to national guidelines, such as the proceedings of JNC VII; Report of the Joint National Committee on the Prevention, Detection, Evaluation, and Treatment of High Blood Pressure (May 2003); and the Third Report of the National Cholesterol Education Program Expert Panel on Detection, Evaluation, and Treatment of High Blood Cholesterol in Adults—Adult Treatment Panel III (2001). In July 2004, NCEP published an update to *ATPIII: Implications of Recent Clinical Trials for the National Cholesterol Education Program Adult Treatment Panel III Guidelines*. The ATP III update has been endorsed by the National Heart, Lung, and Blood Institute, the American Heart Association, and the American College of Cardiology. Based on a review of five clinical trials of cholesterol-lowering statin treatment that were conducted since the release of ATP III, the update offers options for more intensive cholesterol-lowering treatment for people at high risk and moderately high risk for a heart attack.
- Many cardiovascular problems respond well to nonpharmacologic measures. Educate patient to modify lifestyle risk factors. Elderly people respond well to modifications, such as decreased salt intake and weight loss.
- Medications—start low, go slow; elderly people often start at one-half usual adult dose
- Medication compliance is a major problem with chronic cardiac disorders; consider dosing regimens, cost, and side effects to improve outcome
- There are many classes and many drugs in each class of cardiovascular drugs. Be knowledgeable about two or three drugs from each class and prescribe these drugs.
- Pharmacologic intervention is lifelong; therefore, treatment outcomes will be highly correlated to the quality of the relationship the clinician develops with the patient.

CORONARY ARTERY DISEASE (CAD)

Description
- Also called ischemic heart disease and coronary artery disease
- ISD or CAD resulting from atherosclerotic lesions may reduce blood flow to an artery, thus decreasing myocardial oxygen and may progress to the subsequent chest discomfort associated with angina.
  - Classic—substernal pressure or heaviness associated with exertion or anxiety, resolving with rest
  - Atypical symptoms, silent ischemia are more common in the elderly
  - Angina is a clinical manifestation of myocardial ischemia and CAD
  Types of angina include:
    Stable: in past 60 days, pain duration less than 15 minutes with no change in frequency, severity, duration of anginal episodes during the preceding 6 weeks
    Unstable: recent change in characteristic angina symptoms

Variant: vasospasm, Prinzmetal's transient ST-segment elevation, at rest, with angina symptoms related to coronary spasm usually involving right coronary artery

Etiology

ATHEROSCLEROSIS

- Atherosclerosis is the only common one of three types of arteriosclerosis
- Plaque forms on the intima lining of artery, composed of lipoproteins, cellular components, and extracellular matrix molecules and cause the inner lining of the blood vessels to thicken and the blood vessel to lose elasticity
- First appears as a fatty streak for about 30 years
- Foam cells form and plaque begins to form
- Develop into multilayered plaque with fibrous cap to stabilize it
- As early as the fourth decade, the plaque becomes unstable: The foam cells necrose and rupture underneath the fibrous cap.
- The fibrous cap tears and bleeds to produce a thrombus, which occludes the blood vessel either completely or partially and causes decreased blood flow and ischemia or necrosis.

Incidence and Demographics

- Leading cause of death and disability in the US
- Male/female ratio before age 40, 8:1; after age 70, 1:1
- Male peak age 50–60; female peak age 60–70

Risk Factors

- A complex multifactorial disease with interrelated risk factors
  - Age: male gender
  - Family history of atherosclerosis (especially under age 50)
  - Elevated low-density lipoprotein (LDL) cholesterol
  - Low high-density lipoprotein (HDL) cholesterol
  - Diabetes mellitus, insulin resistance
  - Metabolic syndrome
  - Hypertension
  - Elevated blood homocysteine levels
  - Markers of inflammation such as C-reactive protein
  - Cigarette smoking
  - Sedentary lifestyle
  - High saturated fat and cholesterol diet
  - Obesity

Prevention and Screening

- Modifiable life style changes (see Risk Factors)—diet, exercise, smoking
- Treatment of comorbid conditions—hypertension, diabetes, hyperlipidemia
- Aspirin 325 mg every day decreases risk for CAD in adults at high risk but also increases incidence of bleeding complications; weigh risk of GI bleed and hemorrhagic stroke versus risk for CVD and stroke
- Elevated plasma homocysteine levels can be treated with folic acid 1 mg every day (with B_6 and B_{12}), but it is unclear if it is effective in reducing the risk of CAD.
- ACE inhibitors reduce fatal and nonfatal vascular events in patients at high risk for CAD, especially in diabetics.
- New research from Women's Health Initiative suggests women with history of oral contraceptive use may be at decreased risk of adverse CAD outcomes.

Assessment

History
- Classic presentation of substernal pressure or heaviness associated with exertion or anxiety and relieved with rest
- Dyspnea most common symptom, chest pain is next most common symptoms in patients over age of 85
- Often asymptomatic
- Substernal pain with radiation to multiple locations: left arm, shoulder, forearm and hand, jaw, neck
- Other common symptoms: delirium, syncope, falls, weakness, nausea, anxiety
- Precipitation: exercise, stress, cold temperature, heavy meal, smoking
- Duration 15 to 20 minutes
- Discomfort relieved by rest or nitroglycerin
- Typical pattern of angina for each patient—multiple subjective descriptions: tightness, squeezing, burning, pressure, heaviness
- A change in the patient's typical pattern is indicative of unstable angina

Physical
- Vital signs: elevation in BP, pulse, and respirations
- Holosystolic murmur, mitral valve prolapse may be present
- Transient S_3 or S_4
- Comorbid conditions: DM, HBP, aortic stenosis, peripheral vascular disease

Diagnostic Studies
- Resting ECG between episodes will be normal in more than 50% of patients
- ECG at the time of the pain should show change
- Evidence of CVD are left ventricular hypertrophy or ST-T wave changes consistent with ischemia and evidence of previous Q-wave MI
- ECG unreliable in patients with bundle branch block, Wolf-Parkinson-White syndrome
- Chest x-ray to rule out CHF
- Refer to cardiologist for relevant tests when indicated
  - Exercise stress test: S-T segment depression
  - Exercise thallium imaging: hypoperfusion found in areas with diminished uptake
  - Echocardiogram to evaluate left ventricular function
- CT not recommended

Differential Diagnosis

CARDIAC
- Pericarditis
- MI
- Aortic dissection
- CHF

GASTROINTESTINAL
- GERD
- Esophageal spasm
- Cholecystitis
- Peptic ulcer

RESPIRATORY
- Costochondral pain
- Asthma
- Pneumothorax
- Pulmonary emboli
- Pneumonia

MUSCULOSKELETAL
- Chest wall syndrome
- Shoulder arthropathy

PSYCHOLOGICAL
- Anxiety
- Panic disorders
- Depression

Management

Nonpharmacologic Treatment
- Reduction of modifiable risk factors: weight, smoking, aerobic activity, low saturated fat and sodium diet
- Careful exercise program based on stress test results
- Coronary artery bypass grafting (CABG)
- Percutaneous transluminal coronary angioplasty (PTCA)

Pharmacologic Treatment
- Acute: nitroglycerin sublingual tablets or buccal spray 0.3–0.6 repeat q 5 min; max 3 doses; if unrelieved after 3 doses—ER

TREATMENT OF STABLE ANGINA
- Optimal management of comorbid conditions—hyperlipidemia, diabetes, CHF, hypertension, arrhythmias
- New guidelines suggest treatment in patients with symptomatic chronic stable angina to prevent MI or death and to reduce symptoms:
  - Aspirin or clopidogrel when aspirin is absolutely contraindicated
  - Beta blockers in patients with previous MI or without previous MI
  - Low-density lipoprotein (LDL) cholesterol-lowering therapy with a statin
  - Angiotensin-converting enzyme (ACE) inhibitor
- Agents that should be used in patients with symptomatic chronic stable angina to reduce symptoms only are sublingual nitroglycerin or nitroglycerin spray for immediate relief of angina.
- Calcium antagonists (long-acting) or long-acting nitrates when beta blockers are clearly contraindicated
- Calcium antagonists (long-acting) or long-acting nitrates combined with beta blockers when beta blockers alone are unsuccessful

DRUG SPECIFICS
- Nitroglycerin 0.3 mg to 0.6 mg SL 5 minutes before any activity likely to produce angina
- Nitrates (long-acting)—used to promote coronary vasodilatation
  - Patient education regarding storage and use of nitroglycerin so it will remain effective, when and how to take it, when to go for medical help
  - Monitor for hypotension
  - Drug tolerance develops rapidly and so patient should have a planned drug free interval of 10 to 14 hours on a scheduled basis
  - Isosorbide dinitrate 5–40 mg tid
  - Isosorbide mononitrate 10–40 mg PO bid or sustained-release 60–120 mg qd
  - Nitro-Dur skin patch 0.2–0.8 mg/h, on for 12 h, off for 12 h
- Aspirin 81–325 mg qd
- Hyperlipidemic medication—lower LDL to 100 or lower. See section on hyperlipidemia
- Beta blockers: decreases heart rate, contractility, and oxygen requirements
  - Monitor bradycardia, fatigue, depression, CHF, asthma
  - Metoprolol (Lopressor) 25–200 mg bid, atenolol (Tenormin) 25–200 mg qd
- Calcium channel blockers: coronary vasodilatation with reduction myocardial oxygen
  - Best drug for vasospasm
  - Monitor headache, pedal edema, constipation
  - Avoid verapamil and diltiazem in patients with arrhythmias
  - Coronary spasm: nifedipine XL (Procardia) 30–120 mg qd; verapamil (Calan) 120–320 mg qd; diltiazem (Cardizem) 120–480 mg qd.
  - Avoid short-acting calcium channel blockers

When to Consult, Refer, Hospitalize
- Dial 911 for unstable angina
- Refer to physician any new diagnosis of CAD, continued symptoms, and failure of medical therapy coronary artery bypass grafting

Follow-up
- Individualize follow-up dependent on symptoms and cardiac status (e.g., CAD, left ventricular function, comorbid conditions)
- See patient a minimum every 3 months

Expected Course
- Prognosis depends of the number of vessels diseased, the severity of obstruction, left ventricular function, presence of complex arrhythmias
- Course unpredictable with sudden death occurring in one-half of cases
- Aggressive treatment of hyperlipidemia has been shown to decrease the incidence of further ischemic events

Complications
- MI, CHF, cardiac arrest, death

Myocardial Infarction

Description
- Myocardial muscle oxygen demand is severely compromised by thrombus formation. This leads to subsequent reduction in coronary blood flow if there is a total coronary occlusion (Q wave transmural infarction) or nonocclusion (non–Q wave nontransmural infarction—patent but highly narrowed artery)

Etiology
- CAD—coronary thrombosis secondary to ruptured atherosclerotic plaque
- Coronary spasm

Incidence and Demographics
- Global incidence with mortality 30% to 40%
- Male preponderance fourth through sixth decade, equal by age 70

Risk Factors
- See CAD risk factors

Prevention and Screening
- Aspirin 81 mg day

Assessment

History
- Often presents as nonspecific presentation of illness in elderly
- Elderly patient may have no symptoms—silent MI
- Shortness of breath, CHF
- Pain radiates at rest or with minimal activity
- Classic: oppressive retrosternal chest pain, not relieved by NTG, nausea or vomiting, accompanied by diaphoresis

Physical
- High incidence of mortality within first hour following cardiac event
- May have obvious pain, usually reduced sensitivity to pain in elders—"silent MI"
- Nonspecific presentation, delirium, syncope, weakness
- Vital signs: hypotension, tachycardia, dyspnea
- General appearance: apprehensive, appears ill, ashen color

- Respiratory: shortness of breath, rales
- Heart: S_3, S_4, new mitral regurgitation murmur, arrhythmia

Diagnostic Studies
- ECG diagnostic 85% cases with ST segment elevation, Q waves, inverted T waves
  - Subendocardial infarction: note ST segment depression (may be only finding)
- Cardiac enzymes (See Table 9-1)
  - Creatine kinase (CK): CK-MB$_1$ and CK-MB$_2$ ratio—if MB$_2$ to MB$_1$ ratio more than 1.5, infarction is suggested (more sensitive early marker prior to elevation of CK-MB)
  - Troponin T or troponin I (not found in muscle or blood of healthy person) are more specific than CK-MB. Become positive 4 to 12 hours after onset of MI
  - LDH—LDH1 exceeds LDH2 levels in pathology, less specific than cardiac enzymes
  - Troponin T and troponin 1 confers greater sensitivity

Differential Diagnosis
- Unstable angina
- Aortic dissection
- Pericarditis
- Pulmonary embolism
- Esophageal spasm
- Biliary tract disease
- Gastroesophageal reflux disease
- Pancreatitis
- Chest wall muscle spasm

Management

Nonpharmacologic Treatment
- Acute: immediate emergency room care for evaluation and stabilization
- Post-MI: low saturated fat and sodium; caloric restrict if appropriate
- Post-MI: treat underlying risk factors—hypertension, hyperlipidemia

Pharmacologic Treatment

ACUTE
- Nitroglycerin SL 0.3–0.6 mg q 5 min, total 3 doses
- Chest pain unrelieved—transport to nearest emergency room or chest pain center
- Aspirin 160–325 mg, preferably chewable
- O_2 via nasal cannula at 2 LPM if available
- Thrombolytic therapy may confer benefit if initiated within 3–12 hours after onset of pain

POSTINFARCTION
- Treatment of hyperlipidemia
- Smoking cessation
- Antiplatelet agent
  - Aspirin 81–325 mg qd unless contraindicated
  - Clopidogrel (Plavix) 75 mg PO qd if unable to tolerate aspirin
- Beta blockers improve survival rates
  - With the exception of marked CHF or bronchospasm, improve mortality
  - Monitor bradycardia, fatigue, depression
  - Metoprolol (Lopressor) 25–200 mg bid

Table 9-1: Cardiac Enzymes in the Diagnosis of MI

Lab	Onset	Comment
CK: MB 1 & 2	3–4 hours	Sensitive, not specific
Troponin I & T	3.5 hours	Highly specific
LDH 1 & 2	24 hours	Sensitive, not specific

- Atenolol (Tenormin) 25–200 mg qd
- Calcium channel blockers are not effective and are indicated for secondary prevention
- ACE inhibitors should be considered for all patients
  - In patients with left ventricular dysfunction, improves morbidity
  - HOPE study showed reduction of mortality in patients without CHF
  - Most effective for patients with diabetes, hypertension
  - Monitor cough and renal function including hyperkalemia
  - Rare life threatening—angioedema caused by drug
  - Lisinopril 2.5–10 mg qd, start with small dose titrate up,
  - Many other ACE inhibitors available, effective; HOPE study used Ramipril
- Glycosides—consider use in CHF
- Nitrates
  - Effective for residual ischemia and coronary atherosclerosis
  - Monitor hypotension

When to Consult, Refer, Hospitalize
- Acute: immediate referral to emergency department
- Initial post-MI care and evaluation by cardiologist

Follow-up
- Long-term management, see at least every 3 months

Expected Course
- Two variables dictate course: status of vessel disease and ventricular damage
  - Left main CAD—20% mortality first year: single vessel has 2% mortality; double vessel damage has 3%–4% mortality; triple vessel damage has 5%–8% mortality
  - Left ventricular dysfunction—EF <40% doubles annual mortality rate
- Overall mortality rate 10% in hospital phase, 10% mortality during first year
- 60% deaths first hour

Complications
- Death
- Chronic heart failure
- Ventricular tachycardia or ventricular fibrillation first 24 hours
- Atrial fibrillation and flutter, bradycardia, heart block
- Deep vein thrombosis, pulmonary embolism, mitral regurgitation, cardiogenic shock

MURMURS

Description
- Abnormal sounds made by turbulent blood flow due to partial obstruction (stenosis) or faulty valve closure (regurgitation) (also called insufficiency) and that are distinguishable from normal heart sounds

Etiology
- Atherosclerosis
- High output state from another medical condition (e.g., anemia, thyrotoxicosis, fever, hypertension)
- Innocent murmurs: no evidence of cardiac pathology
- Rheumatic fever is a potential contributor to all murmurs
- Infective endocarditis: regurgitation murmurs
- Other contributing factors include:
  - Aortic stenosis: differentiate between common benign lesion and one with significant obstruction associated with diabetes, hyperlipidemia, CAD

- Aortic regurgitation: high blood pressure, aortic dissection, collagen vascular disease
- Mitral regurgitation: LVH left ventricular hypertrophy, CAD with ischemia
- Mitral stenosis: rheumatic fever

Incidence and Demographics
- Murmurs are extremely common
- Aortic stenosis murmur present in more than 50% of patients older than age 75, usually benign

Risk Factors
- Age

Prevention and Screening
- Periodic routine cardiac examination

Assessment

History
- Low output due to valvular disease may cause delirium, fatigue, CHF, weight loss, debility

Physical
- Objective terms: guide to identifying murmurs
  - Assessment of murmurs
    - Grading of intensity: See Table 9-2
    - Location—area with greatest intensity
    - Radiation—heard in direction of blood flow
    - Pitch—high, medium, low
    - Quality—soft, harsh, rumbling
- Timing—within the cardiac cycle (systolic between S_1/S_2; diastolic between S_2/S_1)
  - Once auscultated, a murmur must be identified as systolic or diastolic
    - S_1 is mitral and tricuspid valve closure
    - S_2 is aortic and pulmonic valve closure
    - The period between S_1 and S_2 is systole
    - The period between S_2 and S_1 is diastole

Diastole	Systole	Diastole	Systole
S_2 A/P close M/T open	S_1 M/T close A/P close	S_2 A/P close M/T open	S_1 M/T close A/P close

- Murmurs that occur after S_1 and before S_2 are systolic murmurs
  - Mitral and tricuspid regurgitation (backflow through an incompetent valve)
  - Aortic and pulmonic stenosis (turbulent flow through a tight opening)

Table 9-2: Grading of Murmurs

Grade	Characteristics
I/VI	Very faint, and may not be heard in all positions
II/VI	Quiet but heard immediately upon placing the stethoscope on the chest
III/VI	Moderately loud
IV/VI	Loud accompanied by palpable thrill
V/VI	Very loud, heard with a stethoscope partly off the chest; accompanied by palpable thrill
VI/VI	Heard with the stethoscope entirely off the chest and accompanied by palpable thrill

Figure 9-1: Standard Chest Ausculatory Points

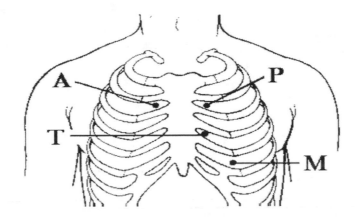

- Murmurs that occur after S_2 and before S_1 are diastolic murmurs
  - Aortic and pulmonic regurgitation (backflow through an incompetent valve)
  - Mitral and tricuspid stenosis (turbulent flow through a tight opening)
- Placement of murmurs (See Figure 9-1)
  - Once murmurs are identified as systolic or diastolic, the likely valve of origin must be identified by location.
  - Murmurs loudest at the second intercostals space, right sternal border are likely aortic murmurs.
  - Murmurs loudest at the second intercostals space, left sternal border are likely pulmonic murmurs.
  - Murmurs loudest at the fourth intercostals space, left sternal border are likely tricuspid murmurs.
  - Murmurs loudest at the fifth intercostals space, midclavicular line are likely mitral murmurs.
- Systolic regurgitant murmur: murmur begins with S_1 and usually lasts throughout systole (pansystolic or holosystolic); caused by blood flow from a chamber that is at a higher pressure throughout systole than the receiving chamber (ONLY associated with VSD, MR, TR)
- Diastolic: early diastolic (caused by the incompetence of the aortic or pulmonary valve—AR, PR); mid-diastolic (caused by turbulence of the tricuspid or mitral valve); or presystolic (caused by flow through the atrioventricular valves during ventricular diastole—TS, MS)
- Continuous murmur: S_1 through S_2; conditions such as PDA
- Innocent heart murmurs (functional, physiologic, benign)
- Left sternal border (LSB) second through fourth left interspaces and apex
  - Grade I-II/VI; low pitch; soft, short, nonradiating, midsystolic
  - Variable loudness—heard best in supine position and diminishes with upright position
- Interpretation of murmurs
- Once timing and placement are identified, the valvular disorder is evident
  - A systolic murmur at the second intercostal space, right sternal border is an aortic murmur occurring when the aortic valve is open—aortic stenosis
  - A diastolic murmur at the second intercostals space, right sternal border is an aortic murmur occurring when the aortic valve is closed—aortic regurgitation
  - A systolic murmur at the fifth intercostals space, midclavicular line is a mitral murmur occurring when the mitral valve is closed—mitral regurgitation

Table 9-3: Types of Murmurs

Systolic Murmur	• Occurs between S_1 and S_2 • Systolic ejection murmur—interval between S_1 and the onset of the murmur (also referred to as crescendo-decrescendo); caused by blood flow through stenotic or deformed semilunar valves or by increased blood flow through normal semilunar valves • Systolic regurgitant murmur—murmur begins with S_1 and usually lasts throughout systole (pansystolic or holosystolic); caused by blood flow from a chamber that is at a higher pressure throughout systole than the receiving chamber (ONLY associated with ventricular septal defect [VSD], mitral, and tricuspid regurgitation [MR and TR])
Diastolic Murmur	• Occurs between S_2 and S_1 • Classified as early diastolic and caused by the incompetence of the aortic or pulmonary valve, atrial and pulmonic regurgitation (AR, PR), mid-diastolic, caused by turbulence of the tricuspid or mitral valve, or presystolic, caused by flow through the atrioventricular valves during ventricular diastole (tricuspid or mitral stenosis TS, MS)
Continuous Murmur	• Occurs with S_1 and continues through the S_2 into diastole • Seen with conditions such as patent ductus arteriosus (PDA), pulmonary artery (PA) stenosis, Blalock-Taussig shunt
Innocent Heart Murmurs (Functional Murmur)	• Murmurs that arise from cardiovascular structures in absence of anatomic abnormalities (80% of children have innocent murmurs sometime throughout childhood usually beginning at age 3 years old); also referred to as functional, benign, or physiological murmurs

- A diastolic murmur occurring at the fifth intercostals space, midclavicular line is a mitral murmur occurring when the mitral valve is open—mitral stenosis

Systolic Murmurs (See Table 9-3)

AORTIC STENOSIS

- Second intercostal space (IC) right of sternum, with patient sitting and leaning forward
- Valve is open when stenotic murmur occurs and is caused by forward flow through stenotic valve
- Begins after S_1 and is a crescendo-decrescendo or diamond-shaped ejection murmur
- Radiation into neck from aortic area
- Medium pitch with intensity variable
- Harsh, loudest at base; musical at apex
- Midsystolic
- Systolic thrill may be present
- Seen frequent in the elderly and associated with a diminished S_2

TRICUSPID REGURGITATION

- Lower LSB
- Begins with S_1; high-pitched, smooth, blowing quality
- Pansystolic regurgitant murmur, increases in intensity with inspiration
- Right ventricular lift
- Always associated with pathology, usually diseased right ventricle from rheumatic heart disease

VENTRICULAR SEPTAL DEFECT

- LSB (third to fifth ICS)
- Radiation wide over precordium but not into axilla
- Loud (particularly base), harsh, pansystolic regurgitant murmur with thrill

Hypertrophic obstructive cardiomyopathy
- LSB
- No radiation
- Murmur increases with Valsalva maneuver, decreases with patient squatting
- Midsystolic

Pulmonic stenosis
- LSB second or third ICS, pulmonary area
- Generally no radiation unless loud and than toward left neck
- Variable intensity, medium pitch
- Midsystolic; begins after S_1 with crescendo-decrescendo contour
- Associated with thrill if significant pathology; usually congenital cause

Mitral regurgitation
- Location-apex; frequently radiates to wide area of chest and to left axilla
- Intensity variable, often loud; does not increase with inspiration
- Pitch is high with a blowing quality
- S_3 usually also heard
- Pansystolic regurgitant murmur frequently accompanied with thrill
- Begins with S_1 (which may be decreased)
- Valve is closed when the murmur occurs; noise caused from backflow through incompetent valve
- Always pathologic

Diastolic Murmurs
- Always indicative of heart disease
- Often heard best with bell of the stethoscope

Mitral stenosis
- Listen with patient in left lateral decubitus position; also with exercise
- Diastolic rumbling murmur that begins after a short period of silence after S_2
- Low in pitch, heard best with bell of stethoscope in light skin contact
- No radiation
- Loudest at apex; best heard after mild exercise

Aortic regurgitation
- Heard at LSB with patient leaning forward and listening with *diaphragm* pressed firmly on the chest
- Early diastolic murmur that begins immediately after S_2 and diminishes in intensity
- Blowing, high-pitched, decrescendo
- Heard with rheumatic heart disease or syphilis

Pulmonary valve insufficiency
- LSB second ICS
- Radiates mid-right sternal border
- High-pitched, loudest base, decrescendo murmur

Continuous murmurs (quality often varies when patient changes position)
- Patent ductus arteriosus
- Coarctation of the aorta
- Peripheral pulmonary stenosis

Diagnostic Studies
- Electrocardiogram to detect underlying heart disease
- CBC to look for signs of infection, anemia
- Chest x-ray to evaluate heart failure, size of heart

Table 9.4: Characteristics of Common Murmurs

Murmur	Grade	Location	Radiation	Pitch	Quality	Timing	Significance
Systolic							
Innocent	I - III, variable	2nd–4th ICS LSBB	None	Medium	Soft	Short early to midsystolic	None
Stenosis							
Aortic	Variable	Aortic	Neck, LSB	Medium	Harsh	Crescendo-decrescendo, midsystolic	Common, cause CHF, angina and syncope
Pulmonic	Variable	Pulmonic area and 3rd ICS LSB	Left shoulder	Medium	Harsh	Crescendo-decrescendo, midsystolic	Rare, pathologic
Regurgitation							
Mitral	Often loud	Mitral	Left axilla	High	Blowing	Pansystolic	Common, pulmonary edema, arrhythmia, CHF
Tricuspid	Variable	Tricuspid	Right of sternum, left MCL	High	Blowing	Pansystolic	Always pathologic
Diastolic							
Stenosis							
Mitral	Variable	Mitral	Little	Low	Rumbling	Begins after short pause after S_2, decrescendo, crescendo	Rare, pulmonary edema, atrial fibrillation
Regurgitation							
Aortic	Often faint	Aortic	Down LSB	High	Blowing	Decrescendo, early systole	LVH, dilation of left ventricle

- Echocardiography—valve pathology and systolic/diastolic function
- Angiography for more thorough evaluation
- Fluoroscopy—demonstrates calcified aortic valve

Differential Diagnosis (See Table 9-4)
- See descriptions of systolic and diastolic murmurs

Management

Nonpharmacologic Treatment
- Patient education on disease entity and lifestyle modifications for underlying disorder
- Valvular surgical repair

Pharmacologic Treatment
- Stabilize hemodynamic deficiencies
- Antibiotics for endocarditis prophylaxis as indicated

How Long to Treat
- Often a chronic condition

Special Considerations
- Geriatrics: aortic stenosis common

When to Consult, Refer, Hospitalize
- Consult or refer if symptomatic (signs of heart failure, growth failure, syncope, cyanosis); diastolic murmur; systolic murmur that is loud (grade III/IV or with a thrill), long in duration, and transmits well to other parts of the body; abnormally strong or weak pulses; abnormal cardiac size or silhouette or pulmonary vasculature on CXR
- If abnormal ECG and symptomatic hospitalization may be necessary

Follow-up
- Asymptomatic patients should be assessed at least annually and at every visit
- Innocent murmurs—no follow-up necessary

Complications
- Chronic heart failure
- Poor activity tolerance; growth and development problems
- Progression of mitral stenosis has potential for thrombus formation and hypoxia
- Progression of mitral regurgitation is associated with dyspnea and orthopnea
- Atrial fibrillation with mitral stenosis and mitral regurgitation
- Stroke and/or TIA
- Bacterial endocarditis

HYPERTENSION

Description
- The following discussion is based primarily on the Seventh Report of the Joint National Committee on Prevention, Detection, Evaluation, and Treatment of High Blood Pressure (JNC VII) 2003.
- Systolic blood pressure (SBP) $\oplus$140 mm Hg and/or diastolic blood pressure (DBP) $\oplus$90
- Hypertension is classified by severity (see Table 9-5)
- Hypertension is classified as either primary (essential) or secondary
  - Primary hypertension 95% of hypertension
  - Isolated systolic hypertension: a subset of primary hypertension
    More common in the elderly
    Defined as systolic greater than 140 with DBP less than 90
    Stronger cardiovascular risk factor than elevated DBP in the elderly

Table 9-5: Classification of Blood Pressure

Category	Classification of Blood Pressure for Adults Aged 18 Years and Older* Blood Pressure, mm Hg	
	Systolic	Diastolic
Normal	<120 and	<80
Prehypertension	120 to 139 or	80 to 89
Stage 1 Hypertension	140 to 159 or	90 to 99
Stage 2 Hypertension	>160 or	>100

*Based on the average of 2 or more readings taken at each of 2 or more visits after an initial screening.

- Secondary Hypertension, 5% of all hypertension, less common in the elderly
  - Sudden onset of hypertension in the elderly is often from secondary cause

Etiology
- Primary hypertension —no known cause
- Isolated systolic hypertension—elevated pulse pressure (SBP – DBP) due to reduced vascular compliance
- Secondary hypertension
  - Renal parenchymal disease
  - Renal vascular disease
  - Cushing's disease
  - Pheochromocytoma
  - Hyperaldosteronism
  - Coarctation of the aorta
  - Sleep apnea
  - Thyroid/parathyroid disease
- Pharmacologic
  - Oral corticosteroids
  - Cocaine
  - NSAIDs
  - Sympathomimetics: decongestants
  - Estrogens
  - Alcohol
  - Cyclosporine
  - Amphetamines
  - Erythropoietin
  - MAO inhibitors

Incidence and Demographics
- 64% of patients over age 60
- Males more than females
- NHANES III study of Americans aged 60 and older: elevated BP found in 60% non-Hispanic white, 71% non-Hispanic African Americans, 61% Mexican Americans
- Diastolic pressure tends to stabilize after age 60, but rising SBP increases rapidly after age 55.

Risk Factors
- Smoking
- Dyslipidemia
- Diabetes mellitus
- Age older than 60 years
- Gender (men and postmenopausal women)
- Family history of cardiovascular disease: women under age 65 or men under age 55
- African American
- Obesity (BMI ⊕30 kg/m^2)
- Stress
- Excessive dietary intake of sodium

Prevention and Screening
- Annual blood pressure screening

Assessment
- Identify severity of hypertension; see Table 9-5
- Signs and symptoms of secondary hypertension
  - Renal parenchymal disease: urinalysis: proteinuria, elevated serum creatinine
  - Renal vascular disease: renal bruits, symptoms variable or absent depending if infarction occurred
  - Cushing's disease: fatigue, weakness, bruising, osteoporosis, truncal obesity, hyperglycemia
  - Pheochromocytoma: episodes of flushing, palpitations, pallor, tremor, profuse perspiration, angina, diaphoresis
  - Hyperaldosteronism: muscle weakness, cramps, paresthesia, decreased serum potassium and magnesium, increased urine potassium and serum sodium
  - Coarctation of the aorta: weak peripheral pulses, CXR
- Target organ damage (TOD)
- Heart
  - Left ventricular hypertrophy: PMI displaced to the left, S_4 gallop
  - Angina/history of MI
  - Prior coronary revascularization
  - Chronic heart failure: S_3, bilateral basilar rales (crackles), peripheral edema
- Brain
  - Stroke or transient ischemic attack: abnormal neuro exam
- Chronic kidney disease
  - Peripheral arterial disease: decreased pedal pulses
- Retinopathy: Scheie Classification
  - Grade 1—slight generalized attenuation of retinal arterioles
  - Grade 2—obvious arteriolar narrowing with focal areas of attenuation
  - Grade 3—Grade 2 plus retinal exudates, cotton-wool spots, and hemorrhages
  - Grade 4—Grade 3 plus optic nerve edema

History
- Known duration and levels of elevated BP
- Symptoms of CVD, heart failure, cerebrovascular disease, peripheral vascular disease, renal disease, diabetes mellitus, dyslipidemia, other comorbid conditions, gout, or sexual dysfunction
- Family history of high blood pressure, premature CVD, stroke, diabetes, dyslipidemia, or renal disease
- Symptoms suggesting causes of hypertension
- History of recent changes in weight, leisure time physical activity, and smoking or other tobacco use
- Dietary assessment including intake of sodium, alcohol, saturated fat, and caffeine
- History of all prescribed and OTC medications, herbal remedies, and illicit drugs
- Results and adverse effects of previous antihypertensive therapy
- Psychosocial and environmental factors that may influence hypertension control

Physical
- Two or more blood pressure measurements (see Table 9-6)
- Verification in the contralateral arm
- Height, weight, and waist circumference
- Funduscopic examination for hypertensive retinopathy: arteriolar narrowing, focal arteriolar constrictions, arteriovenous crossing changes, hemorrhages and exudates, disc edema
- Neck carotid bruits, distended veins, or an enlarged thyroid gland

Table 9-6: Essential Criteria for Measuring Blood Pressure

Criterion	Process
Have patient rest for 5 minutes	Two or more readings taken at each of 2 or more visits after an initial screening
Patient sitting in chair with arm supported	If BP is stage 3, take 3 times at one visit and start management at that visit
Use correct size cuff	Readings 2 minutes apart
Use mercury sphygmomanometer or recently calibrated aneroid	Patient refrain from smoking or caffeine 30 minutes prior to reading
Patient not acutely ill	

- Heart rate rhythm, increased size, precordial heave, clicks, murmurs, and third and fourth heart sounds
- Lung rales and evidence for bronchospasm
- Abdomen bruits, enlarged kidneys, masses, or abnormal aortic pulsation
- Extremities for diminished or absent peripheral arterial pulsations, bruits, and edema
- Neurological assessment

Diagnostic Studies
- General workup
  - Blood chemistry: potassium, sodium, creatinine, fasting glucose
  - Lipids—total cholesterol and HDL
  - 12-lead electrocardiogram
  - CBC
  - Urinalysis
- Additional optional workup JNC VII
  - Creatinine clearance, microalbuminuria, 24-hour urinary protein, blood calcium, uric acid, fasting triglycerides, LDL, glycosylated hemoglobin, TSH, and echocardiography
  - Renal disease suspected: renal and abdominal vascular ultrasound and renal arteriogram if indicated

Differential Diagnosis
- See Etiology

Management
- Goal is lower than 140/90 for most patients but 130/80 for those with diabetes or renal disease

Nonpharmacologic Treatment
- See Box 9-1
- Lifestyle changes are recommended for patients with prehypertension and for ALL patients with hypertension

Pharmacologic Treatment (See Tables 9-7, Figure 9-2, and Table 9-8)
- Because clinical studies have shown proven benefit of diuretics in blood pressure reduction, the JNC VII recommends starting with a diuretic unless patient has compelling indication or comorbid condition affecting choice of medication.
- Diuretics and ace inhibitors are appropriate for initial treatment of hypertension in the elderly
- Many elderly have compelling indications to start with another drug
- Individualized treatment plan should be implemented considering the patient's risk factors, TOD, compelling indications, and concomitant disease
- Most patients will need two or more medications to achieve control

Box 9-1: Life Style Modifications for Prevention and Management of Hypertension

Smoking cessation

Lose weight if overweight, and reduce intake of dietary saturated fats and cholesterol

Limit alcohol intake to no more than 1 oz (30 mL) ethanol (e.g., 24 oz [720 mL] beer, 10 oz [300 mL] wine, or 2 oz [60 mL] 100-proof whiskey) per day or 0.5 oz (15 mL) ethanol per day for women and lighter-weight people

Increase physical activity (30 to 45 minutes most days of the week)

Reduce sodium intake to no more than 100 mmol per day (2.4 g sodium, 6 g sodium chloride, or 1 teaspoon)

Maintain adequate intake of dietary potassium (approximately 90 mmol or 2 g per day), calcium and magnesium

Modified from the Seventh Report of the Joint National Committee on Prevention, Detection, Evaluation and Treatment of High Blood Pressure, NIH, 2003.

DIURETICS (See Table 9-9)

- Target groups: CHF, older patients, blacks, smokers
- Avoid history gout, DM (high dose), hyperparathyroidism, and dyslipidemia
- Thiazide-type diuretics are first-line therapy
- In general, hydrochlorothiazide is preferred over chlorthalidone in elderly because it has a shorter half-life and may have less risk of adverse effects.
- Furosemide (Lasix) is used in patients with renal insufficiency.
- Spironolactone is potassium-sparing diuretic often used for CHF.

BETA BLOCKERS (BB) (SEE TABLE 9-10)

- Target Groups: post-MI, angina, arrhythmias, tremor, hyperthyroid
- First-line therapy
- Avoid asthma, conduction disorders, bradycardia, heart block
- Use with caution in diabetes mellitus (masks symptoms of hypoglycemia)
- Cardioselective beta blockers have greater effect on cardiac receptors than lung receptors as lower doses and are recommended in the elderly
- CHF: carvedilol (Coreg)

Table 9-7: Pharmacological Treatment for Hypertension

BP Classification	Without Compelling Indication	With Compelling Indication
Prehypertension 130–139/85–89	Lifestyle modification	Drugs for compelling indications
Stage 1 140–159/90–99	Diuretic for most; may consider ACEI, ARB, BB, CCB, or combination	Drug(s) for the compelling indications; other antihypertensive drugs (diuretics, ACEI, ARB, BB, CCB as needed)
Stage 2 160 or more/100 or more	Two drug combination for most (usually diuretic and ACEI or ARB or BB or CCB)	

Modified from the Seventh Report of the Joint National Committee on Prevention, Detection, Evaluation, and Treatment of High Blood Pressure, NIH, 2003.
Diuretic: thiazide type
ACEI: angiotensin converting enzyme inhibitor
ARB: angiotensin receptor blocker
BB: beta blocker
CCB: calcium channel blocker

Figure 9-2: Drug Choice for Treatment of Hypertension

Begin or Continue Lifestyle Modifications

↓

Not at Goal Blood Pressure (<140/90 mg/Hg)
130/80 for patients with diabetes or chronic kidney disease

↓

Initial Drug Choices
Start with a low dose of a long-acting once-daily drug, and titrate dose
Low-dose combinations may be appropriate

Without Compelling Indications
Diuretics
May Consider
Beta blockers
ACE inhibitors
Angiotensin receptor blockers
Calcium channel blockers

Compelling Indications
See Table 9-8 for drugs
Diabetes mellitus
Heart failure
Myocardial infarction
High CVD risk
Chronic kidney disease
Recurrent stroke prevention

Not at Goal Blood Pressure

↓

No response or troublesome side effects

↓

Substitute another drug from a different class

Inadequate response but well tolerated

↓

Add a second agent from a different class
(diuretic if not already used)

↓   ↓

Not at Goal Blood Pressure

↓

Continue adding agents from other classes
Consider referral to a hypertension specialist

Modified from the Seventh Report of the Joint National Committee on Prevention, Detection, Evaluation, and Treatment of High Blood Pressure, NIH, 2003.

Table 9-8: Drug Choices for Compelling Indications

Compelling Indication	Diuretic	BB	ACEI	ARB	CCB	Aldo Ant*
Heart Failure	x	x	x	x		x
Post-MI		x	x			x
High CVD risk	x	x	x		x	
Diabetes	x	x	x	x	x	
Chronic Kidney Disease			x	x		
Recurrent Stroke Prevention	x		x			

Modified from the Seventh Report of the Joint National Committee on Prevention, Detection, Evaluation and Treatment of High Blood Pressure, NIH, 2003.
*Aldo Ant: aldosterone antagonist diuretic, spironolactone

Table 9-9: Examples of Recommended Diuretic Therapy

Drug	Dose Range	Side Effects
Hydrochlorothiazide (HCTZ)	12.5–50 mg q AM	Anorexia, nausea, vomiting, cramping, dehydration,
Chlorthalidone	6.25–25 mg qd	hypokalemia, hypercalcemia, hyperlipidemia,
Furosemide (Lasix)	20–80 mg qd	hyperglycemia
Spironolactone	12.5–50 qd	Hyperkalemia, hyponatremia, gynecomastia, GI disturbances, drowsiness

Table 9-10: Examples of Recommended Beta-Blocker Therapy

Drug	Dosage	Side Effects
Metoprolol (Lopressor)	50–100 mg qd or bid	Bradycardia, depression, fatigue, exercise
Atenolol (Tenormin)	25–100 mg qd	intolerance, asthma, sexual dysfunction

ANGIOTENSIN CONVERTING ENZYME INHIBITORS (ACE) (See Table 9-11)
- Target Groups: DM, CHF, post-MI
- Well tolerated; do not cause hyperlipidemia or hyperglycemia
- Avoid use in renal stenosis, elevated creatinine
- Captopril seldom used due to increased incidence of cough, frequency of dosing

ANGIOTENSIN RECEPTOR BLOCKERS (ARB) (See Table 9-12)
- Target groups: identical to ACE, with inability to tolerate ACE due to cough
- Avoid in renovascular disease

CALCIUM CHANNEL BLOCKERS (CCB) (See Table 9-13)
- Target groups: angina, CAD, African Americans, migraine, isolated systolic in elderly, arrhythmia (non-dihydropyridine)
- Contraindicated in conduction disorders
- Three types of calcium channel blockers
- Dihydropyridine—prototype nifedipine, now many others including amlodipine
  - Do not affect cardiac conduction system

Table 9-11: Examples of Recommended Ace Inhibitor Therapy

Drug	Dosage	Side Effects
Prinivil (Lisinopril, Zestril)	2.5–40 mg qd	Hyperkalemia, angioedema, headache, dizziness, fatigue
Ramipril (Altace)	1.25–20 mg qd	

Table 9-12: Examples of Recommended Angiotensin Receptor Blockers

Drug	Dosage	Side Effects
Losartan (Cozaar)	25–100 mg qd	Rare side effects: dizziness, insomnia, muscle cramps, leg pain,
Valsartan (Diovan)	40–320 mg qd	hyperkalemia

Table 9-13: Examples of Recommended Calcium Channel Blocker Therapy

Drug	Dosage	Side Effects
Dihydropyridines		Edema, fatigue, palpitations, dizziness, GI upset, flushing
Nifedipine (Procardia XL)	30–90 mg PO qd	abdominal pain, drowsiness
Amlodipine (Norvasc)	2.5–10 mg qd	
Verapamil (Calan SR)	120–480 mg qd	Constipation, edema, bradycardia, headache, fatigue, CHF, AV block
Diltiazem (Cardizem LA)	120–360 mg qd	Edema, headache, bradycardia, fatigue, AV block, flushing, nausea, CHF, liver abnormalities

- Nondihydropyridine calcium channel blockers
  - Verapamil—affects cardiac conduction system
  - Cardizem has characteristics of both Verapamil and dihydropyridine calcium channel blockers
- Avoid beta blocker and nondihydropyridine calcium channel blocker combination
- Research has shown that short-acting nifedipine increases cardiac morbidity

Special Considerations
- Monitor for side effects of medications particularly orthostatic hypotension and dehydration in frail elderly and those with comorbid disease and polypharmacy

When to Consult, Refer, Hospitalize
- Refer as needed for secondary causes of hypertension
- Consult physician when no response to first-line therapy
- Hypertension emergencies
- Refer for target organ damage/clinical cardiovascular disease

Follow-up
- Follow up 4 to 6 weeks until BP controlled, every 3 to 6 months depending on clinical situation
- Routine visits 3 to 6 months depending on patient clinical situation
- SBP >180 or DBP >110 and follow-up in 48 to 72 hours

Complications
- Stroke, CAD, CHF, target organ damage, aortic dissection

HYPERLIPIDEMIA

Description
- A laboratory measurement of blood lipids showing elevation of cholesterol and/or triglycerides
- Lipids are carried in lipoproteins, which are classified by density
  - High-density lipoproteins facilitate the transfer of cholesterol from the periphery to the liver
  - Low-density lipoproteins facilitate transfer of cholesterol from the liver to the periphery
- This discussion based on the Third Report of the National Cholesterol Education Program (NCEP) Expert Panel on Detection, Evaluation, and Treatment of High Blood Cholesterol in Adults (Adult Treatment Panel III); see References, available at www.nhlbi.nih.gov/guidelines/cholesterol.
- The third report emphasizes importance of LDL, with recommendations to further decrease LDL levels and recognizes diabetes and peripheral arterial disease as well as clinical CAD as high-risk equivalents for coronary heart disease.
- While the NCEP panel emphasizes LDL, triglycerides are known to be an independent risk factor for CVD.

Etiology

- Genetic hyperlipidemia
- Diet: excessive carbohydrate intake, weight gain; increased saturated fat or alcohol intake
- Diseases: diabetes mellitus, hypothyroidism, pancreatitis, renal disease, liver disease
- Medications: oral contraceptives, diuretics, beta blockers corticosteroids

Incidence and Demographics

- See CVD, metabolic syndrome
- Total cholesterol levels increase and achieve plateau in middle age and decline slightly after age 70

Risk Factors

- Hyperlipidemia is a major risk factor for cardiovascular disease
- See assessment

Prevention and Screening

- Low-fat diet
- Annual screening for hyperlipidemia indicated up to age 65
- Meta-analyses have not found cholesterol to be a risk factor for CVD for persons over age 75.
- Consider general health, comorbidities, and life expectancy when counseling regarding screening and treatment of cholesterol over age 75, remembering statins seem to confer protective qualities beyond lowering of LDL

Assessment

- Determine the patient's overall risk status for CVD
  - LDL level
  - Presence of CVD
  - Determine if patient has CVD risk equivalent:
    Presence of clinical forms of atherosclerotic disease
    Type 2 diabetes
    Multiple risk factors that confer a 10-year risk for CVD greater than 20% (use Framingham calculation found online at www.nhlbi.nih.gov/guidelines/cholesterol/risk)
  - Count number of risk factors
    Age: male, age ≥45 or female, age ≥55
    Family history of premature CVD: CVD in male first-degree relative less than 55 years OR CVD in female first-degree relative less than 65 years
    Current cigarette smoking
    Hypertension: blood pressure ≥140/90 OR patient is presently taking antihypertensive medication
    Low HDL cholesterol (less than 40)
    Negative risk factor: high HDL, greater than 60

History

- CVD risk factors
- Comorbid disease
- Medications
- Family history

Physical

- Xanthomas
- Obesity
- Funduscopic exam: Scheie Classification
  - Grade 1—broadening of arteriolar light reflex, minimal A/V crossing changes
  - Grade 2—obvious broadening of arteriolar light reflex and A/V crossing changes

- Grade 3—copper-wire arterioles and more marked A/V crossing changes
- Grade 4—silver-wire arterioles and severe A/V crossing changes
- Look for signs of comorbid disease, complications of hyperlipidemia

Diagnostic Studies

- Complete fasting lipid profile: total cholesterol, HDL, LDL, triglycerides (see Table 9-14)
- Liver function tests
- Routine blood chemistries
- Urinalysis

Differential Diagnosis

- See Etiology

Management

- Intensity of treatment depends on the patient's overall risk status for CVD (see Table 9-15)

Nonpharmacologic Treatment

- Diet—all patients with hyperlipidemia should be started on Step 2 diet
  - Diet produces variable results, especially long term
  - Step 1 diet: reduces total fat to 30% of total calorie intake and saturated fat to 10%, cholesterol to 300 mg/d
    Reduces serum cholesterol by 3%–14%
  - Step 2 diet: further reduces saturated fat to 7% and cholesterol to 200 mg/d
    Additional 3%–7% benefit compared with Step 1
  - Caloric restriction
  - Increase dietary fiber—oatmeal, oat bran, raw fruits and vegetables
  - Weight loss in overweight patients

Table 9-14: Classification of LDL, Total, and HDL Cholesterol

LDL Cholesterol	<100	Optimal
	100–129	Near optimal
	130–159	Borderline high
	160–189	High
	190 +	Very high
Total Cholesterol	<200	Desirable
	200–239	Borderline high
	240+	High
HDL Cholesterol	<40	Low
	60+	High
Triglycerides	<200	Normal
	200–400	Borderline high
	400–1000	High
	1000+	Very high

Table 9-15: Treatment Decisions Based on Risk Category

Risk Category	Initiate Lifestyle Changes	Initiate Drug Therapy	LDL Goal
CVD and CVD Risk Equivalent	100	130	100
Two or More Risk Factors	130	160	130
Fewer Than 2 Risk Factors	160	190	160

- Exercise
  - All patients should be started on appropriate exercise program

Pharmacologic Treatment (See Tables 9-16 and 9-17)
- HMG CoA reductase inhibitors ("statins")
  - Generally well tolerated
  - Contraindication: liver disease
  - Most are metabolized by P-450 (CYP) 3A4, except Pravachol
    Drug interaction with cyclosporine, erythromycin, itraconazole, ketoconazole
    Use caution in combination with fibric acid, increased risk of rhabdomyolysis
  - Monitor for adverse reactions
    Muscle pain and elevated CPK may indicate rhabdomyolysis, which may lead to renal dysfunction
    Elevated liver function tests (LFTs); monitor liver function tests prior to initiation of therapy then every 6 to 12 weeks for a year, then periodically
- Fibric acids
  - Generally well tolerated

Table 9–16: Effect of Medications on Lipids

Drug Type	LDL	HDL	Triglycerides
HMG CoA	-20% to -50%	+5% to 15%	-10–25%
Fibric acids	-10% to -25%	+10% to +15%	-20–50%
Bile acid sequestrants	-15% to -30%	+3% to 5%	+5–30%
Niacin	-10% to 25%	+15% to +35%	-20–50%
Selective cholesterol absorption inhibitor	-15% to -20%	+2% to 4%	-4–6%

Table 9-17: Recommended Lipid Drug Therapy

Drug	Dose
HMG CoA	
Atorvastatin (Lipitor)	10–80 mg PO qd
Cerivastatin (Baycol)	0.4 mg PO qd
Fluvastatin (Lescol)	20–40 mg PO qd
Lovastatin (Mevacor)	10–80 mg PO qd
Pravastatin (Pravachol)	20–40 mg PO qd
Simvastatin (Zocor)	5–80 mg PO qd
Bile Acid Sequestrant	
Cholestyramine (Questran)	4 g bid–24 g divided
Colestipol (Colestid)	5 mg bid–30 g divided
Fibric Acid	
Gemfibrozil (Lopid)	600 qd–1200 divided
Fenofibrate (Tricor)	67–200 mg PO qd
Nicotinic Acid derivative	
Niacin	100 mg qd–3.0 g divided
Nicotinic Acid (Niaspan) extended release	500 mg qd–2.0 g
Selective cholesterol absorption inhibitor	
Ezetimibe (Zeta)	10 mg PO qd

- Adverse reactions: hepatotoxicity, cholelithiasis, dizziness, dyspepsia, bloating, diarrhea, myalgia
- Contraindicated in renal or hepatic dysfunction
- Bile acid sequestrants
  - Not absorbed systemically
  - May safely be used in combination with other lipid-lowering medications
  - Interfere with absorption of other drug: (take 1 hour before med or 4 hours after) and fat soluble vitamins
  - Few able to tolerate due to unpalatability
  - Side effects: constipation, flatulence, nausea, bloating abdominal cramps, malabsorption
- Nicotinic acid
  - Use with caution in DM, CHF, peptic ulcer, gout; monitor for liver toxicity
  - Liver function tests, blood glucose, uric acid prior to initiation
  - Low dose, titrate slowly to avoid flushing, pretreat with aspirin one-half hour prior dose
  - Long-acting has less flushing but more liver toxicity
  - Side effects: flushing, pruritus, impaired glucose tolerance, hyperuricemia, nausea, abdominal pain, diarrhea hypotension, nausea

When to Consult, Refer, Hospitalize
- Patients with the following conditions may require physician consultation and/or referral: diabetes mellitus (especially if poorly controlled), existing CVD, poorly controlled hypertension, chronic renal insufficiency
- Dietitian: poor dietary compliance

Follow-up
- Assessment of adverse reactions to medication, diet assessment, compliance with exercise routine, 24-hour recall of diet
- Monitor CPK and LFTs as described above
- Visits: 8 weeks initially, until lipid control is achieved; then every 6 months

Expected Course
- Dependent on etiology, CAD

Complications
- CAD progression
- Stroke

ARRHYTHMIAS
Atrial Fibrillation

Description
- Acute or chronic arrhythmia that is characterized by a nonsynchronized irregular atrial and ventricular activity; untreated rates vary from atrial rate of 200 to 600 minute with ventricular rate of 80 to 180 minute. This is an irregularly irregular rhythm in which conduction varies from atrium to the ventricular.
- Pulse deficit is the difference between apical rate and radial pulse rate.
- Can be life-threatening in elders due to risk of embolism (CVA) and inability to tolerate tachycardia (increases risk of CHF)
- Often starts as acute episodic, later becomes chronic
- Associated with increase in mortality in otherwise healthy patients, thus should never be considered as benign condition even though no organic heart disease may be found

Etiology

- Rheumatic heart disease
- Cardiomyopathy
- Hypertension
- Acute myocardial infarction
- Pulmonary embolus (PE)
- Chronic heart failure
- Pericarditis
- Hyperthyroidism
- Idiopathic

Incidence and Demographics

- The most common chronic arrhythmia
- Increases with age, steep increase after age 70
- Male preponderance
- High reoccurrence of episodes
- Approximately 4% of population over 60 have sustained atrial fibrillation

Risk Factors

- Patients with atrial fibrillation are at increased risk for stroke
- Profile for those most at risk of stroke includes
  - Age over 65 years
  - Previous TIA or stroke
  - High blood pressure
  - Heart failure
  - Thyrotoxicosis
  - Clinical coronary disease
  - Mitral stenosis
  - Prosthetic heart valve
  - Diabetes

Prevention and Screening

- Avoid excessive alcohol, caffeine, and nicotine
- Treat comorbid conditions
- Assess and aggressively respond to triggers that comprise hemodynamic stability

Assessment

Evaluate for hemodynamic stability
- Shock, severe hypotension, pulmonary edema, myocardial ischemia

History

- Variable symptoms from asymptomatic to severe
- Palpitations
- Angina
- Fatigue
- Decline in activity level
- Marked dyspnea
- Dizziness
- Syncope

Physical

- Tachycardia
- Irregular pulse: marked deficit between apical rate and radial pulse rate
- Pallor
- Orthostatic blood pressure
- Assess comorbid conditions:
- Peripheral edema
- Jugular venous distension
- Tachypnea
- Thyromegaly
- CNS disturbance: decreased mental acuity

Diagnostic Studies

- Serum electrolytes
- ECG—confirmatory with absent p waves, irregular ventricular rate, and rhythm 100 to 160 beats
- Cardiac event monitor
- Echocardiogram

- Thyroid function tests
- Ventilation perfusion scan: rule out pulmonary embolus

Differential Diagnosis
- Atrial flutter
- Sinus tachycardia

Management
- Initial treatment directed toward slowing ventricular response to 60 to 100 beats/minute; restoring sinus rhythm when feasible, and decreasing risk of CVA from embolism
- Chronic treatment goal is rate control and prevention of CVA from embolism

Nonpharmacologic Treatment
- Treat underlying disorders
- Invasive therapy for refractory cases
- Cardioversion to normal sinus rhythm
- Patients on warfarin require extensive patient education regarding diet, signs and symptoms of bleeding, and monitoring and dosing

Pharmacologic Treatment
- Acute
  - Managed in hospital setting under care of cardiologist
- Chronic
  - Digoxin (Lanoxin) (started by physician) is usually used to slow rate if patient cannot be converted to normal sinus rhythm
  - Digoxin: 0.125–0.25 mg qd
    Monitor for toxicity: fatigue, anorexia, weakness, and nausea
    Drug levels 6–8 hours after last dose or prior to dose
    Digoxin control of ventricular response is less effective with activity
  - Active individuals consider beta blocker or calcium channel blocker
  - Beta blockers: metoprolol (Lopressor) 50–100 mg qd; atenolol (Tenormin) 25–100 mg qd (side effects bradycardia, fatigue, depression, impotence)
  - Calcium channel blockers: verapamil (Calan) 120–480 mg qd; diltiazem (Cardizem) 90–360 mg qd (side effects: constipation, dizziness, headaches)
  - Use caution with medication as some have depressing effect on the AV node
- Antithromboembolic therapy
  - Warfarin
  - Monitor PT/INR on a regular basis to assure therapeutic range (usually INR of 2 to 3)
  - Monitor for bleeding: stool OB, UA, CBC with platelets, signs and symptoms including intracerebral bleed
  - Numerous drugs affect INR—need to be aware of what patient is taking (including herbal supplements and OTC drugs); acetaminophen is an underrecognized cause of overanti-coagulation. Taking more than 4 regular strength tablets daily greatly increases the risk of a prolonged INR.
  - Diet also effects INR, increase vitamin K, vegetables *decrease* INR
  - Despite careful monitoring, in the majority of cases there is no known cause found for under- or overanticoagulation

How Long to Treat
- Anticoagulation therapy is indefinite unless situations arise that would contraindicate therapy

Special Considerations
- In order to take warfarin safely, patients must keep regular office appointments, have blood work done regularly, and be reliable in taking their medication correctly.

- Frail and demented elderly and patients unable or unwilling to take warfarin, consider ASA 325 mg qd

Follow-up

Expected Course
- Prognosis dependent on heart disease
- Exercise and activity levels may be limited

Complications
- CHF
- Stroke
- Peripheral arterial embolism.
- Pharmacologic: bradycardia, torsades de pointes
- Warfarin therapy confers increased risk of intracranial hemorrhage

CHRONIC HEART FAILURE (CHF)

Description
- A common clinical syndrome that arises from impairment of the heart's ability to effectively meet the metabolic demands of the body; formerly called chronic heart failure
- Syndrome may be chronic with episodic exacerbations or acute with mild, moderate or severe symptoms
- Major complication of heart disease with serious life-threatening outcomes that need aggressive management
- Life expectancy—5-year survival rate is 50%

Etiology
- Basic causes are from
  - Myocardial damage due to ischemic heart disease, myocarditis, or cardiomyopathy
  - Ventricular overload due to
    Pressure overload as in hypertension, coarctation of aorta, aortic stenosis, or pulmonary stenosis
    Volume overload as from mitral regurgitation, aortic regurgitation, ventral septal defect (VSD), atrial septal defect, patent ductus arteriosus
  - Restriction and obstruction to ventricular filling
    Mitral stenosis, cardiac tamponade, constrictive pericarditis, restrictive cardiomyopathies, atrial myxoma
  - Cor pulmonale and other problems such as AV fistula, thyrotoxicosis, or myxedema

Incidence and Demographics
- Common syndrome, increasing in incidence
- Most common in elderly patients
- Male preponderance until age 75, then equal occurrence
- Frequent hospital-admitting diagnosis

Risk Factors
- Factors precipitating CHF in patients with underlying heart disease include:
  - Progression or complications of basic causes
  - Patient noncompliance with medications
  - Excess salt intake
  - Stress
  - Obesity
  - Arrhythmias

- Cardiac muscle damage
- Blood problems
- Increased volume
- Decreased volume
- Anemia
- Electrolyte imbalance
- Drugs
  NSAIDs
  Beta blockers
  Steroids
  Digitalis toxicity
  Alcohol

Prevention and Screening
- Treat underlying cause if possible
- Monitor for and treat risk factors

Assessment
- Usually begins with left-sided failure, which causes pulmonary signs, then right-sided failure (systemic signs)
- Both left and right failure are usually present

History
- General: diminished exercise capacity, weakness, fatigue, anorexia, nocturia
- Respiratory: cough, at first nonproductive at night, progressing to frequent cough productive of pink frothy sputum
- Dyspnea on exertion (DOE), orthopnea, paroxysmal nocturnal dyspnea (PND)

Physical
- General: cyanosis, hypotension/hypertension
- Respiratory: basilar rales, frothy pink sputum
- Cardiac: S_3 gallop rhythm, elevated jugular venous pressure (JVD), cardiac enlargement
- Extremities: dependent edema
- Abdomen: hepatomegaly
- CNS: delirium

Diagnostic Studies (See Table 9-18)
- Chest x-ray: pleural effusions, pulmonary edema, cardiomegaly and to rule out pneumonia
- Electrolytes CBC, TSH
- Urinalysis
- ECG: possible left ventricular strain
- Echocardiogram: ejection fraction (EF) determines severity and diagnoses failure as systolic or diastolic, which determines appropriate treatment

Table 9-18: NY Heart Association Functional Classification of CHF

Class	Activities That Are Tolerated
Functional Class 1	Ordinary physical exertion does not limit activity
Functional Class 2	Ordinary physical activity presents slight limitations Patient experiences fatigue, dyspnea, angina
Functional Class 3	Comfortable at rest; physical activity presents marked limitations
Functional Class 4	Symptoms at rest; any physical activity presents marked limitations

Differential Diagnosis

- Chronic obstructive pulmonary disease
- Cirrhosis
- Pulmonary emboli
- Acute MI
- Pneumonia
- Asthma
- Chronic venous insufficiency
- Nephrotic syndrome

Management

Nonpharmacologic Treatment

- Identify and treat underlying disease
- Control precipitating factors
- Control leg edema with elastic pressure stockings and elevation of legs
- Sodium and fluid restriction
- Daily weights
- Patient education—goal identification to balance activity with metabolic restriction
- Importance of medication and diet compliance
- Other options—surgical—valve replacement and cardiac transplant

Pharmacologic Treatment (See Table 9-19)

- Patient frequently needs a 3 to 4 drug regimen to control symptoms
- Diuretics—reduces preload and left ventricular filling
- ACEI is cornerstone therapy; prevents progression of left ventricular dysfunction
- ARB is used if patient unable to tolerate ACEI
- Beta blockers: improve ventricular function and reduce postinfarction mortality
- Cardiac glycoside (digoxin): improves contractility in systolic failure
- Vasodilators: reduce after load, used if patient is unable to tolerate ACEI or ARB
- Anticoagulants: prevent thrombus formation

How Long to Treat

- Acute episodes: until resolution and stabilization of symptoms
- Chronic condition: indefinite

When to Consult, Refer, Hospitalize

- Physician consult for initial assessment and management
- Hospitalize if acute pulmonary edema
- In chronic disease: refer if exacerbation is not responsive to treatment
- Consider referral for:
  - ABG
  - Cardiac catheterization: important for determining primary etiology
  - Endomyocardial biopsy: only useful with myocarditis or infiltrative disease

Follow-up

Expected Course

- Patient usually experiences a steady decline after diagnosis
- Acute: generally responsive to initial treatment
- Chronic: EF good indicator of morbidity and mortality
- Poor prognosis if EF less than 20%.

Complications

- Electrolyte disturbances
- Adverse reactions to medications
- Arrhythmias, especially atrial fibrillation
- Death

Table 9-19: Drug Treatment in Chronic Heart Failure

Drugs	Treatment Regimen	Common Side Effects
Diuretics		
Furosemide	Initial: 20–80 mg qd May need large doses in acute CHF, then decrease dosage as tolerated for maintenance	Electrolyte disturbances, orthostatic hypotension, dizziness, weakness, GI upset.
Hydrochlorothiazide	Mild symptoms 12.5–50 mg qd Not usually effective in CHF	Anorexia, nausea vomiting, cramping
Zaroxolyn	2.5–5 mg 1 h prior furosemide Generally, once or twice week	Marked electrolyte imbalance, CNS effects
Spirolactone	25–50 mg qd or in divided doses	Hyperkalemia
Angiotensin Converting Enzyme Inhibitors (ACE)		
Lisinopril	2.5 mg qd, titrate to 20 mg qd	Renal impairment, angioedema, hypotension Cough (common), dizziness, weakness Hyperkalemia—use with caution in renal impairment
Enalapril	2.5 mg bid, titrate to 10 mg bid	
Quinapril	10 mg qd	
Angiotensin Receptor Blockers (ARB)		
Losartan (Cozaar)	25–100 mg PO qd	Rare side effects: dizziness, insomnia, muscle cramps, leg pain, hyperkalemia
Valsartan (Diovan)	40–320 mg qd	
Beta Blockers (BB)		
Carvedilol	3.25 PO bid; titrate SLOWLY to 25 mg bid	Bradycardia, depression, fatigue
Metoprolol	25 mg bid, titrate to 100 mg bid	
Cardiac Glycosides		
Digoxin	0.125 mg PO qd	Monitor drug levels GI—Anorexia, nausea CNS, apathy weakness, headache Cardiac—arrhythmia
Vasodilators		
Hydralazine	10 mg qid; target dose 300 mg daily Requires 8–2 hour nitrate-free period before starting	GI side effects, hypotension, headaches, Tachycardia
Isosorbide dinitrate	5–10 mg tid; target dose 160 mg daily	Same as above

PERIPHERAL VASCULAR DISORDERS
Peripheral Arterial Disease (PAD)

Description
- Obstruction or narrowing of the major arteries, usually in the lower extremities, that may be acute or chronic and is frequently a result of atherosclerosis
- Intermittent claudication is the most common symptom of peripheral arterial disease

Etiology
- Acute thrombus leading to embolus
- Chronic atherosclerotic lesions
- Inflammatory component: thromboangiitis obliterans (Buerger's disease), giant cell arteritis

Incidence and Demographics
- Elderly
- Male preponderance

Risk Factors
- Age greater than 40
- Tobacco usage
- Hyperlipidemia
- Diabetes mellitus
- Hypertension

Prevention and Screening
- Life style modification—stop smoking
- Identification and treatment of comorbid conditions

Assessment

History
- Acute: pain, paresthesia, paralysis, pallor, pulselessness
- Chronic: intermittent claudication—lower extremity aching, fatigue, tiredness occurring with activity and relieved by cessation of activity
- Aorta: back or abdominal pain
- Femoral: hip, buttock, calf pain
- Peripheral vascular disease progresses from silent, asymptomatic disease, to intermittent claudication, to rest ischemia, then to ulceration or gangrene

Physical
- Pallor, pulseless extremity
- Severity determined by amount of time required for venous filling and return of color
- Cool extremity, dependent rubor
- Absent or decreased hair loss of extremity
- Bruit femoral artery

Diagnostic Studies
- Doppler ultrasound
- Angiography for acute or surgical candidates

Differential Diagnosis
- Musculoskeletal strains
- Osteoarthritis
- Acute arterial spasm
- Acute deep vein thrombus

Management

Nonpharmacologic Treatment
- Acute arterial occlusion: avoid elevating affected extremity; protect extremity, and refer for heparin therapy immediately
- In chronic disease, smoking cessation counseling and/or program is crucial
- Control comorbid diseases, such as hyperlipidemia, diabetes mellitus, hypertension
- Initiate prescribed exercise program
- Educate patient about signs and symptoms that require medical attention, care of feet

Pharmacologic Treatment
- Acute: heparin 5000 units IV

- Embolectomy, thrombolytic therapy
- Chronic
  - Indicated for intermittent claudication
    Cilostazol (Pletal) 100 mg bid antiplatelet/vasodilator, contraindicated in CHF
    Pentoxifylline (Trental) 400 mg tid
  - Antiplatelet therapy
    Aspirin 325 mg
    Clopidogrel (Plavix) 75 mg qd when aspirin not tolerated

When to Consult, Refer, Hospitalize
- Acute arterial occlusion
- Arteriosclerosis obliterans
- Recurrent thromboembolism merits
- New onset, severe symptoms: possible vascular surgery

Follow-up

Expected Course
- Chronic: symptoms differs with slow progression to rapid deterioration

Complications
- Gangrene
- Amputation

VENOUS DISORDERS
Superficial And Deep Venous Thrombosis

Description
- Deep venous thrombosis (DVT): acute formation of blood clot(s) in the deep venous system of the lower extremity or pelvic veins
- Superficial: acute inflammation and clot formation with associated redness and tenderness along superficial vein

Etiology
- DVT—three primary predisposing factors
  - Venous stasis—obesity, CHF, prolonged immobility, arrhythmias (especially atrial fibrillation)
  - Hypercoagulability—postoperative state, some malignancies, dehydration, acute or chronic inflammation, abrupt discontinuation of anticoagulants, inherited coagulation deficits, estrogen usage
  - Injury to venous wall intima—PVD, varicose veins, trauma (especially hip fractures)
  - Effect of predisposing factors increased by advanced age and prior history of DVT
- Superficial
  - IV therapy
  - Trauma
  - Bacteria infection

Incidence and Demographics
- Common approximately 1 to 2 million cases per year
- Female preponderance
- High incidence with total hip replacement

Risk Factors
- DVT
  - Orthopedic surgery
  - Immobility
  - Rheumatoid disease—lupus
  - High-altitude elevation

- Carcinoma
- Venous catheters
- Superficial
  - Aseptic procedures
- Coagulation defects
- Polycythemia vera

Prevention and Screening
- Administration of short-term low molecular weight heparin, such as Lovenox after hip surgery
- Postsurgical mechanical leg compression

Assessment

History
- DVT
  - Frequently asymptomatic
  - Possible unilateral leg pain or tenderness and swelling
  - Pain specific to limb or calf
- Superficial
  - Saphenous vein frequently involved
  - Acute episode with define time frame
  - Local redness, tender cord
  - Swelling
  - Dull pain over inflamed vein
  - Fever

Physical
- DVT
  - Signs unreliable
  - Reproducible tenderness with calf compression
  - Positive Homans' sign: pain in calf with dorsiflexion of foot. Note that a negative Homans' sign does not conclusively rule out DVT.
  - Leg circumference greater compared to uninvolved leg
  - Swelling calf or thigh
  - Cool extremity with weak distal pulses
- Superficial
  - No significant swelling of extremity
  - Isolated induration, redness, and tenderness along vein

Diagnostic Studies
- Laboratory
  - Anticoagulation therapy baseline: platelets, PT, APTT, hemoglobin, LFTs, occult blood; monitor platelets daily with heparin
- Referral for testing
  - B-mode ultrasound combined with Doppler flow detection: highly sensitive
  - Contrast venography: most sensitive and specific contrast venography most effective
- Superficial
  - Culture and sensitivity if superficial vein appears infected

Differential Diagnosis
- Cellulitis
- Musculoskeletal strain
- Lymphedema
- Acute arterial occlusion
- Ruptured Baker's cyst

Management

Nonpharmacologic Treatment
- DVT
  - Initial hospitalize with bed rest, anticoagulation; after stabilization prompt mobilization
  - Intermittent pneumatic compression followed by graded pressure stockings
  - Filtering devices: umbrella in vena cava traps emboli; useful if anticoagulants are contraindicated and for recurrent emboli

- Posthospitalization
  Leg exercises
  Avoidance leg crossing
  Bed—elevation of legs
  Educate patient regarding signs and symptoms
- Calf DVT—outpatient management
  - Superficial
    Leg elevation when patient is sitting
    Local heat
    If septic, hospitalization often required

Pharmacologic Treatment
- DVT
  - Anticoagulation therapy: acute treatment and prophylaxis
    - Baseline laboratory tests: platelets, APTT, PT, INR, LFTs, hemoccult, Hgb
    - Heparin IV on inpatient basis
      Does not dissolve thrombi, stops propagation, allows natural fibrinolysis
      Heparin side effects: thrombocytopenia, bleeding—use caution with liver disease
      Heparin and warfarin concurrent with heparin starting day 3; Keep INR at 2.5
    - Low molecular weight heparin effective treatment for uncomplicated DVT
    - Thrombolytic agents may be given in ER
    - Aspirin not beneficial
- Superficial
  - Aseptic: NSAIDs
  - Septic: appropriate antibiotic 6 weeks, sometimes excision of vein

How Long to Treat
- DVT
  - Single episode: 3 to 6 months
  - Indefinite: CHF, recurrent embolism, DVT, or PE
- Superficial
  - Aseptic inflammation subsides 1 to 2 weeks

When to Consult, Refer, Hospitalize
- Refer acute DVTs
- Refer recurrences or complications

Follow-up
- See regularly to get blood work and management of warfarin dosage

Expected Course
- Good once danger of PE has passed
- Superficial: untreated condition may become septic, which increases mortality

Complications
- DVT
  - Pulmonary embolism
  - Chronic venous insufficiency
- Superficial
  - Septic thrombophlebitis, osteomyelitis

Venous Insufficiency

Description
- Venous valve incompetency with venous engorgement and edema of the lower leg that is often chronic but non-inflammatory

Etiology

- Leg trauma
- Incompetent venous valves
- High venous pressure

Incidence and Demographics

- Female predominance
- Onset late adulthood

Risk Factors

- Prior history of pregnancy, deep vein thrombosis
- Prolonged immobility, particularly standing
- Family tendency
- Age
- Obesity

Prevention and Screening

- Early aggressive treatment thrombophlebitis
- Moisturizers to areas of xerosis with avoidance of scratching
- Avoid prolonged standing and immobility
- Compression elastic stockings with ambulation
- Weight loss if appropriate
- Avoidance of restrictive lower extremity garments

Assessment

History

- Fatigue, aching, heaviness in lower extremities
- Lower extremity edema worsens with prolonged standing
- Mild pruritus lower extremity, scratching

Physical

- Hyperpigmentation distal extremity brown, brawny, thickened skin, red
- Ulceration, if present, distal often medial aspect
- Edema of lower extremities
- Eczema
- Varicosities may be present
- Recurrent stasis ulcers, weeping, crust formation

Differential Diagnosis

- Cellulitis
- Chronic renal disease
- Lymphedema
- Acute phlebitis
- Fungal infection
- Atopic dermatitis
- Severe contact dermatitis
- Neurodermatitis

Management

Nonpharmacologic Treatment

- Elastic stockings prior to ambulation
- Elevation of foot of bed
- Avoid prolonged positions or inactivity
- Ulcers—see Dermatology Chapter 6

Pharmacologic Treatment

- Diuretic therapy, generally not recommended unless edema is causing ulcers
- Steroid creams: hydrocortisone cream, triamcinolone 1%, or Valisone

- Cordran tape
- Zinc oxide ointment with ichthammol

How Long to Treat
- Chronic condition
- Treat exacerbations until resolution

When to Consult, Refer, Hospitalize
- Refractory conditions, ulcers that will not heal

Follow-up

Expected Course
- Chronic, recurrent with frequent exacerbation with poor compliance to preventive measures

Complications
- Bacterial infection
- Thrombophlebitis
- DVT
- Stasis ulcers

CASE STUDIES

Case 1. A 68-year-old male is following up after consultation with an orthopedist for a recent fractured thumb. Orthopedist noted that the patient had a blood pressure reading of 166/104.
PMH: Chart shows that the patient had, at the last office visit, BP 144/92. Laboratory work was ordered. Review of chart shows labile blood pressure readings for the prior 2 years, which decreased after weight loss undertaken to treat hyperlipidemia. States he follows low-salt, low-fat diet and exercises 2 to 3 times a week; nonsmoker.
Medications: Lipitor 10 mg qd; ibuprofen (Motrin) 400 mg PO tid
FH: Diabetes type 2 and CAD

    1. What cardiac risk factors does he have?

Lab findings on previous visits:

BUN 22	Cholesterol 230
Creatinine 0.8	Triglycerides 250
Na+ 136	LDL 148
K+ 4.0	HDL 32
Glucose 162	

    2. What additional problem does this lab identify? Is this a significant coronary risk factor?

    3. Is his hyperlipidemia well controlled?

Physical: Vital signs current visit: BP: 160/102; Pulse: 98; Resp: 16; Weight: 205 lb Height: 5'9"
Cardiac: RRR, no murmur, no carotid bruits or pedal edema, no renal bruits
Resp: vesicular sounds throughout all lung fields
Funduscopic: Clear disc, obvious arteriolar narrowing with focal areas of attenuation
UA: trace glucose and protein
ECG sinus rhythm

    4. What is the significance of these findings?

    5. What stage hypertension does he have?

    6. How would you manage this patient's hypertension? List steps.

Case 2. A 73-year-old white female complains of increasing shortness of breath and cough productive of frothy sputum over the last 24 hours. She has had trouble sleeping due to a cough she attributes to allergies and has felt tired for the past 3 months. Two days ago she celebrated her 73rd birthday.

PMH: Two years ago she had an episode of weakness and dizziness. At that time, her EKG showed changes indicative of a mild MI. She was placed on atenolol (Tenormin) 100 mg and has remained stable. Has mild hypertension, hyperlipidemia; menopause 10 years ago. Smoking history: 20 years one-half pack a day; quit 5 years ago.

Lab: chest x-ray showing mild cardiomegaly, otherwise unremarkable. An echocardiogram showing EF 40%, moderate left ventricular dysfunction.

    1. What is the most likely diagnosis?
    2. What factor(s) most likely have precipitated this?
    3. What is most likely the basic cause(s)?
    4. What over-the-counter drugs should you specifically ask about?

Exam: BP: 142/94, Pulse: 88; Resp: 22; Temp: 98.8; Wt: 180
Ht: 5'4" General Appearance: appears mildly short of breath
Resp: tachypnea, occasion nonproductive cough, bi-basilar rales (crackles)
Extremities: 2+ edema extending half way up lower legs

    5. What other physical exam do you need to do and what would you look for?

Medications: Atenolol (Tenormin) 100 mg PO qd, lovastatin (Mevacor) 20 mg qd, aspirin 81 mg qd

    6. What medications would you start today?
    7. What lab work would you need to check before starting these medications?
    8. What adverse reactions would you monitor for?

Case 3. A 70-year-old Caucasian female presents for routine follow-up of lipids.

PMH: Her last visit she was started on a low-saturated fat diet. Medical history significant for osteoporosis and hypercholesteremia. Ex-smoker with 15 pack years, quit 7 years ago. Occasional ETOH with glass of wine once a week.

Medications: Fosamax 10 mg qd; calcium and vitamin D supplements

Exam: General appearance: alert, oriented, NAD; Wt.: 130 lbs; Height: 5'5"
BP: 138/82
Cardiac: RRR, no murmurs; no edema, peripheral pulses present
Resp: Vesicular breath sounds throughout all lung fields
Abdomen: soft, no hepatosplenomegaly or masses

Labs:	Last visit	This visit
Cholesterol, total	275	230
Triglycerides	118	104
HDL	62	56
LDL	189	140

Basic metabolic, CBC, and LFTs unremarkable

    1. What is your assessment?
    2. What cardiac risk factors does this patient have?
    3. What other risk factors should you assess?
    4. What is your plan?

REFERENCES

Ahmed, A. (2003). American College of Cardiology/American Heart Association chronic heart failure evaluation and management guidelines: Relevance to the geriatric practice. *J Am Geriatr Soc, 51,* 123–126.

ALLHAT Collaborative Research Group. (2002). Major outcomes in high-risk hypertensive patients randomized to angiotensin converting enzyme inhibitor or calcium channel blocker vs diuretic. The antihypertensive and lipid lowering treatment to prevent heart attack trial. *JAMA, 288,* 2981–2997.

American College of Cardiology. Available at: www.acc.org.

American Heart Association. Available at: www.amhrt.org.

Appel, I. J. (2002, December 18). The verdict from ALLHAT—Thiazide diuretics are the preferred initial therapy for hypertension. *JAMA, 288,* 3039–3042.

Aronow, W. S. (2002). Should hypercholesterolemia in older persons be treated to reduce cardiovascular events? *J Gerontol A Biol Sci Med Sci, 57,* AM411–413.

Chobanian, A. V., Bakris, G. L., Black, H. R., et al. (2003, December). Seventh report of the Joint National Committee on Prevention, Detection, Evaluation, and Treatment of High Blood Pressure. *Hypertension, 42*(6), 1206–1252.

Expert Panel on Detection, Evaluation and Treatment of High Blood Cholesterol. (2001). Executive Summary of the Third Report of the NCEP Expert Panel in adults. *JAMA, 285*(10), 2486. Accessed at: www.nhlbi.nih.gov.

Falk, R. H. (2001). Atrial fibrillation. *NEJM, 344,* 1067–1078.

Gibbons, R. J., et al. (2002). Guideline update for the management of patients with chronic stable angina: A Report of the American College of Cardiology/American Heart Association Task Force of Practice Guidelines. *J Am Coll Cardiol, 41,*159–168. Accessed at: www.acc.org.

Go, A. S., et al. (2003, November 26). Anticoagulation therapy for stroke prevention in atrial fibrillation: How well do randomized trials translate into clinical practice? *JAMA, 290,* 2685–2692.

Joint National Committee. (2003). The Seventh Report of the Joint National Committee on Prevention, Detection, and Treatment of High Blood Pressure. NIH, NHLBI (NIH No. 03-5233).

Khan, M. G. (2003). *Cardiac drug therapy* (6th ed.). London: W. B. Saunders.

Levy, P. J. (2002). Epidemiology and pathophysiology of peripheral arterial disease. *Clinical Cornerstone, 4,* 1–15.

Massie, B. M. & Amidon, T. A. (2003). Heart. In L. M. Tierney, Jr., S. J. McPhee, & M. A. Papadakis (Eds.), *Current medical diagnosis and treatment* (pp. 312–408) (42th ed.). NY: Lange Medical Books/McGraw-Hill.

National Cholesterol Education Program. (2001). Third Report of the Expert Panel on Detection, Evaluation, and Treatment of High Blood Cholesterol in Adults (Adult Treatment Panel III). Bethesda, MD: Author.

National Heart, Lung, and Blood Institute. (2003). Seventh Report of the Joint National Committee on Prevention, Detection, Evaluation, and Treatment of High Blood Pressure (JNC 7) Express. (NIH Publication No. 5233). Bethesda, MD: National Institutes of Health.

Redfield, M. M., et al. (2003). Burden of systolic and diastolic ventricular dysfunction in the community: Appreciating the scope of the heart failure epidemic. *JAMA, 289,* 194–202.

Sander, G. E. (2002). High blood pressure in the geriatric population: Treatment considerations. *The American Journal of Geriatric Cardiology, 11,* 223–232.

Snow, V., et al. (2004). Primary care management of chronic stable angina and asymptomatic suspected or known coronary artery disease: A clinical practice guideline from the American College of Physicians. *Annals Internal Medicine, 141*(7), 562–567.

Snow, V., et al. (2004). Evaluation of primary care patients with chronic stable angina: Guidelines from the American College of Physicians. *Annals of Internal Medicine, 141*(1), 57–64.

Sonnenblick, E. H. (2000). Detecting and treating heart failure: An update on strategies. *Consultant, 40*(1), 170–176.

US Preventive Services Task Force. (2002, January 15). Aspirin for the primary prevention of cardiovascular events: Recommendation and rationale. *Ann Intern Med, 136,* 157–160.

Yusuf, S., et al. (2000). Effects of an angiotensin converting enzyme inhibitor, ramipril, on cardiovasculare events in high risk patients: The Heart Outcomes Prevention Evaluation (HOPE) Study Investigators. *NEJM 342,* 145–153.

Wald, D. S., et al. (2002, November 23). Homocysteine and cardiovascular disease: Evidence on causality from a meta-analysis. *BMJ, 325,*1202–1206.

White, H. D. (2003, September 6). Should all patients with coronary disease receive angiotensin converting enzyme inhibitors? *Lancet, 362,* 755–757.

Wing, L. M. H., et al. (2003, February 13). A comparison of outcomes with angiotensin converting enzyme inhibitors and diuretics for hypertension in the elderly. *NEJM, 348,* 583–592.

Tsikouris, J. P. & Cox, C. D. (2001). A review of class III antiarrhythmic agents for atrial fibrillation: Maintenance of normal sinus rhythm. *Pharmacotherapy, 21,* 1514–1529.

Zepf, B. (2001). Diagnosis and treatment of venous stasis ulcers. *American Family Physician, 64,* 1452.

GASTROINTESTINAL DISORDERS 10

GERIATRIC APPROACH

Normal Changes of Aging
- Most clinically important changes:
  - Decreased intestinal motility
  - Decreased hydrochloric acid
  - Fewer taste buds
- Effects of aging GI system on absorption and metabolism of medications:
  - Decreased absorption of some medications in an elderly GI tract
  - Metabolism of drugs in GI tract affected by decreased activity of the cytochrome P450 system functions in the GI tract and liver causing increased frequency of drug interactions and drug toxicity
- Decreased immune function in GI tract leads to increased susceptibility to infection
  - Elderly have decreased production of antibodies and other specialized immune cells in the intestinal wall and decreased cytokine activity; this puts elderly at risk for GI infectious diseases (especially food-borne illnesses) and for all infections.
- See Table 10-1 for specific changes.

Clinical Implications
History
- Elderly less likely to feel pain with abdominal conditions
- Elderly are more likely to present with nonspecific complaints.

Physical
- Tend to have a less acute presentation
- Weight loss an important sign

Assessment
- Stool for occult blood: False-positives can be caused by ingestion of iron, aspirin, cimetidine, iodine, or large portions of rare red meat, raw broccoli, turnips, radishes, parsnips or cauliflower. False-negatives can occur from vitamin C ingestion and intermittent bleeding (sensitivity is only 50%).

Treatment
- All patients with stools positive hemoccult require GI referral
- A diet is often an important part of management of GI and other problems. For acute problems, this involves fluid replacement to keep up with fluid loss, starting with ice chips, clear liquids, such as Pedialyte Gatorade, tea, ginger ale, and gradually progressing to soups and crackers and other bland foods as tolerated, including the Braty diet: bananas, rice, applesauce, toast, yogurt.
- For management of many chronic problems, the elderly often need to increase the amount of fiber in their food and increase their fluid intake.

Table 10-1: Summary of Physiologic Aging Effects on GI Tract

Part of System	Effect of Aging	Implications	Contributing Factors
Oropharynx	Impaired neuromuscular coordination	Dysphagia Choking Aspiration	Neuromuscular diseases, such as stroke
Esophagus	Decreased motility	Increased risk of indigestion and GERD	Concurrent medications, obesity, hiatal hernia, diabetes mellitus (DM)
Stomach	Decreased lower esophageal sphincter of stomach (LES) function No change in baseline gastric acid secretion Decreased response to acid Blood flow decreased	Delayed emptying Impaired gastric mucosal protection, decreased response to injury Protects gastric mucosa Increased risk of GERD and PUD	DM, alcohol, medications, tobacco CHF, atherosclerosis Decrease blood flow
Liver	Decreased liver size, blood flow, and perfusion; increased susceptibility to stress	Altered drug metabolism, increased risk of drug interactions	Alcohol, medication use, herbal remedies
Pancreas	Decreased exocrine reserve	Usually not a problem, increased risk of DM	DM
Gallbladder/ Biliary Tree	Less complete emptying due to decreased contractility	Increased risk of cholelithiasis	Obesity, multiparity
Small Bowel	No significant changes	Decreased nutrient absorption	Vascular disease
Colon	Decreased mucosa cell growth, increased transit time	Increased susceptibility to carcinogens, constipation	Colon cancer, diverticulosis, and altered bowel habits
Anal Sphincter	Decreased resting and maximum squeeze pressures in the anal canal	Fecal incontinence	Dementia, neurologic diseases

THERE ARE A FEW CLASSES OF GI DRUGS UTILIZED FOR A MULTITUDE OF GI PROBLEMS
- Antacids
  - Liquid more effective than tablet form
  - Antacids can decrease absorption of other medications (e.g., fluoroquinolones, tetracycline, ferrous sulfate) and need to separate dosing by 2 hours
  - Various preparations are available over the counter:
    - Maalox and Mylanta (antacids) or Gaviscon (antacid with alginic acid) 15 to 30 cc qid, taken 1 hour after meals and before bed as needed
    - Calcium carbonate can cause constipation; milk-alkali syndrome
    - Sodium bicarbonate causes elevated sodium levels; fluid retention
    - Aluminum products cause constipation; CNS adverse effects
    - Magnesium hydroxide causes diarrhea; hypermagnesemia
    - Bismuth subsalicylate (Pepto-Bismol) for nausea and diarrhea: 524 mg (tablets or liquid) every 30 to 60 minutes up to 8 doses in 24 hours or qid with meals and HS for traveler's diarrhea
    - Will cause black stool
    - Radiopaque
- H_2 receptor antagonists: suppress gastric acid secretion (some available OTC at reduced doses)
  - Ranitidine; (Zantac) 75–150 mg qd bid; 300 mg qd
  - Famotidine (Pepcid) 10–40 mg qd bid
  - Nizatidine (Axid) 150–300 mg PO qd bid
- Proton pump inhibitors (PPI): suppress gastric acid secretion to a greater degree than H_2 blockers
  - Omeprazole (Prilosec) 20 mg qd
  - Lansoprazole (Prevacid) 15–30 mg qd
  - Pantoprazole (Protonix) 20–40 mg PO qd
  - Rabeprazole (Aciphex) 20 mg PO qd
  - Esomeprazole (Nexium) 20–40 mg PO qd
- Prokinetic agents: increase LES tone and promote gastric emptying
  - Metoclopramide (Reglan) 5–10 mg qid; used less frequently because of potential for central nervous system side effects (e.g., drowsiness, confusion, depression, extrapyramidal reactions)

COMMON PRESENTING SYMPTOMS
Constipation

Description

SLOW-TRANSIT CONSTIPATION
- Two or more of the following symptoms are present for at least 12 months
  - Decrease in the frequency of stools to less than 2 per week
  - Straining, hard stools, or feeling of incomplete evacuation (on more than one in four occasions)

RECTAL–OUTLET DELAY
- Feeling of anal blockage on greater than one in four occasions and
- Prolonged defecation (more than 10 minutes) or need for manual digitations in the past 12 months

Etiology

MULTIFACTORIAL
- Decreased colonic motility due to aging
- Poor dietary intake of fiber and fluids
- Behavioral habits, such as change in environment with travel or schedule
- Decreased activity, immobility

- Irritable bowel syndrome
- Dementia, does not recognize urge
- Psychogenic
- Neurologic dysfunction causing a change in colonic motility, as in diabetes, spinal cord injury, stroke, multiple sclerosis, and Parkinson's disease
- Metabolic disorders, such as hypothyroidism, hyperparathyroidism, hypokalemia, hypercalcemia, and uremia
- Obstruction, partial or complete
- Anorectal pain from fissures, hemorrhoids, abscesses, or proctitis
- Medications: opiate analgesics, calcium channel blockers, anticholinergics, diuretics, aluminum-based antacids, calcium and iron supplements, NSAIDs, antihistamines, antipsychotic and antiparkinson agents, and laxative abuse

Incidence and Demographics
- Very common, especially in the elderly
- More common in women most likely due to increased self-reporting

Risk Factors
- Immobility
- Lack of fiber in diet
- Increasing age
- Comorbid problems and medications

Prevention and Screening
- Regular physical activity, increase daily fiber and fluid intake
- Avoid all unnecessary medications that may predispose to constipation
- Establish time each day to defecate and do not ignore the urge to defecate

Assessment

History
- Change in pattern, character, and color of stool; fecal and urinary incontinence, anorexia, abdominal or rectal pain, hemorrhoids, weight loss, and laxative use
- Medications, diet, fluid intake

Physical
- Distention, abdominal tenderness, palpable stool in the colon, and decreased bowel sounds may be present. Check for obstruction.
- Digital rectal exam to assess sphincter tone, masses, and impacted stool; stool for guaiac, hemorrhoids, fissures, abscesses, rectal prolapse, rectocele
- In the frail elderly, physical exam may reveal fever, delirium, abdominal distention, urinary retention, decreased bowel sounds, arrhythmias and tachypnea, weight loss

Diagnostic Studies
- Stool for occult blood
- CBC to check for leukocytosis and anemia
- Electrolytes, calcium, BUN, creatinine, and glucose
- Thyroid function tests to rule out hypothyroidism
- Flat plate and upright abdominal films to evaluate for obstruction

Differential Diagnosis
- See Etiology

Management
- Must be individualized; start with mild, increase dose, add another medication as needed

Nonpharmacologic Treatment
- Fiber: 15 g/day (e.g., 2 tbsp bran powder bid mixed with fluids or sprinkled over food)
- Ensure adequate fluid intake with fiber or will worsen constipation
- Fluid: 1.5–2 liters/day
- Physical exercise
- Bowel training program
- Avoid medications that precipitate constipation, especially opioids

Pharmacologic Treatment

INITIAL TREATMENT OF MILD CONSTIPATION
- Hydrophilic colloids or bulk-forming agents
  - Take daily to increase fiber intake; must take adequate fluids or obstruction may occur
  - Psyllium (Metamucil, Fiberall) 3–4 grams 1 to 3 times daily; methylcellulose (Citrucel) 2 grams 1 to 3 times daily; polycarbophil, 1 gram 1 to 4 times daily
- Surfactants: stool softener, not a stimulant, no dependency
  - Take daily, should produce soft stool in 1 to 3 days
  - Useful instead of hydrophilic agents if patient has low fluid intake
  - Docusate sodium (Colace) 50–200 mg daily; docusate calcium (Surfak) 60–120 mg daily

MORE SEVERE CONSTIPATION
- Osmotic laxatives sorbitol is as effective and less expensive than lactulose
  - Lactulose 15–30 cc (10–20 g) PO qd bid
  - Sorbitol 15–30 cc (70% solution) PO qd bid
  - Effective in 12–48 hours
  - Both may cause bloating and hypernatremia
- Stimulant laxatives
  - Used for acute constipation and chronic laxative dependent patients
  - Should result in a bowel movement in 0.5 to 3 hours rectally, 6 to 8 hours orally
    Senna 1–2 of 187 mg tablets at HS or 1 of 652 mg suppository at HS
    Cascara 325 mg tablet at HS
    Bisacodyl 5 mg tablet at HS or 10 mg suppository
  - May cause dependency. Many elderly have become stimulant dependent. Patients on opioids are usually dependent on a stimulant laxative.
  - Do not use if obstruction is a possibility, may cause rupture
- Enemas may be necessary; use instead of stimulant for rectal outlet delay or if obstruction/impaction is a possibility
  - Results in 2 to 30 minutes
  - Sodium phosphate (Fleets) prepared 4.5 oz. squeeze bottle
    May cause fluid retention and hyperphosphatemia
    Use with caution in those with renal failure and underlying bowel disease
  - Warm tap water 750 to 1000 cc for suspected high impaction
    May cause water toxicity and hypervolemia

How Long to Treat
- Many elderly require long-term routine medication plus a PRN medication

When to Consult, Refer, Hospitalize
- Emergently hospitalize for signs and symptoms of acute abdomen or obstruction
- Refer to gastroenterologist
  - Treatment failure
  - Stool positive for occult blood

- Weight loss
- Unexplained change in bowel pattern

Follow-up

Expected Course
- With treatment, resolves in several days if no significant underlying problem
- Elderly frequently need chronic management of constipation

Complications
- Bowel obstruction, fecal impaction, chronic constipation, rectal prolapse, abdominal pain, painful bowel movements

Diarrhea

Description

TWO TYPES OF DIARRHEA:
- Acute diarrhea: sudden onset, lasting less than 3 weeks
  - Inflammatory—invades mucosa
  - Noninflammatory
- Chronic diarrhea: lasts 3 weeks or longer

Etiology
- Acute diarrhea: acute gastroenteritis caused by viral, bacterial, or protozoal/parasitic infection, or drug
- Chronic diarrhea: can be due to many causes including osmosis, secretion, inflammation, malabsorption, motility disorder, and infection

Incidence and Demographics
- Common, almost universal experience

Risk Factors
- Foreign travel
- Ingesting contaminated food or water
- Institutional living, others in living arrangement having infectious gastroenteritis
- Recent course of antibiotics
- Lactose intolerance
- Medications: antibiotics, laxatives, or antacid use
- GI surgery
- Medical diseases such as hyperthyroidism

Prevention and Screening
- Careful food preparation, good hand washing, properly clean fresh fruits and vegetables prior to eating; drink bottled water when traveling to foreign countries

Assessment

History

SUDDEN ONSET, ACUTE SYMPTOMS OF DIARRHEA
- Obtain description of the diarrhea and any associated symptoms: GI, fever, malaise
  - Noninflammatory diarrhea: watery stool, periumbilical cramping, bloating, nausea, and vomiting
  - Inflammatory diarrhea: bloody stool, fever, left lower quadrant pain, cramping, urgency, and tenesmus

SYMPTOMS OF CHRONIC DIARRHEA
- Obtain description of long-term bowel pattern, contributing factors such as certain foods or stress, family history, and stool characteristics (bloody, watery, with mucous)

Physical
- Fever, weight loss may be present
- There may be signs of dehydration: tachycardia, orthostatic hypotension, confusion, poor skin turgor, and dry mucous membranes, decreased urine output
- Abdominal exam may reveal hyperactive bowel sounds and generalized tenderness
- Signs of peritonitis may be seen with severe inflammatory diarrhea
- Rectal exam, stool guaiac may be positive

Diagnostic Studies
- None indicated for diarrhea less than 48 hours and no systemic signs and symptoms
- Stool cultures, ova and parasites, clostridium difficile (C. *difficile*) toxin
- Stool for fecal leukocytes: present in inflammatory diarrhea
- Stool for occult blood
- CBC to look for anemia, leukocytosis, and eosinophilia; may be present in parasitic infections and inflammatory bowel disease
- Electrolytes; evaluate for dehydration and electrolyte abnormalities
- BUN and creatinine; elevations may be indicative of dehydration

CHRONIC DIARRHEA:
- Sigmoidoscopy or colonoscopy to diagnose colitis
- Vitamin B_{12}, folate, vitamin D, albumin, cholesterol, iron, iron-binding capacity, prothrombin time to evaluate for malabsorption
- 24-hour fecal fat collection to diagnose steatorrhea

Differential Diagnosis
- Infectious agents (viral, bacterial, parasitic)

GASTROINTESTINAL DISEASE
- Fecal impaction
- Ileus
- Bowel obstruction
- Malabsorption
- Celiac Sprue
- Inflammatory bowel disease
- Irritable bowel syndrome
- Ischemia secondary to mesenteric atherosclerosis
- Acute appendicitis
- Cholecystitis

SYSTEMIC DISEASE
- Diabetic neuropathy
- Hyperthyroidism

NEOPLASIA
- Obstruction
- Secretory tumors

Management

Nonpharmacologic Treatment
- GI diet, see Clinical Implications, treatment
- Avoid high-fiber foods, milk products, fats, alcohol, and caffeine

Pharmacologic Treatment
- Antidiarrheal agent use is controversial
  - Causative pathogen needs to be eliminated from the body
  - Never use in patients with high fever, bloody diarrhea, or leukocytosis; retained stool may lead to systemic toxicity
  - Antidiarrheal agents can be used in mild to moderate diarrheal illness if it is necessary to control the diarrhea for a short time for a specific purpose.
    Loperamide (Imodium): 2 mg after each loose stool for a maximum of 8 mg in 24 hours, use for 2 days only
    Bismuth subsalicylate (Pepto-Bismol): 2 tablets or 30 mL 4 times daily, maximum 8 doses/day

- Empirical antibiotic treatment while awaiting stool culture results for patients with moderate to severe fever, bloody stools, tenesmus, or the presence of fecal leukocytes. Fluoroquinolones are the drug of choice because they provide good coverage for most invasive bacterial pathogens.
  - Ciprofloxacin 500 mg bid for 5–7 days
  - Levofloxacin 500 mg daily for 5–7 days
  - Alternate treatment: doxycycline 100 mg bid
  - Macrolides and penicillins are no longer recommended because of resistance

IF GIARDIA OR *C. DIFFICILE* IS SUSPECTED

- Metronidazole (Flagyl) 250 mg tid for 7 days. (Avoid alcohol use during and for 48 hours after treatment.)
- Antiemetics if patient vomiting, nausea enough they are not taking in adequate fluids
  - Antiemetics listed below belong to the phenothiazine class, which are anticholinergics and have the standard anticholinergic precautions and adverse reactions.
    - Promethazine (Phenergan): by mouth or by rectal suppository
    - Prochlorperazine (Compazine) by mouth or by rectal suppository

How Long to Treat

- Depends on underlying cause
- For acute diarrhea due to an infection generally treat 5 to 7 days

When to Consult, Refer, Hospitalize

- Any patient with bloody diarrhea, fever, acute abdominal pain and leukocytosis should be referred and evaluated immediately in an acute-care setting.
- Anyone who has not had resolution of diarrhea within 3 weeks needs to be referred to a gastro-enterologist for evaluation.
- Hospitalize elderly if unable to take adequate fluids

Follow-up

Expected Course

- Acute diarrhea should resolve in 24 to 48 hours
- Inflammation of the bowel due to a drug reaction may last for several weeks.
- Acute diarrhea may be prolonged if patient does not adhere to GI diet.

Complications

- Dehydration, electrolyte imbalance, sepsis, shock, malnutrition, anal fissures, and hemorrhoids

Dysphagia

Description

- Difficulty in swallowing (oropharyngeal dysphagia) and passing food from the mouth down the esophagus to the stomach (esophageal dysphagia)

Etiology

- Oropharyngeal—common in the elderly
  - Neurologic disorders—brain stem CVA, dementia, mass lesion, Parkinson's, MS, myasthenia gravis
  - Muscular disorders—myopathies, polymyositis, hypothyroidism
  - Motility disorders—upper esophageal sphincter dysfunction
  - Structural defects—diverticulum, malignancy, surgery radiation
- Esophageal dysphagia
  - Mechanical obstruction
    Esophageal stricture (from GERD)
    Carcinoma

- Motility disorder

  Achalasia: syndrome where there is a lack of lower esophageal peristalsis

  Esophageal spasm (spastic motor disorders of the esophagus); normal peristalsis interrupted by simultaneous nonperistaltic contractions; underlying cause not known.

  Scleroderma
- Esophagitis

  Most commonly medication induced (alendronate, risedronate, tetracycline, quinidine, potassium chloride, and ferrous sulfate)

Incidence and Demographics
- Extremely common

Risk Factors
- Comorbid medical and surgical conditions that increase with age

Assessment
- Oropharyngeal
  - Coughing, choking, and regurgitation that occurs immediately upon initiating swallowing
  - Liquids are more difficult to swallow than soft foods
  - May have neurologic signs and symptoms, such as dysphonia, dysarthria
- Esophageal dysphagia
  - Mechanical dysphagia

    Primarily for solids; recurrent, predictable, may worsen as lumen narrows

    Patient may have sensation of food sticking after swallowed
  - Motility disorders

    Dysphagia for both solids and liquids, episodic, unpredictable, and nonprogressive

    May have chest pain

History
- Assess alcohol and tobacco use, weight loss, malnutrition, bleeding
- Medical history for diseases that may cause dysphagia

Physical
- Depends on suspected etiology
- Weight
- Observe patient swallowing
- Neurological exam: check for gag reflex, tongue movement, and upper palpate mobility

Diagnostic Studies
- CBC, liver functions tests, BUN, albumin, thyroid function tests
- Stool guaiac
- Referral to specialist for more extensive diagnostic testing
  - Endoscopy: standard test for the diagnosis and management of esophageal diseases because it allows for biopsy and a definitive tissue diagnosis; done first if mechanical obstruction suspected
  - Barium swallow or upper GI series; done first if a motility problem is suspected

Differential Diagnosis
- See Etiology

Management
- Depends on underlying cause

Nonpharmacologic Treatment
- Speech, swallowing evaluation and treatment

Pharmacologic Treatment
- Depends on underlying cause

When to Consult, Refer, Hospitalize
- Always refer patients with new symptoms of dysphagia to a gastroenterologist.
- Refer to speech therapy for evaluation and management

Acute Abdomen

Description
- Acute onset of severe pain. An acute abdomen requires emergency management.
- Differentiate between chest pain and abdominal pain; cardiac pain can extend from jaw to epigastric area

Etiology
- Acute abdomen—5 groups of symptoms and signs
  - Pain
    Capsular distention of the outer membrane that often surrounds an organ, such as the liver
    Rebound tenderness cased by peritoneal irritation
  - Shock—(tachycardia, decreased blood pressure, decreased or increased temperature, pallor diaphoresis) often means pancreatitis, hemorrhage, vascular insufficiency
  - Vomiting often means obstruction of bowel or biliary duct
  - Muscular rigidity often means visceral perforation, mucosal ulceration
  - Abdominal distension often means obstruction of large bowel

Incidence and Demographics
- Extremely common as part of other medical problems

Risk Factors
- Other medical problems

Assessment
History
- Determine the onset, progression, migration, character, intensity, and localization
  - Monitor over time, 2 to 3 hours for changes
  - Have patients rate their pain on a scale of 1 to 10
  - Determine if pain interferes with sleep; factors that precipitate or relieve the pain; relationship of pain to meals, specific foods, urination, defecation, exertion, and inspiration
- Blood in the stool, urine or emesis may be present
- Social history including alcohol and intravenous drug use
- Gynecological history: evaluate for bleeding, HRT use particularly unopposed estrogen, hysterectomy, and/or oophorectomy
- Any new medications or medications that may cause constipation
- Previous abdominal surgery

Physical
- Assess for restlessness and body positioning
- Abdominal exam: perform with knees flexed
- Observe for any surgical scars or distention
- Bowel sounds: High-pitched tinkling sounds suggest a dilated bowel with air and fluid under tension. Rushes of high-pitched sounds indicate intestinal obstruction. Absent bowel sounds indicate an ileus or peritonitis.
- Palpate for localized tenderness, rigidity, guarding, and rebound tenderness (an indication of peritonitis). Check for CVA tenderness.
- Evaluate for hepatosplenomegaly and fluid wave (ascites).
- Rectal exam: Rectal wall pain can be an indication of appendicitis or abscess.

- Pelvic exam: if there is no obvious GI explanation for acute abdominal pain and a GYN cause is suspected in a postmenopausal woman

Diagnostic Studies
- CBC with differential may show leukocytosis or anemia.
- Serum electrolytes, glucose, BUN, and creatinine
- Liver function tests may be abnormal (AST, ALT, Alk phos, bilirubin, PT, PTT).
- Amylase and lipase may be elevated.
- Urinalysis to rule out infection and hematuria
- Check stool for blood.
- ECG: rule out referred pain from cardiac etiology
- Chest x-ray: to evaluate for heart, lung, and mediastinal disease
- Flat plate and upright abdominal film: evaluate for bowel obstruction, paralytic ileus, perforation (free air in peritoneal cavity), and biliary or renal stones

Differential Diagnosis

DIFFUSE PAIN
- Generalized peritonitis
- Gastroenteritis
- Metabolic disturbances
- Psychogenic illness

RIGHT UPPER QUADRANT
- Cholecystitis
- Cholelithiasis
- Hepatitis
- Hepatic abscess
- Right lower lobe pneumonia
- Subphrenic abscess

RIGHT LOWER QUADRANT
- Appendicitis
- Cecal diverticulitis
- Ureteral calculi
- Ovarian cyst/torsion

LEFT UPPER QUADRANT
- Splenic enlargement/hematoma
- Left lower lobe pneumonia
- Pancreatitis
- Cardiac disease

LEFT LOWER QUADRANT
- Diverticulitis
- Ureteral calculi
- Ovarian cyst/torsion

EPIGASTRIC OR MIDLINE
- Gastritis
- Cardiac disease
- Peptic ulcer disease
- Pancreatitis
- Abdominal aortic aneurysm

Management
- Varies depending on etiology

Special Considerations
- Signs and symptoms in the elderly may be more subtle as they often do not have classic presentation.

When to Consult, Refer, Hospitalize
- Refer for immediate surgical evaluation in cases of acute abdominal symptoms and signs.
- Refer to gastroenterologist if less acute.

COMMON GI DISEASES
Gastroesophageal Reflux Disease (GERD)

Description
- Reflux of gastric contents into the esophagus producing a variety of symptoms

Etiology

- Lower esophageal sphincter (LES) dysfunction: The LES works in combination with the diaphragm to maintain a physiological barrier against gastric contents entering the esophagus. Transient, spontaneous relaxation in LES tone allows reflux to occur.
- Acidic reflux then causes irritation of the esophageal mucosa due to decreased esophageal mucosal resistance to acid.
- Ineffective esophageal clearance of reflux caused by decreased saliva production and esophageal peristalsis occurs typically during sleep.
- Delayed gastric emptying: gastroparesis (common in diabetics)
- Sliding hiatal hernia (protrusion of the stomach through the diaphragm into the esophagus): may predispose patients to GERD

Incidence and Demographics

- Affects approximately one-third of the US adult population
- Common in the elderly

Risk Factors

- Agents that decrease LES tone: anticholinergics, meperidine, morphine, theophylline, calcium channel blockers, nitrates, diazepam, barbiturates, nicotine, alcohol, caffeine, mints, chocolate, citrus and spicy foods, and foods high in fat
- Eating large meals or lying down within 3 hours after eating
- Wearing tight clothing around the chest or abdomen
- Obesity
- Anxiety
- Smoking

Assessment

History

- Typical symptoms: heartburn (pyrosis) described as a burning retrosternal discomfort radiating upward towards the neck that occurs 30 to 60 minutes after meals
- Symptoms exacerbated by lying supine or bending over; improve sitting up or taking antacids
- Regurgitation of a sour or bitter taste into the mouth is common
- Atypical symptoms: dysphagia, odynophagia (painful swallowing) chest pain, hoarseness, cough, sore throat, nausea, and asthma

Physical

- Abdominal exam may have mild epigastric tenderness, otherwise abdominal exam is normal.
- Stool negative for occult blood

Diagnostic Studies

- Not indicated if typical symptoms of heartburn and regurgitation are present and symptoms are relieved by treatment
- Endoscopy: best study to document GERD and diagnose complications

Differential Diagnosis

- Esophageal motility disorders
- Peptic ulcer disease
- Esophageal tumor
- Cholelithiasis
- Angina pectoris
- Pill- and radiation-induced esophagitis
- Infectious esophagitis

Management

- Goals are to relieve symptoms, heal esophagitis, and prevent complications

Nonpharmacologic Treatment

- Lifestyle modification is the key component to management.
- Elevate head of bed on 6-inch blocks or use wedge under mattress

- Avoid eating 2 to 3 hours before lying down, and eat smaller more frequent meals.
- Lose weight if overweight
- Avoid tight fitting clothing
- Avoid substances that cause symptoms, including foods high in fat, citrus and spicy foods, mints, chocolate, caffeine, and alcohol; stop smoking
- Consider changing medications that decrease LES tone if appropriate.
- Surgical intervention for severe disease

Pharmacologic Treatment (See Clinical Implications treatment)
- Antacids and alginic acid; antacids neutralize gastric acid, and alginic acid (incorporated into Gaviscon) acts as a barrier
  - First-line treatment of mild intermittent symptoms
- H_2 receptor antagonists: suppresses gastric acid secretion; symptomatic improvement occurs in approximately 80% within 6 weeks
  - First-line treatment of moderate symptoms and second-line treatment of mild, intermittent symptoms that are not relieved by lifestyle modification or antacids within 2 to 3 weeks
- Proton pump inhibitors: suppress gastric acid secretion to a greater degree than H_2 blockers
  - First-line treatment of severe symptoms, erosive esophagitis confirmed by endoscopy and second-line treatment of moderate symptoms if H_2 blocker not effective within 6 weeks
- Prokinetic agents: increase LES tone and promote gastric emptying
  - Second- to third-line treatment of moderate to severe symptoms typically in combination with H_2 receptor antagonists or proton pump inhibitors
  - Use with caution because of potential for CNS side effects

How Long to Treat
- Reevaluate 2 weeks after beginning treatment with H_2 antagonists; if effective, reevaluate at 6 weeks, continue for 8 to 12 weeks
- Reconsider diagnosis if no response to proton pump inhibitor after 8 weeks
- Treat erosive esophagitis with proton pump inhibitor for 12 weeks
- If patient has a good response to therapy, gradually withdraw medication while continuing lifestyle medications.
- Maintenance therapy with H_2 blockers should be considered to prevent relapse that occurs in 80% within 6 months.
- Lifestyle modification should continue throughout treatment and indefinitely to prevent relapse.

When to Consult, Refer, Hospitalize
- Consult with or refer to gastroenterologist when the patient does not respond to treatment, or has symptoms of dysphagia, evidence of blood loss, iron deficiency anemia, or significant weight loss.

Follow-up

Expected Course
- Often a chronic, relapsing condition; however, the majority of patients with GERD respond well to medical therapy without developing complications or requiring surgery.

Complications
- Elderly patients have increased incidence of respiratory complications, including aspiration pneumonitis, asthma, laryngeal granulomas, and subglottic stenosis
- Hemorrhage, esophageal stricture, Barrett's esophagus, adenocarcinoma

Peptic Ulcer Disease

Description
- Symptomatic ulceration in the gastric or duodenal mucosa that extends through the muscularis mucosa and is usually 5 mm or greater in diameter

Etiology
- Nonsteroidal anti-inflammatory drugs (NSAIDs)
- Chronic *H. pylori* infection
- NSAIDs and *H. pylori* are about equal in frequency of causing PUD; hypersecretory states are rare
- Acid hypersecretory states (e.g., Zollinger-Ellison syndrome caused by a gastrin-secreting tumor)

Incidence and Demographics
- In the US, approximately 500,000 new cases and 4 million reoccurrences per year
- The incidence of PUD in NSAID users is about 36%.
- The incidence of PUD in *H. pylori*–infected patients is about 42%.
- Duodenal ulcers are 5 times more common than gastric ulcers.
- Benign gastric ulcers occur more often in the elderly.
- Occurs more often in males than females
- About 5% of gastric ulcers are malignant at time of presentation.

Risk Factors
- Aging: decrease in gastric mucosal protective mechanisms
- Chronic NSAID use (increased risk of gastric ulcers)
- Corticosteroid use
- Smoking
- Stress
- Alcohol use does not appear to cause peptic ulcer disease.

Prevention and Screening
- COX-2 inhibitors that spare gastric mucosal prostaglandin synthesis such as celecoxib (Celebrex), Misoprostol (prostaglandin analog) 100–200 mcg 3–4 times day, given with NSAIDs; neither of these 100% effective in preventing GI bleeding
- Stop smoking
- Stress management

Assessment

History
- Classic symptom is epigastric pain (dyspepsia) described as a gnawing or dull ache that fluctuates throughout the day
- Pain may be relieved after meals or antacids (usually duodenal) and then reoccur 2 to 4 hours later
- Pain may worsen with meals (usually gastric)
- Nausea, anorexia, and weight loss may be present, more often with gastric ulcer
- Ask about medications

Physical
- Abdominal exam may reveal mild, localized epigastric tenderness to deep palpation
- Stool may be positive for occult blood

Diagnostic Studies
- Stools for occult blood
- CBC to exclude anemia from GI blood loss and leukocytosis due to ulcer perforation
- Amylase in patients with significant epigastric pain to exclude ulcer penetration into the pancreas
- Fasting serum gastrin level to screen for Zollinger-Ellison syndrome; consider in patients with multiple recurrent ulcers and in those with ulcer and no *H. pylori* or NSAID use (hold H_2 receptor antagonists for 24 hours and proton pump inhibitors for 1 week because they may falsely elevate levels)

- Upper endoscopy: best test to diagnose peptic ulcer disease; allows for biopsy to detect malignancy (gastric ulcer) and *H. pylori* infection (through rapid urease test or histology)
- *H. pylori* serum antibodies (do not imply active infection, may remain positive as long as 18 months); proton pump inhibitors should be held for 7 days prior to test as may cause a false-negative result
- Urea breath test (*H. pylori* generates urease): diagnoses active *H. pylori* infection; useful in evaluating symptomatic patients who have been previously treated for *H. pylori* (if breath test positive, indicates unsuccessful eradication).
- Fecal antigen assay positive result indicated active infection and may cost less than the urea breath test

Differential Diagnosis
- Gastroesophageal reflux
- Cholecystitis
- Pancreatitis
- Biliary tract disease
- Gastric carcinoma
- Cardiovascular disease

Management

Nonpharmacologic Treatment
- Stop NSAIDs
- Maintain well balanced diet
- Smoking should be discouraged as it slows ulcer healing and increases risk for reoccurrence
- Stress management
- Moderate alcohol consumption is not harmful
- Surgery for refractory ulcers is rarely performed
  - Duodenal ulcer; selective vagotomy
  - Gastric ulcer; ulcer removal with antrectomy or hemigastrectomy without vagotomy

Pharmacologic Treatment
- Proton pump inhibitor OR
- H₂ Blocker
- Treatment for *H pylori*–associated peptic ulcer; eradication of *H pylori* for 10 to 14 days
  - 90% of patients treated with triple therapy are negative for *H pylori* at 6 months
  - Proton pump inhibitor (PPI) bid *AND*
  - Clarithromycin 500 mg PO bid *AND*
  - Amoxicillin 1 g bid OR metronidazole 500 mg PO bid
- Alternate treatment
  - Proton pump inhibitor *AND*
  - Bismuth subsalicylate (Pepto Bismol) 2 tabs qid *AND*
  - Tetracycline 500 mg qid *AND*
  - Metronidazole 250 mg qid
- After *H pylori* treatment regimen completed, continue treatment with proton pump inhibitor or H₂ receptor antagonist
  - In patients with complicated ulcer (bleeding, nausea, and significant pain), initiate treatment with PPI first to relieve symptoms, followed by treatment regimen for *H pylori*
- Treatment for NSAID-associated ulcer
  - Discontinue offending agent if possible
  - H₂ receptor antagonists or PPIs are generally effective
  - Test for *H pylori* infection
- Prevention of NSAID-associated ulcers
  - COX-2 selective agent
  - PPI daily along with NSAID
  - Misoprostol 100–200 mcg qid

How Long to Treat
- Gastric Ulcer: 4 to 6 weeks
- Duodenal ulcer: 4 to 8 weeks
- Maintenance therapy is indicated in the following: elderly for 1 to 2 years; patients who are H pylori negative with recurrent ulcer; patients who have failed therapy to eradicate H. pylori; in those with a history of peptic ulcer complications.
  - H_2 receptor antagonists may be used every night when going to sleep

When to Consult, Refer, Hospitalize
- Refer to a gastroenterologist for endoscopic evaluation in patients with symptoms of GI bleeding (iron deficiency anemia, hematemesis or melena), persistent vomiting, and weight loss; severe epigastric pain that may suggest ulcer penetration or perforation; persistent symptoms after several weeks of treatment or for recurrent symptoms after finishing treatment; all gastric ulcers

Special Considerations
- Silent ulcerations common in elderly and may present with massive hemorrhage or perforation
- Lack of symptoms can be due to diminished perception and regular NSAID use that may mask pain.

Follow-up
- Evaluate effectiveness of therapy 2 weeks after initiation, and again after completion (between 4 to 12 weeks)
- Using a urea breath test, confirm eradication of H pylori in patients that continue to have symptoms or relapse (may require retreatment with different antibiotic regimen).
- Urea breath test or fecal antigen tests used to confirm H pylori eradication
  - PPIs reduce sensitivity, stop 7 to 14 days before test
- Successful H. pylori eradication decreases peptic ulcer recurrence to 20% per year
- All gastric ulcers should be reevaluated by endoscopy with cytology after treatment to document resolution and exclude malignancy.

Complications
- Hemorrhage, ulcer perforation or penetration, gastric outlet obstruction, death

Gastric Cancer

Description
- Cancer of the stomach

Etiology
- Gastric cancer is generally caused by gastric adenocarcinoma.
- Gastric cancer can also be due to a primary gastrointestinal lymphoma.

Incidence and Demographics
- More common in men
- Generally does not occur before age 60
- Decreasing incidence in the United States; this may be attributed to improved diets and eradication of H pylori infection
- High incidence of gastric cancer in South America and Japan

Risk Factors
- H pylori infection
- Chronic atrophic gastritis

Prevention and Screening
- Annual stool checks for occult blood
- Treatment of H pylori infection
- Diets high in fresh fruits and vegetables

Assessment

History
- Dyspepsia, epigastric pain, early satiety
- Occasional complaints of nausea and vomiting

Physical
- Weight loss
- Rare hematemesis and melena
- Rare palpation of a gastric mass
- Left supraclavicular lymph node enlargement is a sign of metastatic spread

Diagnostic Studies
- CBC/diff: assess for iron deficiency anemia
- Stool for occult blood is often positive
- Liver function tests may be elevated indicating metastatic disease
- Upper endoscopy

Differential Diagnosis
- Gastric ulcer   • Gastritis   • GERD

Management
- Surgical resection
- Adjunct chemotherapy and radiation therapy have little added benefit.

Special Considerations
- Pernicious anemia is often caused by chronic atrophic gastritis in the elderly; patients with pernicious anemia may be at a greater risk for developing gastric cancer.

When to Consult, Refer, Hospitalize
- Any elderly person with new onset of dyspeptic symptoms especially associated with weight loss, iron deficiency anemia, and occult blood in the stool should be referred to a gastro-enterologist.

Cholelithiasis/Cholecystitis

Description
- Cholelithiasis is presence of gallstones in the gallbladder
- Gallstones consist predominantly of either cholesterol or calcium
- Cholecystitis is inflammation of the gallbladder

Etiology
- Over 90% of cases are due to cystic duct obstruction by an impacted stone
- Carcinoma or other tumor that compress the gallbladder and/or bile ducts

Incidence and Demographics
- Over 10% of men and 20% of women have gallstones by age 65.
- Gallstones are less common in African Americans.
- Cholecystitis is the most common indication for abdominal surgery in patients over age 55.

Risk Factors
- Genetic predisposition
- Obesity, rapid weight loss
- Diabetes mellitus
- Crohn's disease
- Cirrhosis
- Hyperlipidemia
- Medications that cause cholesterol saturation, such as estrogen and gemfibrozil (Lopid)

Prevention and Screening
- Low-fat, low-carbohydrate, high-fiber diet and physical activity
- Using ursodiol (Actigall) during rapid weight loss may prevent stone formation.

Assessment
- Elderly generally have an atypical presentation, less likely to present as acute cholecystitis

History

CHOLELITHIASIS
- Frequently asymptomatic
- May have nausea and vomiting, right upper quadrant
- Pain is usually precipitated by a large or fatty meal

CHOLECYSTITIS
- Colicky epigastric or right upper quadrant pain, nausea, vomiting, and fever
- Pain may radiate to the right shoulder, scapula, or between the shoulder blades if there is irritation of the phrenic nerve.

Physical
- Right upper quadrant pain, increased pain on inspiration during palpation of the right upper quadrant under the costal margin
- Jaundice may be present if there is biliary obstruction.
- Guarding and rebound tenderness may be present.

Diagnostic Studies

CHOLELITHIASIS
- Abdominal ultrasound
- Flat plate and upright abdominal films may show gallstones

CHOLECYSTITIS
- Leukocytosis, an elevated ALT, AST, GGT, and alkaline phosphatase usually present
- Elevated bilirubin may be seen with or without obstruction.
- Serum amylase may also be elevated, especially if a biliary duct obstruction has occurred at or near the pancreatic duct causing a concomitant pancreatitis.

Differential Diagnosis
- Appendicitis
- Bowel obstruction
- Pancreatitis
- Hepatitis
- Peptic ulcer disease
- Gastroesophageal reflux disease (GERD)
- Carcinoma of the gallbladder or bile ducts
- Irritable bowel syndrome
- Pneumonia
- Thoracic disease
- Angina

Management

Nonpharmacologic Treatment
- Cholecystectomy on a nonurgent basis
- Cholelithiasis—low-fat diet
- Cholecystitis—bowel rest and IV hydration, hospitalize

Pharmacologic Treatment
- Ursodiol (Actigall, a naturally occurring bile acid that inhibits intestinal absorption of cholesterol) 8–10 mg/kg/day PO in divided bid/tid doses in patients who refuse or cannot tolerate surgery

When to Consult, Refer, Hospitalize
- Cholelithiasis requires surgical consult.
- Cholecystitis requires hospitalization with surgical evaluation.

Follow-up

Expected Course
- Uncomplicated cholecystectomy usually followed by complete resolution of symptoms

Complications
- In obese, diabetic, elderly, or immunosuppressed patients, may have severe complications with minimal symptoms
- Gangrene, necrosis, pancreatitis, perforation and peritonitis, liver abscess, suppurative cholangitis, and other complications of surgery
- Mortality rate is markedly increased in the elderly who have an open cholecystectomy for acute cholecystitis.

Irritable Bowel Syndrome

Description
- Chronic, recurrent gastrointestinal disorder characterized by abdominal pain and altered bowel habits in the absence of organic disease
- Symptoms may be constant or intermittent, but must be present for 3 months

Etiology
- Unknown, but may be related to the following:
  - Abnormal intestinal motility described as excessive spastic contractions causing constipation, and/or decreased contractions (replaced by infrequent propulsive movements) causing diarrhea
  - Decreased pain threshold in response to abdominal distension from flatulence
  - Specific food intolerances (lactose, high fat, citrus or spicy foods, dietetic sweeteners, and gas-producing foods such as beans, cabbage, and raw onions)
  - Malabsorption of bile acids
  - Psychological problems are present in approximately three-fourths of patients (anxiety, depression, somatization, personality disorders, etc.)

Incidence and Demographics
- Common, occurs in 15% to 20% of the population between the ages of 20 and 40; persists into old age
- More common in women than men

Risk Factors
- Familial history
- Emotional and physical stress can exacerbate symptoms (e.g., anxiety, excessive worry, major loss, improper diet, overwork, decreased sleep, and poor physical fitness)

Prevention and Screening
- Stress reduction
- Maintain healthy lifestyle by eating a well-balanced, high-fiber, low fat diet; regular exercise; and adequate sleep
- Avoid foods or other substances that exacerbate symptoms (see specific foods listed above)
- Avoid caffeine, tobacco, and alcohol

Assessment

History
- Intermittent, crampy, lower abdominal pain that may radiate to the upper abdomen or chest
- Constipation, a more common symptoms in elderly, is described as small, infrequent, hard stools or straining to defecate.
- Diarrhea (usually 4 to 6 stools per day) described as watery, ribbonlike, with clear mucous in the

stool; diarrhea should not wake patient from sleep. Symptoms of incomplete evacuation and urgency may also be present
- Often alternates between both constipation and diarrhea; increased flatulence and bloating may be present. Symptoms exacerbated by meals and stress, usually relieved by defecation
- History of increased emotional or physical stress, depression, or preoccupation with bowel habits

Physical
- Usually normal, may have mild weight loss
- Lower abdominal tenderness may be present, not pronounced; tender cord may be palpated over the sigmoid colon (left lower quadrant), indicates presence of stool; abdominal tympany if air trapping present; mildly hyperactive bowel sounds may be present; digital rectal exam normal

Diagnostic Studies
- Laboratory evaluation
  - CBC with differential, erythrocyte sedimentation rate (ESR), and thyroid function tests are normal; stool test for occult blood negative
  - In patients with diarrhea, stool studies are negative (culture, ova and parasite, and C *difficile*)
- Diagnostic tests
  - Flexible sigmoidoscopy, colonoscopy, or barium enema with sigmoidoscopy to rule out organic disease All tests are usually normal; however, spastic contractions may be noted during barium enema
  - Small bowel series to rule out Crohn disease when diarrhea predominates
  - Abdominal plain radiograph during an acute episode of abdominal pain to exclude bowel obstruction

Differential Diagnosis
- Inflammatory bowel disease
- Infectious diarrhea
- Thyroid disease
- Diverticulitis
- Colon cancer
- Lactose intolerance

Management

Nonpharmacologic Treatment
- Patients should keep a diary in which foods, symptoms, and daily events are recorded to identify possible exacerbating factors.
- Avoid foods and other agents that worsen symptoms.
- A lactose free diet should be tried for 2 weeks in all patients to exclude lactose intolerance.
- A high-fiber diet (20–30 g/day) is recommended; may cause bloating and flatulence initially but usually resolve in few weeks (increase gradually); use 1 tsp bran powder 2–3 times/day added to food or in 8-oz liquid
- Management of stress through relaxation techniques and behavior modification

Pharmacologic Treatment
- Bulk-forming agents may be better tolerated than bran
  - Psyllium (Metamucil) 1 tbs in 8 oz of fluid up to 3 times/day
  - Methylcellulose (Citrucel) 5–20 mL in 8 oz of fluid up to 3 times/day
- Anticholinergic agents: relieve spasm and abdominal pain
  - Dicyclomine hydrochloride (Bentyl) 10–20 mg qid prn
  - Hyoscyamine sulfate (Levsin) 0.125 mg 1–2 (tabs or tsp) qid orally or sublingually prn
  - May increase constipation and increase risk of confusion in the frail elderly
- Tegaserod (Zelnorm)
  - 5-HT4 receptor agonist used for IBS in women whose primary symptom is constipation
  - Main adverse reaction is diarrhea
- Antidiarrheal agents: used on an as-needed basis

- Treatment for flatulence: simethicone (Phazyme, Gas-X) 125 mg qid prn with meals and at nighttime
- Antidepressants: tricyclic or SSRI in patients with chronic, unremitting abdominal pain
- Anxiolytics: Buspirone
- Other anxiolytics and opioids should not be used chronically in these patients because of their high addiction potential and increased constipation with opioids.

How Long to Treat
- High-fiber diet and avoidance of exacerbating agents should be continued indefinitely.
- Use other agents as needed for symptomatic management.

When to Consult, Refer, Hospitalize
- Refer to, or consult with, a physician or gastroenterologist for initial evaluation or for severe disease, nocturnal diarrhea, fever, and weight loss.
- Refer to a psychologist for counseling and stress management if appropriate

Follow-up

Expected Course
- Most respond well to treatment during the initial 12-month period; however, irritable bowel syndrome is a chronic, relapsing condition that may require prolonged therapy.
- Symptoms usually decrease with age

Complications
- Generally none

Diverticulosis/Diverticulitis

Description
- Diverticulosis is an outpouching in the wall of the gastrointestinal tract.
- Diverticulitis is an inflammation that can vary from a small abscess to peritonitis.
- Size of the diverticula can vary from small to large, number can be one to several dozen
- Diverticula more common in the sigmoid colon than in the proximal colon

Etiology
- Diverticulosis is thought to be result of poor dietary fiber intake over many years that results in hypertrophy, thickening, and fibrosis of the bowel wall from movement of hard stool under increased intraluminal pressures.
- Diverticulitis generally caused by mechanical obstruction from retention of undigested food residues and bacteria in the diverticula

Incidence and Demographics
- 30% at age 60
- More than 50% over age 80
- More common in men than women

Risk Factors
- Low-fiber diet
- Sedentary life style
- Increased age

Prevention and Screening
- High-fiber diet

Assessment
- Classical presentation, such as fever, leukocytosis, or significant abdominal pain may be decreased in the elderly.

History

DIVERTICULOSIS
- Usually no complaints
- May have chronic constipation, abdominal pain, or fluctuating bowel habits

DIVERTICULITIS
- Complaints may vary according to severity of the inflammation and infection
- Crampy left lower or mid abdominal pain that may radiate to the back, or acute pain that is localized to the left lower quadrant. Pain usually exacerbated after meals and improved with bowel movement or passage of flatus. Fever, constipation, loose stool, and/or nausea and vomiting may be present.

Physical

DIVERTICULOSIS
- Usually normal but may have mild left lower quadrant tenderness with a palpable mass

DIVERTICULITIS
- Abdomen is often distended and tympanitic to percussion with diminished bowel sounds
- Rebound tenderness may also be present and may be suggestive of a perforated diverticula.
- Rectal exam may reveal a palpable mass indicating a pelvic abscess.

Diagnostic Studies

DIVERTICULOSIS
- Laboratory is normal

DIVERTICULOSIS
- CBC shows a mild to moderate leukocytosis
- Elevated ESR
- Stool for occult blood is often positive
- Flat plate and upright abdominal film is obtained to look for free air (sign of perforation), ileus, and small or large bowel obstruction. Air in the bladder may indicate a fistula.

DIFFERENTIAL DIAGNOSIS

DIVERTICULOSIS
- Irritable bowel syndrome
- Constipation

DIVERTICULITIS
- See Acute Abdomen

Management

Nonpharmacologic Treatment
- Low-residue diet
- Avoid eating seeds, nuts, and corn
- Surgical management required for abscess or perforation
- Encourage fluid intake
- Keep stools soft

Pharmacologic Treatment
- Mild symptoms: metronidazole (Flagyl) 250–500 mg PO q 8 h plus either ciprofloxacin (Cipro) 500 mg PO q 12 h or trimethoprim-sulfamethoxazole 160/800 (Bactrim DS) PO q 12 h
- Moderate to severe symptoms: requires hospitalization and IV antibiotics

How Long to Treat
- Mild symptoms: 14 days
- Moderate to severe symptoms: length of treatment may vary

When to Consult, Refer, Hospitalize
- Hospitalization with surgical consultation should be obtained in all patients with severe diverticulitis (fever, elevated WBC, rebound tenderness, vomiting, rectal pain) and for those who fail 72 hours of medical management.

Follow-up
Expected Course
- Response to antibiotics should occur in 3 days.
- Diverticulitis recurs in one-third of patients who receive medical management. Recurrent attacks are an indication for elective surgical resection.

Complications
- Perforation, peritonitis, hemorrhage, fistula and bowel obstruction, abscess, septicemia

Colorectal Cancer

Description
- Cancer of the large intestine including the rectum

Etiology
- Most colon cancers are adenocarcinomas that begin as adenomatous polyps (benign epithelial growths).

Incidence and Demographics
- Second leading cause of death due to malignancy in the US with 55,000 deaths annually
- Increased prevalence in developed countries, urban areas, and advantaged socioeconomic groups
- Incidence increases after age 40 with 90% of new cases occurring over age 50
- Higher incidence in people of German, Irish, Czechoslovakian, and French descent

Risk Factors
- Age
- Personal history of adenomatous polyps or neoplasia
- Family history
- Inflammatory bowel disease
- Gynecological cancer

Prevention and Screening
- Annual digital rectal examination in all patients over age 40
- Stool for occult blood yearly beginning at age 50
- Flexible sigmoidoscopy at age 50 with follow-up every 3 to 5 years
- High-risk patients with a first-degree relative with colon cancer, a screening air-contrast barium enema or colonoscopy recommended beginning at 40. Patients with a negative screening colonoscopy may defer further screening for 3 to 5 years
- Diet high in fruits, and vegetables, calcium, folic acid
- NSAIDs and a daily aspirin have also been shown to be beneficial.

Assessment
History
- Often colorectal cancer reaches advanced stages without symptoms.
- Left-sided colon cancers more commonly cause rectal bleeding and altered bowel habits. Obstructive symptoms may occur. Pencil-thin stools may occur and occasionally diarrhea.
- Right-sided colon cancers rarely present with obstructive symptoms. Bleeding is slow and not visible in the stool, therefore anemia is the most common presenting symptom.

Physical
- A mass may be palpated in the abdomen.

- Rectal mass may be palpated on digital exam
- The liver should be evaluated for enlargement, suggesting metastatic disease.

Diagnostic Studies
- Stool for occult blood
- CBC to evaluate for iron deficiency anemia
- Carcinoembryonic antigen (CEA)
  - Normally secreted in the GI tract
  - Use for monitoring colorectal cancer, especially for metastatic disease
  - May also be elevated with any mucosal damage to the GI tract such as inflammatory bowel disease
  - Also secreted by tumors of the lung, pancreas, and liver
  - Highest levels are with metastatic disease to the liver
- Elevated liver function tests raise concern for possible liver metastasis
- Colonoscopy with biopsy confirms diagnosis; also used in screening high-risk patients
- Abdominal CT used to evaluate for metastatic disease in patients with colorectal cancer

Differential Diagnosis
- Rectal polyps
- Hemorrhoids
- Rectal fissures
- Colorectal strictures
- Diverticulosis
- Colorectal infections
- Inflammatory lesions
- Other neoplasms
- Inflammatory bowel disease
- Arterial venous malformations
- Masses outside bowel wall

Management
- Depends on cancer stage (tumor size and extent of bowel wall invasion, lymph node involvement, and presence of metastasis), and type of tumor
- Surgery is the treatment of choice

Nonpharmacologic Treatment
- Referral to surgeon for surgery and/or radiation

Pharmacologic Treatment
- Chemotherapy

When to Consult, Refer, Hospitalize
- If colon cancer is diagnosed or suspected, refer to a surgeon
- Patients with high risk should be followed regularly by a gastroenterologist

Follow-up
- Carcinoembryonic antigen (CEA) is a marker for treatment response in patients who have been diagnosed with colorectal cancer. If treatment response occurs, the CEA level should decrease.

Expected Course
- Depends on the stage of the cancer and type of tumor

Complications
- Complications associated with chemotherapy, radiation, surgery, and/or metastasis, death

Hernias

Description
- A defect in the abdominal wall that allows intra-abdominal contents to protrude
  - Types of hernias, based on their location, are inguinal, femoral, umbilical, and epigastric and incisional

- Inguinal hernias further subdivided into direct (through the inguinal floor) and indirect (through the internal inguinal ring)
- Clinically, all hernias can be described as either reducible (contents can be pushed back into the abdominal cavity); nonreducible, also called incarcerated (contents cannot be pushed back into the abdominal cavity); strangulated (an incarcerated hernia, in which the blood supply of the hernial contents is compromised)

Etiology
- Congenital or acquired defect in the abdominal wall
- Situations or conditions that raise intra-abdominal pressure increase occurrence (e.g., Valsalva, ascites, obesity)

Incidence and Demographics
- Common in middle-aged and elderly persons

Risk Factors
- Constipation
- Prostatic hypertrophy (outflow obstruction causes straining during micturition)
- Chronic cough
- Ascites
- Obesity

Prevention and Screening
- Avoid excessive straining and lose weight if overweight

Assessment

History
- Bulging mass exacerbated by standing or straining; may be asymptomatic or described as dull ache or burning discomfort; dragging sensation may occur with large hernia that extends into scrotum
- Strangulated hernias present with severe pain, fever, nausea and vomiting, abdominal distension, and constipation.

Physical
- Inspection and palpation in both the supine and standing positions, while the patient performs a Valsalva maneuver; abdominal exam to evaluate tenderness, masses, hepatomegaly, and ascites; digital rectal exam to exclude enlarged prostate
- Inguinal: with the index finger, invaginate the scrotum following the spermatic cord to the opening of the external inguinal ring, and if possible, follow the inguinal canal up to the internal inguinal ring; have the patient Valsalva while your index finger is at the external inguinal ring and/or in the inguinal canal.
- Indirect hernia occurs near the internal inguinal ring and often extends into the scrotum. A direct hernia occurs near the external inguinal ring.
- Femoral: palpate medial to the femoral vessels and inferior to the inguinal canal
- Umbilical: palpate the umbilical region in the supine position while the patient raises his head and performs a Valsalva maneuver.
- Epigastric: usually a small mass located midline between the umbilicus and xiphoid cartilage
- Incisional: presents as a bulge through a surgical incision

Diagnostic Studies
- CBC may show leukocytosis if strangulation is present
- Ultrasound may be helpful to diagnose a hernia in patients who report symptoms but have no palpable mass; can differentiate an incarcerated hernia from an enlarged lymph node or other cause

Differential Diagnosis

- Muscle strain
- Arthritis
- Lipoma
- Lymphadenopathy
- Groin abscess
- Hydrocele
- Varicocele
- Testicular tumor
- Undescended testicle

Management

Nonpharmacologic Treatment

- Patients with symptomatic, reducible inguinal hernias, who have relative contraindications to surgery, may wear a truss (keeps hernia reduced); however, this is not always effective.

Pharmacologic Treatment

- None indicated

Surgical Intervention

- Patients with evidence indicating a strangulated hernia must undergo emergent surgery.
- Elective herniorrhaphy (hernia repair) is indicated for all abdominal hernias before incarceration and strangulation occur.
- Uncomplicated hernia repair is often done under local or spinal anesthesia as an outpatient.
- Most elderly can tolerate surgery.

When to Consult, Refer, Hospitalize

- Refer to a surgeon for evaluation

Follow-up

Expected Course

- Risk of reoccurrence after hernia repair

Complications

- Ischemic bowel with a strangulated hernia; bowel obstruction

Hemorrhoids

Description

- Hemorrhoids are venous varicosities of the hemorrhoidal venous plexus that are classified as either internal (above pectinate line) or external (below pectinate line).
- Internal hemorrhoids may prolapse and strangulate, causing thrombosis, an extremely painful condition.

Etiology

- Caused by straining that occurs while lifting or having a bowel movement
- Increased portal venous pressure may contribute

Incidence and Demographics

- Occurs in 50% of adults over age 50

Risk Factors

- Constipation
- Prolonged sitting or standing
- Heavy lifting
- Obesity
- Congestive heart failure
- Portal hypertension
- Rectal surgery
- Loss of muscle tone
- Anal intercourse

Prevention and Screening

- High-fiber diet
- Avoiding constipation and straining to defecate
- Avoid straining while lifting

- Avoid prolonged periods of sitting or standing, change position frequently
- Weight loss if overweight

Assessment

History
- Rectal bleeding (usually painless and bright red)
- Rectal discomfort, itching, burning
- Constipation or straining
- Previous management including surgery

Physical
- External hemorrhoids are a soft and painless mass exterior to the anal verge.
- Internal hemorrhoids may be palpated by digital rectal exam or visualized by anoscopy.
- If thrombosed, hemorrhoids are bluish in color, firm, and tender to palpation.

Diagnostic Studies
- CBC to rule out anemia
- Sigmoidoscopy or colonoscopy may be done to rule out other causes of rectal bleeding.

Differential Diagnosis
- Anal skin tags
- Anal fissure
- Abscess
- Hypertrophied anal papilla
- Prolapse of rectal mucosa
- Rectal polyps
- Rectal or anal carcinoma

Management

Nonpharmacologic Treatment
- Eliminate risk factors when possible
- Avoid direct pressure on hemorrhoid while sitting—donut pillow
- Warm sitz baths 2 to 3 times daily for 20 minutes, witch hazel compresses
- High fiber diet (20–30 g/day) and increased fluid intake (six to eight 8-oz glasses/day, recommend increasing fluids with caution in those with CHF or hyponatremia)
- Witch hazel (Tucks) compresses tid–qid prn
- Surgical treatment—injection sclerotherapy, rubber band ligation, excision

Pharmacologic Treatment
- Bulk-forming laxatives to soften stool and prevent constipation
- Stool softeners to reduce straining during defecation
- Topical hydrocortisone preparations: relieve pain, itching, and inflammation; cream, foam, and suppositories are available
  - Pramoxine HCl 1%, zinc oxide 12.5%, mineral oil (Anusol) and Anusol-HC with hydrocortisone 25 mg prn up to 6 times a day
  - ProctoFoam-HC, Hydrocortisone cream 1%–2.5%
- Local analgesic spray, suppository, or cream: provides pain relief
  - Benzocaine (Hurricane), pramoxine (Anusol) or dibucaine (Nupercainal)

How Long to Treat
- Use topical hydrocortisone preparations for a maximum of 2 to 3 weeks; stool softeners and bulk-forming laxatives may be used indefinitely to prevent reoccurrence

When to Consult, Refer, Hospitalize
- Refer to a colorectal surgeon when symptoms do not respond to conservative treatment within 3 to 4 weeks
- Refer to a gastroenterologist for severe pain, rectal bleeding, strangulation, ulceration, perianal infection, rectal prolapse, or for recurrent symptomatic hemorrhoids

Follow-up

Expected Course
- Patients should follow up for further evaluation if no improvement in symptoms within 2 weeks of initiating treatment, if rectal bleeding is excessive or persists, or if constipation continues.

Complications
- Bleeding, thrombosis, strangulation, secondary infection, ulceration, and anemia

Abnormal Liver Function Tests

Description
- Serum liver chemistries are useful in evaluating liver function. Alanine and aspartate aminotransferase (ALT and AST) evaluate hepatic cellular integrity; bilirubin (direct and indirect), alkaline phosphatase (ALP), and gamma-glutamyl transpeptidase (GGT) assess hepatic excretion; prothrombin time (PT) and serum albumin evaluate hepatic protein synthesis

Etiology
- Elevated aminotransferases (ALT and AST) are typically caused by acute hepatocellular injury.
- These enzymes are found in multiple tissues and are released into the plasma in response to cellular injury.
- AST is found predominantly in the liver; therefore, it is more specific than ALT for evaluating hepatocellular damage.
- ALT is found in liver, cardiac, skeletal, kidney, and brain tissue and elevated levels alone may indicate tissue damage in any of those organ systems (e.g., myocardial ischemia or musculoskeletal injury)
- ALT and AST do not indicate the severity of liver injury as they may be normal in severe disease.
- The highest levels of ALT and AST (usually more than 500 U/L) occur with severe viral hepatitis, drug induced liver injury (e.g., acetaminophen, phenytoin, rifampin), or ischemic hepatitis. Moderate elevations (usually less than 300 U/L) are present in mild acute viral hepatitis, chronic active hepatitis, cirrhosis, and liver metastases. Mild elevation may be present in biliary obstruction, with higher levels suggesting the development of cholangitis (causing hepatic cell necrosis). In alcoholic liver disease, the AST/ALT ratio may be greater than 2.
- An elevated bilirubin (a degradation product of heme) should be fractionated to determine if it is predominantly conjugated (direct, processed by the liver) or unconjugated (indirect, not processed by the liver).
- Elevations in direct bilirubin are usually caused by impaired excretion of bilirubin from the liver due to hepatocellular disease (above), biliary tract obstruction, drugs, or sepsis.
- Indirect bilirubin elevation is caused by hemolysis or ineffective erythropoiesis (increased bilirubin production), Gilbert's or Crigler-Najjar syndromes (impaired bilirubin conjugation due to enzyme deficiency), or when hepatic bilirubin uptake is decreased due to drugs, heart failure, or portosystemic shunting.
- Elevated ALP levels (in the absence of bone disease) usually represent impaired biliary tract function.
- Alkaline phosphatase is an enzyme found in various tissues including the liver, bone, intestine, and placenta (more than 80% from liver and bone).
- Fractionation of an elevated serum ALP can be done to determine the source; however, elevation of other liver function tests is helpful in establishing a hepatic cause.
- Mild to moderate increases (usually 1 to 2 times normal) occur with hepatocellular disorders, such as hepatitis or cirrhosis.
- High serum elevations (up to 10 times normal or greater) can occur with extrahepatic biliary

tract obstruction (usually a gallstone blocking the common bile duct) or intrahepatic cholestasis (bile retention in the liver) as seen with drug-induced cholestasis and biliary cirrhosis.

- The ALP is usually mildly elevated in incomplete biliary tract obstruction and in metastatic and infiltrative liver disease (e.g., leukemia, lymphoma, and sarcoid).
- An elevated ALP is also present in nonhepatic disorders, with the most common being bone disease (Paget's disease and bone metastases).
- Elevated GGT, in liver disease, is useful in differentiating the origin of an elevated ALP (hepatic vs bone) as they both tend to increase in similar hepatic diseases.
- GGT is also a highly sensitive indicator of acute alcohol ingestion and of other agents that stimulate the hepatic microsomal oxidase system, such as barbiturates and phenytoin.
- GGT enzyme is also present in the pancreas, kidney, heart, and brain and elevations may occur in disorders involving those organ systems.
- A prolonged PT is caused by impaired hepatic synthesis of coagulation factors seen in significant liver disease and/or with vitamin K deficiency that may occur with malnutrition, malabsorption (e.g., cholestasis, steatorrhea, pancreatic insufficiency), and warfarin use. If administration of Vitamin K corrects the PT, then a deficiency was present.
- Decreased serum albumin, the primary protein synthesized by the liver, may be caused by chronic liver disease or by other nonhepatic factors, such as malnutrition, hormonal factors, or excessive protein loss (nephrotic syndrome or protein-losing enteropathy).
- Inadequate hepatic protein synthesis may lead to a decreased serum albumin; however, because of its long half-life (14 to 20 days), albumin stores are often adequate. In liver disease, it is often an indicator of a chronic process.

Assessment

History
- Generalized symptoms of fever, anorexia, malaise, weight loss, and pruritus may be present.
- Gastrointestinal symptoms: nausea, vomiting, abdominal pain, dark urine, and pale stools
- Additional history is aimed at identifying potential risk factors: history of hepatitis exposure, gallstones, transfusions, previous surgery, medications (including vitamins and herbs), alcohol and drug use, sexual practices, occupational exposure, and travel history.

Physical (See Table 10-2)
- Skin exam: jaundice (include sclera), spider angiomas, palmar erythema, and ecchymosis
- Abdominal exam: ascites, tenderness (usually right upper quadrant), enlarged gallbladder, hepatomegaly and splenomegaly. The liver may be smaller than normal in advanced liver disease.
- Extremities: asterixis and peripheral edema

Diagnostic Studies
- If the patient is asymptomatic, repeat liver function tests first. If normal, repeat testing in 3 to 6 months is suggested
- If repeat is abnormal, obtain hepatitis serologies to exclude viral hepatitis A, B, and C (see section on viral hepatitis)
- If the patient is symptomatic, further tests are guided by history and physical; consider
  - Mono spot and CMV IgG, IgM titers
  - Abdominal ultrasound: best screening test to evaluate for gallstones; it can also detect biliary tree dilation, biliary obstruction, cholecystitis, and liver parenchymal disease
  - Computed tomography (CT) scan (with IV contrast): best test to evaluate liver parenchymal disease and space occupying lesions (tumor or abscess); can also assess biliary tree dilation and identify obstructing lesion
  - Magnetic resonance imaging (MRI): similar to CT scan but can better visualize vessels without the use of IV contrast

Table 10-2: Interpreting Liver Function Tests

Liver Function Test	Enzyme Found in	Cause of Elevation	Seen in the Following Conditions	Comments
Bilirubin				
Direct (conjugated, processed by liver)		Impaired excretion of bilirubin from the liver	Hepatocellular disease, biliary tract obstruction, drugs	Hemolysis, drugs, heart failure
Indirect (unconjugated, not processed by the liver)		is decreased	Hepatic bilirubin uptake	
Alk Phos	Bone, liver	Impaired biliary tract function (cholestasis) or infiltrative liver disease hepatic excretion	**Mild**—hepatitis or cirrhosis, early cancer; **High**—biliary tract obstruction, cholestasis	Increases with age women > men; Also elevated in bone disease
GGT	Liver, pancreas, kidney, heart brain	Hepatic excretion	Sensitive for acute alcohol ingestion	Differentiates the origin of an elevated ALP between bone and liver
Transaminases	Many tissues	Acute hepatocellular injury—from necrosis or inflammation	**Mild**—biliary obstruction, mild viral chronic or active and alcoholic hepatitis, cirrhosis and liver metastases; **High**—viral hepatitis, drug-induced liver injury	Do not indicate severity of liver injury; Most common cause of elevation is alcoholic hepatitis
ALT	Predominantly liver, more specific test	Celiac disease		
AST	Liver, cardiac, skeletal, kidney, brain			AST twice as high as ALT typical of alcoholic liver injury
Prothrombin Time		Impaired hepatic synthesis of coagulation factors	Significant liver disease	
Albumin	Blood serum	Impaired hepatic protein synthesis; Excess protein loss	Chronic liver disease, malnutrition	May decrease with age

- Endoscopic retrograde cholangiopancreatography (ERCP) and percutaneous transhepatic cholangiography (PTC): usually done after screening with ultrasound, CT, or MRI to further assess cause, location, and extent of biliary tree abnormalities
- Liver biopsy: definitive study to determine the cause and extent of hepatocellular and infiltrative liver disease. Biopsy may be guided using ultrasound or CT.

Management
- Aimed at correcting underlying cause

Nonpharmacologic Treatment
- Avoid drugs and other agents that are hepatotoxic.
- Management will vary depending on etiology

Special Considerations
- Geriatrics: higher incidence of neoplasm in this age group

When to Consult, Refer, Hospitalize
- Consult with, or refer to, a physician or specialist when significantly abnormal liver function tests persist without an identifiable cause or for symptomatic patients in need of specialized diagnostic tests and management.

Viral Hepatitis

Description
- Inflammation of the liver caused by a viral infection that may be acute (less than 6 months duration) or chronic (more than 6 months duration)
- Six types of viral hepatitis have been identified: A, B, C, D, E, and G

Etiology
See Table 10-3.

Incidence and Demographics
- After 60 years of age, there is a decreased incidence of hepatitis A due to decreased exposure and increased immunity.

Table 10-3: Etiology of Viral Hepatitis

Type	Causative Virus	Transmission	Incubation Days	Comments
A HAV	RNA	Fecal-oral route, contaminated food and water, food handlers, crowding, poor sanitary conditions	15–45	Rare complications, not chronic
B HBV	DNA with an inner core protein and outer surface coat component	Infected blood, blood products, via body fluids (saliva)	30–180	Less acute onset, chronic infection common
C HCV	RNA, six major genotypes	Infected blood or blood products, body fluids	15–160	Usually mild, can become chronic
D HDV	Defective RNA virus	Only occurs in persons with HBV	30–180	Only in HBV
E HEV	RNA virus	Contaminated food and water poor sanitary conditions	14–60	Rare in US
G HGV	Recently identified	Transmission similar to HCV	Unknown	Rarely causes hepatitis

- Hepatitis B and C in the elderly mostly due to the increased number of transfusions in this population prior to the screening of blood products

Risk Factors
- Persons receiving blood transfusions and/or blood products
- Patients on hemodialysis
- Foreign travel to endemic areas

Prevention and Screening
- Universal precautions
- Vaccination against hepatitis A and B

Assessment (See Table 10-4)
- Symptoms of viral hepatitis are similar; however, the severity of symptoms may vary among types, ranging from asymptomatic infection without jaundice to fulminant hepatitis (severe form of acute hepatitis indicated by encephalopathy, hypoglycemia, bleeding, and prolonged prothrombin time).
- The elderly tend to have more severe symptoms, including jaundice, mental changes, and prolonged course.

History
- Symptoms appear after the incubation period; varies according to the type of virus involved
- Symptoms are categorized into three phases:
  - Prodromal phase: flu-like symptoms described as low-grade fever, chills, general malaise, fatigue, anorexia, myalgias, and arthralgias. Nausea and vomiting usually occur. Mild but constant abdominal pain in the right upper quadrant is present (occasionally more severe). Pruritus, constipation, diarrhea, dark urine, and clay-colored stools may occur. Most infectious in the 2 weeks before the icteric stage.
  - Icteric phase: If clinical jaundice occurs, it usually presents 5 to 10 days after the onset of symptoms; prodromal symptoms begin to improve. May have enlarged liver, pruritus, abdominal pain, anorexia
  - Convalescent/Recovery phase: symptoms continue to improve; jaundice and abdominal pain resolve

Physical
- General toxicity varies with disease severity
- Jaundice of the skin, sclera, and mucous membranes
- Lymphadenopathy usually present in the cervical and epitrochlear areas
- Abdominal exam: liver tenderness with hepatomegaly in 70%
- Dark urine or clay-colored stools

Diagnostic Studies

LABORATORY EVALUATION
- ALT and AST are elevated; levels peak (400 to several thousand U/L) during the icteric phase, then progressively decrease during the convalescent phase
- Serum bilirubin normal to markedly elevated; clinical jaundice evident at levels more than 2.5
- Alkaline phosphatase may be normal or mildly elevated
- Prothrombin time: if prolonged may indicate serious disease
- CBC may reveal an increased number of atypical-appearing lymphocytes.
- Glucose and electrolytes should be normal.
- Urinalysis may be positive for protein and bilirubin.
- Liver biopsy
  - Performed if the diagnosis is uncertain
  - Gold standard for assessing severity and activity of chronic hepatitis

Table 10-4: Serologic Tests for Viral Hepatitis

Lab Tests	Name	Indicates	Use
HAV			
IgM anti-HAV	IgM antibody to HAV	Acute disease, resolves in 3–6 months	Diagnostic for HAV
IgG anti-HAV noninfectivity,	IgG antibody to HAV	Early infection, peak after 1 month	When persists, indicates previous exposure, and immunity to HAV
HBV			
HBsAg	Hepatitis B surface antigen	Appears first, persists through clinical illness; remains positive in chronic hepatitis and asymptomatic carriers	First evidence of HBV, establishes infection, indicates infectivity
Anti-HBs	Antibody to hepatitis B surface antigen	Appears after HBsAg disappears, present after HBV vaccination	Indicates recovery from HBV infection, not infective and immunity
Anti-HBc	IgM and IgG antibody to hepatitis B core antigen	Appears after HBsAg is detected, IgM anti-HBc may persist for 3–6 months and reappear with flares of chronic HBV. IgG anti-HBc is positive during acute HBV and may persist indefinitely despite recovery	Indicates acute HBV infection; may be negative in chronic infection, may be the only indicator of infection when there is a delay between the disappearance of HBsAg and appearance of anti-HBs (the window period)
HBeAg	Hepatitis B core antigen	Appears during incubation period shortly after the detection of HBsAg	Indicates active viral replication and increased infectivity If persists for 3 months after acute infection suggests increased risk for developing chronic HBV infection
Anti-HBeAg	Antibody to HBeAg	Appears when HBeAg disappears	Indicates decreased viral replication and infectivity
HBV DNA		Parallels presence of HBeAg	More sensitive than HBeAg in detecting viral replication and infectivity
HCV			
Anti-HCV	Antibodies to HCV	Initial screening test, confirm with RIBA test	Indicates acute or chronic HCV infection, not protective
RIBA	Recombinant immunoblot assay	Positive in HCV confirmed with HCV RNA	Indicates current or past infection
HCV RNA	Hepatitis C RNA	Ongoing viremia, detects viral load	Most sensitive test to detect infection
HDV			
Anti-HDV	Antibody to HDV	Detects hepatitis D infection	In persons with HBV
HEV and **HGV**	Serologic markers not widely available	Acute—IgM anti-HAV, HBsAg, IgM anti-HBc and anti-HCV Chronic—HBsAg and anti-HCV	

Differential Diagnosis

- Acute cholecystitis
- Common bile duct stone
- Cirrhosis
- Hepatotoxic agents, such as acetaminophen
- Alcoholic hepatitis
- Ischemic hepatitis
- CMV, herpes simplex
- Coxsackie virus
- Toxoplasmosis
- *Candida, Mycobacteria*
- *Pneumocystis*
- *Leptospira*

Management

Nonpharmacologic Treatment

- Activity as tolerated, avoid overexertion
- Normal-caloric, high-protein diet
- Keep well hydrated
- Avoid hepatotoxic agents (e.g., acetaminophen and alcohol)
- Colloid baths and lotions to decrease pruritus if present
- Antiemetics for nausea and vomiting if needed

Pharmacologic Treatment

- For acute, uncomplicated hepatitis, no pharmacologic treatment is indicated
- Vitamin K IM is indicated if the PT is prolonged more than 1 and one-half times normal
- Avoid sedatives as may cause hepatic encephalopathy
- Both chronic hepatitis B and C are treated with recombinant human interferon alfa and/or nucleoside analogs
- Hepatitis A vaccine
  - Preexposure: hepatitis A vaccine; Havrix or Vaqta with a second dose given at 6 to 12 months; recommended for persons at high risk and persons with chronic liver disease (including HBV and HCV)
  - Postexposure: Immune globulin, given within 2 weeks of exposure, prevents illness in 80% to 90%
- Hepatitis B
  - Preexposure: hepatitis B vaccine; Recombivax or Engerix-B IM given in 3 doses at 0, 1, and 6 months. Recommended for persons at increased risk and persons with chronic liver disease (including HCV).
  - Postexposure: Immune globulin (HBIG) given as soon as possible (within 7 days of exposure), followed by initiation of the HBV vaccination series (above); prevents illness in approximately 75%. Recommended after direct transmucosal or parental exposure with HBsAg-infected blood or body fluids

How Long to Treat

- HBV: interferon: treat for 4 months; approximately 40% respond with relapse uncommon
- HCV: interferon: treat for 6 months, approximately 50% respond; after stopping drug, 30% to 50% of those do not relapse. Prolonged treatment (e.g., 12 to 18 months) is recommended. Ribavirin, taken in combination with interferon, results in higher sustained response rates

Special Considerations

- Report hepatitis A to health department
- Monitor patients on interferon closely for depression, suicidal ideation
- Protect skin while on interferon, can cause photosensitivity

When to Consult, Refer, Hospitalize

- Refer all hepatitis B, C, or D patients
- Hospitalization should be considered for patients over 60 due to severity of illness

Follow-up

Expected Course

- Most patients recover from acute viral hepatitis without any sequelae.
- The elderly are more likely to have a prolonged course and increased mortality.
- Main cause of death is fulminant hepatitis, which is more common with hepatitis B
- Patients over age 50 with acute hepatitis C more likely to progress to chronic hepatitis and cirrhosis
- Chronic carriers of HBsAg and HCV RNA have an increased risk of developing hepatocellular carcinoma

Complications

- Hepatic necrosis, chronic active or chronic hepatitis, cirrhosis, hepatic failure, hepatocellular carcinoma (HBV and HCV)

CASE STUDIES

Case 1. A 68-year-old male presents to your clinic with complaints of burning, epigastric pain after meals associated with nausea, especially when he lies down after eating. He has lost 15 lbs over the past month, which he attributes to poor appetite.

HPI: The patient is a recovering alcoholic. He stopped drinking 8 months ago and has been going to AA meetings on a regular basis. The patient is also a heavy smoker and has frequent episodes of bronchitis. He continues to smoke but has cut back significantly. His past medical history includes treatment for a gastric ulcer 1 year ago. He is not taking any medication.

1. What other questions would you ask this patient?

Exam: Vital signs are stable. No lymphadenopathy. Heart and lung exams are normal. Abdomen is soft, non-tender, normal bowel sounds, no hepatosplenomegaly, no masses, no abdominal bruits. Rectal exam is normal with guaiac negative stools.

2. What laboratory tests would you order?
3. What other studies would you order?
4. What treatment would you provide?

Case 2. A 72-year-old male with HTN is in your office for a follow-up visit. He complains of being constipated.

HPI: The patient states that he's always had a regular bowel movement every morning. For the past month, bowel movements occur every 4 to 5 days only after he uses a laxative. Medications include a calcium channel blocker and 1 aspirin a day.

1. Is a new onset of constipation in a 72-year-old concerning? Or is this a normal change related to the aging process?
2. What other history would you obtain?

Exam: The patient is alert and oriented x 3. Blood pressure and other vital signs are normal. His abdomen is mildly distended but nontender. Bowel sounds are present in all quadrants. No enlarged liver or spleen. No bruises. Rectal exam is normal, no impacted stool. The remainder of his examination is normal.

3. What laboratory tests would you order?
4. What other studies would you order?
5. What treatment would you provide?

Case 3. A 62-year-old, obese white female presents with right upper quadrant pain, nausea, and vomiting. The onset of pain was sudden and occurred after eating at a restaurant. She has had similar episodes in the past but not as severe.

    1. What additional history would you like?

Exam: Temp is 99.5, with remaining vital signs normal. Abdomen is soft. Right upper quadrant pain increases when palpating the right upper quadrant during inspiration, and there is localized guarding. There is no rebound tenderness. Bowel sounds are normal. No hepatosplenomegaly. There are no abdominal bruits. Rectal exam is normal with guaiac negative stool. The remainder of her exam is normal.

    2. What diagnostic tests would you order?

    3. What is the most likely differential?

    4. How would you treat her?

REFERENCES

American College of Gastroenterology. Available at: www.acg.gi.org.

American Liver Foundation. Available at: www.liverfoundation.org.

Blumberg, D., et al. (2002). Treatment of colon and rectal cancer. *J Clinical Gastroenterology, 34,* 15.

Chan, F. K., et al. (2002). Peptic ulcer disease. *Lancet, 360,* 933.

Freston, J. W. (2004). Therapeutic choices in reflux disease: Defining the criteria for selecting a proton pump inhibitor. *American Journal Medicine, 117*(Suppl. 5A), 14S–22S.

Greenwald, D. A. (2004). Aging, the gastrointestinal tract, and risk of acid-related disease. *American Journal Medicine, 117*(Suppl. 5A), 8S–13S.

Huang, J. Q., et al. (2002, January 5). Role of *Helicobacter pylori* infection and non-steroid anti-inflammatory drugs in peptic ulcer disease: A meta-analysis. *Lancet, 359,* 14–22.

Koff, R. S. (2002). Hepatitis A, hepatitis B, and combination hepatitis vaccines for immunoprophylaxis. *Digestive Disease Sciences. 47,*1183.

Metz, D. C. (2004). Managing gastroesophageal reflux disease for the lifetime of the patient: Evaluating the long-term options. *American Journal Medicine, 117*(Suppl. 5A), 49S–55S.

National Institutes of Health Consensus Development Conference. (2002). Management of hepatitis C. *Hepatology 36*(Suppl. 1), S1.

Robinson, M. (2004). The pharmacodynamics and pharmacokinetics of proton pump inhibitors: Overview and clinical implications. *Alimentary Pharmacological Therapeutics, 20*(Suppl. 6), 1–10.

RENAL AND UROLOGIC DISORDERS 11

GERIATRIC APPROACH

Normal Changes of Aging

PRERENAL CHANGES
- Impaired thirst perception predisposes patient to dehydration

RENAL CHANGES (see Table 11-1 for consequences of changes)
- **Renal blood flow decreased** due to sclerosis of pre- and postglomerular arterioles
  - Decrease in renal blood flow by 50% by age 80
  - The kidneys compensate by increased arteriolar resistance to maintain filtration; however, stress can cause the compensatory mechanism to fail.
- **Glomerular filtration rate (GFR) decreased** due to increased number of sclerotic and non-functioning glomeruli
  - After age 40, GFR declines; Most have a decrease of ≥30% GFR by age 70
  - However, one third of older persons, who are free of renal and cardiovascular disease, have well-preserved kidney function.
  - Leads to reduced clearance of toxins, some electrolytes, and medications

POSTRENAL CHANGES IN ELDERS PREDISPOSE TO RENAL DAMAGE (See Table 11-1)
- Females commonly experience mucosal atrophy, increasing risk of incontinence and infection.
- In males, enlargement of the prostate may cause urethral obstruction.

Clinical Implications

History
- Chronic medical conditions, such as diabetes or hypertension, that affect renal function
- Medications for hypertension and other nephrotoxins to which they have been exposed
- Genitourinary symptoms
- Symptoms that are impacted by renal function, such as cardiovascular, respiratory, neurologic, and hematologic
- Fatigue, edema, and change in mental or functional status
- Allergies, especially antibiotics and dyes

Physical
- Complete physical exam
- Detection of prerenal problems (e.g., dehydration skin turgor, condition of mucous membranes, daily weight record)
- Detection of postrenal problems (e.g., BPH, mucosal atrophy)

Assessment (See Table 11-2)
- Assessment Principles
  - Identification of risk of renal insufficiency in elders prior to any surgical procedures is crucial as mortality is as high as 60%.

Table 11-1: Age-Related Changes in the Renal System Due to Decreased Renal Blood Flow and GFR

Function	Age-Related Change Noted by the Eighth Decade	Consequences
Maximum Concentration of Urine	20%–30% decrease	Increased risk of volume loss
Dilutional Capacity	Decreased	May predispose to overhydration and hyponatremia after vigorous fluid administration, causing pulmonary or cerebral edema
Sodium Handling	Impaired	Increased risk of volume, acidosis, and either hypernatremia or hyponatremia
Formation of NH_4^+ (ammonia)	Secretion decreased 20%	Impaired ability to correct acidosis
Synthesis of Renin	Decreased	Serum abnormalities, such as hyperkalemia, hypocalcemia, and elevated parathyroid activity
Renin Response to Volume Loss	Decreased	Inability to autoregulate in effort to maintain acceptable perfusion when renal blood flow decreases

Table 11-2: Possible Implications of Renal Symptoms

Symptom	Possible Implication
Pain or Urgency in Lower Urinary Tract	Acute inflammatory process (can occur even when very small quantities of urine are in bladder)
Pain in Upper Urinary Tract	Usually secondary to distention of a hollow viscus, such as obstruction in a ureter or the urethra, or the capsule of an organ (as in pyelonephritis or nephrolithiasis)
Constant Pain	Usually an infection
Colicky Pain	Obstruction
Urinary Frequency	Excess fluid intake, caffeine, diuretics, hyperglycemia
	Lesions of bladder or urethra
	Detrusor overactivity
Suprapubic Ache	Bladder distention
Perineal Pain	Prostate pain is often perineal and may radiate to the lumbo-sacral spine or to the groin
	Women—prolapse
Weight Loss and Malaise	May be associated with a malignancy (pain is usually a late sign of malignancy)
Urgency	Occurs secondary to trigonal or posterior urethral irritation produced by inflammation, stones, or tumor; most commonly occurs with cystitis, urinary incontinence
Dysuria	Infection or inflammation
Frequency, Hesitancy, Urgency and Strangury (slow, painful urination)	Commonly associated with micturition disorders
Hematuria	Should be considered an indication of malignancy until proven otherwise

- Evaluate renal function prior to procedures or surgery due to increased risk of post-op renal failure.
- Diagnostic tests requiring contrast dyes are seldom used because of adverse reactions.

Treatment
- Avoid administration of nephrotoxic drugs or drugs cleared by the kidneys (digoxin, some calcium channel blockers, NSAIDs, aminoglycoside) that may accelerate and cause side effects.
- Careful administration of most pharmacologic agents due to decreased renal clearance and narrowed therapeutic index; elders are also at increased risk of adverse drug reactions due to altered volume of distribution and impaired renal clearance of medications.

ASYMPTOMATIC BACTERIURIA

Description
- Significant (>100,000 bacteria/mL of urine) bacterial count in urine of a patient who has no symptoms

Etiology
- Most commonly caused by *E coli*
- Other gram-negative bacteria include *Proteus mirabilis*, *Klebsiella pneumoniae*, and *Staphylococcus saprophyticus*.

Incidence and Demographics
- Asymptomatic bacteriuria common in elders (especially in institutionalized elderly: 15% to 50%)

Risk Factors
- Female gender
- Aging
- Incontinence
- Structural abnormalities in urinary tract
- Prostatic hypertrophy
- Asymptomatic calculi
- Indwelling urinary catheters

Prevention and Screening
- Hygiene
- Hydration
- Encourage complete voiding
- Avoid use of catheters, even condom catheters

Assessment

History
- No symptoms

Physical
- Usually no findings

Diagnostic studies
- Urinalysis reveals bacteria without WBCs
- Urine culture may be positive

Differential Diagnosis
- Contaminated specimen
- UTI

Management

Nonpharmacologic Treatment
- Increase fluids to flush urinary tract
- Empty bladder fully and frequently to avoid stasis

Pharmacologic Treatment
- None

- Consider antibiotic therapy if patient is immunosuppressed, as in AIDS or malignancy

When to Consult, Refer, Hospitalize
- Usually not required

Follow-up

Expected Course
- Uneventful

Complications
- UTI, Sepsis

URINARY TRACT INFECTION

Description
- Infection of one or more of the structures of the lower urinary tract
- May involve the ureter(s), bladder and/or urethra

Etiology
- Most commonly caused by *E coli*; many strains now resistant to many drugs
- Other gram-negative bacteria from gastrointestinal tract, such as *P mirabilis, K pneumoniae, Enterobacter*, and *Staphylococcus*
- In institutionalized elderly, staff may inadvertently transfer organisms that colonize perineum due to inadequate infection control measures.

Incidence and Demographics
- Most frequent bacterial infection and most common reason for antibiotic use in the elderly
- Prevalence reported to be 15% to 30% of females and 5% to 15% of males. Prevalence may rise to 50% in institutionalized elderly
- When indwelling catheters are used, biofilm collects on the foreign body and creates medium for bacterial growth.

Risk Factors
- Female gender
- History of prior UTIs
- Diabetes mellitus or other immunocompromised state
- Structural urinary tract abnormalities (structures, stones, tumors, neuropathic bladder)
- Procedures: catheterization, recent surgery
- Relaxation of pelvic supporting structures
- BPH or prostatitis
- Incontinence of urine/stool
- Cognitive impairment
- Altered barriers: use of catheters, age-related changes in genital and urethral mucosa
- Underlying neurologic conditions (stroke)

Prevention and Screening
- Meticulous perineal care
- Avoidance of long-term indwelling catheters in all elders and condom catheters in males whenever possible. In patients who must have indwelling catheters, maintain closed systems.
- Drinking cranberry juice/cranberry capsules may reduce pyuria and bacilluria.
- In postmenopausal women, systemic or topical estrogen therapy markedly reduces the incidence of recurrent UTI.
- For those that can void spontaneously, encourage complete voiding.

Assessment

History
- Burning or pain during voiding, nocturia, frequent small voids, urgency, hematuria and/or cloudy

urine, suprapubic/lower abdominal or low back pain
- Fever, chills
- Nonspecific complaints: fatigue, malaise, weakness, or confusion
- New or worsening incontinence of urine (especially in patients with underlying neurologic impairment or cognitive function)

Physical
- Fever, suprapubic tenderness to palpation
- CVA tenderness if upper-tract infection
- Mental status changes may be the only sign
- Males should have careful GU exam with rectal to evaluate prostate

Diagnostic Studies
- Bacteria and WBCs in adequate clean-caught urine or in-and-out cath specimen
- Urine culture shows greater than 100,000 bacteria/1 mL of urine
- Consider reculture after antibiotics completed
- Repeat or refractory infections: urine culture, renal/bladder ultrasound, or IVP
- Other tests if indicated
  - CBC with differential
  - Serum electrolytes
  - Serum BUN and creatinine
  - Blood cultures in septic appearing patients
- If bladder outlet obstruction suspected, do in-and-out catheter to determine postvoid residual
- Suspicion of obstruction with an upper tract-infection requires emergent ultrasound

Differential Diagnosis
- Urethritis
- Diabetes
- Pyelonephritis
- Renal calculi
- Vaginitis
- Female urethral syndrome
- Chemical vaginitis
- Prostatitis
- Meatal stenosis

Management

Nonpharmacologic Treatment
- Hygiene measures
- Hydration
- Remove bladder catheters as soon as possible
- In patients with indwelling catheters, change catheter prior to initiating antibiotic therapy
- Surgical correction of known anatomic abnormalities
- If no contraindications, may encourage use of cranberry juice or tablets to acidify urine

Pharmacologic Treatment
- If symptoms mild, consider waiting to treat until culture results are available
- Treat moderate symptoms with empiric therapy until culture is available.
- Dysuria (some with involuntarily retention): consider phenazopyridine (Pyridium)
- Antibiotics
  - Quinolones such as ciprofloxacin 250–500 bid, norfloxacin 400 mg bid or ofloxacin 200–400 mg bid
  - Trimethoprim/sulfamethoxazole (TMP/SMZ) DS (160/800 mg) bid
  - Nitrofurantoin 100 mg bid x 10 days
  - Cephalosporins such as Cephalexin or Cefaclor 500 mg qid; Cefadroxil 1g/d or bid

How Long to Treat
- Uncomplicated first UTI in women 3 days; men usually receive 10–14 day courses

- In recurrent infection, longer courses of antibiotics are necessary
- Patients with indwelling catheters treated only until asymptomatic (usually 5–7 days) as it is impossible to sterilize their urine, prolonged antibiotic use promotes resistance

Special Considerations
- Uncomplicated cystitis is rare in men; men require further investigation of symptoms to rule out pathological process
- Vaginal estrogen in postmenopausal women may decrease frequency of UTIs

When to Consult, Refer, Hospitalize
- Consult for recurrent infections, if suspect anatomic abnormality
- Refer men to Urology due to likelihood of concomitant prostatic involvement
- Hemodynamically unstable patients, or those in whom urosepsis is a potential concern, may require hospitalization or intravenous antibiotics.
- Patients with signs/symptoms of fever, nausea, vomiting, confusion, or increased WBC generally require admission for IV antibiotics and close observation.

Follow-up
- Check urine culture to determine susceptibility of bacteria to antibiotic.

Expected Course
- If using correct antibiotic (per culture and sensitivity) signs and symptoms should dissipate at 72 hours
- Bacterial cure rates of 70% to 80% are expected for ambulatory elderly
- Patient may have asymptomatic bacteriuria
- Reculture those with atypical course
- Indwelling catheters increase morbidity for UTI

Complications
- Pyelonephritis, recurrent or relapse of infection, renal abscess, urosepsis

PYELONEPHRITIS

Description
- Infection of renal parenchyma or other portion of upper urinary tract

Etiology
- 75% due to *E coli* organism
- 10% to 15% is due to other gram-negatives (*P mirabilis*, *K pneumoniae*, *Enterobacter*). 10%–15% due to *S aureus* or *S saprophyticus*
- Most common route of infections is ascension from bladder

Incidence and Demographics
- Estimated at 10 to 15 hospitalizations for acute pyelonephritis per 10,000 persons over 70

Risk Factors
- Urinary tract structural abnormalities
- Instrumentation
- Stones
- Catheters
- Diabetes or other immunocompromised states
- BPH
- Fecal incontinence

Prevention and Screening
- Hygiene
- Hydration

- Avoid catheters when possible
- May require prophylactic antibiotics if have frequent UTIs

Assessment

History
- Fever, shaking chills, flank pain, myalgias, abdominal pain, hematuria, dysuria, frequency, urgency, nausea and vomiting

Physical
- Classic: acutely ill, shaking chills, high fever with CVA tenderness
- Subacute: low-grade fever, low back pain

Diagnostic Studies
- Urinalysis—bacteria, WBCs,+ leukocyte esterase on dipstick, also present in UTI
- Urinalysis—proteinuria, casts indicates renal involvement
- Leukocytosis on CBC indicates systemic involvement
- Urine culture and sensitivity
- Urologist may order voiding cystourethrogram, renal scan, cystoscopy

Differential Diagnosis
- Stones in renal pelvis or proximal ureter
- Prostatitis
- TB
- Tumors
- Lower urinary tract infection
- Lower-lobe pneumonia
- Any acute abdominal infection (diverticulitis, cholecystitis, appendicitis, pancreatitis)

Management
- Acute: refer immediately for probable hospitalization
- Subacute: may be treated at home

Nonpharmacologic Treatment
- Fluids
- Nonpharmacologic relief measures for symptoms: sitz baths, warm packs, or heating pads

Pharmacologic Treatment
- Antibiotics
- Oral regimens for outpatient treatment
  - Ciprofloxacin 500 mg q 12 h or other fluoroquinolone for 7 days
  - Amoxicillin/clavulanate 875/125 mg bid or 500/125 mg tid for 14 days

How Long to Treat
- Oral regimens treat 7–21 days, depending on severity of illness
- Chronic pyelonephritis—therapy required for 3–6 months
- If obstruction cannot be eliminated and recurrent UTI is common, long-term therapy is useful

Special Considerations
- Rule out mass lesion if no improvement in 3 days

When to Consult, Refer, Hospitalize
- Inpatient management required if patient appears toxic or is hemodynamically unstable
- Outpatient management if able to tolerate oral therapy, adequate renal reserve, reliable supervision, immediate access to health care services if condition worsens
- Refer for urologic consultation

Follow-up
- Repeat culture 2 weeks after completion of therapy and again at 12 weeks

Expected Course
- Symptoms should resolve within 72 hours of initiation of appropriate therapy

- Advanced age may lead to less favorable outcome
- Recurrence rates as high as 15%

Complications
- Sepsis, chronic renal insufficiency, chronic pyelonephritis

URINARY INCONTINENCE

Description
- Involuntary, accidental loss of urine on a regular basis
- Not a disease state, but a clinical symptom of an underlying disease process

Etiology
- Multiple disorders interact to cause UI
- Age-related changes contribute
- Drugs—sedatives, hypnotics, diuretics, opioids, anticholinergics (antidepressants, antihistamines, psychotropics) and cardiac medications (calcium channel blockers, alpha-adrenergic blockers/agonists, ACE inhibitors, beta-adrenergic agonists)
- *Acute incontinence*—sudden onset, related to an acute process or iatrogenic problem, resolves with resolution of problem
  D—delirium, anything that can cause delirium, depression
  R—restricted mobility, retention (acute)
  I—infection, inflammation (atrophic vaginitis or urethritis), impaction (stool)
  P—pharmaceuticals, polyuria (hyperglycemia, excess fluid intake, volume overload due to venous insufficiency or CHF)
- *Persistent Incontinence*
  - Stress incontinence—normal changes of aging (estrogen deficiency in women) combined with pelvic floor muscle weakness, urethral hypermobility, and bladder outlet or urethral sphincter weakness
  - Urge incontinence—due to detrusor instability without local genitourinary conditions, CNS disorders, such as stroke, dementia, parkinsonism, spinal cord injury: UTI acute or chronic, irradiation of bladder, normal changes of aging
  - Overflow incontinence—due to anatomic obstruction from prostatic enlargement, stricture, cystocele, acontractile bladder from diabetes mellitus, or spinal cord injury; neurogenic bladder from MS and other spinal cord and from anticholinergic medications
  - Functional incontinence—due to physical (immobility) or cognitive disability, environmental barriers

Incidence and Demographics
- Occurs in 30% elderly women and 15% elderly men in community setting
- 60% to 80% of nursing home residents
- Overall affects 12 million adults
- Over 10 billion dollars per year in the US are spent on the management of incontinence
- Underreported because many consider it an inevitable consequence of aging

Risk Factors
- Age
- Depends on type of incontinence

Prevention and Screening
- Kegel exercises for women, regular pelvic examination to detect pathology early
- Monitor prostate for BPH and initiate therapy before symptom presents

Table 11-3: Assessment of the Four Types of Persistent Incontinence

Type of Incontinence	History	Physical	Test
Stress	Leakage of small amounts precipitated by increased intra-abdominal pressure, as in cough	Leaks when upright, not supine, cough test when standing—loose urine atrophic vaginitis	Normal urodynamic studies, minimal postvoid residual if needed to rule out mixed incontinence
Urge	Urgency with loss of large amount of urine; inability to delay voiding. Unrelated to activity or position	Prolapse, atrophic vaginitis	Urodynamic testing shows detrusor instability
Overflow	Leak small amounts of urine, a persistent dribbling, no precipitating factor	Suprapubic dullness to percussion, tenderness, may find prolapse in women, enlarged prostate in men	Postvoid residual >100 ml
Functional	Urinary accidents due to inability to toilet	Dementia, immobility	None

Assessment
- Confirm urinary incontinence, identify type, and identify factors that might contribute or exacerbate problem (see Table 11-3)

History
- Requires specific questions such as "Do you have trouble with your bladder?"
- Urgency, leaking, dribbling, burning, hesitancy, nocturia, hematuria
- Assess exposure to medications and other provoking factors, such as caffeine or alcohol
- Bladder habit pattern/record; fluid intake pattern
- GYN history

Physical
- Complete physical
- Mental status exam
- Exam abdomen for masses, suprapubic tenderness or fullness
- Observe voiding to detect problems with hesitancy, dribbling, or interrupted stream
- Pelvic exam to assess perineal skin, cystocele, uterine prolapse, pelvic mass, perivaginal muscle tone, atrophic vaginitis
- Estimate postvoiding residual by abdominal palpation and percussion and/or bimanual exam
- Rectal exam for perineal sensation, resting and active sphincter tone, rectal mass and fecal impaction; assess consistency and contour of prostate
- Neurological exam with deep tendon reflex, sensation; normal sphincter tone indicates intact neurological system to the bladder
- Musculoskeletal exam for secondary causes, such as weakness, ambulation problems

Diagnostic Studies
- Urinalysis and culture to rule out UTI, glycosuria
- Serum BUN and creatinine may reveal decreased renal function
- Serum glucose to rule out diabetes
- Measure postvoid residual urine (less than 100 mL is adequate)
- Additional tests may include

Table 11-4: Treatment for Specific Causes of Incontinence

Type of Incontinence	Treatments, in Order of Preference
Stress	Pelvic floor muscle training (Kegel)
	Bladder training
	Vaginal cones
	Biofeedback
	Alpha-adrenergic agonists
	Estrogen
	Surgery
Urge	Bladder relaxants
	Estrogen
	Bladder training
	Pelvic floor muscle training (Kegel)
Overflow	Surgical removal of obstruction
	Bladder retraining
	Intermittent catheterization
	Indwelling catheter
Functional	Behavioral interventions
	Environmental changes
	Incontinence undergarments

- Urodynamic testing
- Pelvic ultrasound may reveal source of obstruction
- Other tests as indicated by suspected etiology

Differential Diagnosis
- Type of incontinence
- Urinary tract infection
- Urinary retention/obstruction
- Diabetes mellitus
- Neurologic disease

Management (See Table 11-4)
- Good hygiene, frequent voiding, complete voiding, and Kegel exercises

Nonpharmacologic Treatment
- Increase access to toilet or commode
- Limit use of diuretics
- Dietary modifications (avoid caffeine and alcohol)
- Condom catheters in males (only as last resort)
- Incontinence pads (minimize use)

Pharmacologic Treatment
See Tables 11-5 and 11-6.

How Long to Treat
- Indefinitely or until surgical correction

When to Consult, Refer, Hospitalize
- Consult specialist for patients with stress and urge incontinence who fail to respond to behavioral therapy and initial drug treatment.
- Refer atrophic vaginitis with prolapse to GYN
- Refer overflow incontinence or suspected BPH to urologist
- Refer neurologic abnormalities to neurologist

Table 11-5: Pharmacologic Treatment for Urge Incontinence

Class	Drug	Dosage
Anticholinergic and Smooth Muscle Relaxant	Oxybutynin (Ditropan)	2.5–5.0 mg tid/qid
	OR XL	5–10 mg PO qd
	Tolterodine (Detrol)	1–2 mg bid
	OR LA	2–4 mg PO qd
Estrogen Plus Progestin if Intact Uterus	See GYN Chapter 12	Vaginal

Table 11-6: Pharmacologic Treatment of Stress Incontinence

Class	Drug	Dosage
Alpha-Adrenergic Agonists	Pseudoephedrine (Sudafed)	30–60 mg tid
HRT, See GYN Chapter 12	HRT, see GYN chapter 12	0.3–1.25 mg/d PO or vaginal

(Ouslander & Johnson, 1999)

Follow-up
- Weekly visits until symptom controlled

Expected Course
- Prognosis is poor

Complications
- Physical: recurrent UTI, falls, skin breakdown
- Psychological: depression, social isolation, leads to nursing home placement
- Economic costs

HEMATURIA

Description
- The presence of red blood cells (RBCs) in the urine
- May be microscopic (greater than 3 RBCs/high-power field) or gross (visible to naked eye)

Etiology
- Infection is a frequent cause and can be renal, bladder, or urethral
- Neoplasms anywhere in tract—blood in the urine necessitates a workup for GU cancer
- Glomerulonephritis
- Kidney stones
- Benign prostatic hypertrophy, prostatitis, epididymitis
- Tuberculosis
- Connective tissue diseases (lupus)
- Medications (anticoagulants—heparin, warfarin, aspirin, NSAIDs)

Incidence and Demographics
- Dependent on etiology
- Hematuria due to UTI is common in women

Risk Factors
- Depends on etiology

Prevention and Screening
- Prevention of infections

Assessment

History
- Determine onset and appearance
- Associated systemic symptoms—fever, chills, myalgias, weight loss or gain
- Local symptoms dysuria, nocturia, discharge

Physical
- Vital signs, hypertension may indicate renal disease, fever may indicate infectious etiology
- Genitourinary exam—lesions, tenderness, discharge
- Rectal exam—prostate enlargement, bogginess
- Abdominal exam—note tenderness, organomegaly, masses, bruits, percuss for CVA tenderness
- Extremities—lesions, rashes, edema

Diagnostic Studies
- Urinalysis, urine culture, microscopic exam of urinary sediment
- Renal function studies—BUN, creatinine
- CBC/differentia, ESR—rule out infection, inflammation
- Additional testing may be ordered by GU—IVP, renal ultrasound or cystourethrogram

Differential Diagnosis
- See Etiology

Management
- Dependent on etiology

When to Consult, Refer, Hospitalize
- Unexplained hematuria for invasive testing

Follow-up
- Depends on etiology

EVALUATING RENAL FUNCTION

See Table 11-7.
- GFR is the standard measure of renal function
  - It is best measured by creatinine clearance, from a 24-hour urine
  - Creatinine clearance is not sensitive to early disease
  - It can also be estimated from serum creatinine concentration, a blood test
  - It can be calculated by the following formula:
    (140 – age) x body weight in kg divided by 72 x serum creatinine concentration
    It is then multiplied by 0.85 for women

ELEVATED BUN/CREATININE
- Azotemia is increased urea (nitrogen compounds) in the blood measured by BUN (blood urea nitrogen).
- Prerenal azotemia is high BUN not caused by kidney disease but caused by CHF or volume depletion, as in dehydration; the most common cause of acute renal failure
- Uremia is increased urea in the urine, an older term for azotemia/elevated BUN.
- Uremic syndrome is a term for advanced renal failure (end-stage renal disease), when patient has large amounts of urea in the urine—an older term, from when urea in urine was an important lab test. We now rely on serum BUN and creatinine to assess renal function.
- Urea and creatinine are end products of protein metabolism. Both are used as measures of kidney function; creatinine is more accurate because it is less affected by other factors.

Table 11-7: Interpretation of Renal Function Studies

Test	Normal	Renal Insufficiency	Renal Failure	Uremic Syndrome (End-Stage Renal Disease)	Nephrotic Syndrome
BUN	7–22	Increases after 50% loss of renal function	Increases by 10–20 mg/dL	60–100	Normal
Creatinine	Less than 1.0 for women; less than 1.2 for men	1.5–3	Above 3	5–6	Normal
24-Hour Urine for Protein	Less than 200 mg/24 h	Greater than 200 mg/24 h		Over 3 g/24 h	over 3.5 g/24 h
For Creatinine Clearance	Men 85–125 mL/min; Women 75–115 mL/min	50–90 mL/min	10–50 mL/min	<10 mL/min	
Change in GFR	Men 100–140 mL/min; Women 85–115 mL/min	30–50	Less than 30	Less than 15 mL/min	
	50% of normal	29% of normal		10%–15% of normal	

- Serum creatinine tends to remain stable despite decreased GFR due to decreased muscle mass in the elderly.
- BUN/creatinine ratio is used to help decide if the problem is extra renal (pre- or post-) or from intrinsic renal disease. The ratio decreases when the disease is in the kidney, because creatinine rises more than the BUN. For example, when patient is dehydrated, mainly the BUN rises, the creatinine just a little, but in renal disease the creatinine goes up a lot too. Prerenal failure BUN/creatinine ratio >20:1; in intrinsic renal disease less than 15:1

PROTEINURIA
- The presence of proteinuria means the kidney is leaking protein, usually from glomerular disease; also some nonrenal causes
- Nephrotic syndrome is proteinuria of more than 3.5 g of protein in 24-h urine, with casts in urine, has a variety of causes
- Sediment/casts
- Sediment is what is in the bottom of the test tube after urine has been spun in a centrifuge.
  - The two important constituents of sediment are
    Casts: gel-like substances that form in the renal tubules and collecting ducts. They are an indication of serious renal disease.
    Crystals: not usually important in renal disease

GLOMERULAR DISEASE

Description
- Immune complex-mediated damage to glomeruli that produces thickening of the glomerular basement membrane, and an associated decrease in glomerular surface area, which decreases glomerular filtration rate
- Characterized by diffuse inflammatory changes in the glomeruli and clinically by the nephrotic syndrome
- The nephrotic syndrome is the abrupt onset of hematuria, RBC casts, and proteinuria in association with hypoalbuminemia, hypercholesterolemia, and peripheral edema

Etiology
- Postinfection—poststreptococcal, infections in surgical implants especially salmonella, endocarditis, hepatitis B and C
- Renal vasculitis
- Multisystem disorders—SLE, lymphoma, amyloidosis, carcinoma of lung, bladder, prostate
- Drug reactions—allopurinol, hydralazine, rifampin, captopril, lithium, probenecid, NSAIDs

Incidence and Demographics
- Unknown

Risk Factors
- Unknown

Prevention and Screening
- Early and aggressive treatment of underlying cause

Assessment
History
- Edema
- Malaise, fatigue
- Hematuria, oliguria, or anuria

Physical
- Edema, hypertension

Diagnostic Studies
- Urinalysis will demonstrate proteinuria, hematuria
- Serum creatinine, albumin, and cholesterol
- 24-hour urine to measure proteinuria and creatinine clearance
- Serum protein electrophoresis and immunophoresis
- Total serum complement
- Renal biopsy with ultrasonographic guidance

Differential Diagnosis
- Acute renal failure • Chronic renal failure • Cancer

Management
- Refer to nephrologist for renal biopsy and management

When to Consult, Refer, Hospitalize
- Refer to nephrologist

Follow-up

Complications
- Hypertensive encephalopathy or retinopathy.
- Rapidly progressive glomerulonephritis, acute renal failure, CHF

ACUTE RENAL FAILURE (ARF)

Description
- Rapid reduction of renal function associated with azotemia (elevated BUN)
- Classified by etiology as prerenal, intrarenal, or postrenal
- Commonly, but not exclusively, associated with oliguria (decreased/absent urine)

Etiology

PRERENAL—AMOUNT OF BLOOD FLOW TO KIDNEYS DECREASED, MOST COMMON CAUSE OF ARF
- Hypovolemia from fluid loss due to diarrhea, vomiting, hemorrhage, diuretics, inappropriate fluid restriction
- CHF—decreased cardiac output

RENAL—INTRINSIC ARF
- Acute glomerulonephritis
- Collagen vascular diseases affecting kidney (systemic lupus erythematosus—SLE) scleroderma, Wegener's granulomatosis, polyarteritis nodosa)
- Drugs (ACE inhibitors, allopurinol, ampicillin, trimethoprim and sulfamethoxazole, cimetidine, phenytoin, methicillin, thiazides, NSAIDs, aminoglycosides)
- Infection—acute pyelonephritis, others
- Infiltrative conditions—leukemia, lymphoma, sarcoidosis
- Hypercalcemia
- Vascular obstructions—clots, aneurysms, atheroembolic disease

POSTRENAL—OBSTRUCTIVE ARF
- Ureteral and urethral obstruction due to prostatic hypertrophy, renal stones, urethral stricture

Incidence and Demographics
- Three times as prevalent in the elderly as in adults

Risk Factors
- See Etiology

Prevention and Screening
- Early treatment of above-mentioned conditions

- ACE inhibitors have been demonstrated to decrease progression to renal failure in both diabetic and nondiabetic patients; can also precipitate ARF in dehydrated patients, may also cause elevated potassium
- Blood pressure control is crucial
- Avoid dehydration

Assessment

History
- Patients may remain asymptomatic until GFR is less than 10% of normal
- Early manifestations may include only nocturia because of inability to concentrate urine
- Later—anorexia, fatigue, weakness, edema, pruritus, nausea, vomiting, constipation or diarrhea, shortness of breath, lethargy

Physical
- General—delirium, dehydration
- Vital signs—hypertension, tachycardia, tachypnea
- Skin—ecchymosis, petechiae, rash
- Lungs—crackles
- Look for evidence of infection
- Kidneys may be tender to palpation
- Bladder may be enlarged

Diagnostic Studies
- Daily increase in creatinine
- Urinalysis for sediment (casts) and protein—normal in pre- and postrenal failure
- Urine osmolarity
- Elevated BUN and creatinine
- Prerenal failure BUN/creatinine ratio >20:1; in intrinsic renal disease less than 15:1
- Renal ultrasound

Differential Diagnosis
- Glomerulonephritis
- Systemic vasculitis
- Urinary tract obstruction
- Pyelonephritis

Management

Nonpharmacologic Treatment
- Refer to nephrology for care, often with dialysis

Special Considerations
- Avoid urinary catheters when feasible as they dramatically increase risk of infection

When to Consult, Refer, Hospitalize
- Refer to nephrologist

Follow-up

Expected Course
- If cause corrected promptly, failure can be reversed or progression arrested

Complications
- Pulmonary edema
- Hypertensive crisis
- Hyperkalemia
- Chronic kidney disease
- Death

CHRONIC KIDNEY DISEASE (CKD)

Description
- Decrease in glomerular filtration rate associated with progressive, irreversible damage to both kidneys

Etiology
- Acute renal failure untreated leads to CKD
- Most common causes of CKD
  - Diabetic nephropathy
  - Hypertensive disease
  - Glomerulonephritis
  - Renovascular arteriosclerotic disease

Incidence and Demographics
- Incidence increases with age
- Elderly, over 65, comprise over 33% of the dialysis population
- Males more than females
- Increased incidence in nonwhites

Risk Factors
- Advancing age
- Family history

Prevention and Screening
- Control diabetes and blood pressure
- Avoid use of NSAIDs in the elderly
- Keep patients adequately hydrated
- Avoid/monitor use of contrast dyes for diagnostic testing

Assessment

History
- Symptoms are same as ARF but present less acutely

Physical
- Hypertension
- Peripheral neuropathies with sensory and motor deficits
- In late stages
  - Confusion
  - Breathlessness
  - Intractable hiccups
- Yellow-brown skin

Diagnostic Studies
- Significant proteinuria and urinary casts
- Decreased creatinine clearance
- Plasma sodium concentrations may be normal or slightly reduced
- Metabolic acidosis with CO_2 level between 15 and 20 mmol/L
- Low levels of serum calcium and phosphorus are common
- Potassium may be elevated
- Normochromic normocytic anemia
- Reduced kidney size on ultrasound

Differential Diagnosis
- Urinary tract obstruction
- Vasculitis
- Pyelonephritis

Management

Nonpharmacologic Treatment
- Dietary restrictions required to maintain appropriate fluid and electrolyte balance
- Protein restricted to 20 g to 25 g per day of balanced amino acid protein
- Potassium restriction to 2 g per day may be required
- Phosphate should be limited (eggs, dairy, meat)

DIALYSIS
- Hemodialysis is the mode of choice, is equivalent to 10% to 15% of normal renal function
- Peritoneal dialysis may be better tolerated by those with unstable cardiovascular status. In these individuals, sudden volume or electrolyte shifts can cause hypotension, ischemia, and/or arrhythmias.

TRANSPLANTATION
- In recent years, more elders have been deemed eligible for transplantation, as there have been demonstrated benefits. The major complications are infection, rejection, and cardiovascular disease.

Pharmacologic Treatment
- Diuretics (e.g., furosemide) to remove excess free water if kidneys lose ability to regulate sodium; usually not problematic until late in course
- Acidosis may require treatment with sodium bicarbonate if symptomatic (fatigue, tachypnea, lethargy)
- Hyperphosphatemia may require phosphate binders, such as oral calcium acetate or calcium carbonate, to prevent development of renal osteodystrophy.
- Anemia may require erythropoietin.
- Bleeding—fresh frozen plasma may be used to correct bleeding times. Conjugated estrogens have been used for bleeding as well.
- Aldosterone resistance may require fludrocortisone and potassium-binding resins.

How Long to Treat
- Indefinitely

Special Considerations
- Impairments due to renal failure
- Water balance
  - Lose ability to dilute urine leads to fluid retention and decreased sodium
- Acid base balance
  - Dietary protein metabolism produces hydrogen ion (H+), causing metabolic acidosis.
  - This is compensated by respiratory alkalosis and by taking calcium from bones.
- Altered calcium and phosphate
  - Decreased phosphate excretion leads to increased calcium release from bones, which leads to osteoporosis.
- Sodium
  - Reduced ability to maintain sodium homeostasis
  - Inability to eliminate extra sodium leads to fluid retention, hypertension, and edema.
  - Too little sodium leads to hypovolemia and decreased renal blood flow.
- Potassium—becomes a problem later in CKD
  - Kidney loses ability to excrete K+ leads to elevated potassium level
- Lipid disorders
  - Kidney participates in clearing fat from bloodstream
- Anemia
  - Reduction in production of erythropoietin leads to anemia

When to Consult, Refer, Hospitalize

- Refer to nephrologist when renal failure is suspected
- May require dialysis and/or transplantation
- Refer to urologist if suspected obstruction or other surgically correctable conditions

Follow-up

Expected Course

- If untreated and creatinine rises to >10, death is imminent within 3–5 months
- Patients asking to be taken off dialysis because of poor quality of life is the leading cause of death in dialysis for patients older than 70 years

Complications

- Anemia
- Malnutrition
- CHF
- Infection
- Bleeding
- Death

CASE STUDIES

Case 1. Your 94-year-old demented female patient returned home from the hospital for hip surgery with a Foley catheter. She complains of hip pain but not low back or pain or suprapubic tenderness. She has been incontinent of bowel and bladder for many years. She requires total care. Patient is afebrile.

    1. What lab tests would you order?

Lab: Her creatinine is 1.2 and her BUN is 36.
Urinalysis shows many bacteria, no WBCs

    2. How do you interpret this lab work?
    3. What are your initial interventions?

Lab: The nurse obtains a urine culture and C&S without your order. It shows 10,000 colonies each of 3 microorganisms, which are sensitive to ciprofloxin, sulfa/trimethoprim, and Levaquin.

    4. Would you treat the patient with an antibiotic?
    5. What would the urinalysis show if the patient did have a UTI?
    6. What are the possible complications of a UTI in this patient?

Case 2. When talking to your 74-year-old female patient you discover that she has stopped going downstairs for meals in her senior apartment building. She has also stopped going on trips and does not have enough groceries. She denies any pain or fatigue. Seems reluctant to talk about it. Admits to urinary frequency.

History: Upon questioning, patient is afraid she might not make it to the bathroom in time, so has restricted her activities. Urinates every 1–2 hours so she won't be incontinent and still has occasional accidents in which she loses a large amount of urine.

    1. What is the significance of loss of a large amount of urine?
    2. What risk factors would you inquire about?
    3. What medications can contribute to incontinence?
    4. What treatment is effective for her type of incontinence?
    5. What medications would you consider?

Case 3. An 83-year-old man has been taking ibuprofen for 20 years for DJD. He also has hypertension for which he takes hydrochlorothiazide. His blood pressure today is 160/94. He states that is what it usually is and that is fine with him. Routine screening lab shows BUN of 64 and creatinine of 1.8.

1. What is your initial assessment?
2. What other lab tests would you order? What would you look for?
3. Which diuretic is most effective in patients with renal insufficiency?
4. What complications should you monitor for?

REFERENCES

Barry, M. J., et al. (1992). The American Urological Association symptoms index for benign prostatic hyperplasia. *J Urol*, *148*, 1549.

Brown, J. S., et al. (2000). Urinary incontinence: Does it increase risk for falls and fractures? *J Am Geriatr Soc*, *48*, 721–725.

Burgio, K. L., et al. (2002). Behavioral training with and without biofeedback in the treatment of urge incontinence in older women. *JAMA*, *288*(18), 2293–2299.

Ellerkmann, R. M., & McBride, A. (2003). Management of obstructive voiding dysfunction. *Drugs Today*, *39*(7), 513–540.

Grodstein, F., et al. (2003, August). Association of age, race, and obstetric history with urinary symptoms among women in the Nurses' Health Study. *Am J Obstet Gynecol*, *189*, 428–434.

Lepor, H., et al. (1996). The efficacy of terazosin, finasteride, or both in benign prostatic hyperplasia. Veterans Affairs Cooperative Studies Benign Prostatic Hyperplasia Study Group. *NEJM*, *335*, 533–539.

Liu, C. C., et al. (2004). Relationships between American Urological Association symptom index, prostate volume, and disease-specific quality of life question in patients with benign prostatic hyperplasia. *Kaohsiung J Med Science*, *20*(6), 273–278.

Miller, L. G., & Tang, A. W. (2004). Treatment of uncomplicated urinary tract infections in an era of increasing antimicrobial resistance. *Mayo Clinic Proceedings*, *79*(8), 1048–1053; quiz 1053–1054.

National Association for Continence. Available at: www.nafc.org.

National Kidney Foundation. Available at: www.kidney.org.

Ouslander, et al. (2001). Implementation of a nursing home urinary incontinence management program with and without tolterodine. *Academy American Medical Directors Assoc*, *2*, 207–214.

Tan, T. L. (2003). Urinary incontinence in older persons: A simple approach to a complex problem. *Annals Academy Medicine Singapore*, *32*(6), 731–739.

Yoshimura, N., & Chancellor, M. B. (2002). Current and future pharmacological treatment for overactive bladder. *J Urology*, *168*, 1897–1913.

GYNECOLOGIC DISORDERS 12

GERIATRIC APPROACH

Normal Changes of Aging
- For women, menopause is a normal change of aging.
  - Loss of bone mass puts patient at increased risk of osteopenia or osteoporosis, and fractures.
  - Breast: involution of glandular structures after menopause, breast density decreases with age; glandular breast tissue replaced by fat, with increased risk of breast cancer
  - Urogenital atrophy: thinning of vulva, vagina leading to thin friable tissue, increased pH, less acid environment, and decreased lubrication; cervix atrophy
  - Atrophy of the urethra and bladder trigone, contributes to incontinence

Clinical Implications

History
- Many women accept GYN symptoms as inevitable and are reluctant to seek help
- Often feel pelvic exams and Paps are no longer needed
- Often feel a hysterectomy eliminated any risk of GYN cancer, but are still at risk for ovarian, vulvar, and vaginal cancer

Physical
- Many patients will have arthritis with stiff joints and pain that will make the lithotomy position difficult or impossible; may be able to tolerate the position for only a short amount of time
- If unable to get into the lithotomy position, a limited exam can be done with patient on her back or side with one leg raised and supported. A speculum exam may not be possible but the external genitalia will be accessible to exam.
- Delicate friable tissue will make insertion of speculum difficult and likely to cause bleeding, which will then be difficult to differentiate from abnormal vaginal bleeding
- Use smaller speculum; Pederson and pediatric specula available
- Do initial breast exam with patient sitting

Assessment
- Carefully evaluate the risks of the expected conditions and their treatment vs the benefits of treatment or nontreatment before embarking on an extensive workup in the geriatric patient. Include the patient in the decision-making process.
- Dementia may lead to an inability to tolerate the GYN exam; for example, older women may interpret an exam as rape and have a catastrophic reaction.
- While less common in the elderly, STDs should remain in your differential
- Up to 20% of HIV-positive individuals are now elderly

Treatment
- In general, age alone should not determine whether a patient receives optimal therapy for a GYN cancer. Many elderly can tolerate and benefit from full treatment. A well-informed patient can choose her plan of care.

MENOPAUSE

Description
- Perimenopause defined as the time during which age-related biologic reduction in ovarian function results in gradual end of fertility and absence of menstrual periods
- Menopause defined as the point in which menstrual function stops due to loss of ovarian activity. Only identified in retrospect, after cessation of menses for 1 year
- Many gynecologic disorders in elderly due to hormonal changes of menopause

Etiology
- Estrogen and progestin production wanes, reduces inhibition of hypothalamic pituitary axis, results in gradual rise in follicle-stimulating hormone (FSH)
- Perimenopause confirmed when FSH levels >20 IU/L despite continued menses
- Estrogen production in postmenopausal ovary minimal. Most produced by adrenal glands. The post-menopausal ovary continues to produce androgens.
- Fluctuation in estrogen level responsible for perimenopausal symptoms

Incidence and Demographics
- Average age at perimenopause 47 years, duration of approximately 3.5 years
- Average age of biological menopause 51
- About 10% of women have abrupt cessation of menses; 90% have menstrual changes prior to menstrual cessation.
- About 1% of women experience menopause before age 40 (premature menopause).
- Artificial menopause can occur at any time the ovaries are removed or irradiated before biologic failure occurs.

Risk Factors
- Normal change of aging
- Hysterectomy
- Family history of early or late menopause

Assessment

History
- Symptoms vary in individuals, due to non-ovary production of estrogen, as in obesity
- Menstrual cycle irregularity, hot flushes and sweats (vasomotor instability), sleep disturbances, fatigue, irritability, mood changes, vaginal dryness, urinary complaints
- Hot flushes, also called hot flashes, are the predominant complaint.
  - Sudden transient sensation of heat that spreads through body, especially chest, face, and head
  - Accompanied by increased heart rate and profuse sweating
  - Frequently occur during the night, causing increase in nighttime awakenings and fatigue during day
- Many women have other symptoms, such as decreased libido and depression. These are not a direct effect of menopause, but are due to the above changes.
- Obtain history of hormone use including HRT and oral birth control

Physical
- Cardiac exam—for cardiovascular disease
- Musculoskeletal exam—for osteoporosis
- Pelvic exam
  - Lighter pink vagina, thin with less rugae, smaller labia, dry to little, thin watery discharge
  - Vaginal pH 5.5–7 (a rise over premenopausal levels of approximately 4.0).
  - Cervix is atrophied
  - Uterus and ovaries smaller
  - Leiomyomata or adenomyosis reduced

Diagnostic Studies
- Labs: not generally required
- Fluctuation of FSH, LH, and estradiol levels common until menopause
- Within 1 year of cessation of menses, 3- to 4-fold increase in FSH and 3-fold increase in LH (confirm ovarian failure) with estradiol levels below 20 pg/mL
- Pap, wet prep, maturational index: more parabasal cells and less intermediate and superficial cell (changes consistent with reduced estrogen)
- Abnormal amount of WBCs (greater than 10 per HPF) on wet prep
- Any vaginal specimen with blood should prompt a workup for cervical or uterine bleeding sources; minimal trauma during the examination should not cause vaginal bleeding (except the use of a Cytobrush, which often causes slight spotting)
- Endometrial biopsy recommended if:
  - Cessation of menses for more than 6 months, then vaginal bleeding
  - Bleeding more often than every 3 weeks
  - Bleeding longer than 8 days
  - Increased amount of bleeding with clots

Consequences of Menopause
- Urogenital atrophy
- Thinning of vulva, vagina lead to thin friable tissue, increased vaginal pH, less acid environment; decreased secretions lead to increased risk of infection and dyspareunia
- Atrophy of the urethra and bladder trigone may lead to urinary frequency, urgency, and urge incontinence (may occur months to years later)
- Osteoporosis (also see section in Musculoskeletal Chapter 15)
- Increased bone resorption and decreased bone formation

Differential Diagnosis
- Depression   • Thyroid and other endocrine disorders

HOT FLUSHES
- Pheochromocytoma   • Thyroid tumors
- Cancer   • Pancreatic tumors
- Leukemia

VAGINAL ATROPHY
- Infectious vaginitis (trichomoniasis, yeast)   • Vulvar or vaginal cancer
- Bacterial vaginosis   • Diabetes

Management
- Management goals: symptom relief, prevention of long-term complications

Nonpharmacologic Treatment
- Hot flushes—eliminate precipitating factors, such as hot drinks, alcohol, caffeine, warm environment, stress, tobacco
- Vitamin B complex; vitamin E may be helpful
- Many women try natural remedies such as soy; none have been proven effective
- Kegel exercises to prevent urinary incontinence
- Vaginal lubricants such as KY jelly for coitus; petroleum jelly and other oil-based lubricants increase the risk of bacterial growth

Pharmacologic Treatment
- Perimenopause may be managed with low-dose oral contraceptives
  - These include Alesse, Ortho Tri-Cyclen, Desogen, Loestrin
  - Estrogen dose in oral contraceptives about 4 times greater than menopausal therapy estrogens
  - Prevents inadvertent pregnancy

- Low androgenic progestin recommended
- Progestin alone if estrogen contraindicated
- Transdermal clonidine 0.1 mg/day patch 1 x week for hot flashes and other symptoms

HORMONE REPLACEMENT THERAPY (HRT)
- WHI study has changed what the medical profession thought about HRT
  - Long-term estrogen and estrogen plus progestin increase the risk of breast cancer
  - HRT has no beneficial effect on coronary heart disease (CHD)
  - HRT may increase the risk of CHD among generally healthy postmenopausal women, especially during the first year after the initiation of hormone use
  - HRT increases the risk of thromboembolic events and stroke
- Other research suggests HRT may increase chance of dementia
- Large number of formulations of estrogen and progestin for HRT are available
- See Table 12-1 for some of the more common products.

CURRENT RECOMMENDATIONS
- The US Preventive Services Task Force concluded that the harmful effects of combined HRT exceed the benefits in most women.
- In those individuals who desire to have or continue HRT, treatment regimen should be individualized.
  - Begin HRT at time of menopause
  - Give the lowest dose of estrogen needed to alleviate vasomotor instability
  - Women who have a uterus must take progesterone in addition to estrogen to prevent endometrial cancer; estrogen alone adequate in women without a uterus
  - Use for limited number of years
  - HRT usually given orally as either continuous or cyclic therapy
    Usually begin with cyclic therapy as reduces risk of withdrawal bleeding
    Usually change to continuous therapy after about 1 year
      More convenient regimen
      Less breakthrough bleeding
      Many have better relief of vaginal atrophy with combination HRT

BENEFICIAL EFFECTS OF HRT
- Vasomotor stability and sleep patterns improve
- Urogenital atrophy improves
  - Vaginal estrogen best for prevention or alleviation of symptoms of atrophy
    May be used in addition to oral HRT
- Osteoporosis
  - HRT will stabilize osteoporosis and prevent further deterioration.
  - HRT will not stimulate new bone growth.
  - Adequate calcium and exercise also required
- Colon cancer—HRT decreases the risk of colon cancer

ADVERSE EFFECTS OF HRT
- Estrogen alone greatly increases risk of endometrial cancer; increased risk of breast cancer
- Possible increased risk of CHD; increased risk of thromboembolic events and stroke, dementia
- Common estrogen therapy side effects include nausea, breast tenderness, mood swings, migraines (like menstrual migraines)
- Common progestin side effects include nausea, acne, headaches
- Progestin may also cause PMS-type symptoms (irritability) and breast tenderness until cessation of menses is complete
- Common androgenic side effects of progestin include acne and hirsutism

- Current or history of ovarian or breast cancer, undiagnosed breast mass
- Thromboembolia, unexplained genital bleeding, endometrial cancer (unopposed estrogen)

PRECAUTIONS TO USE OF ESTROGENS OR "RELATIVE CONTRAINDICATIONS"
- Seizure disorder, hypertension, familial hyperlipidemia, migraines, gallbladder disease, past history of thrombosis, breast cancer—high risk

TRANSDERMAL OR VAGINAL ROUTE PREFERRED OVER ORAL ESTROGENS IN THE FOLLOWING:
- Chronic impaired liver function, significant liver disease/liver tumors (increased growth of benign vascular tumors in 1950's studies) because it misses the first-pass effect through the liver and allows for lower doses
- Migraines (risk of stroke, increased migraines due to estrogen use in one third of patients)
- Active or history of thrombophlebitis or thromboembolic disorders
- Vaginal cream used for atrophic vaginitis; does have some systemic effect

HOW LONG TO TREAT
- Treat perimenopause with low-dose oral contraceptives for about 1 year, then switch to HRT (see Table 12-1)
- Recommendation: limit use of HRT to 5 to 7 years as risk of adverse effects rises with duration of use
- Discontinue treatment if patient develops contraindications to use or significant adverse reaction to medication

Special Considerations
Include patient's preferences and needs when selecting HRT

When to Consult, Refer, Hospitalize
- If patient has absolute or relative contraindications for HRT
- Adverse reaction to HRT
- Usual HRT not satisfactory to patient, usually due to break-through bleeding

Follow-up

Complications
- Adverse effects of HRT
- Adverse effects of menopause
- Vaginal atrophy
  - Pelvic prolapse
  - Urinary incontinence
- Osteoporosis
  - Kyphosis
  - Fractures
  - Disability

POSTMENOPAUSAL VAGINAL BLEEDING

Description
- Vaginal bleeding that occurs 6 months or more following menopause
- Not due to hormone replacement therapy

Etiology
- Atrophic endometrium, vaginitis
- Endometrial proliferation
- Hyperplasia

Table 12-1: Hormone Replacement Therapy Choices

Drug Class	Trade	Form	Strength	Starting Dose	Comment
Estrogens					
Conjugated Equine Estrogens	Premarin	Tablet Cream	0.3, 0.625, 0.9 mg 0.625 mg/g	0.625 qd 0.5-2 g every night	Continuous—no uterus Gradually taper to lowest dose to maintain vaginal mucosa
Synthetic Conjugated Estrogens	Cenestin	Tablet Vag cream	0.625, 0.9, 1.25 mg 0.5, 1.0, 1.1, 2.0 g	Cyclic: 0.625, 3 weeks on, 1 week off 0.5-2 g every night	Cyclic Gradually taper to lowest dose to maintain vaginal mucosa
17 Beta Estradiol	Estrace Estrace	Tablet Cream	0.5, 1.0, 2.0 mg 1%	1 mg qd 1 g qd	Gradually taper to lowest dose to maintain vaginal health
	Estring Alora, Climara, Estraderm	Vagina ring Patch	One ring 0.37, 0.5, 0.75, 0.1 mg	q 90 days 0.05/day	Reassess need q 3–6 months Change 1–2 x/week depending on brand
	Vagifem	Vaginal tab	25 mcg	qd for 2 weeks then 2 x week	
Esterified Estrogen	Menest	Tablet	0.3, 0.625, 1.25, 2.5 mg	0.625 qd	
Estropipate	Ogen, Ortho-Est	Tablet	0.625, 1.25, 2.5 mg	0.75 qd	
Ethinyl Estradiol		Tablet	0.02, 0.05 mg	Cyclic: 0.02 q1–2 days 3 weeks on, 1 week off	

Progestins

Medroxyprogesterone Acetate	Amen, Cycrin, Provera	Tablet	2.5, 5, 10 mg	Cyclic: 5–10 mg for 10–14 days; Continuous: 2.5–5 mg qd
Norethindrone Acetate	Aygestin	Tablet	5 mg	2.5–5 qd
Micronized Progesterone	Prometrium	Tablet	100 mg	200–400 mg qd for 10–14 days
	Crinone	Vaginal gel	4% (45 mg/dose); 8% (90 mg/cose)	45 mg qod x 6 doses

Combination

Conjugated Estrogen (Medroxyprogesterone acetate: MPA)	Prempro	Tablet	0.625/2.5 mg, 0.625/5 mg	1 tab qd in EZ dial dispensers
	Premphase	Tablet	0.625 estrogen days 1–14; 5 mg MPA added days 15–23	1 tab q̄ din EZ dial dispensers
Esterified Estrogen (Methyl-testosterone)	Estra test, Estra test HS	Tablet	1.25 mg/2.5 mg, 0.625/1.25 mg	Cyclic: 0.625/1.25 3 weeks on, 1 week off
Estradiol, Norethindrone	Activelle	Tablet	1 mg/0.5 mg	1 qd
17 Beta Estradiol, Norethindrone Acetate	CombiPatch	Patch	0.05/0.14, 0.05/0.25	0.05/0.14 qd Continuous, intact uterus
Ethinyl Estradiol, Norethindrone	FemHRT	Tabs	5 mcg/1 mg	1 qd

- Endometrial or cervical cancer
- Administration of estrogens without added progestin
- Anticoagulant administration

Incidence and Demographics
- Common

Risk Factors
- Endometrial hyperplasia and endometrial carcinoma
- Genitourinary problems
- Gastrointestinal
- Thyroid disease
- Thrombocytopenia
- Blood dyscrasia

Prevention and Screening
- Always combine estrogen therapy with progestin in patients with uterus
- Periodic pelvic exams to assess uterus size

Assessment
- Any postmenopausal bleeding must be evaluated thoroughly due to risk of cancer

History
- Timing, duration, amount
- Usually painless
- May report single episode of spotting or profuse bleeding for days or months
- Vaginal discharge, pain, heat/cold intolerance, bleeding or bruising, weight changes
- Associated activity
- Bowel or bladder symptoms
- Anticoagulants, NSAIDs, aspirin

Physical
- Thyroid nodules, enlargement, tenderness
- Hepatomegaly, abdominal pain, guarding, rebound
- Pelvic: vulvar or vaginal bleeding, lesions, or neoplasms
- Rectal blood, hemorrhoids

Diagnostic Studies
- Cytologic smear of the cervix and vaginal pool
- CBC, TSH
- Transvaginal sonogram of uterus to rule out vaginal wall thickening
- Endometrial biopsy

Differential Diagnosis
- Endometrial polyps
- Hyper/hypothyroidism
- Urinary tract infection
- Atrophic vaginitis
- Cancer
- Endometriosis
- Fibroids
- Thrombocytopenia
- Coagulopathy
- Blood dyscrasia

Management
- Treat any causes identified as indicated

Nonpharmacologic Treatment
- Dilation and curettage should be offered to all postmenopausal women with vaginal bleeding
- Hysterectomy if endometrial hyperplasia with atypical cells or carcinoma is found

Pharmacologic Treatment
- Simple endometrial hyperplasia—cyclic progestin therapy for 21 days of each month for 3 months with repeat D&C

When to Consult, Refer, Hospitalize
- Refer all cases to GYN
- Consider admission for acute management of heavy bleeding

Follow-up
Expected Course
- Dependent on etiology

Complications
- Dependent on etiology

PELVIC PROLAPSE

Description
- Loss of normal pelvic support, allows descent and herniation of these organs
- Symptomology depends upon degree and location of the pelvic prolapse
- May present as
  - Uterine/vaginal prolapse
  - Cystocele: bulge of bladder into vagina
  - Rectocele: bulge of rectum into vagina
  - Enterocele: bulge of small intestine into vagina

Etiology
- Multiparous with vaginal delivery
- Menopause: lack of estrogen
- Aging process: decreased tissue turgor
- Hysterectomy

Incidence and Demographics
- Incidence unknown due to underreporting
- Estimate 15% to 30% of multiparous women have some degree of pelvic prolapse

Risk Factors
- See Etiology

Prevention and Screening
- Rectocele: avoid constipation

Assessment
- Correlate symptoms to clinical findings
- Graded by severity: leading edge of prolapsing organ
  - Mild: descending halfway to the vaginal introitus
  - Moderate: descent to the introitus
  - Severe: prolapse beyond introitus

History
- Pelvic pressure or heaviness
- Complaint of protrusion or bulge through the vagina
- Irritation with walking or exercising secondary to a bulge felt in the vagina
- Feeling of obstruction in the vagina
- Incomplete rectal emptying
- Low back pain
- Chronic pelvic aching

Physical
- Examine in lithotomy and standing positions to evaluate degree of prolapse
- Have patient strain
- Bimanual exam and rectovaginal exam
- Repeat in standing position

Diagnostic Studies
- None

Differential Diagnosis
- Urinary incontinence
- Rectocele: constipation, incontinence of stool

Management

Nonpharmacologic Treatment
- Mild to moderate prolapse
  - Avoid stress to the pelvic floor—heavy lifting, high impact aerobics, repetitive stooping, obesity, chronic cough
  - Kegel exercises
  - Weighted vaginal cones
- Severe
  - Intravaginal pessary if patient does not want surgery or surgery in contraindicated
    - Teach patient correct use, remove and clean monthly
    - If patient unable to use, may have family member insert
  - Surgical repair of the specific defect

Pharmacologic Treatment
- None

How Long to Treat
- Pessary indefinitely
- Surgery curative

Special Considerations
- Patients who are fitted with a pessary occasionally become lost to follow-up and/or demented and the pessary may remain in the patient without cleaning for long periods of time

When to Consult, Refer, Hospitalize
- Consider surgery

Follow-up
- Pessary: see weekly until comfortable with pessary
- Pessary must be removed and cleaned monthly

Expected Course
- Variable

Complications
- Prolapse: bleeding, ulceration infection, pain, organ incarceration, urinary retention
- Pessary: infection incarceration; erosion into bladder, rectum, or abdominal cavity

BARTHOLIN GLAND CYSTS AND ABSCESSES

Description
- Infection of the Bartholin gland (unilaterally or bilaterally), which obstructs the duct and prevents drainage; pain, swelling, abscess formation results with chronic ductal stenosis and residual distension

Etiology
- Most common pathogen *E coli*
- Trauma

Incidence and Demographics
- Uncommon

Risk Factors
- None known

Prevention and Screening
- None known

Assessment

History
- Previous episodes; any prior surgical treatment, such as incision and drainage (I&D)
- Pain on the sides of the introitus, dyspareunia, painful sitting or walking

Physical
- Physical exam may show fluctuant mass at 4 o'clock or 8 o'clock or both; if active infection, there may be pain; size can vary up to more than 4 cm
- Swelling on the sides of the introitus
- Tenderness indicates active infection

Diagnostic Studies
- I&D and wound cultures should be done for gonorrhea, chlamydia, *E coli*

Differential Diagnosis
- Inclusion cysts
- Lipoma
- Fibroma
- Hematoma
- Bartholin's gland cancer (rare)

Management

Nonpharmacologic Treatment
- Cyst needs no treatment if not symptomatic
- Mild—warm soaks can alleviate pain and promote spontaneous ductal opening
- Treatment is to perform I&D or refer for marsupialization to establish new ductal opening; laser incision can also be used.
- Wound catheter can be inserted at time of I&D; suture if needed, or tape into place and let drain over 4 weeks

Pharmacologic Treatment
- None

How Long to Treat
- Warm soaks for a week, if not resolved, refer

When to Consult, Refer, Hospitalize
- Refer to GYN if not resolved by warm soaks

Follow-up

Expected Course
- Recurrent episodes unless patient has treatment

Complications
- Stenosis of the duct outlet with distension may persist
- Reinfection causes recurrent tenderness and enlargement of the duct

ABNORMAL GROWTHS
Benign Growths
Leiomyomas

Description
- Leiomyomas are also known as uterine fibroids, myomas
- Benign uterine smooth muscle and connective tissue growth responsive to estrogens
- Discrete, firm, roundish, often multiple in various anatomic locations: intramural, submucous, subserous, intraligamentous, pedunculated, cervical
- Mostly asymptomatic and found incidentally on examination

Incidence and Demographics
- Occurs in 4% to 11% of women; increases with age (20% of women over 35 and 40% of women over 50)

Assessment

Physical
- Occasionally causes menorrhagia (with degeneration and calcification) and anemia, dysmenorrhea, pelvic pain (enlargement, encroachment on adjacent structures, torsion), bladder, and back or lower pelvic pressure
- Reduces in size and symptoms after menopause
- Enlarged, firm, irregular uterus; mobile, mostly nontender, and negative for other exam findings Clinically useful to note size comparable to gestational size ("10–12 weeks' size"; "umbilicus minus 1 cm") for comparative evaluation over time

Diagnostic Studies
- Labs: HCG, CBC (iron deficiency anemia), screening Paps and other health maintenance as indicated
- Pelvic ultrasonography can identify characteristic fibroid changes (hypoechoic, no cysts, uniform structure); map number and location, measure size, and assess normalcy of adjacent structures (endometrial thickness); helpful to rule out other concerns (ovarian cysts)

Differential Diagnosis
- Endometriosis
- Endometrial carcinoma
- Ovarian cysts
- Uterine cancer
- Leiomyosarcoma (0.5% of fibroids; more common over age 40)
- Abnormal vaginal bleeding
- Adenomyosis
- Cervical cancer
- Ovarian cancer

Management

Pharmacologic Treatment
- No treatment needed if asymptomatic
- Iron replacement therapy if needed
- Chronic pain
  - NSAIDs work well
  - Analgesics with narcotics only if unremitting pain; needs gynecological consultation
  - Reduce size medically (Depo-Provera, Lupron), then surgical excision or hysterectomy

When to Consult, Refer, Hospitalize
- Consult with GYN about options to reduce bleeding (Lupron), surgical excision (hysterectomy), and if endometrial sampling is indicated

GYN Cancer
Abnormal Cervical Cytology/Cervical Cancer

Description
- Hyperplasia of the intraepithelial cells of the cervix
- Malignant transformation of intraepithelial cells of the cervix
- Invasion of the surrounding tissues occurs in 2 to 10 years

Etiology
- About 85% of cervical cancer is squamous cell carcinoma
- Endocervical adenocarcinoma is more rare
- 13% of all cancers in postmenopausal women are GYN cancers; risk increases with age
- Optimal treatment of GYN cancer patients should not be withheld because of age

Incidence and Demographics
- The Pap smear has moved cervical cancer from a top killer (US in the 1940s) to a preventable disease.
- Accounts for about 20% of all GYN cancers
- Current lifetime risk for death by cervical cancer in the US is 0.83%.
- Average age at diagnosis of precancerous lesions is the mid 30s.
- Average age at onset of cervical cancer is 45 to 55.
- 25% of invasive cervical cancers and 41% of deaths occur in women over age 65.
- Underscreening is the number one reason 15,700 women get cervical cancer in the US and why 4900 die from it annually.
- Half of women diagnosed with invasive cervical cancer have never been screened, and another 10% have not had a Pap in 5 years.
- Least likely to be screened: elderly, poor, black, Hispanic, and uninsured women

Risk Factors

ABNORMAL CERVICAL CYTOLOGY
- History of early sex with multiple partners, STDs, HPV, HIV, HSV
- Tobacco: nicotine and other substances bind to cells (cancer cofactor)
- DES exposure

CERVICAL CANCER
- Advanced age
- Those who have not received regular screening (Black, Hispanic, and Native Americans, low socioeconomic status)

Prevention and Screening
- No smoking
- Pap smear to collect cells for analysis. Highest risk area on the uterine cervix for cancer is the "transformation zone" (TZ) where stratified squamous epithelial tissue intersects with columnar epithelial tissue.
- TZ appears well outside the external os in very young women and migrates into the canal as the woman ages or as there is disruption in the cervix (childbirth, invasive procedures, cancer treatment). With hormonal stimulation, the TZ may be more visible (hormonal contraception, pregnancy). In DES-exposed women, the TZ may extend into the vagina.
- All women who are or have been sexually active should have regular cervical cytological screening from the time sexually active or 18 years old
- If 3 or more normal Paps and annual examinations, screen every 3 years. Because of the prevalence of HPV and the false-negative rate of Pap smears, some clinicians will opt to screen women yearly despite this recommendation.

- If not screened for 10 years prior to age 66, screen every 3 years to age 75.
- Women who have had a hysterectomy in which the cervix was removed do not require cytologic screening (<10% yield on vaginal cuff smears) but should continue to have vaginal inspection annually.
- Annual cytology is advised if a hysterectomy was done to treat cervical dysplasia, cervical cancer, or uterine cancer.
- Remember that a hysterectomy may NOT remove the cervix. It is important to visualize the vagina and assess for the presence of a cervix.
- If a woman happens to have 2 cervices, be sure to collect a Pap on each one and to label the Paps appropriately (e.g., right cervix, right Pap)

Assessment

History
- Cervical cancer is asymptomatic until well advanced.
- Later symptoms include pain in lower abdomen pelvis or back, anorexia, urinary frequency
- Irregular or any kind of vaginal bleeding
- Assess the history of cervical cancer screening and management of any abnormalities.
- Note any colposcopy, biopsy, and any past ablative or surgical therapy.

Physical
- On pelvic exam, the cervix may appear normal or may have small ulcerated lesions
- Late signs include weight loss
- If frank cervicitis noted, collect appropriate cultures or screens for common etiologies (trichomoniasis, gonorrhea, chlamydia, mycoplasma, Ureaplasma, herpes simplex, syphilis).
- Collect cervical cytology specimens after treatment of cervicitis, wait at least 4 to 6 weeks
- If frank cervicitis is not cleared up, make note of this finding on the cytology lab form and strongly consider colposcopy and biopsy regardless of the cytologic results.

COMMON COMPLAINTS THAT SUGGEST A CERVICAL PROCESS
- Altered vaginal discharge (without odor or itch)
  - Unusual color or amount: suggests change in cervical mucus production or an inflammatory process that has secondary discharge
  - The most ominous etiology is advanced cervical cancer
- Vaginal bleeding
  - Vaginal bleeding of purely cervical origin is most commonly caused by cervical polyps, which can cause postdouching or postcoital bleeding (but are mostly asymptomatic).
  - Infectious diseases often cause postcoital spotting but also cause bleeding from the endometrium.
  - Advanced cervical cancer can also cause frank bleeding.

Diagnostic Studies
- Paramount lab test is the Pap smear
- Late lab abnormalities include hematuria, anemia
- Recall that false-negatives occur from sampling error and from detection error.

REASONS FOR INACCURATE CONVENTIONAL CYTOLOGY (PAP)
- Lab error (detection error): one third of errors; false-negatives, 5%; false-positives, 3%–10%
- Poor specimen collection technique (sampling error): estimated two thirds of errors; with excellent technique, can miss endocervical cells (ECC) in up to 10%. False-negatives are more common in specimens without ECC.

THIN PREP
- Cervical specimen is placed directly into preservative vial.
- Increases number of cells sampled by removing confounding mucus, blood, and debris

- Reduces inadequate specimens or sampling error by 50%
- Increases detection of LSIL by 65% (screening) but only 6% in high-risk samples

CONVENTIONAL PAPANICOLAOU SCREENING

- Pap cytology is most accurate and very specific for carcinoma or invasive cancer and high-grade lesions.
- Not very specific for low-grade lesions and these are often overdiagnosed

CERVICAL CYTOLOGY CLASSIFICATION

- 1940s Papanicolaou five-class system with the WHO standardized nomenclature
- 1988/1991 Bethesda cytology system changed to correlate more closely with the histologic diagnosis
- Bethesda Pap grading system updated in 2001—now more comprehensive
  - Specimen adequacy
    Satisfactory for evaluation
    Presence or absence of endocervical or transformation zone components or other quality indicators, such as partially obscuring blood or inflammation
    Unsatisfactory for evaluation (specify reason)
    Specimen rejected or not processed (specify reason)
    Specimen processed and examined, but unsatisfactory for evaluation of epithelial abnormalities (specify reason)
  - General categorization—optional
    Negative for intraepithelial lesion or malignancy
    Epithelial cell abnormality
    Other
  - Interpretation/result
    Negative for intraepithelial lesion or malignancy
    Organisms
      Trichomonas vaginalis
      Fungal organisms morphologically consistent with Candida species
      Shift in flora suggestive of bacterial vaginosis
      Bacteria morphologically consistent with Actinomyces species
      Cellular changes consistent with herpes simplex virus
    Other non-neoplastic findings (optional to report)
    Reactive cellular changes associated with:
      Inflammation (includes typical repair)
      Radiation
      Intrauterine contraceptive device
    Glandular cells status posthysterectomy
    Atrophy
    Epithelial cell abnormalities
    Squamous cell
    Atypical squamous cells (ASC)
    ASC of undetermined significance (ASC-US)
    ASC, cannot exclude high-grade squamous intraepithelial lesion (ASC-H)
    Low-grade squamous intraepithelial lesion (LSIL)
    Encompassing: human papillomavirus, mild dysplasia, carcinoma in situ, CIN 2, and CIN 3
    Squamous cell carcinoma
    Glandular cell
    Atypical glandular cells (AGC)

Specify endocervical, endometrial, or glandular cells not otherwise specified
Atypical glandular cells, favor neoplastic
Specify endocervical or not otherwise specified
Endocervical adenocarcinoma in situ (AIS)
Adenocarcinoma
Other (list not comprehensive)
Endometrial cells in a woman 40 years or older
Automated review and ancillary testing (include if appropriate)
Educational notes and suggestions (optional)

Management

Nonpharmacologic Treatment
- Benign with inflammation—follow up in 3 months
- Cryotherapy (freezing) or cauterization—appropriate for noninvasive small lesions without endocervical extension
- Laser excision—appropriate for large visible lesions
- Loop electrosurgical excision procedure (LEEP)—appropriate when CIN is clearly visible
- Cone biopsy (conization) for higher grade or invasive lesions
- Hysterectomy, radiation, or chemotherapy is not indicated unless invasion is suspected.

When to Consult, Refer, Hospitalize
- Refer all abnormal Pap findings to GYN.
- Refer cervical cancer to gynecologic oncologist for management.

Follow-up
- If undetected or untreated, 15% to 20% cervical lesions progress while the rest either stay stable or regress.
- With appropriate management, future cancer risk is less than 5%. Many clinicians use automated cytology procedures if the patient has had therapy.
- After ablative treatment, screening cytology should be repeated at accelerated intervals, commonly every 3 to 4 months for the first year, then every 6 months for the next year, then annually once a pattern of normal readings has been established.
- Most treatment failures show up within 1 to 2 years postprocedure.
- Any recurrent abnormals need colposcopic follow-up and repeat endocervical curettage and biopsy
- After invasion has occurred, death usually occurs in 3 to 5 years without treatment, or in unresponsive cancers

Expected Course
- Invasion pattern moves from the cervix to the uterus then the pelvis, internal lymphs, ureters, bladder, and rectum
- Five-year survival rates vary by stage from 99+% for early to 2% for advanced
- 75% of recurrences occur in first 2 years, carry a poor prognosis (less than 5%)

Complications
- Vaginal fistulas, urinary and fecal incontinence, back pain, leg edema, ureteral obstruction, and eventually renal failure, death

Endometrial Cancer

Description
- Malignant changes of endometrial stroma and glands (adenocarcinoma)

Incidence and Demographics
- The most common invasive GYN cancer
  - Incidence 21/100,000; average age at onset 60; only 5% occur younger than 40 years old

Risk Factors
- Atypical endometrial hyperplasia
- Obesity
- Nulliparity
- Early menarche/late menopause
- Estrogen therapy without progestin
- Diabetes
- Cigarette smoking
- Tamoxifen

Prevention and Screening
- Not proven to be of much clinical value in endometrial cancer
- Annual Pap screening at vaginal cuff site (insensitive for endometrial cancer but rules out cervical changes)
- Mammography advised because of increased risk of breast cancer
- Occult blood stool screening also advised because of increased risk of metastasis to colon cancer

Assessment
History
- 80% to 90% present with painless abnormal bleeding pattern as cardinal sign
- Less common are leukorrhea, pelvic pressure, and symptoms of metastasis

Physical
- All women over age 40 with abnormal Pap finding should have referral for endometrial biopsy.
- Vaginal bleeding occurring after established menopause merits workup
- Assess for tenderness, uterine or adnexal enlargement, cervical lesions, hemorrhoids

Diagnostic Studies
- Pap screen
- CBC
- Ultrasound of endometrial thickness (<5 mm atrophic, >15 mm hypertrophic)
- Endometrial biopsy
- Chest x-ray (most common metastasis site)

Differential Diagnosis
- Endometrial hyperplasia
- HRT-related BTB
- Cervical cancer
- Vaginal cancer
- Hemorrhoids
- Bleeding disorders
- Polyps

Management
Nonpharmacologic Treatment
- Treatment is total abdominal hysterectomy with bilateral salpingectomy and oophorectomy (TAH-BSO)
- Radiation therapy is for later stages.

Pharmacologic Treatment
- Hormone therapy for metastatic or recurrent cancer
- Cytotoxic chemotherapy for palliation

When to Consult, Refer, Hospitalize
- Refer for endometrial biopsy (90% accuracy)

Follow-up
- Every 3 months for 2 years then every 6 months, and annually afterward

Complications
- Recurrence
- Five-year survival rate varies by stage of cancer, from 95% for early to 25% for late
- Death

Ovarian Cancer

Description
- Cancer of the ovary; most ovarian cancers are advanced with extensive spread at the time of diagnosis.

Incidence and Demographics
- Incidence of 12.9 to 15.1/100,000 women; median age 61 with peak age 75 to 79
- Leading cause of death among GYN cancers

Risk Factors
- Inverse relationship between number of lifetime ovulatory cycles and ovarian cancer risk. Conditions that suppress ovulation are protective, such as multiparity, oral contraceptives, anovulatory disorders.
- Increased risk: low parity, delayed childbearing, infertility, late menopause
- Lifetime risk 1.6% without family history, 5% if first-degree relative had ovarian cancer, 7% with 2 or more affected first-degree relatives (3% of these will be BCRA positive, with risk of developing breast cancer >40% in these women)

Prevention and Screening
- Not shown to be effective

Assessment
- 60% to 75% present with advanced disease and metastasis

History
- Few symptoms in early stages
- Nonspecific GI symptoms such as dyspepsia, nausea, early satiety, change in bowel habits, and abdominal fullness
- Presentation is vague: mild, dyspareunia, irregular vaginal bleeding, fatigue, or pelvic pressure

Physical
- Weight loss and anorexia are poor prognostic signs
- Careful abdominal, pelvic, and lymph node examinations
- A palpable ovary in postmenopausal women requires a workup to rule out cancer.
- Physical exam findings occur late in disease; palpable adnexal mass; ascites is a poor prognostic sign

Diagnostic Studies
- Transvaginal sonography and CA 125 assessment
- Pelvic ultrasonography: findings suggestive of cancer; solid, multiple septations; free fluid noted, irregular borders to lesion or papillation
- Abdominal CT with contrast
- Labs: CBC, comprehensive metabolic
- Serum CA 125 is often not elevated until advanced disease; (more than 35 units suggest cancer); false-positives occur with endometriosis, leiomyoma
- Laparoscopy

Differential Diagnosis
- Gastrointestinal or other GYN malignancies
- Chronic pelvic pain syndromes
- Benign ovarian mass
- Hepatic disease (ascites)
- Diverticulitis
- Fibroids

- Endometriosis
- IBS
- Colitis

- Urinary tract disease
- Ovarian cyst

Management

Nonpharmacologic Treatment
- Treatment is TAH-BSO with lymph sampling

Pharmacologic Treatment
- Postoperative chemotherapy is indicated in most cases.

When to Consult, Refer, Hospitalize
- Oncology or GYN consult
- Any ovarian masses should have surgical evaluation.

Follow-up
- Careful follow-up with oncology

Expected Course
- Survival rate decreases with increased age
- Five-year survival varies from 85% for an early cancer, 36% for local spread only, to 18%, for an advanced cancer with metastases
- Those with metastatic disease to breast or colon usually die within 1 year.

Complications
- Death

Vulvar Cancer (Bowen Disease)

Description
- Skin cancer on the vulva

Etiology
- Squamous cell accounts for 85%
- Melanomas account for 5%

Incidence and Demographics
- Only 5% of genital tract cancers; incidence is on the rise
- Primarily postmenopausal; mean age at diagnosis 65
- 30% to 50% of patients HPV+
- In situ disease: 40s
- Invasive disease: 60s

Risk Factors
- Cervical cancer, HPV, smoking, genital warts

Assessment

History
- Symptoms mild, nonspecific
- Persistent itching or pain, raised area on vulva, poorly healing lesion, occasional bleeding, vaginal odor
- Advanced stage: rectal bleeding, urethral obstruction

Physical
- Pelvic exam including palpation of Bartholin glands
- Toluidine blue dye (1%) or dilute acetic acid may make lesion more visible
- Raised area on vulva, leukoplakia, altered skin tones, may be multifocal in nature, ulcerations
- Inguinal lymphs may be palpable, suggests advanced disease

Diagnostic Studies
- Cytologic smear should target focal lesions on vulva, vagina, and cervix (unreliable)
- Vulvar biopsy if qualified or refer to gynecologic specialist for biopsy

Differential Diagnosis
- Atrophic vulvitis (atrophy)
- Tuberculosis
- Vulvar dystrophies
- STDs (syphilis, granuloma inguinale, lymphogranuloma inguinale, herpes)
- Paget's disease

Management
- Treatment is surgical excision; chemotherapy and radiation depend on staging
- Aggressive wound care is essential

When to Consult, Refer, Hospitalize
- Refer to GYN for biopsy

Follow-up
Expected Course
- Five-year survival rate varies by stage from 90% for early to 20% for late
- Squamous cell cancer slow growing and late to metastasize
- Melanomas grow quickly with early metastasis

Vaginal Cancer

Description
- Malignant changes in epithelial layer (90% squamous, 10% adenocarcinoma) of the vagina

Incidence and Demographics
- Most rare of all genital tract cancers
- If lesions on cervix or on vulva, then not classified as vaginal cancer
- May be metastasis from other cancer in body
- Carcinoma in situ: mid 40s to 60s; invasive stage mid 60s to 70s

Risk Factors
- Cervical malignancy, HPV, smokers, DES exposure, multiple partners

Assessment
History
- Abnormal bleeding, dyspareunia, postcoital bleeding
- Pain is a late sign (spread)

Physical
- Exam shows gross lesion "fungating" tumor inside vagina

When to Consult, Refer, Hospitalize
- Refer for colposcopy, biopsy, and surgical management (vaginectomy) to gynecological oncologist

BREAST MASSES

Description
- Benign mammary dysplasia also referred to as fibrocystic changes; majority not risk for breast cancer
- Fibroadenomas are solid benign masses.
- Duct ectasia is a collection of dilated terminal collecting ducts.
- Abscesses represent bacterial colonization.

- Most newly developed breast masses in older women are cancer.
- Retraction is often a sign of malignancy although can also be of benign etiology
- Galactorrhea is milky nipple discharge not associated with lactation.

Etiology
- Breast cancer incidence increases with age
- Fibrocystic changes are the most common benign breast condition; caused by ductal dilation usually 2 mm or less; 20% to 40% enlarge to palpable cysts (usually fluid filled) and may increase and decrease with menstrual cycle
- Fibroadenomas are made of glandular and fibrous tissue, often located in upper quadrant, caused by an inflammatory reaction from ductal irritation, with onset late teens to early 20s
- Galactorrhea can be caused by any lesion or medication (e.g., phenothiazine, oral contraceptives, tricyclic antidepressants, opiates) affecting hypothalamic inhibition of dopamine; about 10% to 12% of breast cancers are associated with nipple discharge
- Physiologic etiologies for galactorrhea include stress, breast stimulation, exercise, eating, and sleep; bilateral nipple discharge can be expressed in up to 80% of asymptomatic women
- Fat necrosis of the breast may occur after substantial trauma

Incidence and Demographics
- Most common ages 30 to 50; up to 50% of women affected
- Cysts and fibroadenomas most common benign breast changes followed by duct ectasia
- Duct ectasia typically occurs in the 40s and is most common cause of nipple discharge.
- Fibroadenomas often occur in younger women within 10 years of menarche
- Cancer—peak age at diagnosis is 45 to 60; occurs in 1 of 8 women

Risk Factors
- Fibrocystic disease: caffeine intake, chocolate, smoking, family history
- Cancer: risk increased with early menarche, late menopause, first pregnancy after age 35, obesity, android fat distribution

Prevention and Screening
- Monthly breast self-exam and periodic clinical breast exam
- Mammography on routine screening schedule unless focal area of concern (dominant mass of different texture, new mass); women older than 40 should have screening mammography every 1 to 2 years

Assessment

History
- Achy, tender, or painless lumpy breasts
- More tender with menses
- Vision problems, headaches
- Any nipple discharge—may be seen in galactocele or ductal ectasia, papilloma, or cancer
- Cold intolerance, weight gain, fatigue

Physical
- Benign multiple breast masses, fluctuating size with menses (cystic, adenosis, fibrosis, ductal hyperplasia) occasionally with unilateral or bilateral nipple discharge
- Fibroadenomas: unilateral mass, often solitary; well-defined, round, rubbery mobile masses
- Fibrocystic disease: multiple masses, tender with menses, fluctuating size, rare nipple discharge
- Nipple discharge typically green to yellow to black in color if physiologic, coming from multiple ducts versus spontaneous, unilateral, and bloody more likely associated with cancer
- Nipple discharge often associated with duct ectasia often thick and cheesy
- Cancer: solitary, hard nonmovable, nontender mass without well-defined margins, skin dimpling, nipple retraction, discharge

- Axillary, supraclavicular and infraclavicular lymph node exam for suspicious nodes
- Abscess: sudden onset, unilateral, tender, fluctuant, erythema, edema, induration, fever
- Visual field defects

Diagnostic Studies
- Breast ultrasonography can identify cystic structures vs solid mass
- Mammograms more useful for older women with less dense breast tissue
- Fine-needle aspiration or biopsy any suspicious area; if bloody fluid obtained, or no fluid or persistent mass, refer for excision
- TSH, prolactin and MRI of sella turcica as needed

Differential Diagnosis
- Breast cancer
- Fat necrosis
- Fibroadenoma
- Benign cyst
- Breast abscess
- Prolactinoma
- Galactocele

Management

Nonpharmacologic Treatment
- Fibroadenoma; excise or aspirate
- Fibrocystic disease: vitamin E supplements, reduce caffeine and chocolate in diet, supportive brassiere, oral contraceptive pills
- Abscesses: warm compresses, discontinue breastfeeding, OTC analgesics
- Monthly breast self-exams encouraged
- Avoid nipple stimulation
- Evening primrose oil

Pharmacologic Treatment
- Vitamin E supplements 400 IU daily, vitamin B_6 25–50 mg daily, magnesium supplements
- Oral contraceptives may or may not relieve symptoms
- Antibiotics for abscess

Special Considerations
- Breast pain in postmenopausal women not on HRT should be worked up for cancer
- Despite limitations for example, reduced mammographic sensitivity, women with implants should continue to be radiographically screened as appropriate for their age and risk factors

When to Consult, Refer, Hospitalize
- Refer to a surgeon for fine-needle aspiration to confirm that cyst is fluid filled, or excisional biopsy, or for suspicious findings as outlined above
- Refer to oncologist for suspicion of cancer

Follow-up
- Reevaluate in 1 to 2 months soon after menses to determine efficacy of therapy and if further work-up required

Complications
- Usually none if benign process

Breast Cancer

Description
- Malignancy of the breast

Etiology
- Precise etiology unknown

- Noninvasive—intraductal tumors including ductal carcinoma in situ (DCIS) or lobular carcinoma in situ (LCIS)
- Invasive—tumor no longer contained within basement membrane
  - Invasive ductal carcinoma originates from epithelial cells lining mammary ducts; subtypes include medullary, papillary, tubular, and colloid
  - Invasive lobular carcinoma arises from mammary lobules

Incidence and Demographics
- 1 in 8 women (lifetime risk)
- Peak age at diagnosis 45 to 65 with more than 75% occurring over age 50
- About 70% are invasive; invasive ductal more common than lobular (96%–97% vs 3%–4%)
- Most common site is upper outer quadrant (49%)

Risk Factors
- Risks include early menarche, late menopause (after 53), nulliparity and first pregnancy after age 35 (1.5 x risk), prior breast cancer (5–10 x risk), obesity (may be linked to hyperinsulinemia or fat cell production of androgens converted to estrogens), android fat distribution, excess alcohol use, tobacco use. Data are mixed on whether estrogen use increases risk.
- 20% family history (autosomal dominant with maternal linkage) relative risk (RR) 2.2 with first-degree relatives, with bilateral disease in premenopausal relatives (10.5 RR), bilateral disease in postmenopausal relatives (5.5 RR)
- 90% of women with breast cancer have NO family history
- BRCA (breast cancer recessive autosomal) carriers have risks for breast and ovarian cancers, usually early onset

Prevention and Screening
- Protection may be conferred by exercise, dietary soy, weight control especially in postmenopausal years
- Tamoxifen as prophylaxis in high-risk women (watch for endometrial abnormalities)

SCREENING FOR BREAST CANCER
- Ages 20 to 39: monthly breast self-exam (BSE) and clinical breast examination every 3 years
- Baseline mammogram between age 35 and 40
- 40 to 49: monthly BSE and annual clinical breast examination; mammography every 1 to 2 years
- 50 and over: monthly BSE and annual clinical breast examination and mammography every year (reduces cancer mortality by 30% to 50% in women aged 50 to 69; over age 70, the data is conflicting; no evidence to benefit women over age 75)
- False-negative rate of 10% to 15% and a false-positive rate of 15% to 20% for screening mammogram
- Clinical breast examination to find changes that may indicate a malignancy soon enough for timely intervention and to teach or to reinforce breast self-examination (BSE)
- Yearly mammogram for women who have had breast cancer

Assessment

History and Physical
- 55% palpable nontender mass; 35% abnormal mammogram without palpable mass
- Persistent nipple itching or burning suggests Paget disease; may present with minimal skin changes and no mass palpable, may have erosion or ulceration
- Exam shows solitary, nontender firm to hard mass without well-defined margins, often fixed position
- Ominous signs are enlarged or tender lymphs, skin color changes, skin erosion, peau d'orange (edema), dimpling, nipple retraction, pain, breast enlargement

12
Gynecologic

Diagnostic Studies
- Fine-needle aspiration
- Mammography
- Ultrasound (US)
- CBC, LFT, CXR, estrogen and progesterone receptor determination (usually ordered once biopsy done), bone scan, CT or US to assess lymph node involvement and metastasis

Differential Diagnosis
- Fibrocystic changes
- Fibroadenoma
- Intraductal papilloma
- Lipoma
- Fat necrosis

Management
- Decision making
  - Risk/benefit analysis
  - Consider life expectancy, comorbidities, treatment risks, patient values, quality of life
  - Older women generally tolerate surgery and radiation well; comorbidity influences surgical morbidity
- Local therapy
  - Breast-conserving therapy (BCT) or mastectomy: treatment patterns influenced by age, patient preferences
  - Modified radical mastectomy for multifocal disease, diffuse suspicious microcalcifications or prior breast irradiation
  - Sentinel node evaluation of axilla (less risk of lymphedema)
  - Local radiation following BCT: benefit less certain in older women
  - Radiation after mastectomy in high-risk women (large tumors, positive nodes)
- Systemic therapy (adjuvant)
  - Tamoxifen for 5 years after surgery: beneficial for estrogen receptor (ER) positive tumors
    Reduces risk of recurrence and improves survival
    Reduces risk of new primary breast cancer
    Marked benefit in women over 70
  - Tamoxifen first-line therapy in women unable to tolerate surgery
  - Consider chemotherapy if high risk of recurrence
  - Decreasing benefit of chemotherapy with increasing age (chemotherapy may be less effective and more toxic in elderly)
    Consider toxicities, comorbidities, preferences in women over 70
    Benefits negligible with major comorbidities

Special Considerations
- Tamoxifen may be given to women at high risk for prevention of breast cancer
- Delayed diagnosis and inadequate treatment associated with poor social support, transportation problems, impaired cognition
- Risk for undertreatment with advanced age, even controlling for comorbidity, functional status, cognitive disorders

When to Consult, Refer, Hospitalize
- Breast mass or abnormal calcifications on mammogram
- Eczema of nipple, new onset nipple or breast retraction, persistent nipple discharge

Follow-up
- Periodic physical examinations (every 3 to 4 months for 3 years, every 6 months for next 2 to 3 years, then yearly)
- Yearly mammogram after BCT

- Routine screening for other cancers (e.g., colorectal, uterine)
- Periodic lab tests: CBC, liver function tests
- Intensive follow-up to detect recurrence after primary therapy is not indicated in asymptomatic persons

Expected Course
- Stage of breast cancer is the most reliable indicator of prognosis
- Localized cancer cure rate is 75% to 90%
- When axillary lymph nodes are involved with tumor, survival is 4% to 50% at 5 years and about 25% at 10 years

Complications
- Increased risk of endometrial cancer, thromboemboli, stroke in postmenopausal women on Tamoxifen
- Exacerbation of postmenopausal symptoms may occur with Tamoxifen (hot flushes, vaginal dryness, cognitive changes)

CASE STUDIES

Case 1. A 69-year-old female comes to your office for her annual physical exam. On exam, you note a lump in the upper outer aspect of the right breast. The lump is about 1 cm, mobile, firm, with regular borders. There is no dimpling, retraction, or other breast or chest wall lesions. There is no tenderness. There is no adenopathy. The remainder of the physical exam is normal. She was not aware of this lump or other changes in her breasts. However, she does not perform regular self-breast exam. Her last mammogram was 3 years ago and last Pap smear was 1 year ago.

Breast History: The patient has no prior history of breast cancer or breast biopsies. Menarche: age 9. The patient is gravida 1, para 1, miscarriages/abortions 0. Age at first full-term pregnancy: 36. Age at Menopause: 54. Hormones: HRT (Prempro): 10 yr

Past Medical History: Hypercholesterolemia, osteopenia

Medications: Prempro, atorvastatin (Lipitor) 20 mg, multivitamin, calcium

Habits: Diet: Generally follows low-fat diet; Exercise: walks three times a week for one-half hour; Alcohol: 3 to 4 drinks/week; Tobacco: none

1. Based on the history and physical, what is your recommendation regarding diagnostic evaluation of the breast lump?
2. The mammogram shows a small mass in the upper outer quadrant of the right breast. The sonogram shows a cystic lesion with a small solid component in the area of the palpable mass. What would be your next recommendation for follow-up of this mass?
3. What aspects of Mrs. Jones' history would be considered risk factors in assessing her risk of breast cancer?

Case 2. A 70-year-old female comes to the clinic because she thinks she is shrinking. She is 5' 2", weighs 98 pounds, has smoked for 30 years, has COPD. Upon questioning, admits to having difficulty holding her urine due to frequency and urgency. She wears pads when she goes out, but she doesn't go out much because she is embarrassed.

1. What consequences of menopause does she have?
2. What other consequence would you evaluate her for?
3. What physical exam is indicated?
4. What diagnostic tests would you order?
5. What is the single most important thing she can do to improve her health?

6. The pelvic exam shows moderate vaginal atrophy. How would you manage the vaginal atrophy?

Case 3. A 78-year-old healthy female has a routine Pap result of CIN II
  1. What does the CIN II mean?
  2. What counseling would you give when you told her about the results?
  3. What would your actions be?
  4. What would her life expectancy be if she were not treated?
  5. What follow-up would the patient need?

REFERENCES

GYN

Anderson, G. L., et al. (2003, October 1). Effects of estrogen plus progestin on risk of fracture and bone mineral density: The Women's Health Initiative randomized trial. *JAMA, 290*(13), 1729–1738.

Anderson, G. L., et al. (2004, April 14). Effects of conjugated equine estrogen in postmenopausal women with hysterectomy: The Women's Health Initiative randomized controlled trial. *JAMA, 291*(14), 1701–1712.

Anderson, G. L., et al. (2003, October 1). Effects of estrogen plus progestin on gynecologic cancers and associated diagnostic procedures: The Women's Health Initiative randomized trial. *JAMA, 290*(13), 1739–1748.

Basil, B., et al. (2001). Cervical carcinoma: Contemporary management. *Obstet Gynecol Clin North Am, 28,* 727.

Chlebowski, R. T., et al. (2004, March 4). Estrogen plus progestin and colorectal cancer in postmenopausal women. *NEJM, 350*(10), 991–1004.

Chlebowski, R. T., et al. (2003, June 25). Influence of estrogen plus progestin on breast cancer and mammography in healthy postmenopausal women: The Women's Health Initiative randomized trial. *JAMA, 289*(24), 3243–3253.

Gull, B., et al. (2000). Transvaginal ultrasonography in women with post menopausal bleeding: Is it always necessary to perform an endometrial biopsy? *Am J Obstet Gynecol. 185,* 509.

Manson, J. E. (2003, August 7). Estrogen plus progestin and the risk of coronary heart disease. *NEJM, 349*(6), 523–534.

Rossouw, J. E., et al. (2002, July 17). Risks and benefits of estrogen plus progestin in healthy postmenopausal women: Principal results from the Women's Health Initiative randomized controlled trial. *JAMA, 288,* 321–333.

Sawaya, G. F., (2003, October 16). Risk of cervical cancer associated with extending the interval between cervical cancer screenings. *NEJM, 349,* 1501–1509.

Shumaker, S. A., et al. (2003, May 28). Estrogen plus progestin and the incidence of dementia and mild cognitive impairment in postmenopausal women: The Women's Health Initiative Memory Study: A randomized controlled trial. *JAMA, 289*(20), 2651–2662.

Speroff, L., Glass, R. H., & Kase, N. G. (1999). *Clinical gynecologic endocrinology and infertility* (6th ed.). Philadelphia, PA: Lippincott, Williams and Wilkins.

Tabor, A., et al. (2002, April). Endometrial thickness as a test for endometrial cancer in women with postmenopausal vaginal bleeding. *Obstet Gynecol, 99,* 663–670.

US Preventive Services Task Force. (2002, November 19). Postmenopausal hormone replacement therapy for primary prevention of chronic conditions: Recommendations and rationale. *Ann Intern Med, 137,* 834–839.

Warren, M. P. (2004, April). A comparative review of the risks and benefits of hormone replacement therapy regimens. *Am J Obstet Gynecol, 190*(4), 1141–1167.

Wassertheil-Smoller, S., et al. (2003, May 28). Effect of estrogen plus progestin on stroke in postmenopausal women: The Women's Health Initiative: A randomized trial. *JAMA, 289*(20), 2673–2684.

Breast Masses

Cauley, J. A., et al. (2003). Lipid-lowering drug use and breast cancer in older women: A prospective study. *J. Women's Health, 23*(9), 749–756.

Chlebowski, R. T., et al. (2003, June 25). Influence of estrogen plus progestin on breast cancer and mammography in healthy postmenopausal women: The Women's Health Initiative randomized trial. *JAMA*, 289, 324–353.

Harris, J. M., Lippman, M., Morrow, Osborne, C. (Eds.). (2000). *Diseases of the breast.* Philadelphia: Lippincott, Williams & Wilkins.

Kimmick, G. G., & Balducci, L. (2000). Breast cancer and aging. *Hematology/Oncology Clinics of North America.* *14*(1), 213–234.

Mandelblatt, J. S., et al. (2000). Patterns of breast carcinoma treatment in older women. *Cancer,* 89(3), 561–572.

Randolph, W. M., et al. (2002, November 19). Regular mammography use is associated with elimination of age-related disparities in size and stage of breast cancer at diagnosis. *Ann Intern Med, 137,* 783–790.

MALE REPRODUCTIVE SYSTEM DISORDERS 13

GERIATRIC APPROACH

Normal Changes of Aging

Male Reproductive System
- Decreased testosterone level leads to increased estrogen/androgen ratio
- Testicular size decreases
- Decreased sperm motility, fertility reduced but still possible
- Increased incidence of gynecomastia

Sexual Function
- Slowed arousal
- Erection less firm, shorter lasting
- Decreased forcefulness at ejaculation
- Longer interval to achieve subsequent erection

Prostate
- By fourth decade of life, stromal fibrous elements and glandular tissue hypertrophy stimulated by DHT (active androgen within the prostate); hyperplastic nodules enlarge in size, ultimately leading to urethral obstruction

Clinical Implications

History
- Many men are overly sensitive about complaints of the male genitourinary system; men are often not inclined to initiate discussion or seek help. It is important to take an active role in screening with an approach that is open, trustworthy, and nonjudgmental.
- Sexual function remains important to many men, even at ages over 80.
- Lack of an available partner, poor health, erectile dysfunction due to medication adverse effect, and lack of desire are the main reasons men do not continue to have sex.
- Nocturia reported in 66% of patients over 65
  - Due to impaired ability to concentrate urine or BPH
  - Frequent cause of insomnia

Physical
- Digital rectal exam (DRE) is almost universally dreaded by men; provide privacy, allow for dignity

Assessment
- In men diagnosed with benign prostate hypertrophy (BPH), periodic evaluation for prostate cancer must continue

Treatment
- A man may not want treatment for BPH because of the fear of erectile dysfunction.

PROSTATE GLAND DISORDERS
Prostatitis

Description
- Inflammation and/or infection of the prostate gland, categorized as acute bacterial or chronic bacterial

Etiology
- Various causes: allergic, auto-immunologic response, infectious, related to instrumentation, UTIs, prostatic abscess or stone
- Acute infection: generally gram-negative bacilli; primarily *E coli*; may also be *Enterobacter, Klebsiella, Proteus, Staphylococcus aureus*
- Infectious causes usually occur by direct invasion from the urethra, typically UTI

Incidence and Demographics
- Chronic bacterial occurs primarily in older men
- Acute bacterial is uncommon

Risk Factors
- Age over 50
- Instrumentation of urinary tract
- Abscess elsewhere in the body
- Recurrent UTIs

Prevention and Screening
- Avoidance of unnecessary procedures

Assessment (See Table 13-1)

History
- Symptoms of dysuria due to compression of the urethra by the inflamed prostate
- Chronic bacterial prostatitis characterized by remissions and exacerbations with recurrent UTIs
- Acute bacterial characterized by acute onset with systemic symptoms and pattern of pain and dysuria
- Current medications (e.g., anticholinergics), other medical illness, and sexual history to assess risk of infection

Table 13-1: Clinical Presentation of Prostatitis

Assess	Acute Bacterial	Chronic Bacterial
Symptoms	Chills, fever, malaise Dysuria Urgency Burning Frequency Hematuria Pain: pelvis, perineum, lower back, scrotum, with defecation, with intercourse	+/– low-grade fever Dysuria Hesitancy Hematuria Hematospermia Pain mild: perineum, scrotal, abdominal, with ejaculation
Physical Findings	Fever Prostate very tender, boggy, warm Urethral discharge	No systemic findings Prostate may be normal, indurated, mildly tender, boggy or irregular +/– prostatic stones Scrotum +/– edema, erythema, and tenderness

Physical
- Abdominal exam: check for tenderness or distended bladder from urinary retention
- Genitalia: urethral discharge
- CVA tenderness to assess kidneys
- Rectal exam
- ***Warning Regarding Prostate Examinations***: Examining the prostate is a part of this exam; however, due to exquisite tenderness and risk of bacterial spread into the bloodstream, it is to be done very gently or, in the case of suspected acute prostatitis, perhaps not at all until treatment has been initiated.
- In the nonacute patient, prostatic massage *is* indicated to carry out the 3-step urinalysis and culture for evaluation of prostatic secretions, and as part of therapeutic treatment.

Diagnostic Studies
- Urinalysis and culture/sensitivity: if pyuria on initial clean-catch wet prep, and positive urine culture, adequate diagnosis for acute bacterial prostatitis
- If initial clean-catch wet prep is negative for bacteria, proceed to prostatic massage and collect post-massage urine for wet prep and culture. If prostatic massage wet prep has at least 10 to 15 WBCs, culture will usually yield gram-negative organisms indicative of chronic prostatitis. Negative culture with WBCs indicates nonbacterial prostatitis. If no WBCs and negative culture, suspect prostatodynia and refer.
- Chronic prostatitis is additionally evaluated with CBC, serum BUN and creatinine, and possible IV pyelogram and/or transrectal ultrasound.
- Bladder cancer screening via urine cytology

Differential Diagnosis
- BPH
- Prostatodynia
- Urethral stricture
- Nonbacterial prostatitis
- Cancer of the bladder or prostate
- Renal colic
- Other infections: abscess, epididymitis, cystitis, urethritis

Management (See Table 13-2)

Nonpharmacologic Treatment
- Avoidance of known irritants: caffeine, alcohol, OTC antihistamine or decongestants
- Hydration maintenance (force fluids)
- Rest and sitz baths 20 minutes 2 to 3 times a day for pain as needed

Pharmacologic Treatment
- Prostate gland difficult to penetrate with antibiotics. First-line treatment with trimethoprim-sulfamethoxazole (Bactrim) or fluoroquinolones
- NSAIDs recommended for both anti-inflammatory effects and pain relief. Choice of medications may be limited due to intolerance/side effects of NSAIDs.
- Stool softeners as needed

Table 13-2: Antibiotic Management of Infections

Treatment	Acute Bacterial	Chronic Bacterial
Antibiotics	Ciprofloxacin 500 mg PO bid Levofloxacin 500 qd Trimethoprim/sulfamethoxazole (Bactrim) DS bid Other antibiotic appropriate to the organism	Cipro 500 mg PO bid Trimethoprim/sulfamethoxazole (Bactrim) DS bid
How Long to Treat	2–6 weeks	1–4 months

When to Consult, Refer, Hospitalize
- Hospitalization indicated for all patients with systemic involvement for IV antibiotics, treatment of possible septicemia
- Refer to a urologist if no improvement within 48 hours of treatment
- Refer to a urologist older patients (older than 50) who are symptomatic, have recurrent prostatitis, or acute bacterial prostatitis, as BPH may be a compounding problem

Follow-up

Expected Course
- Chronic prostatitis: follow-up appointments with urinalysis, culture, and sensitivity every 30 days, sooner as indicated based on response to treatment and changes in symptoms
- Acute prostatitis: reevaluation in 48 to 72 hours, then 2 to 4 weeks later for urinalysis, urine and prostatic secretion cultures to monitor treatment effectiveness and assess for complications. Repeat 1 month after completion of antibiotic course.

Complications
- Potential for serious sequelae including development of prostatic abscess, stones, ascending or recurrent UTIs, epididymitis, urinary retention, renal infection

Benign Prostatic Hyperplasia

Description
- Benign, gradual enlargement of the periurethral prostate gland in which the enlargement mechanically obstructs urination by compressing the urethra
- Differentiate between benign hypertrophy and prostate cancer

Etiology
- Unknown; may be combination of hormonal changes, growth factors
- Medications known to increase symptoms: alpha-adrenergic agonists, anticholinergics, antihistamines, opioids, tricyclics, sedative hypnotics, alcohol

Incidence and Demographics
- Approximately 50% of 50-year-old men, 80% of 70-year-olds, 90% of 85+
- Initially asymptomatic, many develop urinary symptoms by age 60

Risk Factors
- Age
- Presence of androgens

Prevention and Screening
- Most organizations recommend annual DRE examination after the age of 40
- Use of the PSA for screening remains controversial
- Early screening starting in the 40s may allow for earlier treatment, slowing of the progression of hyperplasia and possible reduction of symptoms

Assessment

History
- Assess degree of impairment via the American Urological Association AUA Symptom Index
  - Not emptying bladder completely, frequency, stop and start again several times, urgency, weak stream, push or strain to begin urination, nocturia
- Obstructive symptoms: difficulty starting/stopping stream, hesitancy, dribbling, weakening force/size of stream, sensation of full bladder after voiding, urinary retention
- Irritative symptoms: urgency, frequency, nocturia, urge incontinence, dysuria, suprapubic discomfort
- Medications: anticholinergics (decongestants, antihistamines, tricyclic antidepressants, tranquilizers) impair bladder contractility; sympathomimetics increase outflow resistance

- PMH: explore for other conditions that may be associated with these symptoms—surgery, diabetes, neuromuscular disease (multiple sclerosis), psychogenic disorder, cardiovascular disease (CHF), and hypercalcemia
- General: fever, malaise, back pain, hematuria, pain with voiding indicate possible complication of BPH

Physical

- Abdomen: possible distended bladder on percussion or palpation; CVA tenderness if renal sequelae
- Neurologic: screening exam to note nonprostate etiology for symptoms of neurogenic or myogenic etiology, detrusor muscle impairment, compression of nerves
- Digital rectal exam (DRE) for prostate: intact anal sphincter tone; prostate nontender, firm, smooth and rubbery consistency with blunting or obliteration of midline median sulcus
- Enlargement may be symmetric, nodular, or asymmetric. Any nodules should be considered possibly malignant.

Diagnostic Studies

- Urinalysis: hematuria, glycosuria, or infection
- Urine culture and sensitivity if evidence of infection
- Serum creatinine to assess renal function: may be abnormal if urinary retention and/or obstruction has affected upper urinary tract, as well as with underlying renal disease
- Urine culture and sensitivity if evidence of infection
- Prostate specific antigen (PSA): controversial if patient is asymptomatic, normal is 4 to 7 ng/mL for the elderly; more than 10 ng/mL may be cancer or prostatitis
- Urinary flowmetry studies (flow rate) postresidual urine, and urodynamic studies, transrectal ultrasound (to guide needle biopsy), and abdominal ultrasound done by urologist

Differential Diagnosis

- Prostate cancer
- Prostatitis
- Bladder neck contracture or cancer
- Diseases associated with increased urination (CHF, DM, hypercalcemia)
- Urethral stricture
- Urinary tract infection
- Infectious or inflammatory disease (prostatitis, cystitis, urethritis)
- Neurologic disease

Management

Nonpharmacologic Treatment

MILD SYMPTOMS

- Watchful waiting, monitoring of symptoms
- Avoidance of bladder irritants: coffee, alcohol, medications listed in etiology
- Limit intake of fluids in the evening, avoid large quantities in short time

MODERATE SYMPTOMS

- Treatment initiated when symptoms interfere with quality of life (e.g., frequent nocturia disrupting sleep, incontinence)

SEVERE SYMPTOMS

- Treatment required if patient has refractory retention, recurrent urinary tract infections, recurrent or persistent gross hematuria, bladder stones, or renal insufficiency due to BPH
- Surgical options include transurethral resection of prostate (TURP), transurethral incision of prostate (TUIP), and open prostatectomy via abdominal incision (rarely used)
- Laser surgery and coagulation necrosis techniques performed under ultrasound guidance are newer techniques that are minimally invasive.

Pharmacologic Treatment

- Aggravating medications should be discontinued when feasible

MILD TO MODERATE

- Two classes of medications are available (see Table 13-3)
- Alpha-adrenergic blockers: reduce both muscle tone through effect on alpha-adrenergic nerves in bladder neck and prostatic urethra, so there is decreased resistance to urine flow
- 5 alpha-reductase inhibitors block conversion of testosterone to DHT, decreasing hormonal (androgen) effect on prostate, shrinking prostate size and symptoms, resulting in increased peak urinary flow rate
- Less commonly used drugs include GnRH agonists, progestational antiandrogens, flutamide, and testolactone
- Saw palmetto is an alternative therapy that is controversial but commonly used
- Treat UTI if present

How Long to Treat

- Dependent upon type and severity of symptoms and impact on daily functioning
- Medications may be prescribed until symptoms are no longer manageable and nonpharmacologic treatment may be needed (see Table 13-3)

Table 13-3: Pharmacologic Management of BPH

Drugs	Dosage	Comment
α_1-**Adrenergic Blockers**		
Terazosin (Hytrin)	Always begin with 1 mg PO q h, may increase to 2 mg, then 5 mg up to 10 mg/d to achieve symptom relief or desired flow rate	Drugs of choice for smaller prostate and acute irritative symptoms Improvement dose dependent, 4–6 weeks for maximal therapeutic effect
Doxazosin (Cardura)	1 mg qd, HS, may double every 1–2 weeks to max of 8 mg/d	May cause postural hypotension, dizziness, palpitations, or syncope; first-dose syncope requires first pill be taken while patient is in bed
Alfuzosin HCl (Uroxatral)	10 mg extended-release tablet taken at the same time daily after a meal	May be beneficial for those with concomitant BPH and HTN; can reduce number of medications needed
Tamsulosin HCl (Flomax) alpha-1A blocker	0.4 mg qd 30 min before meal at same time each day; may increase to 0.8 mg after 2–4 weeks	No cardiovascular side effects, postural hypotension not common May cause dizziness, abnormal ejaculation, rhinitis
5 α-Reductase Inhibitor		
Finasteride (Proscar)	5 mg qd No titration needed	Drug of choice for large prostate and those with contraindications or failed treatment with alpha andrenergics Improvement not noted for up to 6–12 months Must be used indefinitely to sustain effect Decreases PSA by up to 50%, blocking effectiveness of PSA as screening tool for CA

Special Considerations
- In presence of concomitant diseases (diabetes mellitus, CV, or neurologic disease), care should be coordinated with regard to medications, ability for self-care, and recommendations for procedural or surgical treatment.
- Must always rule out prostate cancer

When to Consult, Refer, Hospitalize
- Referral to a urologist is indicated for AUA index score of 8 or more, symptoms not responsive to medications, infections (epididymitis, repeat UTIs), obstruction or acute urinary retention, renal disease, or suspicion of malignancy
- Refer if surgical procedure may be indicated

Follow-up
- Annual evaluation with DRE indicated for asymptomatic or minor symptoms, sooner if symptoms warrant

Expected Course
- Without intervention, prostate gland will continue to increase in size, ultimately causing symptoms of obstruction
- Depending upon response to medication, may have prolonged course of milder symptoms, slowing of hyperplasia
- Follow up initially every 2 to 4 weeks until stable
- Individuals on finasteride need follow-up in 6 months

Complications
- Recurrent UTI/sepsis
- Obstruction of urinary flow with urinary retention
- Incontinence
- Azotemia
- Chronic renal failure

Prostate Cancer

Description
- Malignant neoplasm of the prostate gland

Etiology
- Unknown

Incidence and Demographics
- 190,000 new cases per year
- Second most common cause of cancer deaths in men
- One in 5 men develop prostate cancer; average age at diagnosis is 72 years
- About 80% of all clinically diagnosed cases of prostate cancer are men over age 65
- 40% greater incidence in African American men. At all ages, African American men are diagnosed with prostate cancer at later stages and die of the disease at higher rates than white men.

Risk Factors
- Age
- Exposure to chemical carcinogens, history of STDs
- Family history
- Possibly related to prior vasectomy
- Diet high in animal fat
- African American race

- Low vitamin D levels
- Sun exposure
- History of agricultural work

Prevention and Screening
- Annual digital rectal exam (DRE) beginning between ages 40 and 50
- Annual PSA from age 50 is recommended for screening and early detection by some groups; US Preventive Health Services suggests research does not support this due to high number of both false-positives and false- negatives
- Avoid use of androgen supplements

Assessment

History
- Asymptomatic initially
- May include any or all BPH symptoms described above
- With enlargement, frequency, nocturia, dribbling develop
- Bone pain in hips, pelvis, or back occur with advanced metastatic cancer

Physical
- Depending upon stage of the cancer, the prostate on DRE may be normal on the palpable lateral and posterior portion of the gland or may be asymmetrical, generally firmer with hard induration, localized nodule, and obliterated median sulcus.
- Hematuria may be present
- Examine back for spinous process tenderness and lower extremities for neurological abnormalities if metastatic disease is suspected

Diagnostic Studies
- PSA level >4 ng/mL indicates possible cancer
- Normal PSA in 40% of patients with cancer; PSA discredited as good screening examination
- CBC, urinalysis, urine C&S for workup of urinary symptoms
- Acid phosphatase increased with late stage (metastatic) to bone

Differential Diagnosis
- BPH
- Prostatitis
- UTI
- Proximal urethral stone
- Bladder or renal cancer
- Urethral stricture

Management
- Treatment choice based on stage of disease

Nonpharmacologic Treatment
- Asymptomatic with life expectancy <10 years, watchful waiting is option
- If localized, treatment options include watchful waiting, radical prostatectomy, and radiation therapy
- Disseminated disease treated with surgical or chemical castration (hormonal therapy) or chemo-therapy

Pharmacologic Treatment
- LHRH agonist: Leuprolide (Lupron) monthly injection
- Antiestrogen: flutamide 250 mg tid

How Long to Treat
- Follow-up exam and PSA every 3 months first year, then every 6 months for 1 year
- Chest x-ray and bone scan every 6 months for 1 year then as indicated by changes in PSA
- Early stage may be cured with no further treatment needed if localized and surgically removed
- Hormonal treatment is maintained throughout the course of the advanced stages
- Radiation, chemotherapy treatments vary depending upon staging

When to Consult, Refer, Hospitalize
- All patients with PSA >10 or sudden increase in serial PSA even if still within normal limits, abnormalities on DRE, and/or symptomatic are referred to urologist

Follow-up
Expected Course
- PSA should be undetectable after prostatectomy, negligible after radiation
- Rise in PSA after treatment indicates recurrence
- Concurrent with treatment of the cancer is the need for addressing the effects of the diagnosis, sequelae of the disease, and side effects of treatments. These include such things as coping with a chronic terminal illness, loss of self-image or self-esteem, transient or permanent incontinence (2% to 5%), loss of libido, and impotence.

Complications
- Incontinence, erectile dysfunction, pain, pathologic fractures related to bone metastases to regional lymph nodes and bone (axial skeleton most common site), death
- Impotence occurs in 40% postoperatively and 25% to 35% postradiation; hormonal treatment may additionally result in gynecomastia, cardiovascular complications, or hot flashes

PENILE DISORDERS
Phimosis

Description
- Inability to retract the foreskin of uncircumcised penis that had formerly been retractable

Etiology
- Occurs when orifice of the prepuce is too small to allow retraction of the foreskin
- Acquired from trauma, prior infection, or poor hygiene (retained smegma and dirt) that results in inflammation and development of adhesions
- Geriatric patients may develop phimosis with use of condom catheters

Incidence and Demographics
- Elderly at increased risk due to inability to care for self

Risk Factors
- Poor hygiene
- Trauma

Prevention and Screening
- Hygiene of the genitalia with retraction of the foreskin during washing
- Make sure to replace foreskin after washing.

Assessment
History
- May be asymptomatic, with phimosis discovered on examination
- When related to an infectious or inflamed process, patients complain of irritation and tenderness of the glans, discomfort with voiding, or pain on erection
- *If severe enough, outflow of urine may be compromised by an opening that is too small, presenting as a **urological emergency**

Physical
- Glans nonretractable, prepuce pallid, striated, and thickened
- If actively infected: erythema, smegma, and/or exudate and tenderness

Differential Diagnosis
- Penile lymphedema associated with trauma, allergic reaction, insect bite

Management

Nonpharmacologic Treatment
- Treatment of the underlying cause such as infection or inflammation with good hygiene, sitz baths, and warm compresses
- Surgical release or circumcision

Pharmacologic Treatment
- If concurrent infection or inflammation, treatment with topical antifungals or steroids may be sufficient to allow for retraction

How Long to Treat
- Topical treatment for underlying infection or inflammation for 1 to 2 weeks

When to Consult, Refer, Hospitalize
- Refer to urologist for surgical release or circumcision if nonresponsive to topical treatment and hygiene, urinary flow compromised, or asymptomatic phimosis remains

Follow-up

Expected Course
- Resolves with treatment

Complications
- Inflamed prepuce
- Meatal stenosis
- UTI
- Premalignant changes

Erectile Dysfunction

Description
- Inability to achieve or maintain a satisfactory erection more than 25% to 50% of the time
- May be defined by patients as loss of orgasm; premature ejaculation; loss of emission, libido, or erections

Etiology
- Classified as either psychological or organic
- Psychological origin is likely with loss of orgasm when libido and erection are intact and with premature ejaculation concurrent with anxiety, depression, relationship problems, new partner, or emotional disorders
- If patient has nocturnal erections, problem is probably psychological, not organic
- Gradual loss of erections over time is indicative of organic causes
- Medications such as anabolic steroids, digoxin (Lanoxin), antihypertensives, especially centrally acting (reserpine, clonidine, methyldopa), beta-blockers and spironolactone (loss of libido), antidepressants (MAOIs, tricyclics, SSRIs)
- Lifestyle issues of alcohol, drug, and cigarette (or other nicotine) use
- Hormonal and endocrine disorders of the thyroid, kidney, pituitary gland, or testicular function; Addison and Cushing syndrome
- Vascular disorders, such as arterial insufficiency, venous disease, atherosclerosis
- Neurologic disorders: cortical, brainstem, spinal cord, peripheral neuropathies
- Posttreatment of prostate disorders
- Diabetes mellitus, increased with poor glucose control
- Renal failure
- Pain
- Arthritis

Incidence and Demographics

- Widely unreported, estimated that 10% of the male population affected
- 10 to 20 million men in the US; increases with age

Risk Factors

- See Etiology

Prevention and Screening

- Maintaining a healthy relationship, seeking support or counseling
- Avoidance of known stressors that affect sexual relationships
- Close management of chronic diseases, especially diabetes

Assessment

History

- Determine the patient's perception or definition of erectile dysfunction to clarify the problem and symptoms, the timing, circumstances, frequency of occurrence
- Complaints include any of the following: reduced size and strength of erection, lack of ability to achieve or maintain erections adequate for intercourse, rapid loss of erection with penetration, or lack of libido
- Determine nature of patient's relationship, sexual partners, lifestyle, and stress
- Inquire about nocturnal or morning erections: presence reflects intact blood supply, nervous system, and sexual apparatus; reduce likelihood of organic cause
- Associated symptoms indicative of underlying disease: decreased body hair, gynecomastia, neuropathies, anxiety, headaches, vision changes, decreased circulation, excessive dryness or skin changes, changes in testicle size, consistency or shape, and changes in penis, such as rash, discharge, or phimosis
- Review past medical history for other diseases, testicular infections, or insults, medications (Rx, OTC, and herbal), and history of smoking, drug, alcohol use

Physical

- Complete screening physical noting general appearance, generalized anxiety or hyperactivity, vital signs for postural hypotension, dry hair, loss of secondary sex characteristics, spider angiomas, hyperpigmentation, palmar erythema, or goiter
- Chest, abdomen, and extremities for cardiac abnormalities, gynecomastia, aortic or femoral bruits, peripheral vascular deficits
- Genital examination for penile circulation, discharge, fibrosis or lesions; testicles for size, masses, varicoceles or atrophy; DRE for prostate abnormalities, sphincter tone
- Neurologic screening for cortical, brainstem, spinal, or peripheral neuropathies, noting especially bulbocavernosi reflex, cremasteric reflex, pinprick or light touch to genital and perianal area, focal tenderness of spine

Diagnostic Studies

- Key studies to screen for underlying etiology begin with plasma glucose, prolactin, and free testosterone, CBC, U/A, and lipid profile
- Other tests dependent on findings of H & P and results of preliminary tests
- Urologist may include nocturnal penile tumescence and rigidity testing, duplex ultrasonography, penile angiography, nerve conduction studies or a trial injection of prostaglandin E_1, phentolamine, and papaverine intracorporeally to assess vascular integrity, noting penile response

Differential Diagnosis

- See Etiology

Management

Nonpharmacologic Treatment

- Modify lifestyle: stress reduction techniques; stop alcohol, drugs, and cigarettes

- Use of a vacuum constriction device for those with venous disorders of the penis or non-responsiveness to vasoactive injections
- Surgical treatment—penile implants

Pharmacologic Treatment
- Substitute or discontinue medications known to cause erectile dysfunction
- Some antihypertensives that are less likely to cause ED are calcium channel blockers (nifedipine), angiotensin-converting enzyme blockers (lisinopril), selective beta-blockers (atenolol)
- Alternative antidepressants instead of SSRIs (Prozac, Zoloft, Paxil, Celexa)
- Some antidepressants less likely to cause ED are bupropion (Wellbutrin) and venlafaxine (Effexor)
- Treat abnormal hormones as follows:
  - Insufficient testosterone treated with a 3-month testosterone trial (if indicated by androgen deficiency, do not have prostatic cancer) using testosterone injections 200 mg IM q 3 weeks or topical patches of 2.5–6 mg/d
- Hyperprolactinemia treated with bromocriptine initially 2.5 mg bid, up to 40 mg/d
- Phosphodiesterase type 5 inhibitor—do not give if patient on nitroglycerin
  - Sildenafil (Viagra) 25–50 mg 1 hour prior to desired erection (works within 30 min to 4 hours)
  - Tadalafil (Cialis) 2–20 mg
  - Vardenafil HCl (Levitra) 2.5–20 mg
- Controversial oral agents include yohimbine, trazodone, and ginkgo biloba
- Penile injections, such as alprostadil (Caverject), first dose in office setting 1.25– 2.5 mcg with repeat dose after 1 hour if no response. Patient to remain in office until detumescence completed. Partial response may have second injection within 24 hours.
- Use of injections or oral agents require thorough patient teaching on proper use, frequency of use, side effects and risk of priapism, and when to seek medical help, such as erection lasting >6 hours
- Alternatives to alprostadil are papaverine or phentolamine
- Urethral suppository of alprostadil (Muse) in various strength pellets

How Long to Treat
- Variable depending upon treatment methods

Special Considerations
- Age 70+: rarely seek help, most likely have physical problems

When to Consult, Refer, Hospitalize
- Psychotherapist for individual or couples therapy, sex therapy
- Urologist, endocrinologist, cardiologist, neurologist referrals as indicated by diagnosis and requirements for further evaluation or advanced treatment

Follow-up
- Follow-up is varied depending upon diagnosis, underlying etiology, response to treatment, and need for therapy. Patients should be seen initially at shorter intervals to adjust and monitor responsiveness to treatment, then every 3 months.

Expected Course
- Improvement in many patients with oral medications, vacuum devices, suppository and penile implants 15% spontaneously improve
- 20% failure rate with vacuum device, 10% to 30% dissatisfaction with penile implant
- Alprostadil injections have an 85% to 90% response rate, while the urethral pellet method rates are 40% to 60%
- Phosphodiesterase type 5 inhibitors are effective for 70% of patients at maximal dose

Complications
- Variable depending upon underlying etiology and treatment method side effects
- Phosphodiesterase type 5 inhibitors cause hypotension, headache, flushing, nausea, nasal congestion, abnormal vision, cardiovascular events, priapism, prolonged erections

CASE STUDIES

Case 1. An 83-year-old man complains of urinary hesitancy, dribbling, urinary frequency of small amounts, and nocturia 4 times per night. This has been gradually getting worse for the past few months.

1. What is the most likely diagnosis?
2. What physical exam is required?
3. If the symptoms are not troublesome, what is the usual approach?
4. What symptoms would require referral for treatment?
5. What nonpharmacologic treatment may be helpful?
6. Which medications would you consider starting the patient on? What are their main disadvantages?

Case 2. A 78-year-old black man comes to you feeling poorly. He complains of fatigue and low back pain, which has been gradually increasing for the past few months. He has had urinary symptoms, which he attributed to BPH for the past 6 years, gradually worsening so that he is now having hesitancy, dribbling, and a feeling of not emptying his bladder completely. He has never sought treatment for the BPH symptoms because he thought it was an inevitable consequence of aging.

PMH: 50-pack per year smoking, COPD, osteoarthritis, hypertension, and hyperlipidemia. Medications: Combivent inhaler, Tylenol PRN pain, hydrochlorothiazide 25 mg PO qd, atorvastatin (Lipitor) 40 mg PO qd.

1. What do his urinary symptoms indicate?
2. What are the most likely possibilities for a differential diagnosis?
3. What lab work would you order?
4. Which would be most useful to decide between the differential?
5. What risk factors does he have?
6. What would you do?
7. What follow-up is required?

Case 3. A 68-year-old man comes to your office with the complaint of insomnia. Says he is having some problems with his wife. She is not too happy with him. Patient seems reluctant to say what is really bothering him.

1. How would you approach this situation?
2. What normal changes of aging affect sexual function?

History: Patient tells you he has a gradual loss of the ability to maintain an erection for the past year or so. His wife is upset about this and has been nagging him to do something about it. The problem became worse recently, after an argument with his wife.

3. Is this ED psychological or organic?

PMH: Patient has hypertension, diabetes, lipid disorder, osteoarthritis

4. How do these diseases affect ED?
5. What would be your initial approach?

REFERENCES

Barry, Fowler, O'Leary, et al. (1992, November). UAU Measurement Committee. Correlation of the American Urological Association Symptom Index with self-administered versions of the Madsen-Iverson, Boyarsky and Maine Medical Assessment Program Symptoms Indexes. *J Urol, 148,* 1558–1563.

Carson, C. C. (2004). Erectile dysfunction: Evaluation and new treatment options. *Psychosom Med, 55*(5), 664–671.

Chapple, C. R. (2004). Pharmacological therapy of benign prostatic hyperplasia/lower urinary tract symptoms: An overview for the practicing clinician. *British Journal Urology International, 94*(5), 738–744.

DeLuca, G. (2001). Prostatitis. *The American Journal for Nurse Practitioners, 5*(3), 45–54.

Edmunds, M. W., & Mayhew, M. S. (2004). *Pharmacology for the primary care provider* (2nd ed.). St. Louis: Mosby.

Ferri, F. F. (2003). *Ferri's clinical advisor* (6th ed.). St. Louis: Mosby.

Gambert, S. R. (2001). Prostate cancer: When to offer screening in the primary care setting. *Geriatrics, 56*(1), 22–31.

Dambro, M. R. (2004). The 5 minute clinical consult. Philadelphia: Lippincott, Williams & Wilkins.

Lovejoy, B. (2001). Diagnosis and management of chronic prostatitis by primary care providers. *Journal of the American Academy of Nurse Practitioners, 13*(7), 317–321.

Male Sexual Dysfunction Task Force, (1998, July-August). AACE clinical practice guidelines for the evaluation and treatment of male sexual dysfunction. *Endocrine Practice. 4*(4), 219–235.

Meredith, P. V., & Horan, N. M. (2000). *Adult primary care.* Philadelphia: W. B. Saunders.

Raja, S. G., & Nayak, S. H. (2004) Sildenafil: Emerging cardiovascular indications. *Ann Thorac Surg, 78* (4), 1496–1506.

Tierney, L. M., McPhee, S. J., & Papadakis, A. (2005). *Current Medical Diagnosis and Treatment,* (44th ed.). NJ: Appleton & Lange.

Wagenlehner, F. M., & Naber, K.G. (2003). Antimicrobial treatment of prostatitis. *Expert Rev Anti Infect Ther, 1*(2), 275–282.

MUSCULOSKELETAL DISORDERS 14

GERIATRIC APPROACH

Normal Changes of Aging
- Body composition: fat mass increases, bone and muscle mass and strength decrease
- Decreased water content leads to stiffness in tendons, ligaments, and cartilage
- Endocrine changes affecting bones and muscle
  - Adrenopause—reduced dehydroepiandrosterone (DHEA) levels may play part in increased adiposity and decreased lean muscle mass
  - Andropause
    - Reduction of total and free testosterone in men
    - Decreased testosterone in postmenopausal women has been associated with increased fracture risk.
  - Menopause increases bone resorption, increasing the risk of osteopenia and osteoporosis.
  - Growth hormone (GH) and insulin-like growth factor I (IGF-I) levels decrease; lower levels may assist in increasing adiposity, decreasing lean muscle mass and strength
  - Parathyroid hormone—PTH levels increase; higher levels associated with increased bone resorption, increased osteoblast activity

Clinical Implications

History
- Age, previous/current occupation, military service, athletics
- Onset of problem (insidious or sudden? progression of symptoms?)
- Timing: when does pain occur? worse at night? with rest? with activity? with weather?
- Mechanism of injury (e.g., fall, twisting motion, how much force was involved?)
- Symptoms associated with pain: certain movements, positions, activities, any locking, catching, or giving way of a joint?
- Does the pain or symptom interfere with function (ADLs and IADLs)?
- Previous pain, injury, or surgery in same area?
- Previous treatment? Self-treated or another provider?; include any medications, OTCs, herbs
- Concomitant medical problems, medications

Physical
- Assess for inflammation, joint pattern, systemic disease
- Compare sides to assess for abnormalities
- Inspection—note signs of underlying pathology (e.g., vascular changes of skin, poor healing of wounds, presence of deformity or malalignment, gait)
- Movements—check unaffected side first: first active, then passive ROM (painful movements last); check ADL/transfer, ambulation/gait
- Tenderness to palpation, with active/passive movement (normal ROM may be decreased)

- Palpate for crepitus, grinding, catching of joints
- Manual muscle testing against resistance to assess strength, rate on scale of 1/5 to 5/5
- Provocative tests specific to area

Assessment
- Intra-articular processes will produce decreased range of motion, swelling, and inflammation
- Involvement of small joints (elbows, wrist, metacarpal phalangeal joints, and ankles) may indicate an inflammatory joint process rather than mechanical
- False-positive rheumatoid factor and elevated sedimentation rates are common. Order these tests to make a specific diagnosis based on history and physical exam.
  - Consider deconditioning when evaluating a musculoskeletal problem.
  - Immobility, for any reason, causes a rapid decrease in muscle strength very quickly; any decrease in activity will cause a corresponding decrease in strength.
  - Reduced muscle mass and strength is associated with increased risk of physical frailty, falls, fractures, decreased function
  - Exercise can improve functional performance in elderly and increase muscle strength
  - Consider depression in the patient with chronic pain

Treatment
- Normal changes of aging may delay healing of musculoskeletal injuries
  - Physical modalities of rest, ice, heat, compression, elevation, massage, and exercise may need to be modified due to changes in muscle mass, bone density, visual disturbances, or decreased sensory acuity but are essential to management of musculoskeletal conditions in the elderly.
- Medications
  - Acetaminophen is usually first-line pain medication for most musculoskeletal pain or injuries
    Acetaminophen at 3000 to 4000 mg per day divided on regular basis
    Maximum dose of acetaminophen is 4000 mg in 24-hour period
    Use with caution in presence of liver disease and alcohol use
  - Nonselective NSAIDs
    Useful for short-term relief of pain in chronic arthritis, acute injury
    Adverse effects more common in the elderly
    Side effects include GI bleed, renal failure, liver failure, CHF, edema, confusion, and elevated blood pressure. Use with extra caution in patients with these conditions.
    Patients with history of peptic ulcer disease or GI bleed have 10 times more risk of GI bleed
    When used long term, use lowest dose, monitor for:
      Symptoms of blood loss/GI bleed, heart and renal failure
      CBC for anemia and renal failure every 3–6 months
    Ibuprofen: 400–800 mg with food tid–qid
    Nabumetone (Relafen): 1000–1500 mg, may be give qd or divided bid with food .
  - Selective COX-2 inhibitors
    COX-2 inhibitors less risk of GI side effects and bleeding in those with risk
    Celecoxib (Celebrex) 100–200 mg qd bid, sulfa allergy a relative contraindication
    Valdecoxib (Bextra) 10–20 mg PO qd, sulfa allergy a relative contraindication
  - Narcotics may be safely used for noncancer pain not amenable to other treatment. Use lowest effective doses. Use with extreme caution regarding confusion, drowsiness, and constipation.
      Oxycodone generally fairly well tolerated; start at low doses and frequency: 5 mg at HS. May give bid–qid, use for shortest possible duration
      Propoxyphene increased risk of delirium in elderly; use with caution for those taking antidepressant or anxiolytics, excessive alcohol use, addiction risk, or suicidal
      Monitor use of OTC medications, particularly with regard to prescribed medications and dosages of acetaminophen, NSAIDs, or aspirin

Other adverse effects include respiratory and cardiac depression, dizziness, nausea, vomiting, diaphoresis

Almost always causes constipation; start bowel regime (see GI, constipation), try stool softener with osmotic agent or stimulant. Avoid hydrophilic colloid or bulk-forming agents, particularly if inadequate fluid intake is an issue

Encourage fluids, increased dietary fiber, and mobility for all elderly on narcotics

Neurontin and Ultram (tramadol) also used as adjuvant drugs

- Use muscle relaxants (cyclobenzaprine, methocarbamol, metaxalone) with caution, if at all, as they may cause dizziness and falls.
- Alternative treatments for pain: behavioral interventions

Try heat/ice to affected areas

Consider physical activity/movement to decrease pain

ARTHRITIS AND OTHER DISEASES
Osteoporosis

Description
- Osteoporosis: Bone resorption occurs faster than bone formation, causing increased bone porosity in the trabecular bone (larger marrow spaces) and thinning of cortical bone.
- Bone mineral density (BMD) at least 2.5 standard deviations (SD) below peak bone density (30-year-old control); represented as T score of negative 2.5 or lower
- Osteopenia: BMD T score of negative 1 to 2.4

Etiology
- Hormone deficiency—estrogen, androgen
- Cushing's syndrome or steroid use
- Malignancy (multiple myeloma, leukemia)
- Chronic hyperthyroidism, hyperparathyroidism
- Rheumatoid arthritis
- Vitamin D deficiency, excess; vitamin A excess
- Chronic heparin use

Incidence and Demographics
- Approximately 20 to 25 million women
- 5 to 6 million men
- Primarily affects postmenopausal women (over 50) and men over 70
- 21% of postmenopausal women have osteoporosis
- About 40% of women over 50 have had a fracture due to osteoporosis

Risk Factors
- Menopause, early menopause (natural or surgical)
- Inadequate calcium intake; premenopausal intake important
- Genetic predisposition (positive family history)
- Petite frame, low weight (less that 127 pounds), tall height
- Caucasian or Asian ethnicity
- Advancing age
- Decreased physical activity, immobilization
- Smoking
- Excessive alcohol intake

Prevention and Screening
- Nutritional diet with adequate intake of calcium and vitamin D

- Regular weight-bearing exercise/resistance exercise
- Smoking cessation
- Avoiding high alcohol intake
- Dual energy x-ray absorptiometry (DXA) scan of axial skeleton for screening and diagnosis recommended for all women 65 and older and for women 60 and older with increased risk, those who have lost height, discrepancy between height and arm length

Assessment

History
- Fracture after age 40 (spine, hip, wrist)
- Loss of height
- Back pain (from vertebral fracture)
- Diet, exercise, medications
- Articular stiffness, developing into pain with motion; pain relieved by rest

Physical
- Usually no finding specific to osteoporosis, especially early
- Kyphosis with bulging abdomen is common in more advanced osteoporosis
- Fracture is the most common presenting sign
- Documented decrease in height over time

Diagnostic Studies
- Bone densitometry (DXA scan)
- Osteoporosis shows on regular x-rays after more than 30% of bone is lost
- To rule out secondary causes of osteoporosis: comprehensive metabolic panel, CBC

Differential Diagnosis
- Osteoarthritis
- Paget disease
- Metastatic bone disease
- Rheumatic disease
- Fibromyalgia
- Gout
- Multiple myeloma
- Acute injury

Management

Nonpharmacologic Treatment
- Regular weight-bearing exercise (20–30 minutes/day 6–7 days/week)
- Fall prevention management and education
- Calcium supplementation (1500–2000 mg/day) or adequate dietary intake
- Adequate vitamin D intake (400–800 IU/day)
- All pharmacological treatments for osteoporosis require optimal calcium and vitamin D intake to be effective

Pharmacologic Treatment
- Bisphosphonates: alendronate (Fosamax) 70 mg or risedronate (Alendronate) 35 mg PO once weekly. Must take on empty stomach in AM and remain sitting or standing for one-half hour before eating, or it will not be absorbed or will cause severe esophagitis; intravenous pamidronate (Aredia) may be appropriate for individuals unable to tolerate oral bisphosphonates OR
- Calcitonin nasal spray (Miacalcin) 200 units/day intranasal, alternating nostrils; use as analgesic for compression fractures and for patients unable to take bisphosphonates due to GI distress OR
- Selective estrogen receptor modulators (SERMs): raloxifene (Evista) 60 mg/day PO for post-menopausal women
- Zoledronate (Zometa) is a third-generation bisphosphonate given IV over 15 minutes every 6–12 months (myalgia and fever common)
- Parathyroid hormone teriparatide (Forteo) 20 mcg SC qd for a maximum of 2 years. May be more effective than bisphosphonates but is more expensive and must be given SC.

How Long to Treat
- Indefinitely or until treatment is contraindicated due to patient's condition

When to Consult, Refer, Hospitalize
- Refer to rheumatologist if patient does not respond to treatment
- Refer to orthopedist for suspected fracture; hospitalize for any hip fracture

Follow-up

Expected Course
- Improvement or maintenance of bone density evident by DXA 1 to 2 years after initiation of therapy
- Benefit continues to be seen after 10 years of treatment with no new adverse effects
- Follow-up monitoring (DXA) may improve adherence to treatment plan
- Monitor height

Complications
- Major cause of morbidity in the elderly
- Fracture (vertebral most common, associated with chronic pain; hip most disabling and has greatest mortality); see section on fractures for more information
- Impaired gait
- Chronic pain syndrome
- Inability to perform basic activities of daily living has major impact on quality of life

Arthritis

See Table 14-1.

Osteoarthritis

Description
- Degenerative disorder of the movable joints characterized by destruction of cartilage and bone hypertrophy, formation of osteophytes and subchondral cysts. There is no systemic involvement.
- Hypertrophy of bone at the articular margins
- Inflammation absent or minimal

Table 14-1: Characteristics of Osteoarthritis and Rheumatoid Arthritis

Characteristics	Osteoarthritis	Rheumatoid Arthritis
Radiographic Appearance	Joint space narrowing, osteophytes, subchondral bone sclerosis, subchondral cysts	Evidence of osteoporosis with/without subchondral bone destruction (bone and cartilage involvement in later stages), joint deformities
Morning Stiffness	Lasts <30 minutes	Lasts >1 h
Joint Involvement	Usually weight-bearing (spine, hips, knees), or distal finger joints (DIP)	Multiple small joints, symmetric joint involvement (esp. of hands); rare in spine
Laboratory Findings	ESR <20–40 mm/h; RF negative	Serum RF abnormal (usually elevated) ESR usually elevated (*not definitive diagnosis)
Clinical Findings That May Be Present	Joint pain, bony tenderness and hypertrophy, crepitus, may have some deformity; no palpable warmth, occasional fluid in joint	Joint deformity, muscle atrophy, extra-articular soft tissue nodules (rheumatoid nodules) acute: red, warm, swollen, and tender

Etiology
- May be a combination of mechanical and genetic factors
- May be secondary to injury or repetitive use

Incidence and Demographics
- Most common form of arthritis; affects more than 20 million people in US
- Up to 90% of US population older than 40 years has radiographic evidence of osteoarthritis
- Incidence increases with advancing age
- Asian, Pacific Islanders have lower prevalence rate than other races
- Native Americans have greatest prevalence

Risk Factors
- Advancing age
- Repetitive joint use
- Trauma
- Obesity
- Family history

Prevention and Screening
- Moderate physical activity
- Maintain ideal body weight, avoid obesity

Assessment

History
- Gradual onset of joint pain and stiffness that often worsens with activity and is relieved by rest
- Morning stiffness common but usually lasts less than 30 minutes
- Weather changes may affect symptoms
  - More advanced symptoms include:
  - More joints involved
  - Joint instability, especially with osteoarthritis of knees
  - Coarse crepitus felt in joint
  - Bony enlargement of joint with decreased range of motion
  - May have decreased sensation

Physical
- Localized to affected joints, not a systemic disease
- Bony hypertrophy of joint, tenderness at joint line; limited range of motion
  - Distal interphalangeal (DIP) joint swelling: Heberden's node
  - Proximal interphalangeal (PIP) joint swelling: Bouchard's node
- Soft-tissue swelling may be present; decreased ROM
- Crepitus with movement
- Joint effusion, if present, usually mild

Diagnostic Studies
- Plain radiographs: presence of osteophytes, asymmetric joint space (narrowing), subchondral bone, sclerosis, and cysts
- Presence of radiographic changes does not correlate with presence or severity of symptoms
- Laboratory findings: SED rate almost always normal; primary use is ruling out inflammatory condition; no specific laboratory tests for osteoarthritis

Differential Diagnosis
- Gout
- Fibromyalgia
- Osteoporosis
- Multiple myeloma
- Acute injury
- Rheumatoid arthritis
- Polymyalgia rheumatica
- Trauma

Management
- Goals are to relieve symptoms, maintain/improve function, avoid adverse effects of medication

Nonpharmacologic Treatment
- Physical activity/therapy is the cornerstone of treatment
- Occupational therapy
- Heat/cold to affected joint
- Non–weight-bearing exercise. Arthritis self-help and water aquatics courses
- Ambulation aids (canes, braces, walkers) or assistive devices to facilitate function
- Weight loss programs if appropriate

Pharmacologic Treatment (See Clinical Implications)
- Glucosamine 750 mg and chondroitin 600 mg have been shown to be effective
- Acetaminophen up to 4000 mg/day in divided doses is first-line therapy for pain
- Topical analgesic creams such as capsaicin 0.025% bid/salicylate creams
- NSAIDs can be very effective, especially in those with severe disease; use COX-2 inhibitors in those at risk for bleeding
- Intra-articular corticosteroid or hyaluronic acid injections may be helpful

Surgical Treatment
- Consider when other modalities are not sufficient to manage pain and facilitate function

When to Consult, Refer, Hospitalize
- Patients with functional impairment need for intra-articular corticosteroid injections or moderate to severe pain should be considered for joint replacement. Refer to orthopedic surgeon.

Follow-up

Expected Course
- Gradual progressive worsening
- Limitation of activity, difficulty with ADLs

Complications
- Decreased quality of life
- Chronic pain
- Adverse effects of pain medications
- Injury to specific joints: cervical and lumbar radiculopathy, rotator cuff tears, meniscus and quadriceps rupture, and impingement syndromes

Rheumatoid Arthritis

Description
- Chronic, inflammatory, systemic disease with symmetric bone erosions, small joint destruction, and progressive limitation in function

Etiology
- Probably autoimmune, but no specific inciting factor yet identified
- Genetic, environmental factors affect progression and extent of disease

Incidence and Demographics
- Prevalence in general population is 1% to 2%
- Prevalence about 2.5 times greater in females
- Usual age of onset is between fourth and fifth decades, but may begin at any age
- Persists and progresses in old age

Risk Factors
- Susceptibility is genetically determined

Assessment

History
- Usually insidious, gradual onset over several weeks, diagnosed after symptoms have been present for 6 weeks
- May have acute flares superimposed over chronic progressive course

SYSTEMIC SYMPTOMS
- Prodromal symptoms of malaise, fatigue, weight loss, low-grade fever, anorexia, weakness, may persist indefinitely

JOINT INVOLVEMENT
- Stiffness and pain in smaller joints
- Hands: proximal interphalangeal (PIP), metacarpophalangeal (MCP)
- Wrist, elbow, ankle, and metatarsophalangeal (MTP) joints of foot
- Involvement usually symmetrical, in 3 or more joints
- Morning stiffness lasts longer than 1 hour

Physical
- Acute inflammation of joint with redness, heat, swelling, and tenderness to palpation may occur
- Often less acute presentation with symmetric joint swelling with stiffness
- Stiffness, in AM, after inactivity, and after strenuous activity is a good measure of activity of the disease
- Subcutaneous nodules over bony prominences or extensor surfaces, especially inguinal, epitrochlear, are mobile and nontender.
- As disease progresses, damage to joints progresses and joint deformities become more pronounced.

Diagnostic Studies
- No single test is adequate to make diagnosis
- Positive serum rheumatoid factor (RF) in about 85% of cases (also positive in infection, old age, other autoimmune diseases)
- CBC frequently shows anemia of chronic disease; elevated platelet count may be present in severe disease
- ESR (erythrocyte sedimentation rate) correlates with degree of synovial inflammation
- CRP (C-reactive protein) may also be used to monitor inflammation
- Synovial fluid shows sterile leukocytosis
- Gammaglobulinemia—elevated IgM and IgG
- X-ray will show joint erosions and narrowing of joint spaces

Differential Diagnosis
- Systemic lupus erythematosus (SLE)
- Rheumatic fever
- Septic joint
- Psoriatic arthritis
- Ankylosing spondylitis
- Osteoarthritis
- Gout

Management
- Goals are early diagnosis and early treatment to prevent or limit irreversible joint damage, maximize mobility, and limit pain.
- Course of therapy depends on disease severity; consultation with or referral to rheumatologist is appropriate.

Nonpharmacologic Treatment
- Patient education (Arthritis Foundation self-help courses)
- Physical and occupational therapy to strengthen muscles, improve joint ROM and function, protect joint(s)

- Regular exercise program, except rest during flares
- Assistive devices (canes, splints) to facilitate function

Pharmacologic Treatment
- NSAIDs are used first, while diagnosis is being confirmed
  - Have not been shown to alter disease course but may offer symptom relief
- Methotrexate is considered by many to be treatment of choice
  - Beneficial effect in 2 to 6 weeks
  - Common adverse effect is gastric irritation
  - Serious adverse effects are interstitial pneumonitis, hepatotoxicity, and bone marrow suppression
- Biologic agents (disease-modifying antirheumatic drugs [DMARDs]); tumor necrosis factor (TNF) inhibitors are new drugs that may replace methotrexate as first-line therapy
  - Leflunomide (Arava), etanercept (Enbrel), and infliximab (Remicade) may cause hypersensitivity reaction, severe infections or sepsis, and autoimmunity (lupus-type syndrome)
  - Work faster than methotrexate, good response in 60%
  - Are extremely expensive, insurance unlikely to cover
- Antimalarials—hydroxychloroquine
  - Good for mild disease, 25% to 50% will respond, takes 3 to 6 months to have effect
  - Comparative low toxicity: serious—pigmentary retinitis, requires ophthalmology exams; also may cause neuropathies, myopathies
- Corticosteroids
  - Prednisone PO or methylprednisolone IM
  - For acute flares; failure to respond to other medications
  - Do not alter course of disease

How Long to Treat
- Lifelong therapy is indicated

When to Consult, Refer, Hospitalize
- Refer to rheumatology for management; patients in long-term care facilities are referred when symptoms are not controlled
- Physical therapy

Follow-up
- Frequent follow-ups are indicated until symptoms are controlled, then regular evaluations at 3- to 6-month intervals
- Laboratory testing as indicated by medication side effect profile

Expected Course
- Destruction of joints begins to appear within a few months of disease onset
- Variable course; however, 10-year survival rate is poor
- For some patients, the acute inflammation resolves, but patient left with deformities of joints with severely decreased functional ability

Complications
- Severe systemic effects—pleuritis, pericarditis, vasculitis
- Musculoskeletal—muscle wasting, contractures, carpal tunnel syndrome
- Patients may sustain substantial joint damage and develop poor functional status
- Adverse effects of medications, especially GI bleed and to hepatic and renal systems

Gout

Description
- Disease resulting from hyperuricemia in which there is deposition of uric acid or monosodium urate crystals in supersaturated extracellular fluids (particularly in and around joints and tendons)

- Three classic stages: asymptomatic hyperuricemia; acute intermittent gout; chronic tophaceous gout
- Pseudogout is calcium pyrophosphate dihydrate crystal deposition disease (CPPD)

Etiology
- Underlying pathology is hyperuricemia (serum urate more than 7.0 mg/dL) due to overproduction and/or underexcretion of urate
  - Overproduction: high intake of purine-rich foods (organ meats, shellfish, peas, lentils, beans); hemolytic diseases, psoriasis, glycogen storage diseases, severe muscle exertion
  - Underexcretion: reduced renal function, lactic acidosis, ketoacidosis, certain diuretics, dehydration, certain drugs (ethambutol, cyclosporine), lead nephropathy
    - Combined overproduction/underexcretion: alcohol abuse, hypoxemia

Incidence and Demographics
- Affects 2.1 million in US
- Higher incidence in men; occurs in postmenopausal women
- Slightly higher incidence in African American males than Caucasian
- High incidence in Pacific Islanders
- Peak incidence is fifth decade

Risk Factors
- Heredity
- Obesity
- Thiazide diuretics

Prevention and Screening
- Correct/control underlying etiology
- Avoid foods high in purines
- Maintain normal body weight

Assessment

History
- Classic: sudden attack of red, hot, swollen, exquisitely tender joint is common; if this occurs in first MTP joint, it's known as podagra
- More commonly: chronic joint pain in more than one joint
- Foot, ankle, knee are most common sites; wrist, elbow, fingers also may be affected

Physical
- During acute attack, joint is red, hot, swollen, exquisitely painful; fever, chills, malaise may accompany acute attack
- Tophi (sodium urate crystals deposited in soft tissue) present in chronic tophaceous gout; usually after 2 to 3 to 10 years from onset of acute intermittent gout; may be confused with nodules from rheumatoid or osteoarthritis
- Joint swelling, restricted movement in late/chronic stages due to arthritis

Diagnostic Studies
- Joint aspiration: fluid shows presence of urate crystals on polarized light microscopy, increased WBC
- Serum uric acid more than 7.0 mg/dL supports diagnosis but is not specific
- Elevated ESR in acute gout
- Excision of nodule shows gouty tophus
- X-ray shows punched-out lesions in subchondral bone, usually first seen in first MTP joint ("Mickey Mouse" ears); tophi may be seen if at least 5 mm in diameter

Differential Diagnosis
- Septic joint
- Pseudo gout
- Acute rheumatic fever
- Rheumatoid arthritis
- Osteoarthritis

Management

Nonpharmacologic Treatment

ACUTE

- Rest
- Local application of cold, use with caution in patients with peripheral vascular disease or peripheral neuropathy

CHRONIC

- Dietary modification—avoid purines and alcohol
- Fluid intake ≥3 liters/day
- Weight loss in obese patients

Pharmacologic Treatment

- Asymptomatic hyperuricemia is rarely treated
- Use all gout medications with caution, especially in patients with renal insufficiency or dehydration

ACUTE

- NSAIDs are the treatment of choice
  - Indomethacin is not recommended for use in geriatric patients since it produces the most central nervous system side effects
  - See Clinical Implications treatment, treat until pain resolved. COX-2 inhibitors not FDA approved for gout.
- Colchicine may be used
  - Dose is 0.5 mg–0.6 mg PO qh until pain is relieved or nausea or diarrhea appears; total dose not to exceed 8 mg
  - Diarrhea or abdominal cramping frequently occurs. Bone marrow suppression and myoneuropathy may occur.
  - Used for patients who are not good candidates for NSAIDs, such as individuals on anti-coagulants, congestive heart failure, renal insufficiency
  - Drug has very narrow therapeutic index, monitor closely
- Corticosteroids PO or injection may be used for patients unable to take oral NSAIDs

CHRONIC

- Treat chronic gout to keep uric acid level within normal limits to minimize urate deposition in tissues
- Avoid or decrease dose of diuretics
- Colchicine 0.6 mg PO 1–2 times a day
- Allopurinol is for chronic gout only
  - 100 qd PO, increase up to 600 mg qd, divided >300 mg/d
  - Do not use to treat acute gout or asymptomatic hyperuricemia
  - Adverse events include fatal skin reactions, hypersensitivity reactions, renal and hepatotoxicity

How Long to Treat

- Acute symptoms treated until symptoms are relieved
- Lifelong therapy begun if
  - Repeated attacks of disabling gout
  - Chronic gout
  - Presence of tophi

When to Consult, Refer, Hospitalize

- Consult for any complicated presentation, renal disease, underlying metabolic pathology
- Refer for joint aspiration, unclear diagnosis

Follow-up

Expected Course
- Decrease in frequency, severity of attacks with appropriate treatment

Complications
- Kidney stones, renal obstruction, and infection
- Joint destruction, chronic arthritis of multiple joints with decreased mobility
- Complications frequent from medications used to treat

Polymyalgia Rheumatica

Description
- Polymyalgia rheumatica (PMR) is a syndrome characterized by aching and morning stiffness in the proximal joints (shoulder and pelvic girdles) associated with an elevated sedimentation rate
- Giant cell arteritis (GCA) is a systemic inflammation of medium and large arteries. When it affects the temporal arteries, it is called temporal arteritis (TA). TA may lead to blindness. See EENT Chapter 7 for details.
- PMR, GCA, and TA appear to be related disorders. PMR responds to low-dose steroids; while GCA and TA require high-dose therapy.

Etiology
- Genetic predisposition
- Cellular, immune, and humeral mechanisms involved

Incidence and Demographics
- PMR is relatively common in the elderly
- Occurs in persons aged 50 years or older
- Average age at onset is 70
- Women affected twice as often as men; Caucasians more than African Americans

Risk Factors
- Family history

Prevention and Screening
- None

Assessment

History
- Onset is usually gradual, but may be abrupt
- Fatigue, anorexia, and weight loss may be early symptoms
- Stiffness, malaise, aching, depression may be present
- Shoulder girdle first to be affected; may start unilateral, then become bilateral
- Pelvic girdle often affected; patients have difficulty standing up without pushing up with arms
- Gelling after inactivity and early morning stiffness are prominent

Physical
- Weakness of proximal joints
- Difficulty and pain with movement of joints
- Low-grade fever may be present

Diagnostic Studies
- Sedimentation rate is essential for diagnosis. Must be 40–50 mm/h
- May have anemia and elevated LFTs, especially alkaline phosphatase
- Not associated with rheumatoid factor, antinuclear antibodies, or other autoantibodies

Differential Diagnosis

PMR IS A DIAGNOSIS OF EXCLUSION:

- Rheumatoid arthritis
- Polymyositis
- Chronic infection
- Malignancy
- Hypothyroidism
- Hyperthyroidism
- Myeloma/leukemia

Management

Nonpharmacologic Treatment

- Exercise to maintain and augment function

Pharmacologic Treatment

- High initial dose prednisone; prednisone 10 mg to 20 mg qd may be required for life
- Clinical response should be within 3 days, if no response, reevaluate diagnosis

How Long to Treat

- Continue prednisone for 6 months to 2 years
- Taper depending on ESR
- Disease flares are common as prednisone is decreased

Special Considerations

- If signs and symptoms are consistent with TA, start 60 mg prednisone immediately and refer for temporal artery biopsy; untreated TA can cause blindness
- A PMR patient on low-dose prednisone can develop TA

When to Consult, Refer, Hospitalize

- Patient should be referred to rheumatologist for confirmation of diagnosis and management

Follow-up

- Monitor ESR closely, monthly and after each change in prednisone
- Monitor for signs and symptoms indicative of temporal arteritis

Expected Course

- PMR generally resolves after about a year

Complications

- PMR can lead to TA, which can cause blindness
- Anticipate and manage side effects of prednisone, including hyperglycemia, edema, osteoporosis

INJURY/OVERUSE SYNDROMES
Neck Pain

Description

- Injury or damage to structures in the neck may cause occipital headache, neck, trapezius, rhomboid, or parascapular pain.

Etiology

- Most common causes
  - Osteoporosis or osteoarthritis
  - Trauma, especially whiplash
  - Neck strain or spasm
  - Falls
  - Significant kyphosis

Incidence and Demographics

- 50% of those over age 50 will have neck pain at some time
- 80% of those over age 55 have some evidence of degenerative disk disease on cervical spine x-rays

Risk Factors
- Age
- Previous trauma or injury, degenerative joint disease
- Osteoporosis

Assessment

History
- Identify onset or precipitating events or trauma
- Acute or chronic
- Associated neurological symptoms: paresthesia, weakness, dizziness or vertigo, drop attacks, visual or hearing impairments, particularly with neck movement
- Impact on function and sleep
- Previous attempts at pain management

Physical
- Do not test range of motion if fracture suspected (e.g., any trauma)
- Asymmetric range of motion of neck
- Distal muscle wasting
- Decreased reflexes
- Sensory impairment
- Neurological and muscular skeletal exam may reveal level of cervical lesion
  - C-5: weakness of shoulder abductors and elbow flexors
  - C-6: weakness of wrist extensors
  - C-7: weakness of finger abductors

Diagnostic Studies
- X-rays: rule out tumor, findings of degenerative changes may not correlate with severity of symptoms
- MRI to confirm positive neurological findings if herniated disk or cord compression is suspected
- Electromyogram to confirm diagnosis of radiculopathy

Differential Diagnosis
IMPORTANT TO RULE OUT:
- Tumor, metastasis
- Meningitis
- Rheumatoid arthritis
- Polymyalgia rheumatica
- Compression fracture
- Torticollis
- Ankylosing spondylitis
- Cervical herniated nucleus pulposus

Management

Nonpharmacologic Treatment
- Heat
- Soft cervical collar short term for whiplash
- Exercises for neck strengthening as tolerated
- Surgery for decompression if indicated

Pharmacologic Treatment
- See Clinical Implications for pain management
- Use muscle relaxants with caution in the elderly
- Refer for consideration of injecting trigger points with local anesthetic or cortisone

Special Considerations
- Surgical decompression for myelopathy is 75% to 80% effective

When to Consult, Refer, Hospitalize
- Emergently immobilize neck and refer to ED if acute traumatic fracture is suspected
- Refer to neurosurgery for focal neurologic deficits with suspected cord or nerve root compression

- Refer for corticosteroid injection
- Physical therapy for exercises

Follow-up

Expected Course
- Most pain responds to 4 to 6 weeks of conservative treatment

Complications
- Chronic pain, limited ROM, weakness, pain, decreased function of upper extremities

Low Back Pain

Description
- Low back pain (LBP): aching or sharp pain in lower lumbar, lumbosacral, or sacroiliac area
- Sciatica—symptom of pain that radiates down one or both buttocks/legs, often but not always caused by herniated disk
- Herniated disk: rupture of nucleus pulposus through annulus fibrosis of intervertebral disk; compresses spinal cord or irritates associated nerve root; more often unilateral but may have central herniation
- Spinal stenosis is narrowing of the spinal canal, usually from osteoarthritis
- Cauda equina is the collection of spinal roots descending from the lower spinal cord; compression of these is a medical emergency

Etiology
- Musculoskeletal most common
  - Muscle/ligament strain
  - Osteoarthritis
  - Degenerative disk disease
  - Disk herniation
  - Spinal stenosis
  - Vertebral compression fracture

Incidence and Demographics
- One of the most common complaints in primary care
- Most back pain in older patients has its onset before age 65

Risk Factors
- Physical deconditioning
- Poor body mechanics
- Cigarette smoking
- Obesity
- Scoliosis
- Depression
- Degenerative joint disease
- Osteoporosis

Prevention and Screening
- Regular exercise program
- Maintain ideal body weight
- Proper body mechanics and posture

Assessment
- Key is to assess for neurological compromise from herniated disk

History (See Table 14-2)
- Onset of back pain, any precipitating events, chronic or acute
- Impact on function, mobility and ADLs

Table 14-2: Differences Between Simple LBP and LBP Due to Herniated Disk

Clinical Problem	History	Physical Examination
Simple Low Back Pain	Pain in back, buttocks, and/or thigh Onset usually after exertion No history of trauma, infection, malignancy Pain relieved by lying supine	Paravertebral tenderness, muscle spasm Loss of normal lumbar lordosis common No neurologic deficit
Low Back Pain due to Herniated Disk	Initially, back pain severe Chronic herniation usually results in leg pain greater than back pain Often, + history of trauma, forced flexion Central herniation results in bilateral leg weakness, bowel/bladder dysfunction (cauda equina syndrome)	L5-S1 (most common): pain in posterior thigh, posterior/lateral calf, heel; weak plantar flexion of foot; diminished ankle reflex L4-5: pain in lateral thigh, anterior calf and dorsum of foot; weak dorsiflexion of foot L3-4: pain in anterior and lateral thigh, medial calf and foot; weak quadriceps; diminished patellar reflex

- Stiffness usually associated with muscular injury
- Paresthesia or sciatica (burning pain in buttock and leg) is associated with herniated disk or radiculopathy
- Gait disturbance along with back pain suggests spinal stenosis
- Pain at night unrelieved by rest suggests tumor, compression fracture, ankylosing spondylitis, or malignancy
- Bilateral leg weakness, saddle area anesthesia, or bladder and bowel incontinence indicate a cauda equina process from tumor, epidural abscess, or massive disk herniation

Physical
- With the patient on his/her back, raise one leg with knee absolutely straight, until pain is experienced in the thigh, buttock, and calf. Record angle at which pain occurs. A normal (pain-free) value would be 70 to 90 degrees, higher in people with lax ligaments.
- Then perform sciatic stretch test: Dorsiflex foot at the point of discomfort. Test is positive if additional pain results.
- Flexing the knee will relieve the buttocks pain, but this is restored by pressing on the lateral popliteal nerve.
- Severe root irritation is indicated when straight raising of the leg on the unaffected side produces pain on the affected side.

Diagnostic Studies
- X-ray: order when new onset and to rule out acute compression fracture as treatment options are different; x-ray not often necessary for simple LBP but useful for identifying degenerative changes, vertebral alignment, bone tumor, disk space height
- MRI: most useful for identifying herniated nucleus pulposus, diskitis
- Bone scan: helpful for identifying metabolically active processes such as tumor, occult fracture, infection, abscess
- Serum studies usually not helpful but ESR elevated in infection; HLA-B27 elevated in ankylosing spondylitis

Differential Diagnosis

METABOLIC DISORDERS
- Osteoporosis secondary to compression fractures
- Osteomalacia
- Paget disease

CANCER
- Metastatic prostate
- Multiple myeloma
- Lymphoma

AUTOIMMUNE CONNECTIVE TISSUE DISORDERS
- Rheumatoid arthritis
- Psoriatic arthritis
- PMR
- Ankylosing spondylitis
- Reiter's syndrome

NONMUSCULOSKELETAL ORIGIN
- Abdominal aortic aneurysm
- Renal stones
- Peptic ulcer
- Ovarian cysts, tumors
- Endocarditis
- Infection
- Pancreatic disease

Management
- Most simple LBP responds to conservative treatment
- 80% or more of patients with LBP due to herniated disk also respond to conservative treatment

Nonpharmacologic Treatment
- Relieve pain to facilitate function and maintain activity
- Avoid bed rest, which causes deconditioning
- Modified activity as tolerated, no heavy lifting, avoid activities that provoke pain
- Heat and massage
- Physical therapy for muscle conditioning exercises
- In certain instances, braces may reduce symptoms for vertebral compression fractures but may be uncomfortable and restrict respirations in the elderly
- Chiropractic manipulation use with caution in elderly with osteoporosis
- Resumption of normal activities with careful body mechanics, back exercises

Pharmacologic Treatment (see Clinical Implications treatment)
- Short term
  - Tylenol, NSAIDs
  - Use muscle relaxants with caution
- Long term—see Pain Management in Chapter 4

How Long to Treat
- Most episodes resolve within 4 to 6 weeks of conservative treatment; if patient in severe pain, reevaluate in 24 to 48 hours

When to Consult, Refer, Hospitalize
- Refer for vertebroplasty immediately if evidence of cauda equina syndrome, acute fractures. This is an image-guided, minimally invasive, nonsurgical therapy used to strengthen a broken vertebra by injecting an orthopedic cement mixture through a needle into the fractured bone.
- Refer for spinal instability, neurological deficit
- Hospitalize for suspected abscess, tumor, abdominal aneurysm
- Obtain consult for patients who do not respond to 6 to 8 weeks of conservative treatment
- Physical and occupational therapy

Follow-up
- Provide patient education about body mechanics, conservative therapy, use of medications and their side effects

Table 14-3: Common Problems of Joints, Organized by Joint and Problem

Joint	Bursitis	Tendinitis	Strain/ Sprain	Entrapment Neuropathies	Other Local Conditions
Shoulder	Subacromial Subdeltoid	Rotator cuff Bicipital	Deltoid muscle strain	Impingement syndrome	Adhesive capsulitis Rotator cuff strain, tear
Wrist		De Quervain's	Radiocarpal muscle strain	Carpal tunnel	Ganglion cyst
Elbow	Olecranon	Medial, lateral epicondylitis		Cubital tunnel	
Hip	Trochanteric Iliopsoas Ischial				Spontaneous fractures
Knee	Prepatellar Infrapatellar Pes anserine	Iliotibial band Patellar	Collateral ligament sprains		Meniscus tear Quadriceps rupture
Ankle	Retrocalcaneal	Achilles Posterior tibialis Peroneal	Ligaments of ankle sprain		

Expected Course
- Most acute LBP resolves in 4 to 6 weeks with conservative care
- Remitting and recurring symptoms are common

Complications
- Few complications if diagnosed and treated, though recurrence is common
- Can develop a chronic pain syndrome that can be difficult to manage
- With neurologic deficit, can have permanent nerve damage if compression of nerve root not relieved in timely manner
- Depression

SPECIFIC JOINT PROBLEMS

- Elderly have many complaints of joint pain, stiffness
- Arthritis often initially presents with single joint involvement but will progress to multiple joints.
- Specific joint problems may be a complication of a generalized arthritis, such as RA, OA, and gout.
- If the patient consistently has a specific joint problem, consider the following options:
- Bursitis, tendinitis and muscle strain, and ligament sprain will be discussed as a group (see Table 14-3).
- Impingement syndromes and other problems will be discussed individually.
- See Chapter 4 for discussion of fractures.

Bursitis

Description
- Inflammation of bursal sac, which is a synovial fluid-filled sac that cushions and reduces friction in joints.

Etiology
- Trauma
- Infection (septic)
- Chronic overuse
- Inflammatory arthritis

Risk Factors
- Chronic pressure on bursa (kneeling, resting point of elbow on hard surface, overhead activity)
- Chronic arthritis

Prevention and Screening
- Avoidance of activities that apply pressure to bursae

Assessment
History
- Sudden or gradual onset of localized swelling; sometimes painful but swelling alone may cause patient to seek treatment

Physical
- Localized fluctuant swelling
- Sometimes red, warm, and/or painful to touch
- No loss of ROM
- If cellulitis, tissue breakdown evident in local area, consider septic bursitis

Diagnostic Studies
- Fluid aspiration analysis to evaluate for infection (elevated WBC, presence of organisms on Gram stain, culture), hemorrhage (elevated RBC), gout (presence of characteristic crystals)

Differential Diagnosis
- Septic joint
- Joint effusion
- Acute rheumatoid arthritis flare
- Osteoarthritis
- Gout

Management
Nonpharmacologic Treatment
- Temporary rest or immobilization of affected joint
- Aspiration of bursal sac

Pharmacologic Treatment
- Antibiotics if infected (*Staphylococcus aureus* most common pathogen), cephalexin 250–500 mg qid PO for 2–3 weeks
- NSAIDs
- Local corticosteroid injection: not performed unless infection and cellulitis is ruled out
- Retrocalcaneal injection not recommended due to risk of Achilles tendon rupture

How Long to Treat
- Antibiotics used for 7–14 days for infected bursa
- NSAIDs for 1–3 weeks until swelling subsides

When to Consult, Refer, Hospitalize
- Any local skin infection, marked cellulitis, signs of systemic illness associated with bursitis necessitate parenteral antibiotics, possible hospitalization
- Surgical drainage may be necessary if infection does not respond to antibiotics, local aspiration
- Refer if not trained to aspirate bursa

Follow-up
- Provide patient education about need to rest joint
- To ensure that there is no evidence of acute infection

Expected Course
- Symptoms usually improve within 2–3 days of aspirating/injecting bursa (if not infected)
- If infected, localized erythema should improve within 10 days

Complications
- Chronic bursitis

Tendonitis

Description
- Tendons are collagen fibrils, sheathed in connective tissue, which provide the elasticity and strength to transmit the forces of muscle to bone.
- Overuse syndrome

Etiology
- Continued stress on tendons due to repetitive motion
- Trauma

Risk Factors
- Weak muscles
- Repetitive motion
- Increasing age

Prevention and Screening
- Strengthening of muscles

Assessment

History
- Pain initially activity-related then continues at rest with progression of problem
- Difficulty using joint
- Numbness and tingling are NOT usually associated
- Shoulder—rotator cuff, bicipital tendinitis
  - Progressive pain with certain activities (usually overhead) that may progress to constant pain
  - Pain worse with lifting, pushing objects away
  - Difficulty lying on affected side
  - Decreased range of motion
- Elbow—medial, lateral epicondylitis
  - Lateral—pain with resisted wrist extension and power grip
  - Medial—pain with resisted wrist flexion and pronation
- Wrist—de Quervain tenosynovitis
- Insidious onset of burning, aching pain over radial aspect of wrist and base of thumb
- Pain often worse with grasping movements

Physical—all tendonitis
- Local inflammation over the affected tendon, acute swelling
- Affected tendon is very tender to touch
- Symptoms reproduced by passive or active ROM
- Shoulder—rotator cuff, bicipital tendinitis
  - Tenderness over inflamed tendon(s)—palpated in bicipital groove
  - May have weak abduction
  - Painful arc (pain between 70 and 120 degrees of abduction)
- Elbow epicondylitis
  - Lateral (tennis elbow)—swelling, tenderness just distal to and slightly anterior to lateral epicondyle
  - Medial (golfer's elbow)—pain and tenderness over medial epicondyle
- Wrist—de Quervain tenosynovitis
  - Pain with passive, active thumb extension
  - May have visible thickening of tendon

Differential Diagnosis
- Fracture
- Ligament sprain
- Bursitis
- Nerve impingement
- Arthritis

Management

Nonpharmacologic Treatment
- Heat
- Physical therapy, including early passive ROM, ultrasound, stretching exercises as tolerated
- Splint affected joint: wrist—de Quervain's tendinitis—radial gutter splint for 3 weeks
- Elbow, knee band: tighten over muscle, displaces stress from tendon to muscle

Pharmacologic Treatment
- NSAIDs are mainstay of treatment
- Local corticosteroid injection may be considered
- Shoulder tendinitis symptoms should improve after 2 weeks of conservative therapy; if not, refer for physical therapy.

When to Consult, Refer, Hospitalize
- Refer to Orthopedics if NSAIDs not effective

Follow-up
- Provide patient education about removing underlying cause of the problem to avoid recurrence

Expected Course
- Noticeable improvement should occur within 6 weeks of treatment

Complications
- Chronic tendinitis with loss of ROM of joint
- Muscle weakness

Muscle Strain

Description
- Tearing of muscle fibers resulting in varying degrees of pain, swelling, and decreased function; graded I-III
  - Grade I: stretching, tearing of muscle fibers but fascia remains intact
  - Grade II: tearing of muscle fibers resulting in significant hemorrhage
  - Grade III: rupture of muscle, damage to fascia
- Common problem of chest wall, neck, wrist (radiocarpal), and shoulder (deltoid)

Etiology
- Excessive stress placed on any muscle (strain)

Incidence and Demographics
- Common problem, many instances self-treated
- Most common presentation to the office is chest pain due to muscles strained from coughing or unaccustomed activity

Risk Factors
- Lifting or moving objects
- Unaccustomed activity

Prevention and Screening
- Appropriate stretching, warm-up exercises prior to activity

Assessment

History
- Sudden onset of muscle pain associated with activity
- Bruising, swelling, and loss of function may occur with more severe injury
- Gradually increasing muscle pain may occur with repetitive use of specific muscle/group

Prevention and Screening
- Maintain activity, balance, coordination

Assessment

History

- Trauma—usually forced hyperextension or flexion
- Fall, twisting, or sudden pulling of a muscle
- Hearing or feeling a "pop" at joint not uncommon, followed by pain, swelling, and ecchymosis
- Pain with movement
- Decreased ROM

Physical

- Localized tenderness, swelling, ecchymosis; pain with resisted muscle contraction and passive stretching of muscle
- Assess neurovascular status
- Numbness/tingling are unusual more than a day or two after injury
- Pain with active and passive ROM
- Tenderness over joint but no point tenderness

Diagnostic Studies

- X-ray if fracture suspected (point tenderness over bony prominences or bony deformity)
- MRI may be useful to identify extent of muscle involvement but usually not necessary

Differential Diagnosis

- Tendinitis
- Fracture
- Tumor

Management

Nonpharmacologic Treatment

- Remember with the mnemonic RICE
  - **R**—rest (non–weight-bearing)
  - **I**—ice (20 minutes qid until swelling has resolved)
  - **C**—compression (elastic bandage)
  - **E**—elevation for 48 to 72 hours
- Splinting, weight bearing as tolerated, ROM and strengthening exercises
- Grade III injuries may require casting, surgery
- After 24 to 48 hours, use heat
- Physical therapy to regain strength, mobility
- Increase activity slowly and gradually to avoid reinjury

Pharmacologic Treatment

- NSAIDs are mainstay of treatment; use for 10 to 14 days, use with caution in elderly, particularly those on anticoagulant therapy; see Clinical Implications

Special Considerations

- Patients should not return to full activity until they are pain-free

When to Consult, Refer, Hospitalize

- Refer for any injury involving muscle weakness, neurovascular compromise, or suspected fracture

Follow-up

Expected Course

- Varies with degree of injury
- Grade I strains resolve in 2 to 3 weeks; Grade II sprains require 6 to 8 weeks
- Grade III may require 8 or more weeks of treatment
- If pain is not resolving in 2 to 3 weeks, consider x-rays to rule out occult stress fractures

Complications

- Permanent deformity, loss of strength, gait disorders, falls

Ligament Sprain

Description
- Overstretching and /or partial tearing of ligaments, usually around the ankle or knee
- Standard grading indicates extent of damage:
  - Grade I: stretching but no tearing of ligaments; no joint instability
  - Grade II: partial (incomplete) tearing of ligament; some joint instability but definite endpoint to laxity
  - Grade III: complete ligamentous tearing; joint unstable with no definite endpoint to ligamentous stressing

Etiology
- Excessive stress placed on any ligament

Incidence and Demographics
- Common injury; often accompanies fracture

Risk Factors
- Unaccustomed activity
- Sudden forceful stretching of a joint—loss of balance

Prevention and Screening
- Appropriate stretching, warm-up exercises prior to activity
- Maintain activity, balance, coordination
- Avoidance of high-heeled shoes
- Joint strengthening exercises

Assessment

History
- Sudden onset of pain associated with activity; bruising, swelling, and loss of function may occur with more severe injury
- Gradually increasing pain may occur with repetitive use

Assessment

History
- Fall, twisting, or sudden pulling of a joint
- Hearing or feeling a "pop" at joint not uncommon, followed by pain, swelling, and ecchymosis
- Trauma-twisting injuries, determine if inversion or eversion
- Pain with weight bearing immediately after injury suggests fracture

Physical
- Localized tenderness, swelling, ecchymosis; pain with resisted muscle contraction and passive stretching of muscle
- Rule out joint instability
- Assess neurovascular status
- Assess the distal and proximal joints for secondary injuries sustained in fall

Diagnostic Studies
- X-ray if fracture suspected (point tenderness over bony prominences or bony deformity)
- Ankle: x-ray if:
  - Bony tenderness with palpation over medial or lateral malleolus, tarsal navicular, or base of fifth metatarsal
  - Unable to bear weight immediately after injury or during exam

Differential Diagnosis
- Tendinitis
- Fracture
- Tumor

Management
- Same as for muscle strain

Carpal Tunnel Syndrome

Description
- Entrapment neuropathy in which there is soft tissue pain due to entrapment or compression of peripheral nerves because of trauma or structural abnormalities
- Carpal tunnel syndrome of wrist: compressive neuropathy of the median nerve beneath the transverse carpal ligament
- Another entrapment neuropathy is impingement syndrome of the shoulder; see below for shoulder problems.

Etiology
- Multiple causes, including any process that encroaches on peripheral nerves
  - Rheumatoid arthritis
  - Osteoarthritis
  - Metabolic disorders (hypothyroidism, gout, diabetes mellitus)
  - Alcoholism
  - Tumors (including ganglion cyst)
  - Connective tissue disorders (amyloidosis, hemochromatosis)

Incidence and Demographics
- Affects approximately 1% of US population
- Most common in women aged 30 to 50 years
- Women affected more often than men

Risk Factors
- Repetitive wrist flexion/extension, use of vibratory tools or machinery
- Colles fracture

Prevention and Screening
- Proper ergonomics
- Treatment of underlying problem

Assessment

History
- Initially burning or aching pain, numbness, tingling that wakes patient at night and resolves after shaking the affected hand ("wake-and-shake")
- As disorder progresses, symptoms affect thumb, index and long fingers, may radiate into arm
- Patient may report dropping objects

Physical
- Painless thenar muscle-wasting is late finding; usually no visible abnormality
- Tinel's sign: positive if symptoms are reproduced by tapping the median nerve at the wrist
- Phalen's sign: positive if symptoms reproduced within 60 seconds of wrist flexion

Diagnostic Studies

ELECTROMYOGRAPHY/NERVE CONDUCTION STUDIES—EMG/NCS
- Mild to moderate symptoms should be present for 6 months for EMG/NCV studies to be accurate
- Electromyography/nerve conduction velocity (EMG/NCV) studies are confirmatory
- Plain x-rays if any history of trauma to rule out fracture

Differential Diagnosis
- Cervical radiculopathy (C6, C7)
- Brachial plexopathy
- Carpal navicular fracture

Management

Nonpharmacologic Treatment
- Splinting (cock-up wrist splint at night)
- Vitamin B_6 (pyridoxine) 50–100 mg bid PO
- Ergonomic modification of work, hobby
- Surgical release if conservative methods fail

Pharmacologic Treatment (see Clinical Implications treatment)
- Acetaminophen up to 4000 mg/day PO in divided doses
- NSAIDs
- Corticosteroid injection into carpal tunnel (not nerve)

How Long to Treat
- Depends on severity of symptoms
- Generally, allow 6 months from onset of symptoms before obtaining EMG/NCS

When to Consult, Refer, Hospitalize
- Refer to orthopedic surgeon who specializes in hands if patient's symptoms not improved with splinting, NSAIDs

Follow-up

Expected Course
- Mild cases usually respond to conservative measures
- Patient may require surgical release of nerve if burning, numbness, tingling persist or increase; loss of grip/pinch strength is persistent; or evidence of muscle atrophy

Complications
- Irreversible nerve damage, thenar muscle atrophy

OTHER LOCAL CONDITIONS
Shoulder–Rotator Cuff Tear, Adhesive Capsulitis

Description
- The rotator cuff is formed by four scapulohumeral muscles that function in countertraction to abduction by the deltoid; tendinitis and tears are common to this region.
- Adhesive capsulitis (or frozen shoulder) occurs as a result of immobility of the shoulder resulting from pain due to trauma or neuropathy (can occur within weeks).

Etiology
- Trauma, arthritic, infectious, or degenerative conditions

Incidence and Demographics
- Chronic shoulder pain and fracture due to falls are often found in older adults
- Rotator cuff tear—age usually more than 50 years
- Adhesive capsulitis more common in women than men after age 50

Risk Factors
- Repetitive overhead activity (occupational, recreational)
- Rheumatoid arthritis
- Osteoarthritis
- Previous shoulder injury

Assessment

History
- Rotator cuff tear
  - Pain in the shoulder girdle; pain may radiate into deltoid area

- May have felt "pop" or "something give" in shoulder
- Inability to raise arm overhead; weakness or inability to externally rotate arm
- Inability to sleep on affected side
- Adhesive capsulitis
  - May or may not have history of trauma
  - Progressive loss of motion
  - Pain varies from minimal to severe

Physical
- Rotator cuff tear
  - Weakness or inability to externally rotate shoulder
  - Limited abduction, forward flexion of shoulder
  - Inability to maintain resisted abduction at 90 degrees
- Adhesive capsulitis
  - Marked restriction in active and passive ROM
  - Pain over anterior joint, rotator cuff
  - Patient often uses scapular muscles to "increase" abduction

Diagnostic Studies
- Plain x-ray: useful for evaluating fracture, deformity, presence of osteophytes, calcific tendinitis
- MRI: can show tendinitis, rotator cuff tear, ligamentous, cartilage injury, impingement syndrome

Differential Diagnosis
- Bursitis
- Tendinitis
- AC separation
- Septic joint
- Gout
- Chondroclavicular disease

Management

Nonpharmacologic Treatment
- Physical therapy to maintain, improve ROM, strengthen muscles
- Passive ROM exercises, progress to active, resistive exercises as healing continues
- Ice or heat for rotator cuff tear
- Surgical intervention indicated for complete rotator cuff tear, displaced fracture

Pharmacologic Treatment
- NSAIDs—see Clinical Implications Treatment
- Local corticosteroid injection

When to Consult, Refer, Hospitalize
- Refer for any fracture, suspected rotator cuff tear, rheumatoid arthritis, AC separation with deformity, dislocation or chronic instability, adhesive capsulitis, corticosteroid injection
- Consult for rotator cuff tendinitis if symptoms do not resolve within 4 to 8 weeks

Follow-up

Expected Course
- Rotator cuff—pain will gradually decrease; withhold exercise temporarily if pain reoccurs
- Adhesive capsulitis—treatment with corticosteroid injections and exercise has demonstrated quicker recovery than analgesics alone

Complications
- Permanently decreased ROM, muscular weakness, chronic pain

CASE STUDIES

Case 1. A thin, petite 75-year-old Asian woman comes to clinic for sudden onset of thoracic back pain 2 days ago when she coughed.
1. What pertinent history is it important to ask?
2. What would you expect to find on PE?
3. How would you treat this patient?
4. How soon should the pain be relieved?
5. What follow-up?

Case 2. A 68-year-old woman complains of hip and knee pain for many years. She is over-weight and unable to walk more than a half block because of pain. She spends her day in a recliner eating snacks and watching television. She has become incontinent because she cannot make it to the toilet on time. Every once in a while she thinks her knee is going to give out from under her. She notes loud cracking noises when she stands up. Her knees are enlarged with decreased ROM.
1. What history would you expect?
2. Which of her symptoms are indicative of advanced disease?
3. What is the most likely diagnosis?
4. What nonpharmacologic treatment would you institute?
5. What pharmacologic treatment would you order?
6. What lab tests must be monitored if the patient is placed on an NSAID?
7. When should you refer?

Case 3. A 78-year-old man complains of low back pain (LBP) for past 5 days. Pain is in his lower lumbar area radiating into the left buttock. Pain is worse when sitting up in hard chair; he has not been able to go out to the park and play checkers with his friends.
PMH: Has had episodes of LBP for past 5 years. Patient worked as a truck driver, delivering packages before he retired. Has not been active recently due to COPD from smoking, gets SOB easily, and cannot walk long distances.
1. What risk factors does he have for low back pain?
2. What symptoms would prompt an emergency referral?
3. What simple physical maneuver will be the most useful?
4. What is your most likely diagnosis?
5. If patient is compliant with therapy, how soon can he expect to have pain resolve?

REFERENCES

Arthritis Foundation. Available at: www.arthritis.org.

Arthritis Foundation. (2000). *Primer on the rheumatic diseases* (12th ed.). Atlanta, Georgia: The Arthritis Foundation.

Bone, H. G., et al. (2004, March 18). Ten year's experience with alendronate for osteoporosis in postmenopausal women. *NEJM, 350*, 1189–1199.

Colyar, M. (2004, July 12). Bone density testing. *Adv Nurse Pract*, (7), 24–25.

Crowther, C. L. (2003). *Primary orthopedic care* (2nd ed.). St. Louis, MO: Mosby.

Felson, D. T., et al. (2000). Osteoarthritis: New insights. Part I: The disease and its risk factors. *Ann Intern Med, 133*, 635–646.

Felson, E. T. et al. (2000). Osteoarthritis: New insights. Part II: Treatment approaches. *Ann Intern Med, 133*, 726–727.

Kohlmeier, L. (1999). Osteoporosis update: Prevention and treatment. *Drug Benefit Trends, 11*(7), 43–44, 47–50, 53–54.

The Medical Letter. (2002). Drugs for prevention and treatment of postmenopausal osteoporosis. *Treatment Guidelines, 1*(3), 13–18.

National Osteoporosis Foundation. Available at: www.nof.org.

Nelson, H. D., et al. (2002, September 17). Screening for postmenopausal osteoporosis: A review of the evidence for the US Preventive Services Task Force. *Ann Intern Med, 1367,* 529–541.

NIH National Institute of Arthritis and Musculoskeletal and Skin Diseases. Available at: www.niams.nih.gov.

NIH Consensus Development Panel on Osteoporosis Prevention, Diagnosis, and Therapy. (2001). Osteoporosis prevention, diagnosis and therapy. *JAMA, 285,* 785–795.

Salvarani, C., et al. (2002). Polymyalgia rheumatica and giant cell arteritis. *NEJM, 347,* 261.

US Preventive Services Task Force. (2002). Screening for osteoporosis in postmenopausal women: Recommendations and rationale. *Ann Intern Med, 334,* 1519–1525.

NEUROLOGICAL DISORDERS 15

GERIATRIC APPROACH

Normal Changes of Aging

- Decreased brain weight
- 20% decrease in blood flow to the brain with changes in autoregulation
  - Contributes to risk of orthostatic hypotension and increased potential for falls
- Loss of neurons with a general decrease in dendritic connections
- Changes in neurotransmitters in specific areas
- Decrease in spinal cord motor neurons
- Increased risk of hypothermia or hyperthermia due to impaired skin vasodilation and vasoconstriction
- Decreased thirst drive may be due to decreased endorphins or decreased response to them

COMMON NORMAL CHANGES OF AGING FOUND ON PHYSICAL EXAM

- Decreased vibratory sensation and proprioception
- Decreased/absent Achilles reflex; other reflexes in arms and legs decreased less often
- Increased postural sway
- Gait slowed, forward flexed and mildly unsteady, decreased arm swing
- Pupils size unequal, pupil reaction decreased or absent
- Increased rigidity in legs

AGE-ASSOCIATED MEMORY IMPAIRMENT

- Generally there is no change in thinking, behavior, or intellectual function, except decreased speed of processing
- A number of elderly experience minor changes in short-term or recent memory
- Patient notices and complains about memory loss in everyday activities
- Poor recall of specific items infrequently used, such as names of people, street addresses, vocabulary
- Items recalled later when they stop trying
- Worse under stress, then improves; not progressive or disabling

Clinical Implications

History

- Assess impact of symptoms and illness on function and ability to perform ADLs and IADLs
- Validate history with family member, caregiver, and medical records as appropriate

Physical

- A complete neurological examination consists of cranial nerves, motor, sensory, reflexes, autonomic, cognitive, and behavioral evaluation
- Format of the neuro exam is unchanged for the elderly but may take longer
- Include functional assessment in complete history and physical of the elderly and when appropriate

Assessment
- Neurological problems range from chronic to acute and fatal
- Consider cardiac or metabolic etiology or adverse medication reactions particularly for global complaints, such as syncope, weakness, or change in cognition without focal neurological symptoms
- Generalized weakness or change in cognition may also suggest a more global problem, such as dementia, delirium, or depression
- Focal findings suggest a space-occupying lesion of brain or spinal cord, or a peripheral compressive neuropathy

Treatment
- Acute or sudden onset of symptoms such as headache, unilateral weakness, aphasia, visual changes or change in level of consciousness require immediate consult, referral, or hospitalization, as do deficits resulting from head or spine trauma.
- Symptoms developing over weeks or months, such as headaches, memory loss, or weakness, can generally be evaluated and treated in the office without patient diagnostic testing as appropriate.
- Refer to neurology if unusual presentation or no response to adequate trial of standard therapy

Dementia, delirium, and dizziness can be found in Chapter 4

STROKE AND TRANSIENT ISCHEMIC ATTACK

Description
- Strokes are ischemic or hemorrhagic
- Ischemic stroke is an interruption in blood flow to brain causing neuronal death or infarction; further classified as thrombotic, embolic, or lacunar
- Hemorrhage accounts for less than 10% of strokes; the bleed may be intraparenchymal or subarachnoid
- Transient ischemic attack (TIA) is a temporary interruption in cerebral vascular blood flow; the deficit lasts less than 24 hours, usually 2 to 4 hours. There is no infarcted tissue or residual deficit.
- Presenting signs and symptoms, management, and prognosis depend on the type and location of the stroke (see Table 15-1).

Etiology

ISCHEMIC STROKE
- Lack of blood flow to brain due to hypoxia, decreased cardiac output, etc.

THROMBOTIC STROKE
- Caused by atherosclerotic plaque leading to occlusion of an intracranial vessel
- Most common in the posterior cerebral circulation

EMBOLIC STROKE
- Caused by atherosclerotic debris from the heart, aorta, or carotids that flow into internal carotids and occlude smaller vessels of cerebral circulation
- Usually the anterior cerebral circulation

LACUNAR INFARCTS
- Less than 5 mm, occur in internal capsule, basal ganglia, or thalamus
- Due to slow progressive occlusion of the penetrating arterioles
- TIAs may be thrombotic, embolic, or lacunar in nature

HEMORRHAGIC STROKE
- Intracerebral hemorrhage
- Spontaneous bleeding into parenchyma from microaneurysm of vessel; most commonly occurs in the basal ganglia
- Due to hypertension, hematological disorders, or anticoagulation therapy

Table 15-1: Location and Signs and Symptoms of Intracranial Lesions

Location	Signs and Symptoms
Frontal Lobe	Intellectual and cognitive decline
	Personality change
	Contralateral grasp reflex
	Expressive aphasia
	Focal motor seizures, contralateral weakness
	Loss of sense of smell (anosmia)
Temporal Lobe	Seizures (may be partial without loss of consciousness)
	Emotional and behavioral change
	Auditory hallucinations
	Visual field cuts
	Receptive aphasia
Parietal Lobe	Contralateral sensory loss
	Loss of tactile discrimination (astereognosis)
	Contralateral field cuts
	Alexia, agraphia, apraxia, acalculia
	Right-left confusion
Occipital	Homonymous hemianopsia
	Visual agnosia
	Cortical blindness
Cerebellum and Brain Stem	Ataxia and incoordination, nystagmus, vertigo
	Cranial nerve palsies
	Nausea/vomiting
	Motor and sensory deficits (unilateral or bilateral)
	Increased intracranial pressure

SUBARACHNOID HEMORRHAGE
- Bleeding from a ruptured aneurysm in the Circle of Willis or arteriovenous malformation

MISCELLANEOUS
- Anemias
- Subclavian steal syndrome—occlusion of the subclavian artery proximal to the vertebral artery; blood is "stolen"; risk factors for embolization may be present (e.g., atrial fibrillation, rheumatic heart disease, mitral valve disease)
- More common in men
- Inflammatory arterial disorders (e.g., giant cell arteritis, systemic lupus erythematosus)

Incidence and Demographics
- Acute stroke afflicts 730,000 Americans per year
- Stroke the third leading cause of death
- Incidence is higher in men than women
- Incidence increases in women over age 75
- Incidence doubles for each decade over age 55
- One-fourth of stroke victims die
- 50% of survivors will have some disability
- 15% to 30% will require nursing home placement

Risk Factors
- Previous cerebrovascular disease, stroke, or TIA
- Risk highest in the month after TIA

- Age
- Conditions that predispose to emboli: rheumatic heart disease, atrial fibrillation, infective endocarditis, valve disease, ulcerated plaque, cardiomyopathy, coronary artery disease
- Other risk factors for vascular disease: hypertension, dyslipidemia, diabetes mellitus, smoking
- HIV/AIDS infection

Prevention and Screening

PRIMARY PREVENTION
- Management of hypertension
    - Treat as directed by Seventh Report of the Joint National Committee on Prevention, Detection, Evaluation, and Treatment of High Blood Pressure
    - Screen normotensive patients for hypertension and risk factors every 2 years
- Lipid lowering
    - Important to lower LDL levels to below 100 if arthrosclerotic disease is present, 130 if high risk
    - HMG-CoA reductase inhibitors (statins) also contribute to plaque stabilization, reduce inflammatory markers, and have an antiplatelet effect
- Anticoagulation therapy
    - Warfarin for high-risk patients with atrial fibrillation or prosthetic cardiac valves
- Antiplatelet therapy
    - Aspirin 81–325 mg qd for stroke prevention
    - Clopidogrel is minimally more effective than aspirin and much more expensive
    - The combination of aspirin and clopidogrel causes increased bleeding risk without added benefit; however, studies are in progress evaluating this combination.
    - Aspirin remains the drug of choice for primary prevention, with clopidogrel used if the patient cannot tolerate aspirin.
- Screening for asymptomatic carotid stenosis by auscultation of carotid bruits or carotid ultrasound remains controversial with insufficient evidence to recommend for or against
- High-risk patients over age 60 with other risk factors for vascular disease may benefit from screening and subsequent endarterectomy
- All patients will benefit from diet and exercise counseling and smoking cessation.
- Educate patients and families about strokes, warning signs, and need for immediate care of stroke symptoms.

Assessment

History
- Onset, duration, and progression of symptoms most important in determining etiology and management
- Resolution of symptoms in minutes to hours is a TIA
- Onset during sleep with progression suggests thrombotic
- Sudden onset with activity suggests embolic or hemorrhagic
- Detailed description of symptoms or deficits including visual changes, aphasia, motor weakness, paresthesias may give clue to location of stroke or lesion
- Review of systems: headache, seizure, loss of consciousness, vertigo, vomiting, syncope, and cardiac symptoms
- Lack of headache excludes hemorrhagic stroke
- Loss of consciousness is associated with hemorrhage or posterior circulation thrombosis
- Vertigo usually suggests vestibular disease but may occur with vertebrobasilar artery insufficiency
- Vomiting is most often associated with increased intracranial pressure usually due to hemorrhage but may occur with vertebrobasilar insufficiency
- Syncope suggests arrhythmia or other cardiac etiology
- Syncope, dizziness, or vertigo alone is not indicative of a TIA

- Past medical history: cardiac disease, peripheral vascular disease, diabetes, and previous neurologic conditions such as seizure, head trauma, dementia, and brain tumors gives clues to etiology and possible differential diagnosis
- Review all medications, particularly those that can alter level of consciousness or cause bleeding

Physical
- Complete neuro exam, including level of consciousness, cognitive ability (apraxia, agnosia, aphasia, amnesia), motor and sensory function (contralateral deficits), cranial nerve exam including funduscopic and visual field deficits, reflexes (hyperreflexia or Babinski on affected side)
- Cardiovascular exam for presence of hypertension, atrial fibrillation, heart murmurs, carotid bruits, abdominal aneurysm
- Symptoms of carotid TIA: weakness of contralateral arm, leg, or face, individually or in combination; numbness or paraesthesia may occur alone or in combination with motor deficit; may be dysphagia or monocular visual loss, carotid bruit; DTRs may be hyperreflexic during attack; may see atherosclerotic changes on funduscopic exam. Signs and symptoms disappear as TIA resolves.
- Symptoms of vertebrobasilar TIA: vertigo, ataxia, diplopia, dysarthria, dimness or blurry vision, perioral numbness, weakness or sensory complaints on one or both sides of body, or drop attacks due to bilateral leg weakness

Diagnostic Studies
- CT scan to rule out small hemorrhage, infarct, or tumor
- MRI if posterior circulation involved
- Lumbar puncture if CT negative for hemorrhage and SAH suspected
- Carotid duplex for evaluation of symptomatic carotid stenosis if patient surgical candidate for endarterectomy
- Carotid studies are useless for evaluation of posterior circulation
- Angiography remains the "gold standard" for assessing carotid stenosis, as well as identifying aneurysms, arteriovenous malformations, and vasculitis
- Electrocardiogram, chest radiograph, echocardiogram
- Holter monitor to rule paroxysmal arrhythmias
- CBC, ESR, coagulation studies, RPR, FBS
- Serum chemistries and lipids

Differential Diagnosis
- Subarachnoid or intracerebral hemorrhage
- Cerebral aneurysm or AVM
- Intracranial tumor
- Migraine with aura
- Seizure (Todd paralysis)
- Hyperventilation
- Encephalopathy
- Intoxication
- Hypoglycemia
- Syncope
- Vertigo
- Postural hypotension

Management
- Suspected hemorrhagic stroke, increased intracranial pressure or ischemic stroke with onset of deficits of less than 3 hours must be transported by ambulance to the emergency department for immediate evaluation and management

Nonpharmacologic Treatment
- Provider should perform accurate assessment and referral for emergency care
- Management of acute ischemic stroke is supportive
- Educate patients and families about stroke, need for same immediate response as heart attack
- Post-acute phase: physical therapy, occupational therapy, and speech therapy should be started as soon as possible

- Emotional support of patient and family
- Referral for home health services
- Management of poststroke complications: see Special Considerations

Pharmacologic Treatment
- Tissue plasminogen activator (TPA) must be administered in a hospital within 3 hours of onset of symptoms of ischemic stroke, after hemorrhagic stroke is excluded
- Patients awaking with focal deficits are not appropriate for TPA because duration of deficits is unknown
- Medical management of post-acute stroke as well as TIAs involves anticoagulation or antiplatelet agents and treatment of underlying heart disease, hypertension, diabetes, and hyperlipidemia
- Aspirin 325 mg each day
- If unable to tolerate aspirin, give clopidogrel (Plavix) 75 mg q day
- Warfarin: used for patients with symptoms on antiplatelet medication or those with atrial fibrillation or prosthetic heart valves. See Cardiovascular Chapter 9 for details.
  - Consider risk of falls, ability to comply with a complex medication regime, and INR monitoring when initiating warfarin therapy
- Evaluate and treat depression

How Long to Treat
- Continue antiplatelet or anticoagulation as long as they are not contraindicated (increase risk of GI or intracerebral bleeding)

Special Considerations
- The nurse practitioner is an important member of the multidisciplinary team required for rehabilitation of the post stroke patient
- Members of the team will include as needed PT, OT, speech therapy, nutritionist, social worker, physicians, mental health specialists
- Stroke patients have many problems, depending on the location of the stroke including immobility, impaired balance, falls, skin breakdown, incontinence of bowel and bladder, constipation, impaired vision, dysphagia, aphasia with inability to communicate, poor judgment, infections such as skin, pneumonia, UTIs
- Depression is very common post stroke and makes it difficult for the patient to participate in rehabilitation; aggressive treatment is necessary

When to Consult, Refer, Hospitalize
- Refer all acute stroke patients to neurology
- Emergently hospitalize all patients with focal neuro deficits of less than 3 hours for TPA if not contraindicated
- Emergently hospitalize patients with sudden, severe headache, decreasing level of consciousness, or vomiting, and focal neuro deficits
- Consult with neurologist as needed for management of TIAs and post-acute stroke
- Cardiology referral for management of heart disease
- Post-stroke rehabilitation may be in home or nursing facility
- Psychiatric referral for depression if needed

Follow-up

Expected Course
- Variable, most stroke recovery occurs early; the longer deficits last, the more unlikely they are to resolve although improvement may be seen for 6 months
- Physical therapy improves functional recovery
- Older age, coma, and early acute CT changes are associated with poor prognosis

- Patients with risk for cerebrovascular disease should be monitored every 3 to 6 months for symptoms of TIA, hypertension, and counseled regarding stroke prophylaxis, diet, exercise and smoking cessation

Complications
- Increased risk of second stroke
- Poorer prognosis and increased incidence of infection, myocardial infarction, renal failure, and delirium with advancing age
- 27% of stroke patients die within 1 year, and 53% at 5 years
- Incidence of dementia increases by 10% within a year of stroke
- TPA has a 6% increased risk of intracerebral hemorrhage but a 4% decrease in mortality at 3 months
- Antiplatelet and anticoagulation therapy has risk of intracerebral bleed or GI bleed

PARKINSON DISEASE

Description
- Neurodegenerative disease characterized by bradykinesia (slow movement), rigidity, and resting tremor caused by destruction of substantia nigra and nigrostriatal tract; results in damage to dopanergic neurons, leaving active unopposed acetylcholine neurons intact
- Imbalance of dopamine and acetylcholine results in loss of refinement of voluntary movement

Etiology
- Unknown, although genetics, endogenous toxins, and exogenous toxins (including manganese, carbon monoxide, and the illicit drug MPTP) have been implicated

Incidence and Demographics
- Prevalence 60 to 187 per 100,000 with 20,000 to 50,000 new cases per year
- Ethnic and gender incidence is the same
- Less prevalent in Africans and African Americans than in Asians, Europeans, and Caucasian Americans
- New onset is only 1% of those over age 65, but many Parkinson patients survive beyond age 65

Risk Factors
- Age
- Heredity
- Possible environmental factors

Prevention and Screening
- None, although elderly patients may benefit from periodic assessment of mobility, cognition, function, and fall risk

Assessment

History
- Focused, detailed history of chief complaint, including time frame and progression, aggravating and alleviating factors, such as stress or rest
- Complete review of neuro symptoms including weakness, paresthesia, tremor, diplopia, aphasia, mood and cognitive changes
- Past medical history including neurological disorders, exposure to environmental toxins, illicit drug use
- Family history of Parkinson disease, other movement disorders, or dementia
- Medications, including over the counter anticholinergics, antihistamines, decongestants, or cough and cold preparations
- Functional assessment: difficulty with ADLs and IADLs, mobility including stair climbing (patients with progressive supranuclear palsy will have problem descending stairs) and rising from chair

- Falls and injuries
- Review of systems for associated autonomic dysfunction, including perspiration, continence, constipation, and postural hypotension
- Assess for depression and mental status; may use Geriatric Depression Scale and Folstein Mini-Mental Status Exam or other tools
- Interview family or caregiver

Physical
- General: manner, affect, dress and hygiene, speech may be soft and monotone
- Cranial nerve exam: extraocular movements, fourth cranial nerve palsy with progressive supra-nuclear palsy, wide palpebral fissures, impaired swallowing
- Motor exam: no weakness; tapping over bridge of nose produces sustained blink response (Myerson sign)
- Bradykinesia: slowness of voluntary movement and difficulty initiating movement, difficulty rising from chair, shuffling gait, problems with turns and stopping movement
- Stooped, flexed posture with knees and hips flexed, hands held in front, close to body, loss of postural reflexes
- Freezing or difficulty initiating movement or changing direction
- Rigidity: cog wheeling, resistance to passive movement
- Tremor: mouth and lips, resting tremor present in one limb, limbs on one side, 4 limbs, or may be absent in 20% of Parkinson patients; see slow tremor of 4 to 6 cycles per second, most prevalent at rest
- Tremor may increase with emotional stress and decrease with voluntary activity
- "Masked facies": fixed facial expression, drooling, soft voice
- Incoordination of rapid alternating movements
- Deep tendon reflexes are unaffected, no Babinski
- Seborrhea
- Orthostatic hypotension

Diagnostic Studies
- Consider head CT if diagnosis not clear and stroke or space occupying lesion is suspected

Differential Diagnosis
- Benign essential tremor
- Progressive supranuclear palsy
- Depression
- Dementia
- Cerebrovascular disease
- Brain tumor
- Adverse effects of anticholinergic medications, particularly antipsychotics
- MPTP induced Parkinson disease
- Carbon monoxide poisoning
- Normal pressure hydrocephalus
- Huntington's disease
- Creutzfeldt-Jakob disease
- Shy-Drager syndrome

Management
- There is no cure for Parkinson disease; current therapy is aimed at managing symptoms to preserve independence and mobility
- The Hoehn and Young Scale can be helpful for staging the disease and guiding pharmacological and supportive therapy
  - Stage I: unilateral involvement
  - Stage II: bilateral involvement but no postural abnormalities
  - Stage III: bilateral involvement with mild postural instability, patient leads an independent life
  - Stage IV: bilateral involvement with postural instability, patient requires substantial help
  - Stage V: severe, fully developed disease, patient is restricted to bed and chair

Nonpharmacologic Treatment
- Patient and family education regarding progressive nature of disease and complex pharmacologic treatments
- Nutritional counseling regarding low-protein diet and diet management of constipation
- Compression stockings for postural hypotension
- Physical, occupational, speech therapy with appropriate assistive devices for ambulation and ADLs
- Fall precautions and home safety evaluation; install rails, raised toilet seats, tub chairs
- Encourage walking, social activities, and interaction
- Emotional support
- Surgical intervention
- May consider deep-brain stimulation to reduce symptoms

Pharmacologic Treatment
See Table 15-2.

DOPAMINE PRECURSOR
- Carbidopa/levodopa
  - 25 mg carbidopa/100 mg levodopa 3 times a day or 10 mg carbidopa/100 mg levodopa 3–4 times a day, titrate up by 1 tablet every 2–7 days as needed and tolerated, not to exceed 200 mg carbidopa and 8000 mg levodopa a day
  - "On-off" phenomena occurs in 40%–50% of patients after 2–3 years
  - Patients will experience inconsistent effect from the same dose
  - "Wearing-off" symptoms appear before next dose is due
  - Use lowest doses possible; consider addition of dopamine agonists

DOPAMINE AGONISTS
- Pergolide (Permax): 0.5 mg first 2 days titrate by 0.1–0.15 mg/day every 3 days up to 3 mg/day divided in 3 doses
- Pramipexole (Mirapex) 0.125 mg 3 times a day titrate up to 1.5 mg 3 times a day over 7 weeks
- Ropinirole (Requip) 0.25 mg 3 times a day titrate up weekly by 1.5 mg/day up to a total dose of 24 mg/day. Maintenance dose is 3–24 mg/day. Discontinue slowly over 1 week.

MAO-B INHIBITOR
- Selegiline (Eldepryl): 5 mg twice a day

ANTICHOLINERGIC AGENTS
- Benztropine (Cogentin): 1–2 mg/day
- Amantadine (Symmetrel): 100 mg twice a day

COMT INHIBITOR
- Tolcapone (Tasmar): 100–200 mg 3 times a day
  - Use with caution secondary to potential for hepatic injury
  - Do not initiate therapy in those with known liver disease or elevated LFTs
  - Monitor LFTs every 2 weeks for first year, then every 4 weeks for 6 months, then every 8 weeks.
  - Discontinue if no improvement on tolcapone

How Long to Treat
- Medication combinations and dosages must be individualized and adjusted during the course of the disease.

Special Considerations
- Prescribe Parkinson's medications with caution, particularly for those with comorbid heart, renal, or liver disease.
- Avoid anticholinergics, tend to be poorly tolerated in those over age 60 years, have increased risk of side effects including confusion, agitation, arrhythmias, and urinary retention

Table 15-2: Treatment Algorithm for Parkinson Disease

Stage or Problem	Therapeutic Alternatives
Mild Disease (Stage I and II)	Selegiline for neuro protection Anticholinergics if tremor predominant Amantadine Group support, exercise, education, nutrition
Functionally Impaired (Stage III) Age ≥60 years Stage IV or V	Dopamine agonist Sustained-release carbidopa/levodopa Immediate-release carbidopa/levodopa Dopamine agonists
Poor Symptom Control	Increase carbidopa/levodopa dose Add or increase dopamine agonist dose Add COMT inhibitor

Suboptimal Peak Response	Begin combination dopaminergic therapy
	    Add levodopa to dopamine agonist
	    Add dopamine agonist to levodopa
	    Increase dose of levodopa/carbidopa or dopamine agonist
	Add COMT inhibitor as levodopa adjunct switch dopamine agonists

Wearing Off	Begin combination of dopaminergic therapy
	    Add levodopa to dopamine agonist
	    Add dopamine agonist to levodopa
	    Increase frequency of levodopa dosing
	Increase dose of levodopa/carbidopa (sustained or immediate release)
	Add COMT inhibitor and decrease levodopa dose
	Change to sustained-release carbidopa/levodopa
	Add liquid levodopa/carbidopa
	Add selegiline if not already taking

On–Off	Begin combination dopaminergic therapy
	    Add levodopa to dopamine agonist
	    Add dopamine agonist to levodopa
	Add COMT inhibitor
	Modify distribution of dietary protein

Freezing	Increase or decrease carbidopa/levodopa dose Add dopamine agonist Increase or decrease dopamine agonist dose Discontinue selegiline Gait modification, assistance device
No "On" Time	Manipulate time and dose of levodopa Add COMT inhibitor Avoid dietary protein Increase GI transit time

Modified from Young, L. R. (2004). Antiparkinson agents, in M. W. Edmunds, & M. S. Mayhew (Eds.), *Pharmacology for the primary care provider* (2nd ed). St. Louis, MO: Mosby.

When to Consult, Refer, Hospitalize
- Refer to neurologist for confirmation of diagnosis and guidance with medical management
- Neurosurgical consultation for those with severe symptoms refractory to medications or cannot tolerate medications; may consider deep-brain stimulation to reduce symptoms

Follow-up

Expected Course
- Progressive, See Hoehn and Young scale for staging

Complications
- Related to immobility and falls, hip fractures are common
- Pneumonia may occur in Stage 5
- Aspiration of food
- 30% have coexisting dementia with a poorer prognosis
- Depression and social isolation occur

MULTIPLE SCLEROSIS

Description
- Progressive neurodegenerative disease characterized by demyelination and inflammation of the neuronal sheath in the brain and spinal cord

Etiology
- Autoimmune disease; possible causes may be genetic, viral, immunologic, or environmental

Incidence and Demographics
- Prevalence 250,000 to 300,000 in the United States
- More common in persons of western European lineage who live in temperate zones
- Age of onset usually 15 to 55 years; 2–3:1 women to men, may be related to estrogen-progesterone levels
- Late onset of MS in the sixth or seventh decade usually severe and rapidly progressive

Risk Factors
- Familial 1% to 3% increased risk in first-degree relatives (15 times greater than general population)
- Climate or place of residence, established by residence in the first 15 years of life
- Urban dwelling, upper socioeconomic status, Western European descent

Assessment

History
- Neurological history: paresthesia, weakness and spasticity, ataxia fatigue, visual changes, vestibular disturbances, trigeminal neuralgia, optic neuritis, bowel and bladder dysfunction
- Time frame with exacerbations and remission
- Past medical history: systemic lupus erythematosus, Lyme disease, cerebral and spinal tumors, AIDS, seizures, peripheral neuropathy, head or spinal trauma

Physical
- Complete neurologic exam
  - Cranial nerve exam
    Optic neuritis: decreased visual acuity, abnormal pupillary response, hyperemia–edema of optic disk
    Internuclear ophthalmoplegia: cranial nerve 6 palsy or weakness of the medial rectus muscle with lateral gaze nystagmus
  - Sensorimotor exam
    Decreased strength, increased tone, clonus, positive Babinski
    Decreased proprioception and vibratory sensation
    Positive Romberg
    Electrical sensation down the back into the legs is produced with neck flexion

Diagnostic Studies
- MRI to visualize characteristic lesions
- Cerebrospinal fluid analysis for immunoglobins and oligoclonal bands
- Visual, auditory, and sensory evoked potentials

Differential Diagnosis
- Stroke
- Cerebral or spinal tumors
- Ischemic optic neuropathy
- Systemic lupus erythematosus
- Lyme disease
- Peripheral neuropathy
- Seizure disorder
- AIDS
- Intoxication
- Amyotrophic lateral sclerosis

Management
- Aimed at delaying progress, managing chronic symptoms, and treating acute exacerbations
- Has changed recently with the advent of immune modulators

Nonpharmacologic Treatment
- Physical and occupational therapy
- Mental health services for assistance with coping strategies

Pharmacologic Treatment
- Complex, neurologist required
- Immune modulators
  - Interferon beta-1a (Avonex), interferon beta-1b (Betaseron), interferon alfa-2b (Intron), glatiramer (Copaxone), peginterferon alfa-2a (Pegasys), and interferon beta-1a (Rebif) are all available
- Acute exacerbations
  - Prednisone 60–80 mg/day for 1 week, taper over 2–3 weeks
- Spasticity
  - Baclofen: 40–80 mg/day in divided doses, start with 5 mg 2–3 times a day and titrate up every 3 days

How Long to Treat
- Use corticosteroids only for acute exacerbations, not for maintenance

When to Consult, Refer, Hospitalize
- Refer all patients with suspected MS to neurologist for confirmation of diagnosis and management
- Ophthalmology
- Continence specialist or urologist for bladder dysfunction
- Mental health referral for coping or depression

Follow-up

Expected Course
- Progressive with exacerbations and remissions
- Prognosis has changed dramatically with the advent of immunomodulators

Complications
- Hydronephrosis and renal failure secondary to urinary retention
- Falls
- Depression

ESSENTIAL TREMOR

Description
- Rhythmic, involuntary movement usually of distal upper extremities; head is also frequently affected
- Usually not present at rest, occurs with sustained posture or movement

Etiology

- Unknown, familial with an autosomal dominance inheritance, although 50% have no family history

Incidence and Demographics

- May occur any time from childhood to later life
- Prevalence and severity increase with age
- Senile tremor is not a separate process

Risk Factors

- Age
- Heredity

Prevention and Screening

- None

Assessment

History

- Time of onset, duration, frequency
- Alleviating or exacerbating factors
  - Alleviating: rest, alcohol
  - Exacerbating: movement, emotional stress
- Associated neurological symptoms: weakness, paresthesias, slowed movement
- Past medical history: head trauma, stroke, Parkinson disease, multiple sclerosis, psychiatric illness, asthma, and hypothyroidism
- Family history of tremor
- Function: problems with ADLs and IADLs or social life because of embarrassment
- Medications: antipsychotic, anticholinergics, theophylline, beta agonists

Physical

- Neuro exam is normal except for tremor
- Tremor may be demonstrated with rapid alternating movements
- Mild cogwheeling may be present in tense, anxious patients
- Cogwheeling is not pathopneumonic for Parkinson disease
- Normal posture and gait

Diagnostic Studies

- Usually not needed; consider electromyography if unusual presentation or difficult case
- Imaging to identify underlying pathology if abnormal neuro exam
- Thyroid function studies if hypothyroidism suspected

Differential Diagnosis

- Physiologic tremor
- Parkinson's disease
- Medication-induced tremor
- Posttraumatic tremor
- Dystonia or torticollis
- Cerebellar lesions
- Demyelinating disorders

Management

Nonpharmacologic Treatment

- Reassure that disability only related to tremor; although this can be severe and disabling, most are relieved that they do not have Parkinson disease
- Counsel regarding genetic nature
- Refer to International Tremor Foundation
- Explain medical treatment; improvement often unpredictable

- Alcohol sometimes most effective treatment but improvement may be short
- Severe and disabling cases: contralateral thalamotomy or high-frequency unilateral thalamic stimulation

Pharmacologic Treatment
- Beta-adrenergic blockers
  - Propranolol: start with 10–20 mg three times a day, or 60 mg of sustained release each, increase each week up to 240 mg/day
  - Metoprolol (more cardioselective for beta-1 receptors), although not approved for tremor, has been successfully used in asthma and COPD patients
- Primidone: 50 mg/day, may gradually increase to 125 mg twice a day

How Long to Treat
- Stop medications if they are not alleviating symptoms

Special Considerations
- May be more severe and disabling in older patients
- Primidone may be poorly tolerated in older patients

When to Consult, Refer, Hospitalize
- Consider neurology consultation or referral if cause for tremor unclear
- Neurosurgical evaluation for thalamotomy or thalamic stimulation if medication not effective and tremor is disabling

Follow-up

Expected Course
- Often may require no treatment if not disabling
- May be exacerbated during predictable situations and require only intermittent medication

Complications
- Social withdrawal due to embarrassment or inability to perform ADLs and IADLs
- Complications secondary to medication or surgery

SEIZURES

Description
- A transient alteration in behavior, function, and/or consciousness that results from an abnormal electrical discharge of neurons in the brain
- Epilepsy or seizure disorder refers to chronic recurrent seizures
- Most older adults have partial seizures that may quickly generalize to tonic-clonic

Etiology
- A seizure is a symptom of an underlying disorder
- Primary epilepsy cause is unknown but is believed to be related to abnormalities of neurotransmission
- New onset of primary epilepsy is extremely rare in the elderly, but patients with primary epilepsy can continue to have seizures into old age.
- Secondary epilepsy due to injury to cerebral cortex

Incidence and Demographics
- 84/100,000 persons with new onset seizure disorder a year are over age 70 years

Risk Factors
- Trauma, use of medications that lower seizure threshold, alcohol intoxication or withdrawal, chronic illness that predisposes to metabolic abnormality, certain triggers: flashing lights/television, emotional stress, hormonal imbalance, fever

Table 15- 3: Classification of Seizures

Class	Category	Description
Partial Seizures		Only part of one cerebral hemisphere is affected
	Simple partial seizures	Focal symptoms without impaired consciousness
	Complex partial seizures	Impaired consciousness accompanies symptoms
Generalized Seizures		Affect the general cerebral cortex
	Absence (petit mal)	Impairment of consciousness
	Atypical absence	Impairment of consciousness with change in postural tone
	Myoclonic seizures	Single or multiple myoclonic jerks
	Tonic-clonic (grand mal) seizures	Sudden loss of consciousness, tonic rigid phase followed by clonic jerking

Prevention and Screening
* Head trauma and fall prevention, home safety counseling

Assessment (see Table 15-3)

History
* Interview witness also if possible—this is the most important diagnostic information
* Detailed history of event includes
  * Seizure activity (generalized or partial), loss of consciousness, incontinence
  * Prodromal symptoms, such as aura, confusion, or focal neuro symptoms
  * Postictal state: antegrade amnesia, level of consciousness
* Prior seizure history including type, frequency, duration
* Triggers: stress, sleep deprivation, drug and alcohol ingestion or withdrawal
* Seizure medications: any changes, missed doses, and levels
* Medications: Ciprofloxacin, metronidazole, theophylline, stimulants, antipsychotics, bupropion can lower seizure threshold
* Diuretic, antihypertensives, diabetic medicines can cause metabolic disturbances that can cause seizure
* Past medical history: Previous intracranial lesions, trauma, stroke, migraines, diabetes, HIV, dementia, psychiatric illness
* Family history of seizure

Physical
* Assess for head trauma
* Neuro exam may be normal even with structural lesions
* Focal deficits may be worse immediately after seizure
* Evaluate cardiovascular and pulmonary status
* Blood pressure and pulse will be elevated during and immediately after a seizure

Diagnostic Studies

FIRST-TIME SEIZURE
* Metabolic panel, toxicology if appropriate
* CBC
* MRI
* EEG may determine seizure type and guide treatment and prognosis; does not need to be repeated
* Serologic test for syphilis

- Check drug level at time of seizure if possible

Differential Diagnosis

SECONDARY CAUSES FOR SEIZURE: CONSIDER THESE UNDERLYING ETIOLOGIES:

NEUROLOGIC DISORDERS
- Head trauma
- Brain tumor
- Stroke
- Encephalitis

METABOLIC DISORDERS
- Electrolyte imbalance
- Hypoglycemia

OTHER
- Alcohol withdrawal
- Medications/withdrawal
- Fever

DISORDERS THAT MAY APPEAR TO BE SEIZURES (SEE ALSO CHAPTER 4 SPELLS)
- Syncope
- Transient ischemic attack
- Panic attacks or psychosis
- Drug intoxication
- Migraine
- Multiple sclerosis
- Postural hypotension

Management

Nonpharmacologic Treatment
- Educate patient and family about seizure disorder and cause
- First seizures without cause do not have to be treated with anticonvulsants
- Educate family about acute seizure management; to protect patient from injury, place on left side to maintain airway if possible; do not place objects in mouth
- Patients with known recurrent seizures do not need to go to emergency department for every seizure, only if seizure lasts more than 2 minutes or breathing is impaired (aspiration)
- Advise regarding state driving regulations
- Advise regarding swimming alone or operating dangerous equipment
- Teach about side effects and toxic effects of medications, not to discontinue seizure meds abruptly, what may precipitate seizure
- Avoid seizure triggers: sleep deprivation, alcohol, stress, low-grade fever, and infection
- Wear medic alert bracelet

Pharmacologic Treatment

ANTICONVULSANTS: PHENYTOIN, PHENOBARBITAL, CARBAMAZEPINE, AND VALPROIC ACID
ARE FIRST-LINE CHOICES
- 40% to 50% of patients can be maintained seizure free on a single agent
- Phenytoin: initially 100 mg 3 times a day, maintenance dose 300–600 mg/day divided
- Phenobarbital: 60–100 mg/day
- Carbamazepine: initially, 200 mg twice a day, increase by less than 200 mg/day in divided doses 3–4 times a day up to 1200 mg
- Valproic acid: initially 15 m/kg/day, increase at 1-week intervals by 5–10 mg/kg/day until seizures are controlled or side effects prevent further increase in dose; maximum dose 60 mg/kg/day, divide total daily doses over 250 mg

CONSIDERATIONS
- Anticonvulsants are metabolized in the liver and involve the cytochrome P450 enzyme system; care must be used when administering these medications with multiple other medications
- Lower, less frequent doses may be needed for those with hepatic and renal dysfunction
- Anticonvulsants have small therapeutic ranges
- Some patients may do well at the lower or upper range; elderly are often controlled by subtherapeutic levels of drug

- Levels should be drawn when adjusting therapy and change in seizure frequency
- Liver enzymes must be monitored

How Long to Treat
- Consider discontinuing seizure medications in those without seizures for over 2 years
- Obtain an EEG before stopping medication
- 40% will have a reoccurrence, most within the first year
- Must consider risk factors of seizure reoccurrence and medications for each individual patient; consult with neurologist

Special Considerations
- New onset seizures must be evaluated in those with previous history of stroke or dementia; there may be new intracranial lesions, such as tumor or hematoma
- Survivors of neurosurgery or brain trauma usually do not develop epilepsy. It is common practice to administer an anticonvulsant at the time of neurosurgery or head trauma. This treatment is appropriate at the time when the brain is swollen and cerebral blood flow is compromised. However, there is no evidence that prophylactic anticonvulsant therapy prevents epilepsy; therefore, it is not necessary to maintain these patients on long-term anticonvulsants.

When to Consult, Refer, Hospitalize
- Referral to neurology for first-time seizures, when considering discontinuing therapy, seizures refractory to adequate trials of monotherapy
- Status epilepticus is a medical emergency defined as 2 or more seizures without complete recovery or a seizure lasting over 30 minutes
- The primary care provider witnessing status epilepticus must activate 911 and be prepared to initiate emergency procedures. Intravenous (IV) access and administration of IV benzodiazepines (lorazepam) should be initiated as protocols permit.

Follow-up

Expected Course
- Variable; after one seizure, patient may not have another or others may have intractable seizures

Complications
- Status epilepticus, airway obstruction, injury during seizure activity

HEADACHE

Description
- Head pain that arises from extracranial structures: the muscles, skin, arteries, or from the posterior fossa; the dura, intracranial arteries, and cranial nerves at the base of the brain
- The brain itself is not sensitive to pain

PRIMARY HEADACHES
- Tension headaches are described as squeezing, bandlike pain; onset usually gradual and lasts days to years; is present when awaking and associated with anxiety or depression; no aura or associated neuro symptoms
- Migraines may be preceded by aura lasting hours to days of scotoma, paresthesia, and unilateral weakness; the headache is usually unilateral, associated with photophobia, sonophobia, and nausea and vomiting
- Unusual for new onset primary headache syndromes to occur after age 50

SECONDARY HEADACHES ARE A SYMPTOM OF AN UNDERLYING DISORDER
- New-onset headache in the elderly may be a symptom of a serious illness requiring emergent intervention, especially in the presence of other neurological signs and symptoms

Etiology

TENSION HEADACHE
- Essentially unknown cause
- Studies have not supported "muscle tension" or increased muscle contractions
- Depression, anxiety, or stress may play a role

MIGRAINES
- Believed to be caused by vascular constriction and dilation possibly triggered by circulating estrogens, alcohol, and serotonin

SECONDARY HEADACHES ARE MOST COMMON IN THE ELDERLY
- Neurologic causes include subarachnoid hemorrhage, trauma, brain tumors, and encephalitis
- Common diseases outside the CNS that cause headache include:
  - giant cell arteritis, sinusitis, intoxication, cervical spine arthritis, visual disturbances, fever, hypothyroidism, carbon monoxide poisoning, or infection

Incidence and Demographics
- Incidence of primary headaches declines in the sixth to tenth decade
- Migraines usually decrease in frequency with age, unusual to begin after age 50

Risk Factors
- Depends on etiology

Prevention and Screening
- None

Assessment

History
- Problem focused organize to evaluate secondary causes
- Time frame of syndrome as well as individual headaches including onset, duration, frequency, quality, location, intensity, change in pain, provoking and alleviating factors
- Review of systems to include
  - Neurologic: aura, paresthesia, paralysis, vertigo, mood, sleep changes
  - Visual symptoms: photophobia, diplopia, scotoma, tearing
  - Ear, nose or throat symptoms, may indicate sinusitis
  - Gastrointestinal: nausea, vomiting, diarrhea, and constipation
- Constitutional symptoms: fever, chills, weight changes, appetite changes
- Suspect tension headaches with gradual onset lasting days to years without neurological symptoms; may be associated with anxiety, depression, and stress
- Suspect migraine with history of aura and neuro symptoms that resolve, then actual headache accompanied by photophobia and/or nausea and vomiting, usually a pattern and precipitating events
- History of head trauma, previous and current medical and nonpharmacologic management, diagnostic testing, and referrals
- Family history of headache
- Functional history: Is headache interfering with ADLs and IADLs?
- History of sudden onset, change in character, associated neuro symptoms, fever, neck pain, rash, or weight loss suggests a serious headache and potential emergency
- (Also see brain tumor and stroke for pertinent history of these secondary causes of headache)

Physical
- Primary—neurologic usually normal
- Focused physical exam as directed by history to rule out secondary causes of headache
- Funduscopic exam to rule out papilledema

- Neuro deficits suggest a secondary cause, such as subarachnoid hemorrhage (SAH), CVA, tumor, or subdural hematoma
- Temporal artery tenderness and visual changes particularly in patients over 50 suggest giant cell arteritis
- Rash over cranial nerve V with corresponding pain indicates herpes zoster

Diagnostic Studies

- Lifelong history consistent with tension headache with normal physical exam usually does not require further diagnostic evaluation
- Brain CT if new headache in the elderly
- Immediate CT if
  - Sudden, severe headache
  - Progressive headache
  - Headache with exertion, straining, sexual activity, or coughing
  - Change in mental state, focal neuro deficits, or fever
- ESR to rule out giant cell arteritis
- Other diagnostic testing as directed by history and physical exam to rule out infectious, metabolic, or autoimmune process
- Electroencephalogram is not useful in screening or diagnosing headaches

Differential Diagnosis

- Subarachnoid hemorrhage
- Cerebral aneurysm
- Brain tumor
- Giant cell arteritis
- Subdural hematoma
- Cervical spine arthritis
- Posttraumatic headache
- Meningitis
- Encephalitis
- Brain abscess
- Hydrocephalus
- Sinusitis
- Referred pain from ear, eyes, teeth
- TMJ
- Viral syndrome
- Drug induced
- Caffeine withdrawal
- Depression and anxiety
- Intoxication

Management

Nonpharmacologic Treatment

- Primary
- Relaxation techniques, biofeedback, stress reduction

Pharmacologic Treatment

PRIMARY

- Analgesics: Acetaminophen 650–1000 mg 4 times a day as needed or NSAIDs
- Use NSAIDs with caution; see Musculoskeletal Chapter 14

SECONDARY

- Manage and treat the underlying cause
- Avoid opioids if level of consciousness needs to be monitored
- Acetaminophen for pain and fever if not contraindicated

How Long to Treat

- Treat acute attacks until headache resolves
- Opioids can be used to treat intractable pain

When to Consult, Refer, Hospitalize

- Sudden, severe headache or headache with change in level of consciousness or focal deficits, refer to emergency department for imaging and evaluation

- Neurosurgeon if tumor, aneurysm, or AVM suspected
- Neurologist for headaches that do not respond to medical management
- Surgeon or ophthalmologist for temporal artery biopsy if GCA suspected
- Ophthalmologist if a visual disorder is suspected cause or contributing factor
- Psychologist or psychiatry for relaxation therapy or psychotherapy or when depression suspected that does not respond to trial of antidepressants
- Interdisciplinary pain center for chronic, intractable pain, interfering with daily life

Follow-up

Expected Course
- Tension headaches may be lifelong
- Migraines usually decrease in frequency or stop as the patient ages
- Secondary headaches depend on cause

Complications
- Unrecognized or mistreated serious headaches from secondary causes can lead to death

BRAIN TUMORS

Description
- Primary brain tumors: abnormal growth of cells arising from structures or tissues within the cranium (see Table 15-4)
- May be malignant or benign
- Secondary brain tumors most often metastasize from the lung, breast, kidney, or gastrointestinal tract

Etiology
- The exact cause of brain tumors is unknown.
- Gliomas of supporting glial tissues account for 46% of all central nervous system tumors, higher grade has poorer prognosis
- Meningiomas develop from the covering of the brain and are rarely malignant.

Incidence and Demographics
- Incidence of primary brain tumor is 8 per 100,000 in the United States
- Greatest incidence in those 60 to 70 years old
- Gliomas more common in men; meningiomas and pituitary adenomas most common in women

Risk Factors
- Meningiomas increase with age
- Primary cerebral lymphoma associated with AIDS

Prevention and Screening
- None, no recommended screening for relatively rare disease

Assessment

History
- Focused, complete neuro history including weakness, slurred speech, or word-finding difficulty, visual changes including diplopia or field cuts, hearing loss, cognitive changes, drowsiness, seizures, headache
- Tumors are suspected in patients with progressive deficits
- Deficit may suggest the location of the tumor
- Headache associated with tumor is dull and aching, increases over weeks
- Headaches are usually secondary to hydrocephalus or posterior fossa tumors stretching pain sensitive structures

Table 15-4: Primary Brain Tumors

Tumor	Structure	Treatment and Prognosis
Astrocytoma (Grade I, II Glioma)	Glial tissue	Total excision usually not possible May respond to radiation Variable prognosis
Glioblastoma Multiforme (Grade III, IV Glioma)	Glial tissues	Total excision not possible, reoccur Radiation and chemotherapy may slow growth Poor prognosis
Oligodendroglioma	Cerebral hemispheres	Successful surgical treatment Slow growing
Ependymoma	Glioma usually of the fourth ventricle	Presents with signs of increased intracranial pressure, shunt Surgical resection if possible Radiation therapy
Craniopharyngioma	Sella tunica Depresses optic chiasm	Surgical resection usually incomplete Bitemporal field cuts Endocrine dysfunction
Meningioma	Dura or arachnoid mater	Surgical excision, difficult to completely remove posterior fossa tumors Cure with complete resection
Acoustic Neuroma	Nerve sheath Vestibular branch of eighth cranial nerve at the cerebellar pontine angle	Excision usually good outcome May have residual ipsilateral hearing loss, imbalance, facial weakness or numbness
Primary Cerebral Lymphoma	Reticuloendothelial system Immunocompromised patients	Shunt Prognosis depends on CD4 count

- New onset seizures in adulthood suggest a tumor, possibly temporal lobe
- Review of systems include HEENT, loss of sense of smell or field cuts suggest pituitary adenoma, or craniopharyngioma, unilateral hearing loss consider acoustic neuroma
- History of nausea and vomiting with deficits or headache suggest increased intracranial pressure
- Assess for symptoms of Cushing syndrome (see Endocrine Disorders) if pituitary adenoma suspected

Physical
- Complete neurological exam may reveal focal cranial nerve or motor deficits
- Other systems as indicated by history
- If pituitary adenoma is suspected, will need complete endocrine assessment; elevated blood pressure may be present
- Metastatic brain tumor: if primary tumor site unknown, will need to evaluate for lung, breast, kidney, or colon cancer

Diagnostic Studies
- CT scan
- Magnetic resonance imaging for suspected posterior fossa lesions and intrasellar lesions
- Angiography of intrasellar lesion with normal hormone levels to differentiate pituitary adenoma from an aneurysm

- Pituitary adenoma: ACTH, thyroid function test, and serum glucose and electrolytes
- Metastatic brain tumors: chest x-ray, mammogram, colonoscopy as appropriate to locate primary tumor if unknown

Differential Diagnosis
- Subdural hematoma
- Arteriovenous malformation
- Aneurysm
- Abscess
- CVA
- Hydrocephalus
- Pseudotumor cerebri

Management

Nonpharmacologic Treatment
- Neurosurgical referral for excision
- Emotional support of patient and family
- Refer to social services, home health services, and spiritual counseling as needed

Pharmacologic Treatment
- Radiation and chemotherapy by neuro-oncologist
- Medical management of endocrine complications of pituitary adenoma
- Dexamethasone for cerebral edema: 4–20 mg q 6 h
- Anticonvulsant therapy for seizure management (see Seizures and Epilepsy)

How Long to Treat
- Defer to neurosurgeons, neurologists, oncologists, and endocrinologists

Special Considerations
- Malignant brain tumors
- Those under 45 live 3 times longer than those over 65
- Prognosis decreases with lower premorbid function

When to Consult, Refer, Hospitalize
- All patients with space occupying lesions on imaging must be referred to neurosurgery.
- Coordinate primary care with neuro-oncology team
- Pituitary adenomas with abnormal endocrine function tests refer to endocrinologist
- Social work, home health services, hospice as needed

Follow-up

Expected Course
- Depends on type of tumor, location, age of patient
- Supratentorial meningioma expect complete cure
- Glioblastoma 6- to 18-month life expectancy (see Table 15-4)

Complications
- New focal deficits as result of damage to normal brain tissue during surgery
- Usually complications associated with surgery and anesthesia
- Usual adverse effects of radiation and chemotherapy
- Death

TRIGEMINAL NEURALGIA

Description
- "Tic douloureux" is a paroxysmal lancinating pain of the face, usually unilateral. Pain originates near mouth and shoots to nose, eye, or ear

Etiology
- Compression of the fifth cranial nerve root, usually by a blood vessel

Incidence and Demographics
- Most common in middle-aged to older women

Risk Factors
- Triggers for pain are touch, movement, drafts, chewing

Prevention and Screening
- None

Assessment

History
- Focused history if chief complaint of facial pain
- Establish time frame, description of episode, any triggers and pain management
- Review of systems to identify any neuro deficits, such as weakness, numbness, diplopia indicating a space-occupying lesion
- Any ear, nose, throat, or dental symptoms indicating sinusitis, dental abscess, or otitis
- History of fifth cranial nerve herpes zoster or multiple sclerosis

Physical
- Examine head, eyes, ears, nose, throat, mouth and neck, cranial nerves
- Complete neuro exam if cranial nerve abnormalities
- No physical findings with classic trigeminal neuralgia except possibly poor dental hygiene or lack of shaving or make up on affected side

Diagnostic Studies
- CT or MRI if neuro deficits
- ESR if giant cell arteritis suspected

Differential Diagnosis
- Fifth cranial nerve tumor
- Multiple sclerosis particular in young or bilateral pain
- Sinusitis, otitis, dental abscess, TMJ
- Herpes zoster, pain may present before vesicular rash
- Postherpetic neuralgia

Management

Nonpharmacologic Treatment
- Avoid triggers
- Surgical decompression, radiofrequency rhizotomy, gamma radiosurgery

Pharmacologic Treatment
- Carbamazepine 100 mg twice daily, increase by 200 mg daily up to 1200 mg daily in divided doses, use lowest effective dose
- Phenytoin 100–300 mg/day
- Gabapentin 100 mg three times a day titrate up to 1800 mg divided/day, adjust for renal insufficiency
- Baclofen 50–60 mg/day in divided doses
- Start with lowest possible dose of medications, titrate up slowly

How Long to Treat
- Attempt to decrease or discontinue dose every 3 months

When to Consult, Refer, Hospitalize
- Refer to neurology for confirmation of diagnosis and coordination of plan of care
- Refer to neurosurgery if fifth cranial nerve tumor or for surgical decompression if intractable pain with adequate trials of medication, or unable to tolerate meds
- Surgery is inappropriate for trigeminal neuralgia secondary to multiple sclerosis

Follow-up

Expected Course
- Monitor CBC and liver function if on anticonvulsant medication
- Attempt to wean and discontinue medications

Complications
- Secondary to medications, use with caution, these are not simple analgesics
- Cranial nerve paralysis secondary to fifth cranial nerve tumor

BELL PALSY

Description
- Acute onset of isolated, unilateral peripheral or lower motor neuron facial weakness due to inflammation of the seventh cranial nerve
- Paresis typically progresses over 7 to 10 days; most patients expect full recovery in 6 months

Etiology
- Unknown, although reactivation of Herpes simplex virus has been implicated
- Cases are often preceded by an upper respiratory infection
- There is an acute inflammatory response causing swelling of the facial nerve and entrapment in the foramen of the temporal bone

Incidence and Demographics
- 20 to 30 per 100,000 individuals a year
- Median age is 40 years
- No gender or race predilection
- 10% have a familial association

Risk Factors
- Diabetes mellitus
- Hypothyroidism
- AIDS
- Lyme disease
- Syphilis
- Sarcoidosis

Prevention and Screening
- None

Assessment

History
- Focused history with complete history of present illness; most important to establish time frame— sudden onset over hours to a few days suggests neuritis, progressive weakness over weeks indicates a tumor or other space-occupying lesion
- Past medical history, including any recent upper respiratory infection, otitis, facial trauma, and history of chronic illness, including diabetes, thyroid disease, multiple sclerosis, sarcoidosis, and AIDS
- Review of systems including visual pain and tearing, altered hearing or otalgia, altered taste, skin rash, history of tick bite or outdoor exposure, other neuro symptoms

Physical
- Complete HEENT exam including all cranial nerves
- Bell's palsy indicated by complete unilateral peripheral seventh nerve paresis or paralysis, with flattening of the forehead furrows, inability to completely close the ipsilateral eye, flattening of the nasolabial fold, drooping of the mouth

- A central seventh palsy or only drooping of the mouth indicating damage only to the lower branch of the facial nerve indicates an upper motor neuron lesion (stroke or tumor)
- Inspect eye for corneal abrasion, tearing
- Inspect ear canal and TM for otitis or vesicular lesions
- Vesicular lesions indicate cephalic herpes zoster
- Palpate parotid glands for masses
- Check for lymphadenopathy and thyroid enlargement
- Inspect skin for rash, particularly bull's eye lesion or erythema migrans of Lyme disease, although rash may not be present
- Complete neuro exam if indicated by history or presence of other cranial nerve abnormalities, although neuritis of multiple cranial nerves is not uncommon

Diagnostic Studies
- EMG and nerve conduction studies 5 to 10 days after onset of symptoms if complete paralysis or no improvement to guide prognosis and treatment; if over 90% neural degeneration, surgical decompression may be indicated
- X-ray if temporal bone fracture suspected
- MRI if tumor or space-occupying lesion suspected
- MRI also allows visualization of the facial nerve and temporal bone structures
- Complete blood count, chemistry panel, thyroid function tests if indicated by history to rule out associated chronic diseases
- ESR if giant cell arteritis suspected
- Lyme titer if indicated
- Syphilis and HIV serology if indicated by history and physical
- Audiology if hearing not improving after 1 week or acoustic neuroma suspected
- Cerebrospinal fluid analysis only if meningitis is suspected

Differential Diagnosis
- Tumor
- Stroke or TIA
- Herpes zoster
- Temporal bone fracture
- Giant cell arteritis
- Lyme disease
- HIV
- Infections
- Diabetic neuropathy
- Hypothyroidism
- Sarcoidosis
- Parotid gland obstruction or mass
- Multiple sclerosis or other demyelinating conditions
- Diabetic neuropathy
- Hypothyroidism
- Sarcoidosis

Management

Nonpharmacologic Treatment
- To protect eye—artificial tears during the day, lubricant ointment at bedtime, patch eye
- No evidence that surgical decompression improves outcomes

Pharmacologic Treatment
- Medical treatment of Bell palsy remains controversial
- 60% recover completely without treatment
- 10% may have permanent disfigurement and long-term consequences without treatment
- Possibly effective
  - Prednisone 60–80 mg qd (divided doses) for 4–5 days, then taper over 10 days
  - Acyclovir 400 mg 5 times/day for 10 days

How Long to Treat
- Eye protection until patient can close and protect eye
- Steroid and antiviral therapy for 10 days

Special Considerations
- Poor prognosis is associated with complete paralysis, pain, or hyperacusis at presentation
- These characteristics combined with increased age and comorbidities should guide decision to treat with steroids and antiviral agents

When to Consult, Refer, Hospitalize
- Ophthalmology if corneal abrasion or significant, prolonged decreased lacrimation
- Neurology if other neurologic deficits present or recurrent paresis or paresis lasting over 6 months

Follow-up
Expected Course
- Facial weakness will generally get worse over 10 days, then begin to improve over 2 to 3 weeks with expected complete improvement in 6 months or less

Complications
- Incomplete recovery or recurrent paresis or paralysis
- Corneal abrasion

CASE STUDIES

Case 1: A 72-year-old female falls 3 times in the last 2 months without serious injury. Reports difficulty getting out of chair and poor balance. She feels stiff and slow. She is otherwise healthy without significant past medical history. She takes 2 Tylenol a day for aches.
1. What other history is needed?
2. What assessment tools would you use?
3. What part of the neurologic exam should be normal?
4. What abnormalities do you expect to find on neuro exam?
5. What is your most likely diagnosis?

Case 2: A 66-year-old male presents in the office for follow-up after evaluation in the emergency department for left hemiparesis lasting 30 minutes. Reported negative head CT, chemistry panel, CBC and toxicology screen. He has history of "borderline" hypertension and takes no medications except over-the-counter ibuprofen.
1. What was the event he had?
2. What other history do you want to obtain?
3. What physical findings might you expect?
4. What further diagnostic tests would be indicated?
5. How will you initially manage this patient?

Case 3: A 78-year-old female presents with left-side headache for 2 days. She has no relief with 1000 mg acetaminophen every 6 hours. She has a history of headaches since age 16. Past medical history is significant for hypertension controlled with Atenolol 25 mg a day.
1. What other history is important?
2. What systems will you examine?
3. What diagnostic testing?
4. What is your differential diagnosis?

REFERENCES

Albers, G. W., et al. (2004). Antithrombotic and thrombolytic therapy for ischemic stroke: The seventh ACCP conference on antithrombotic and thrombolytic therapy. *Chest 26*(Suppl. 3), 483S–512S.

American Medical Directors Association (AMDA). (2002). Parkinson's disease in the long term care setting. Columbia, MD: American Medical Directors Association.

American Parkinson Disease Association. Available at: www.apdaparkinson.org.

Antithrombotic Trialists' Collaboration (2002). Collaborative meta analysis of randomized trials of antiplatelet therapy for prevention of death, myocardial infarction, and stroke in high risk patients. *BMJ, 324*, 71–86.

Brodie, M. J., et al. (2000). Management of epilepsy in adolescents and adults. *Lancet, 356*, 323.

Brott, T., & Bogousslavsky, J. (2000). Treatment of acute ischemic stroke. *NEJM, 343*, 710–722.

Coull, A. J., et al. (2004). Population based study of early risk of stroke after transient ischemic attack or minor stroke: Implications for public education and organization of services. *BMJ, 328*, 326–328.

Goodin, D. S., Frohman, E. M., Garmany, G. P. Jr., et al. (2002, January 22). Disease modifying therapies in multiple sclerosis: Report of the Therapeutics and Technology Assessment Subcommittee of the American Academy of Neurology and the MS Council for Clinical Practice Guidelines. *Neurology, 58*(2), 169–178.

Grogan, P. M., & Gronseth, G. S. (2001, April 10). Practice parameter: Steroids, acyclovir, and surgery for Bell's palsy (an evidence-based review): Report of the Quality Standards Subcommittee of the American Academy of Neurology. *Neurology, 56*(7), 830–836.

Heart Protection Study Collaborative Group. (2004). Effects of cholesterol lowering with simvastatin on stroke and other major vascular events in 20,536 people with cerebrovascular disease or other high-risk conditions. *Lancet, 363*, 757–767.

Johnson, S. C., et al. (2002). Transient Ischemic Attack. *NEJM, 347*, 1687.

National Parkinson Foundation. Available at: www.parkinson.org.

NIH National Institute of Neurological Disorders and Stroke. Available at: www.ninds.nih.gov.

Smith, S. C. Jr., et al. (2004). Principles for national and regional guidelines on cardiovascular disease prevention: A scientific statement from the World Heart and Stroke Forum. *Circulation, 109*(25), 3112–3121.

Straus, et al. (2002). New evidence for stroke prevention. *JAMA, 288*, 1388–1395.

HEMATOLOGIC DISORDERS 16

GERIATRIC APPROACH

Normal Changes of Aging
- Hematopoiesis is slowed and the presence and number of progenitor cells decline

Clinical Implications

History
- Fatigue, weakness, dizziness, drowsiness, irritability, and loss of libido are symptoms of all anemias.
- The diseases of the blood in the geriatric population are usually insidious and often go undetected.

Physical
- Pallor or sometimes jaundice of the skin, gums, and mucosal surfaces, and splenomegaly are all signs of anemia.

Diagnostic Studies
- Most anemias in the elderly tend to present with normocytic, normochromic anemia. MCV increases slightly with age; therefore, categorization by MCV is less accurate than in younger adults.
- An elevated reticulocyte count, indirect hyperbilirubinemia, and elevated LDH are diagnostic of hemolytic anemia.
- A low reticulocyte count, elevated indirect bilirubin, and elevated LDH suggest ineffective erythropoiesis.
- Macrocytosis in the elderly strongly suggests vitamin B_{12} and folate deficiency.
- Infection in the elderly should not be excluded if the white blood cell count is normal or low or the neutrophil response is blunted. Look for change from patient's baseline.

Assessment
- Anemias are classified by their morphology or structure.
- 60% of all anemias are seen in people over age 65.
- Do not assume that anemia in patient with chronic inflammatory disease is "anemia of chronic disease"
- Nutritional deficiencies are major causes of anemia for the elderly
- Do not begin treatment for B_{12} deficiency without assessing and treating folate deficiency.
- Malignancies in the elderly tend to present insidiously. Taking action to diagnose them early will improve the overall treatment and prognosis.
- Important to identify the type of leukemia for appropriate treatment

ANEMIAS—LOW RED BLOOD CELLS

Definitions (See Tables 16-1 and 16-2 for lab values)
- Anemia: a reduction in the total number of circulating red blood cells; measured by red blood cell count (RBC) or hematocrit (HCT), % of red blood cells (RBCs), or a decrease in the quality or quantity of hemoglobin (Hgb)
  - Hematocrit is calculated from the MCV and RBC

Table 16-1: Normal Ranges for RBC Studies

Test	Females	Males
Hematocrit	36%–48%	40%–53%
Hemoglobin	12–16 g/dL	13.5–17.7 g/dL
RBC (10^6/ul)	4.0–5.4	4.5–6.0
MCV	80–100 fl	80–100 fl
MCH	26–34 pg	26–34 pg
MCHC	31%–37% g/dL	31%–37% g/dL
Reticulocyte Count	0.5%–1.5% of RBC	0.5%–1.5% of RBC
Serum Iron	50–170 µg/dL	65–175 µg/dL
TIBC	250–450 µg/dL	250–450 µg/dL
Ferritin	10–120 ng/mL (avg. 55)	20–250 ng/mL (avg. 125)

Table 16-2: Blood Values Helpful in Differentiating Anemias

Anemia	MCV	Appearance of Red Cell
Chronic Disease	Normal	Normochromic, normocytic, or microcytic
Aplastic	Normal	Normocytic, normochromic
Drug Induced	Normal	Normocytic, normochromic
Iron Deficiency	<80 fl	Normocytic or microcytic, hypochromic
Posthemorrhagic	Normal	Normocytic, normochromic
Vitamin B_{12}	>100 fl	Macrocytic, hyperchromic
Folate Deficiency	>100 fl	Macrocytic, hyperchromic

- Mean corpuscular (cell) volume (MCV) represents the size of the RBC and is calculated from either the hemoglobin, hematocrit or RBC; used in differentiation of types of anemia
  - Macrocytic anemia: anemia with elevated MCV, (e.g., vitamin B_{12}, folate deficiency)
  - Microcytic anemia: anemia with decreased MCV (e.g., iron deficiency, which is also a hypochromic anemia)
  - Normocytic anemia: anemia with normal MCV, (e.g., anemia of chronic disease, aplastic anemia)
- Mean corpuscular hemoglobin (MCH) represents the average amount of Hgb in the cells
  - Hypochromic (low MCH): erythrocytes containing decreased level of hemoglobin, causing the cells to appear "paler" on smear (e.g., iron deficiency)
  - Hyperchromic (high MCH): containing increased level of hemoglobin, causing the cells to appear "darker" on smear. These anemias are rare.
- Mean corpuscular hemoglobin concentration (MCHC): ratio of the weight of hemoglobin to the volume of the cell expressed as a percent; normal means the cell has the proper amount of hemoglobin for its size
- RDW: Red blood cell distribution width, a statistical index of the variation in red cell widths; elevated value indicated abnormal RBCs
  - Anisocytosis: measure of variation in red cell size; occurs frequently in leukemias and most anemias, may indicate severity
  - Poikilocytosis: variation of red cells from their normal shape
- Reticulocyte count: immature red blood cells in the peripheral blood, increased in a severe anemia, shows bone marrow is functioning

- Iron Studies
  - Total iron binding capacity (TIBC): an indirect measure of transferrin, the amount of iron that can be bound to transferrin; decreased in anemia of chronic disease
  - Ferritin: represents iron storage in the serum. May be elevated during infection or chronic inflammation and decreased in iron deficiency
  - Transferrin: iron transport protein, binds with free iron, marker of nutritional status

NORMOCYTIC ANEMIAS
Anemia Of Chronic Disease

Description
- The anemia of chronic disease is felt to be a consequence of long-term disease with a major inflammatory component.
- A diagnosis made from excluding active blood loss or production abnormalities associated with iron or folate intake

Etiology
- Inflammatory process

Incidence and Demographics
- The most common anemia in the elderly
- The second most common anemia in the world
- Incidence parallels the rate of chronic inflammatory disease

Risk Factors
- Renal disease, liver disease, endocrine disorders, rheumatoid arthritis, infection, and some forms of cancer

Assessment

History
- Chronic disease
- Fatigue, dyspnea on exertion, irritability, listlessness

Physical
- Signs of the underlying disease
- Signs of anemia—depending on severity—pallor, tachycardia, tachypnea on exertion

Diagnostic Studies
- CBC, reticulocyte count, iron studies (serum iron, TIBC, ferritin); studies pertinent to underlying disorder
- Characteristic labs: Hgb usually 8–12 g/dL, Hct 25%–35%, MCV 75 to 85 as Hgb falls <10, often low serum iron, low total iron-binding capacity (TIBC) and normal or increased ferritin (TIBC is increased and ferritin decreased in iron deficiency), serum erythropoietin normal or in end-stage renal disease, low

Differential Diagnosis
- Fe deficiency anemia
- Multifactorial anemia
- Chronic renal insufficiency
- Liver disease (usually alcohol related)
- Posthemorrhagic anemia
- Endocrine disorders: hypothyroidism
- HIV infection

Management

Nonpharmacologic Treatment
- Treat underlying disease
- Ensure appropriate nutrition
- Transfusion only in severe symptomatic cases

Pharmacologic Treatment
- Recombinant erythropoietin (Epogen, Procrit) in symptomatic patients at 30,000 units once weekly may be effective. Epogen is very expensive.
- Iron supplements with erythropoietin and otherwise as indicated by iron studies

How Long to Treat
- Treatment required as long as underlying disease and anemia persist

Special Considerations
- A similar profile as iron deficiency may eventually develop with patient becoming mildly microcytic and hypochromic as Hgb falls <10 g/dL.
- Anemia of renal disease relates to severity of renal failure, due to decreased erythropoietin production

When to Consult, Refer, Hospitalize
- Refer if diagnosis is questionable
- Refer to confirm underlying cause (e.g., rheumatologist for collagen/vascular problem or oncologist for cancer, nephrologist for renal disease, infectious disease specialist for infections)

Follow-up
- Frequent monitoring of BP, CBC, iron studies with recombinant erythropoietin therapy
- CBC should improve in 2 to 4 weeks on Epogen; do not continue Epogen if not effective

Expected Course
- Anemia will improve as the underlying disease improves or progress as underlying disease progresses or remain static
- Patient can often tolerate fairly low HCT and Hgb, as low as 30/10, if they develop gradually.

Complications
- Possible exacerbation of cardiopulmonary disease, particularly in the elderly (anemia results in less oxygen delivered to tissues; heart rate and cardiac output increase to compensate, heart may begin to fail)

Aplastic Anemia

Description
- Intrinsic bone marrow dysfunction with defective red blood cell synthesis
- Produces pancytopenia: anemia, neutropenia, thrombocytopenia
- Normochromic, normocytic anemia

Etiology
- 50% idiopathic; 20% drug or chemical exposure; 10% viral
- Chloramphenicol is noted for this, but occurs only in 1:40,000–1:25,000 courses of chloramphenicol
- Autoimmune suppression, tumor or fibrotic marrow, drugs, radiation, infection

Incidence and Demographics
- Not common in United States
- Rate equivalent in men and women

Risk Factors
- Family history, viral illnesses, thymus tumors, some medications, radiation

Prevention and Screening
- Hepatitis A and B vaccination; avoid radiation exposure, avoid causative agents

Assessment

History
- Insidious onset
- Fever, fatigue, weight loss, weakness

- Dyspnea, palpitations
- Rectal bleed, epistaxis

Physical
- Pallor, petechiae, bruises, sore throat
- No hepatosplenomegaly, bone tenderness/pain, or lymph node enlargement

Diagnostic Studies
- CBC with differential, peripheral smear, bleeding studies, iron studies, urinalysis, bone marrow, liver function
- Lab results: normochromic, normocytic anemia, total iron binding capacity (TIBC) normal
- Hematuria, bone marrow shows hypoplasia, fatty infiltration
- Pancytopenia is pathognomonic

Differential Diagnosis
- Leukemia
- Hypersplenism
- Systemic lupus erythematosus (SLE)
- Myelodysplasia
- Sepsis

Management

Nonpharmacologic Treatment
- Education and supportive care
- A well-balanced diet decreases risk of infection
- Manage underlying cause

Pharmacologic Treatment
- Immunosuppression therapy, oxygen
- Mild cases: RBC and platelet transfusions, antibiotics
- Severe: bone marrow transplant possible, although many centers defer transplants for patients over 35

How Long to Treat
- Lifelong treatment may be required unless effective bone marrow transplant is curative

Special Considerations
- Other forms of drug-induced anemia are similar in morphology of the RBC but will not have the pancytopenia and will be less severe than aplastic anemia

When to Consult, Refer, Hospitalize
- Refer immediately to hematologist when diagnosis is suspected; work closely with hematologist throughout therapy

Follow-up

Expected Course
- Often favorable outcome depending on age and treatment response
- Untreated cases are fatal

Complications
- Infection, leukemia, heart failure, hemorrhage

HYPOCHROMIC ANEMIAS
Iron Deficiency Anemia

Description
- Microcytic, hypochromic anemia due to decreased iron stores, poor iron utilization, or poor iron reutilization, iron deficient due to chronic blood loss
- Posthemorrhagic anemia due to acute blood loss, may not be iron deficient

Etiology
- Hemorrhage, occult malignancy, decreased absorption

Incidence and Demographics
- Seen in 7% to 10% of adult population
- Prevalent in all ages and populations in the United States

Risk Factors
- Inadequate diet (institutionalization, elderly)
- Impaired absorption (achlorhydria, gastric surgery, celiac disease)
- GI bleeding, (neoplasm, duodenal/gastric ulcers, gastritis from medicines, diverticulosis, ulcerative colitis, hemorrhoids, arteriovenous malformations)
- Disorders of hemostasis

Prevention and Screening
- Adequate diet
- Dietary supplements if patient has risk factors

Assessment

History
- Initially asymptomatic
- Easily fatigued, dyspnea on exertion, irritable, listless
- Palpitations, infection history, neuralgia
- Diet low in iron
- Drug/chemical exposure

Physical
- Angular stomatitis, ulcerations or fissure of the mouth
- Chronic atrophy of the nasal mucosa
- Pallor
- Dry skin and mucous membranes
- Nails thin and flat
- Splenomegaly

Diagnostic Studies
- CBC with differential, iron studies
- Laboratory findings: low Hct; MCV and MCH; RDW >15, serum ferritin level <10 ng/mL in women and <20 ng/mL in men; increased TIBC
- Bone marrow aspiration if diagnosis in doubt, absent for iron stain
- Special tests to determine underlying bleed

Differential Diagnosis
- Thalassemia
- Infection
- Cancer
- Chronic diseases
- Hypothyroidism
- Renal Failure

Management

Nonpharmacologic Treatment
- Correct underlying cause
- Symptomatic care on treatment side effects (constipation, nausea, cramps, diarrhea)
- Dietary consideration: no dairy or antacid within 2 hours of oral iron; increase dietary iron intake
- Normal dietary intake meets only daily losses, not therapeutic; RDA iron = 10 mg/day for men and 15 mg/day for women

Pharmacologic Treatment
- Oral iron supplements; oral iron therapy is safer and less costly than IM or IV iron
- Parenteral iron if poor absorption or inability to tolerate oral iron

Other
- Blood transfusion is not recommended for iron supplementation

How Long to Treat
- Anemia should resolve within 2 months
- Treat iron deficiency until iron stores are replaced, often takes 6 months of treatment

When to Consult, Refer, Hospitalize
- Refer if patient is not responsive to treatment
- Refer if underlying cause is not determined

Follow-up

Expected Course
- Increase in Hgb of 1 g/week expected
- Cure expected
- Regular follow-up recommended

Complications
- May have unidentified underlying source of bleeding
- Prolonged course of treatment may be required because of noncompliance
- Excessive iron levels can be harmful to the elderly

MACROCYTIC ANEMIAS
Vitamin B$_{12}$ Deficiency

Description
- Macrocytic anemia in which MCV is more than 100 and blood level of Vitamin B$_{12}$ is less than 200 pg/mL

Etiology
- Pernicious anemia
- Malabsorption conditions (GI parasites, GI surgery, Crohn's), chronic alcoholism, strict vegetarians (rare)
- Elderly stomachs less acidic, B$_{12}$ needs acid to be absorbed

Incidence and Demographics
- Onset between age 50 and 60; median age at diagnosis = 60
- Women slightly more than men

Risk Factors
- Age
- Chronic alcoholism
- GI surgery
- Crohn's disease
- Family history pernicious anemia

Prevention and Screening
- Adequate dietary intake
- Avoid risk factors if possible

Assessment

History
- Insidious onset
- Alcohol consumption
- GI surgeries or disorders, anorexia
- Peripheral numbness
- Personality changes, memory loss
- Should be considered in the differential diagnosis of dementia

Physical
- Characteristic beefy red, shiny tongue; may be sore
- Abdominal tenderness, organomegaly
- Numbness, sensory ataxia, limb weakness, spasticity

Diagnostic Studies
- CBC with differential, peripheral smear, and serum B_{12} levels
- Laboratory results: serum B_{12} levels <200 pg/mL; Hct decreased; MCV markedly elevated; decreased reticulocyte count
- On smear, see a large, nucleated embryonic type of cell that is a precursor of erythrocytes in an abnormal erythropoietic process

Differential Diagnosis
- Folic acid deficiency
- Myelodysplasia
- Liver dysfunction
- Side effects of medications
- Alcoholism
- Bleeding/hemorrhage
- Hypothyroidism

Management

Nonpharmacologic Treatment
- Education and supportive therapy
- Maintain good health, hygiene

Pharmacologic Treatment
- Initial: 1000 mcg of vitamin B_{12} IM weekly for 4 weeks
- Maintenance: 1000 mcg monthly

How Long to Treat
- Lifetime

Special Considerations
- B_{12} deficiency may cause peripheral neuropathy and dementia in the absence of anemia
- If patient presents with abnormal neurologic signs, the symptoms might be irreversible, even with treatment
- Might have hypokalemia in first week of treatment
- Do not begin treatment for B_{12} deficiency without assessing for and treating folate deficiency also, as treatment of B_{12} deficiency may mask the symptoms of folate deficiency, while the damage from low folate will continue

When to Consult, Refer, Hospitalize
- Refer as needed for underlying cause; refer for follow up endoscopy every 5 years to rule out malignancy

Follow-up

Expected Course
- Response rapid; good prognosis if treatment within 6 months of neuro signs

Complications
- Stomach cancer
- Permanent CNS signs/symptoms

Folic Acid Deficiency

Description
- Macrocytic, normochromic, anemia due to lack of folic acid

Etiology
- Folic acid–deficient diet
- Malabsorption syndromes

Incidence and Demographics
- All races and age groups
- Malnourished people
- Most common between ages 60 and 70 years

Risk Factors
- Elderly
- Alcoholics
- Patients with malabsorption syndromes
- Hemodialysis patients

Prevention and Screening
- Adequate intake of folic acid (RDA = 200 mcg/day)
- Avoid medications that interfere with folic acid absorption (e.g., trimethoprim, phenytoin, oral estrogen, or progesterone supplements)
- Monitor level if patient is on above medications

Assessment

History
- Indigestion, constipation, diarrhea, anorexia, lethargy
- Fatigue, weakness, headache, dizziness, dyspnea on exertion
- There may be no complaints of neurologic deficits
- Renal failure on hemodialysis

Physical
- Pallor
- Atrophic glossitis (red, shiny tongue), stomatitis
- Mild confusion, depression, apathy, intellectual loss
- Tachycardia, wide pulse pressure, heart murmur
- Peripheral neuropathy

Diagnostic Studies
- CBC, RBC, serum folate, serum B_{12}, TIBC, LDH
- Abnormal laboratory results: serum folate <3 ng/mL RBC folate <150 ng/mL, Hct decreased, Hgb normal, RDW elevated
- TIBC normal, LDH and MCV elevated, MCHC normal, Schilling test normal, serum B_{12} normal

Differential Diagnosis
- Vitamin B_{12} deficiency
- Myelodysplastic syndromes
- Pernicious anemia

Management

Nonpharmacologic Treatment
- Education and supportive therapy
- Good oral hygiene

- Folate rich diet—good sources of folic acid include green leafy vegetables, red beans, wheat bran, fish, bananas, asparagus
- Need for frequent rest

Pharmacologic Treatment
- Folic acid replacement: 1 mg PO qd for 2–4 weeks or until folic acid serum evaluations are normal, or can administer chronically if there is suspicion that the patient will not be able to maintain an appropriate diet or has a clinical situation demanding increased intake of folate, such as chronic hemodialysis

How Long to Treat
- Treat until anemia corrected, usually about 2 months until folic acid stores replenished
- Duration of treatment depends on elimination of underlying cause

Special Considerations
- Folate acid body stores can be depleted in about 4 months

When to Consult, Refer, Hospitalize
- Not usually needed
- Refer patients that do not improve with therapy

Follow-up

Expected Course
- Good prognosis

LEUKEMIAS—LOW WHITE BLOOD CELLS

Description

LEUKEMIAS: THE LEUKEMIAS ARE A COLLECTION OF DISORDERS INCLUDING:
- Malignancy of the hematopoietic progenitor cells (acute lymphoblastic leukemia [ALL])
- Acute myelogenous leukemia [AML]
- Clonal malignancy of B lymphocytes (chronic lymphocytic leukemia [CLL]), and an overproduction of myeloid cells (chronic myelogenous leukemia [CML])
- These diseases produce a variety of bone marrow and white blood cell abnormalities that may be imminently fatal or may remain asymptomatic for years. They are characterized by specific laboratory findings and symptom presentation.

MALIGNANT PROLIFERATION IS SEEN OF
- Immature lymphocytes in acute lymphoblastic leukemia (ALL)
- Myeloid cells in acute myelogenous leukemia (AML) or acute nonlymphocytic leukemia (ANLL)
- Mature-appearing lymphocytes (CLL)
- Immature granulocytes (CML)
- Mature B cells with prominent projections (hairy cell leukemia)

Etiology
- Unknown; theorized to be caused by exposure to chemicals and/or ionizing radiation, genetic factors (chromosomal abnormalities), viral agents

Incidence and Demographics
- CLL: most common form of leukemia in Western countries; middle-aged and elderly
- Hairy cell leukemia, rare disease of old age

Risk Factors
- Chemical and/or radiation exposure; chromosomal abnormalities; immunodeficiency; cigarette smoking

Prevention and Screening
- None known

Assessment

History
- General: fever, malaise, weakness, bruising, bleeding, weight loss
- CLL: might be asymptomatic, dyspnea on exertion

Physical
- Lymphadenopathy
- CLL: hepatosplenomegaly, lymphadenopathy, sustained absolute lymphocytosis, bone marrow + lymphocytes

Diagnostic Studies
- CBC with differential and platelet, chemistries as baseline
- Bone marrow aspiration and biopsy
- Consider: chest x-ray, ultrasound or CT scan, coagulation profile

Differential Diagnosis
- Aplastic anemia   • Viral diseases   • Myelodysplasia syndromes

Management

Nonpharmacologic Treatment
- Patient and family education and supportive therapy
- Good diet, compliance with treatment, management of side effects, chronic effects of diagnosis

Pharmacologic Treatment
- Chemotherapy, infection prevention medications

Other
- Hospitalization required for induction of chemotherapy
- Binet staging A–C for CLL
- Avoid activities that might cause injury; avoid medications that affect platelets (e.g., aspirin, etc.)

How Long to Treat
- Goal is remission

Special Considerations
- Patients with leukemia are prone to other infections

When to Consult, Refer, Hospitalize
- Refer to hematologist upon suspicion of diagnosis and consult with frequently throughout therapy

Follow-up

Expected Course
- CLL: depends on stage at diagnosis; median survival about 9 years

Complications
- Infections, bleeding, side effects of chemotherapy and/or radiation, relapses

MULTIPLE MYELOMA

Description
- Malignant disease of the plasma cells characterized by replacement of bone marrow, bone destruction, and paraprotein formation

Incidence and Demographics
- Peak incidence during the seventh decade of life
- Median age is 60 years
- Slightly higher incidence in men and occurs twice as much in blacks than in whites

Risk Factors
- Exposure to radiation, asbestos, benzenes, herbicides, and insecticides
- Repeated antigenic exposure to the reticuloendothelial system
- Family history

Assessment

History
- Bone pain of the back, chest, or extremities
- Weakness and fatigue
- Pathologic fractures
- Abnormal bleeding

Physical
- Pallor
- Palpable liver and spleen
- Radiculopathy

Diagnostic Studies
- CBC with differential, liver and renal functions, chemistry profile, erythrocyte sedimentation rate (ESR), immunoelectrophoresis (M band occurs in >90%), urinalysis, and urine electrophoresis
- Bone marrow aspiration and biopsy
- Lab results: elevated creatinine and calcium, proteinuria, normochromic, normocytic/microcytic, increased sedimentation rate, bone marrow with infiltrates of plasma cells

Differential Diagnosis
- Metastatic carcinoma
- Connective tissue diseases
- Chronic infection
- Lymphoma
- Benign gamma clonopathy
- Polyclonal hypergammaglobulinemia

Management

Nonpharmacologic Treatment
- Psychosocial considerations for patient and family, monitoring

Pharmacologic Treatment
- Minimal disease—palliation
- Chemotherapy

How Long to Treat
- Aim is to cure with minimal toxicity

When to Consult, Refer, Hospitalize
- Referral to specialist for suspected cases

Follow-up

Expected Course
- Median survival is 3 years without transplant. This number is variable depending on "tumor burden"

Complications
- Prone to frequent infections especially from encapsulated organisms
- Hypercalcemia
- Renal insufficiency
- Fractures/pain

HODGKIN LYMPHOMA

Description
- Malignant disease characterized by lymphoreticular proliferation and presence of Reed-Sternberg cells

Incidence and Demographics
- 3.5/100,000; bimodal age distribution (15–34 [peak at 20] and over 50 [peak at 70])
- Male: female: 8:1

Risk Factors
- Immunodeficiency, autoimmune diseases, HIV, first-degree relatives with Hodgkin's

Prevention and Screening
- None

Assessment

History
- Persistent fever, night sweats, persistent dry cough
- Unexplained pruritus
- Substernal discomfort
- Supraclavicular, cervical, or axillary adenopathy
- Weight loss >10%, anorexia

Physical
- Painless lymphadenopathy, mediastinal adenopathy node biopsy will show characteristic Reed-Sternberg giant cell

Diagnostic Studies
- CBC with differential, liver and renal functions, chemistry profile, chest x-ray
- Lymph node biopsy (needle aspiration is not sufficient)
- Lab results: normochromic, normocytic/microcytic, increased sedimentation rate, increased serum alkaline phosphatase and LDH, lymphocytopenia, mild leukocytosis, thrombocytosis

Differential Diagnosis
- Non-Hodgkin lymphoma
- Leukemia
- Toxoplasmosis
- Cat scratch disease
- Drug reaction
- AIDS/HIV

Management

Nonpharmacologic Treatment
- Psychosocial considerations for patient and family, monitoring
- Radiation

Pharmacologic Treatment
- Chemotherapy

Other
- Treatment is determined by stage of disease

How Long to Treat
- Aim is to cure with minimal toxicity

When to Consult, Refer, Hospitalize
- Referral to specialist for suspected cases

Follow-up

Expected Course
- Prognosis is good depending on classification at diagnosis

Complications
- Leukemia, chemotherapy and radiation side effects including secondary malignancies, sterility and gonad dysfunction, infections, anemia

NON-HODGKIN LYMPHOMA

Description
- Malignant disease of the lymphoreticular system with absence of giant Reed-Sternberg cells

Etiology
- Unknown, suggestions: virus, immunodeficiency, exposure to ionizing radiation or chemicals

Incidence and Demographics
- Median age is 50 years
- Most common neoplasm between ages 20 and 40

Risk Factors
- Incidence increases with age

Prevention and Screening
- Avoid potential etiological factors

Assessment

History
- Persistent cough, chest discomfort
- Fever, night sweats, weight loss possible
- Skin lesions, testicular mass possible
- If abdomen involved: chronic pain, fullness, easily satiated

Physical
- Early systemic findings usually absent
- Painless peripheral lymphadenopathy

Diagnostic Studies
- Lab results: mild anemia, elevated LDH and ESR, absence of giant Reed-Sternberg cells
- Lymph node aspiration and biopsy
- CBC with differential, sedimentation rate, UA, LDH, BUN, creatinine, liver function tests
- Chest x-ray, bone marrow evaluation

Differential Diagnosis
- Infectious mononucleosis
- CMV
- Other malignancies
- STD
- Tuberculosis
- HIV
- Toxoplasmosis

Management

Nonpharmacologic Treatment
- Patient and family education and supportive therapy

Pharmacologic Treatment
- Radiation therapy, chemotherapy

Other
- Treatment depends on histologic findings

How Long to Treat
- Intermediate and high-grade lymphomas should be treated with cure in mind; others are cared for with palliative therapy

Special Considerations
- International Prognostic Index to categorize into risk groups
- Prognosis not as good as with Hodgkin disease

When to Consult, Refer, Hospitalize
- Immediate referral to hematologist when diagnosis is suspected

Follow-up
Expected Course
- Response to treatment depends on classification at diagnosis; usually progressive

Complications
- Chemotherapy and radiation side effects
- Recurrence

DRUG-INDUCED NEUTROPENIA

Description
- A diagnosis of exclusion in patients receiving known or potentially bone marrow–suppressing drugs, such as alkylating chemotherapeutic drugs, antimetabolites, colchicine, and agents that interfere with the synthesis of RNA or DNA

Etiology
- Drugs interfere with the cell division process in the marrow

Incidence and Demographics
- Occurs anytime and at any age, but the elderly seem to be more vulnerable

Risk Factors
- Exposure to any of the following is likely to cause neutropenia
  - Ionizing radiation
  - Alkylating agents
  - Antimetabolites
  - Colchicine
  - Anthracycline derivatives
- Long-term exposure to the following may cause neutropenia
  - Analgesics
  - H$_2$ blockers
  - Antihistamines
  - Antimicrobial agents
  - Anticonvulsants
  - Antithyroid agents
  - Phenothiazines or other tranquilizers
  - Sulfonamides as antibacterial agents, diuretics, or hypoglycemic agents

Prevention and Screening
- Awareness of toxicities and screening of WBC as needed based on toxicities of drug therapies

Assessment
History
- Drug

Physical
- None

Diagnostic Studies
- CBC with differential and platelet, chemistries, bone marrow aspiration and biopsy

Differential Diagnosis

- Leukemia
- Aplastic anemia
- Endotoxemia
- Myeloproliferative disorders
- Vitamin B or folate deficiencies
- Idiopathic

Management

Nonpharmacologic Treatment

- Patient and family education and supportive therapy

Pharmacologic Treatment

- Stop offending drug
- Support with cytokine therapy (e.g., granulocyte colony–stimulating factor [GCSF])

When to Consult, Refer, Hospitalize

- Refer to hematologist

Follow-up

Expected Course

- Response to treatment with return of normal WBC to normal after stopping the offending drug and or with support of GCSF

HEMOSTASIS—DRUG-INDUCED THROMBOCYTOPENIA

Description

- Decrease in platelet count below 150,000 in response to a drug

Etiology

- IgG mediated response to drug or drug metabolites

Incidence and Demographics

- Can occur at any age and in response to a variety of different agents

Risk Factors

- New or continued exposure to
  - Quinine and quininelike drugs
  - Valproic acid
  - Heparin
  - Antimicrobials: cephalosporins, penicillin, trimethoprim, sulfa agents
  - Anti-inflammatory drugs
  - Cardiac drugs, such as digoxin
  - Antiarrhythmic drugs, such as procainamide and amiodarone
  - Diuretics
  - H_2 antagonists
  - Antihistamines
  - Antineoplastic drugs

Prevention and Screening

- High index of suspicion when new thrombocytopenia occurs
- Appropriate screening of platelet counts when using drugs well known to cause thrombocytopenia, such as antineoplastic agents

Assessment

History

- Excessive bruising, bleeding hours or days after injury, hematuria, hemorrhage, or hematoma after minor injury

Physical
- Bruises, deep tissue bleeding, intracerebral hemorrhage

Diagnostic Studies
- CBC with platelet count and differential, PT/PTT/bleeding time, factor VIII, IX, and vitamin K levels
- Laboratory results: platelet count normal, PT normal, PTT greatly prolonged, bleeding time usually normal (prolonged in hemophilia A 15%–20%) factor VIII low in H-A, factor IX low in H-B

Differential Diagnosis
- Von Willebrand's
- Vitamin K deficiency or malabsorption
- Other platelet disorder
- Disseminated intravascular coagulation (DIC)

Management

Nonpharmacologic Treatment
- Patient and family education and supportive therapy
- Early treatment of any trauma and/or spontaneous bleed; avoid aspirin, NSAIDs
- Activities restricted in relation to amount of thrombocytopenia

Pharmacologic Treatment
- Stop the offending agent if possible
- Platelet transfusion support

How Long to Treat
- Until platelet count is steadily above 20,000

When to Consult, Refer, Hospitalize
- Refer to hematologist at time of diagnosis of thrombocytopenia, hospitalize for platelet count below 20,000

Follow-up
- As needed

Expected Course
- Patients will fully recover once offending drug is removed from the regimen

Complications
- Spontaneous bleeding in the brain

CASE STUDIES

Case 1. An 83-year-old white male presents with a chief complaint of fatigue for the past few months, which is gradually getting worse. He now is too tired to walk to the dining room in his assisted-living residence.

PMH: Patient has hypertension, history of PUD with GI bleed, smoker, depression, hyperlipidemia, rheumatoid arthritis, chronic hepatitis C, renal insufficiency.

Current medications: paroxetine (Paxil) 40 mg OD; atorvastatin (Lipitor) 20 mg OD, naproxen (Naprosyn) 250 mg PO bid, amlodipine (Norvasc) 5 mg qd, omeprazole (Prilosec), and lisinopril (Zestril) 10 mg

PE: BP 164/84; some pallor; conjunctive slightly pale

   1. What types of anemia is this patient at risk for? What puts him at risk?

Lab: CBC done 1 month ago; results: RBC 3.34, Hgb 10.6, Hct 31.8, MCV 95.5, MCHC 34.5, RBC morphology normal.

   2. How would you classify/describe this anemia?

3. Does the lab work tell you which kind of anemia he has?
4. What additional tests are needed?
5. What is your diagnosis?
6. What treatment do you recommend?
7. Will an iron supplement be helpful? Why?

Case 2. An 88-year-old African American female is noted to have anemia on routine screening. Last CBC was done a year ago and her H&H were 11 and 34. Patient is wheelchair bound, lives in nursing home, a picky eater, likes sweets, and eats 1 to 2 servings of fruit/vegetables daily. Patient recently had an acute exacerbation of her COPD and was treated with prednisone PO for 2 weeks. Patient was noted to have diarrhea last week.
PMH: diabetes mellitus, osteoarthritis, COPD, aortic stenosis, CHF, constipation
Medications: metformin (Glucophage) 500 mg bid, nabumetone (Relafen) 500 PO bid, Combivent inhaler, furosemide (Lasix) 40 mg, Senokot qd
CBC: hemoglobin 9.6, hematocrit 28.9, MCV 80
Iron studies: Ferritin low with increased TIBC
    1. Classify/describe the anemia
    2. What anemias present as microcytic hypochromic?
PE: Pulse is 100, 20; BP 130/80; cardiac exam shows tachycardia, murmur of atrial stenosis. Abdomen diffusely tender. Lungs, distant lung sounds. Peripheral neuropathy present, 2 plus pedal edema
    3. What do you learn from the physical exam?
    4. What risk factors for anemia does the patient have?
    5. What lab tests would you order? Why?
    6. The stools for occult blood come back positive. What is your diagnosis?

Case 3. The family brings their 94-year-old mother into clinic because she seems more confused and tired recently.
PMH: Irritable bowel syndrome, lactose intolerance, S/P cholecystitis, history asthma, macular degeneration, history of alcoholism
Current medications: dicyclomine (Bentyl) 10 mg tid, Metamucil 1 scoop qd, LactAid with meals, omeprazole (Prilosec) 20 mg qd
PE: patient confused, has peripheral neuropathy
Lab: RBC 5.23, Hgb 10.1, Hct 31.8, MCV 104.0, MCH 23.1, MCHC 29.7
    1. Classify/describe this anemia
    2. What diagnoses are you considering?
    3. What additional information do you need?
Lab: The B_{12} level is less than 250 and the folate level is 4 ng/mL
    4. What is your diagnosis now?
    5. What risk factors does she have for B_{12} deficiency?
    6. Why is it necessary to screen for folate deficiency before treating B_{12} deficiency?
    7. What is your treatment plan?
    8. Will the peripheral neuropathy resolve?

REFERENCES

Allen, L. H. (2004). Folate and vitamin B_{12} status in the Americas. *Nutritional Review*. 62(6 pt 2), S29–33; discussion S34.
Andreoli, T. E. (Ed). (2001). *Cecil essentials of medicine* (5th ed.). Philadelphia: W. B. Saunders.

Beghe, C., et al. (2004, April 5). Prevalence and outcomes of anemia in geriatrics: A systematic review of the literature. *Am J Med, 116* (Suppl. 7A), 3S–10S.

Blackwell, S., & Hendrix, P. C. (2001). Common anemias: What lies beneath. *Clinician Reviews, 11*(3), 52–64, 121–122.

Blackwell, S., & Hendrix, P. C. (2001). Less common anemias: Beyond iron deficiency. *Clinician Reviews, 11*(4), 57–65.

Braunwald, E., et al. (Ed). (2001). *Harrison's principles of internal medicine* (15th ed.). New York: McGraw-Hill.

Dambro, M. R. (2004). *The 5 minute clinical consult.* St. Louis: Lippincott, Williams & Wilkins.

Dodd, J., Dare, M., & Middleton, P. (2004). Treatment for women with postpartum iron deficiency anemia. *Cochrane Database Syst Rev, 18*(4), CD004222.

Ferri, F. F. (2003). *Ferri's clinical advisor* (6th ed.). St. Louis: Mosby.

Goodnough, L. T., et al. (2000). Erythropoietin, iron, and erythropoiesis. *Blood, 96,* 823.

Lee, G., Foerster, J., Lukens, J., Paraskevas, F., & Rodgers, G. (2003). *Wintrobe's clinical hematology* (11th ed.). Baltimore: Lippincott, Williams and Wilkins.

Paulman, P. M., Prest, L. A., & Abboud, C. (1998). Selected disorders of the blood and hematopoietic system. In R. B. Taylor (Ed), Family medicine: Principles and practice (5th ed.). New York: Springer.

Petz, L. A., & Garratty, G. (2003). *Immune hemolytic anemias* (2nd ed.). New York: Churchill-Livingston.

Provencio, M., et al. (2004). Prognostic factors in Hodgkin's disease. *Leuk Lymphoma, 45*(6), 1133–1339.

Tierney, L. M., McPhee, S. J., & Papadakis, A. (2005). *Current medical diagnosis and treatment* (44th ed.). NJ: Appleton & Lange.

Young, N. S. (2002). Acquired aplastic anemia. *Ann Intern Med, 136,* 534.

**16
Hematologic**

ENDOCRINE DISORDERS 17

GERIATRIC APPROACH

Normal Changes of Aging
- Reduced ability to maintain homeostasis, progressive loss of reserve capacity
- Occasionally, function of the system maintained by increase in secretion of one hormone to offset decrease in another hormone
- Alteration frequently is undetected unless the patient is under stress

Specific Endocrine Function
- Thyroid gland becomes more fibrotic, nodular, and smaller, but generally circulating hormone levels remain within normal limits.
- Parathyroid hormone levels increase, apparently to maintain calcium concentration
- Testicular testosterone secretion decreased: to compensate, pituitary luteinizing (LH) increased
- Adrenal production of cortisol unaffected
- Adrenal production of aldosterone and dehydroepiandrosterone (DHEA) decline
- Pancreatic function does not change significantly
- Postprandial glucose levels increase 5 mg/dL/decade after age 20 due to
  - Increased fat and decreased muscle mass
  - Decreased insulin sensitivity
  - Sedentary lifestyle

Clinical Implications
History
- May present with no symptoms at all or as an abnormality in a system other than the endocrine system
- Patient presents with nonspecific signs and symptoms or a functional decline
- Medications being administered for other problems can mask or change symptoms of existing illnesses and cause confusion

Physical
- Gynecomastia in elderly men is usually due to decreased testosterone levels but also may be secondary to medications
- Endocrine disorders in the elderly patient often only detected with laboratory testing
- There are no age-adjusted normal ranges for endocrine test results

Assessment
- Endocrine dysfunction usually has multisystem effects
- Disorders ranging from hypertension to depression may originate from endocrine problems
- Regulation of hormone secretion is through negative feedback system
- Basically, three types of hormones
  - Steroids, such as cortisol (adrenal cortex), estrogen, progesterone (ovaries), and testosterone (testes)

- Amino acid tyrosine, such as thyroxine (thyroid) and catecholamines (adrenal medulla)
- Proteins, peptides, such as insulin (pancreas)

Treatment
- A key goal is to enhance or improve the individual's cognitive and physical function level
- Consider other medical conditions when treating an endocrine problem
- Medications: Start low and go slow; too rapid increase in levothyroxine can precipitate angina
- Patients may need to carry or wear Medic alert identification

DISORDERS OF THE PANCREAS
Diabetes Mellitus

Description
- Metabolic syndrome characterized by disorder in metabolism of carbohydrate, protein, and fat; results in high blood glucose level
- Fasting glucose level recommended for diagnosis of DM in the elderly

American Diabetes Association Diagnostic Criteria

DIABETES MELLITUS
- Fasting glucose levels 126 or higher on 2 occasions
- Classic symptoms plus random glucose 200 or higher
- OGGT (oral glucose tolerance test)—glucose of 200 or more at 2 hours

IMPAIRED GLUCOSE TOLERANCE (COMMON IN THE ELDERLY)
- OGGT—glucose 140–200 at 2 hours

Assessment
- Differentiate between types of DM by clinical history

History

BOTH TYPE 1 AND 2
- Polyuria, polydipsia, polyphagia, fatigue, slow healing wounds, chronic skin infections, and recurrent infections (especially Candida and urinary tract infections)
- More prominent macrovascular changes than microvascular, such as peripheral vascular insufficiency, cardiovascular/cerebrovascular disease, and atherosclerosis
- History related to neurogenic and micro/macro vascular changes
  - Eyes: blurred vision, visual impairment
  - Cardiovascular: postural dizziness
  - GI: abdominal pain, nausea, vomiting, constipation, nocturnal diarrhea
  - GU: nocturia, bladder dysfunction, recurrent UTIs, impotence, recurrent vaginal infections
  - Neuro: confusion, altered level of consciousness, paresthesia, cold extremities

Physical
- Skin infections, including cellulitis, and lower extremity ulcers
- Visual changes, ptosis, funduscopic exam: microaneurysms with soft (cotton wool spots) and hard exudates, deep retinal hemorrhages, neovascularization, cataracts, glaucoma
- Oral and dental exam, oral Candida infections
- Cardiovascular: orthostatic hypotension, resting tachycardia, silent myocardial infarctions
- Abdominal: gastroparesis, incontinence, residual urine
- Peripheral vascular: decreased circulation, cool extremities, decreased pulses, edema, capillary refill greater than 3 seconds
- Neurologic: decrease sensation of pain, proprioception, vibration, light touch; absent lower extremity reflexes, dysfunction in extraocular movements, weakness, ataxic gait

Follow-up

Complications
- Retinopathy, glaucoma, cataracts, blindness
- Nephropathy and renal failure, leads to dialysis
- Cardiovascular disease with lipid abnormalities, atherosclerosis, silent MIs
- Peripheral neuropathy, foot and skin ulcerations, gangrene of lower extremities
- Infections
- Cerebrovascular disease, stroke
- Hyperglycemic hyper osmolar nonketotic coma

Diabetes Mellitus Type 1

Description
- Absolute deficiency or failure to produce insulin. Type 1 diabetes mellitus is very rare in the elderly and will be discussed only briefly.
- Without insulin therapy, ketoacidosis occurs rapidly

Etiology
- Destruction of beta-cells in pancreatic islets and absolute deficiency and/or failure to produce insulin

Incidence and Demographics
- Type 1 accounts for 10% to 12% of cases in US; generally occur in puberty, between ages 8 and 14
- Can develop in adulthood, rare onset in geriatric patients
- Due to improvements in treatment, more Type 1 diabetics are living to older age

Assessment

History
- Acute onset, weight loss, dehydration, ketotic episodes

Physical
- Ill looking, fruity odor to breath, ketoacidosis
- Weight loss, thin

Management
- Insulin therapy: See Table 17-1

When to Consult, Refer, Hospitalize
- Refer to endocrinologist to develop initial treatment plan

Diabetes Mellitus Type 2

Description
- Metabolic disease causing hyperglycemia, characterized by resistance to the action of insulin in target tissues, decrease in insulin receptors, and/or impairment of insulin secretion
- Diabetes has been shown to be an important risk for cardiovascular disease, including hypertension and coronary artery disease. Management of cardiovascular disease is important in the treatment of diabetes.

Etiology
- Formally called non–insulin-dependent, NIDDM, adult or maturity onset, type 2, non-ketotic
- Genetically and clinically a heterogeneous disorder with familial pattern
- Insulin resistance with failure of adequate compensatory insulin secretion
- Influenced by environmental factors, see Risk Factors
- No HLA or islet cell antibodies

Table 17-1: Insulin Products

Preparation	Brand	Onset (hrs)	Peak (hrs)	Duration (hrs)	Administration
Rapid					
Insulin Analogue	Humalog	<25	1.0	3.5–4.5	SC before meals
Short					
Regular (R)	Humulin R	0.5	2–4	6–8	SC, IM, IV before meals
Intermediate					
NPH	Humulin N	1–2	6–12	18–24	SC, at least bid
Long					
Ultralente	Humulin L	1–3	6–12	18–24	SC, q 12 h
Long					
Insulin Glargine	Lantus	1.1	none	24+	SQ, qhs

Incidence and Demographics
- Increases dramatically with increased age
- Approximately 20% of elderly over 75 have DM
- Increased prevalence in Native American tribes, particularly Pima and Navajo; Mexican American of southwest US; South Africa; and Indian (south Asian)

Risk Factors
- Obesity/inactivity >20% ideal body weight or body mass index (BMI) >27 kg/m^2
- Diet: high refined carbohydrate and fat diet, low fiber
- Family history of diabetes, mostly type 2
- Previously impaired glucose tolerance
- Age
- African American, Asian American, Hispanic American, Native American or Pacific Islander
- metabolic syndrome (syndrome X): cluster of disorders including hypertension, insulin resistance, truncal obesity, abnormal lipid levels, hyperinsulinism
- High-density lipoprotein cholesterol ≤35 mg/dL and/or triglycerides >250 mg/dL

Prevention and Screening
- Adults over 45 years screened every 3 years, more often with increased risk factors or borderline glucose
- Nonspecific recommendations for geriatric patients; many providers screen yearly
- Education regarding obesity, diet, exercise

Assessment

History
- Insidious onset
- No dehydration, no ketoacidosis
- May have polyuria and polydipsia
- History of macrovascular disease: MI, CAD, TIAs, strokes, hypertension, hyperlipidemia

Physical
- Obesity, predominantly upper body fat with high waist to hip ratio
- Chronic skin infections and candidal vaginitis in women
- Usually discovered on routine exam with elevated glucose level
- Mildly hypertensive

Diagnostic Studies
- Other tests indicated

- Urinalysis for protein, glucose and ketones, microalbuminuria screening at initial diagnosis
- BUN and urine and serum creatinine
- Serum cholesterol and lipid profile
- Glycosylated hemoglobin A_{1c} (HgA_{1c})—index of glycemic control over 2 to 3 months (5.5% to 7% good control)
- EKG and chest x-ray for coronary and pulmonary pathology
- Consider stress test

Differential Diagnosis
- Diabetes mellitus type 1
- Impaired glucose tolerance
- Diabetes insipidus
- Pancreatitis or pancreatic disease
- Secondary effects of corticosteroid, thiazide, phenytoin, nicotinic acid or severe stress from trauma, burns or infection
- Pheochromocytoma
- Cushing syndrome
- Liver disease

Management

Nonpharmacologic Treatment
- Establish treatment goal
- For healthy elder, goal is fasting glucose less than 120
- In frail, forgetful patients, hypoglycemia may precipitate falls, with potentially significant injury more likely; less strict control is indicated
- Patient education about condition and management to include diet, exercise, and medication
- Nutrition counseling for weight reduction: loss of 5 to 10 lbs increases insulin sensitivity
  - 3 meals with 3 snacks with emphasis on balanced diet, avoid simple sugars and refined carbohydrates
  - General diet guidelines 30% calories from protein, 20% fats, and 50% from carbohydrates. Cholesterol 300 mg per day, fiber 25 g/1000 calories
- Exercise recommended daily, at least 30 minutes every other day, to tolerance; exercise should be regular
- Avoid alcohol, avoid smoking
- Foot care plan, use properly fitting shoes at all times
- Identification bracelet or necklace
- Annual influenza vaccine
- Referral to local support groups and American Diabetes Association

Pharmacologic Treatment
- Step Approach, See Table 17-2
- Begin oral antidiabetic agent with a low dose, increase dosage every 1 to 2 weeks on basis of glycemic control
- With failure to respond to first oral antidiabetic agent, switch to second agent
- If second oral antidiabetic agent fails, try combination

OBESE PATIENT
- Step one: mild disease: alpha glucosidase inhibitors or metformin
- Step two: add thiazolidinedione or sulfonylurea
- Step three: insulin

NON-OBESE PATIENT
- Step one: mild disease: sulfonylurea
- Step two: metformin or thiazolidinedione
- Step three: insulin

Table 17-2: Oral Antidiabetic Agents

Generic & Lass	Brand Name	Duration of Action	Dose	Administration	Precautions/Side Effects
Second-Generation Sulfonylureas—Increase endogenous insulin through stimulation of beta cells					
Glipizide	Glucotrol	12–18 h	2.5–10 mg qd tid	Take ° hour before meals	Good for postprandial hyperglycemia
	Glucotrol XL	24 h	2.5–10 mg qd	Take with breakfast	Risk of hypoglycemia
Meglitinides—Increase endogenous insulin					
Repaglinide	Prandin	Fast, short	0.5–4 mg bid–qid	Take before meals	Caution renal, liver disease. elderly, malnourished Greater risk of hypoglycemia
Biguanides—Decrease hepatic glucose production; Increase action on muscle glucose uptake					
Metformin	Glucophage	Short–intermediate acting	500–1000 qd bid	Start with evening meal Take with meals	Contraindicated with creatinine >1.5 in males, >1.4 females
	Glucophage XR	Long acting	500 mg qd bid	Take once a day	Use with caution in renal or liver disease, CHF, alcohol use, and elderly over age 80 Risk of hypoglycemia, diarrhea, lactic acidosis
Nateglinide	Starlix	Short acting	60–120 mg tid, give within 30 min before meals	120 mg tid	Quick onset, which may be useful in individuals with irregular eating schedules; do not take if a meal is skipped. Use with caution in severe renal disease. May be used as an adjunct with metformin
Thiazolidinediones—Reduce Insulin Resistance					
Pioglitazone	Actos	24 h	15–45 mg qd	Timing not critical	Headache, myalgia, edema
Rosiglitazone	Avandia	24 h	2–8 mg qd bid	Actos may be used in combination with insulin, sulfonylureas, or metformin	Caution in renal, hepatic disease, CHF Used alone does not cause hypoglycemia
Alpha-Glucosidase Inhibitors—Delays CHO digestion & decrease PP glucose					
Acarbose	Precose	Very short acting	50–100 mg 3 x/day	Take with first bite of meal	GI side effects
Miglitol	Glyset	Very short acting	25–100 mg 3 x/day		Used alone does not cause hypoglycemia

OTHER
- Treat hypertension (B/P >135/85) with ACE inhibitor unless contraindicated
- Treat proteinuria, nephropathy with ACE inhibitor
- Consider aspirin 81–325 mg PO qd to reduce risk of diabetic atherosclerosis
- Treat hyperlipidemia

Special Considerations
- Hypoglycemia
  - Plasma glucose concentration <50 mg/dL
  - Cause: overmedication, poor or irregular nutrition, increased activity
  - Risk factors: kidney or liver disease, alcohol or sedative use, cognitive disorder
  - Classic symptoms: shakiness, tremors, nervousness, headache, sweating, weakness, dizziness, hunger, irritability, anxiety, visual changes, rapid heart rate, palpitations. Typically last 15 to 30 minutes; less likely in the elderly
  - Elderly more likely to have CNS symptoms: headache, mental dullness, clumsiness, fatigue, confusion, visual disturbances, loss of consciousness, convulsions, coma
- Treatment
  - If able to take by mouth, simple carbohydrate plus protein
  - Coma or mental confusion, administer intravenous injection of 25–50 g glucose in 50% solution
  - Follow blood sugars closely
- Complications
  - Brain damage and tissue death from prolonged low glucose level
  - Elderly are susceptible to falls and fractures
- Hyperglycemic hyperosmolar nonketotic state
  - Syndrome: extreme hyperglycemia ($\oplus$600), hyperosmolality, severe volume depletion
  - High mortality rate
  - Often precipitated by severe illness, such as infection
  - Usually hospitalized—require IV insulin, fluid replacement, treatment of underlying illness

When to Consult, Refer, Hospitalize
- Endocrinologist referral for uncontrolled hyperglycemia
- Diabetic educator for further teaching for all patients
- Registered dietitian for further nutritional teaching
- Ophthalmologist for at least yearly checkups
- Podiatrist for routine foot care in elderly and foot problems as indicated
- Hospitalize for severe infections, hyperglycemic hyperosmolar nonketotic state

Follow-up

Expected Course
- When first diagnosed or when adjusting medications see weekly, then biweekly, monthly
- Well-controlled diabetics, see every 6 months
- Annual urine protein, FBS, lipid profile, creatinine, EKG, full physical exam with funduscopic, neurologic exam, complete foot inspection
- If treated with medication, obtain hemoglobin A_{1c} every 3 to 6 months; goal <7%

THYROID DISORDERS
See Table 17-3.
- Nonthyroidal illnesses, such as active hepatitis, cirrhosis, nephrotic syndrome, infections, malnutrition, and severe acute illness, can affect thyroid functioning serum tests.

Table 17-3: Thyroid Function Tests

Condition	Test	Comments
Hypothyroidism	TSH elevated	Most sensitive screen for primary hypothyroidism
	Free T_4 decreased	Confirmatory test, also excellent, may be normal in mild early, hypothyroidism
	Antithyroglobulin and antithyroid peroxidase antibodies	Elevated in Hashimoto's thyroiditis
Hyperthyroidism	Serum TSH decreased or undetectable	Most sensitive screen for primary hyperthyroidism
	T_4 usually elevated	If normal and hyper is suspected, order T_3
	T_3 (RIA) elevated	Confirmatory
	Antithyroglobulin and antimicrosomal antibodies	Elevated in Graves disease
Nodules	123 I uptake and scan used to detect nodules	Cancer is usually "cold spots" less reliable than fine-needle aspiration
	Fine-needle aspiration (FNA)	Best diagnostic method for evaluating if a nodule is cancerous
	Ultrasound	Solid vs cyst

Hypothyroidism

Description
- Decreased circulating thyroid hormone due to dysfunctions in thyroid or pituitary glands

Etiology
- Primary: inability of thyroid gland to produce hormone
  - Hashimoto's and other autoimmune thyroiditis
  - Ablation of gland due to surgery, radiation, radioactive iodine, treatment of hyperthyroidism (Graves disease)
- Secondary: lesions in pituitary gland—lack of pituitary TSH
  - Pituitary adenoma
- Tertiary: TRH deficiency from hypothalamus
  - Certain drugs, such as lithium, amiodarone, alpha interferon, coexisting autoimmune disorders
  - Iodide deficiency

Incidence and Demographics
- Primary: thyroid dysfunction > secondary > tertiary
- Females more than males
- Increasing frequency in patients older than 60
- Older than 60 years, incidence 10%

Risk Factors
- Family history of thyroid or autoimmune disorders
- There is some evidence that subclinical hypothyroidism confers increased risk of coronary heart disease

Prevention and Screening
- Routine screening is not recommended in healthy young old patients
- Periodic TSH screening in patients treated for hyperthyroidism

- Some recommend screen geriatric patients yearly, especially those with vague symptoms, such as fatigue
- TSH should be ordered as part of the workup for change in mental status

Assessment

History
- Fatigue, lethargy, memory loss, depression, weakness, arthralgias, myalgias, constipation, cold intolerance

Physical
- Weight gain
- Face: dull expression, swollen
- Skin: dry skin, coarse dry hair, brittle nails, hair loss, temporal thinning of eye brows
- Eyes: periorbital edema
- Ears: decreased auditory acuity
- Mouth: swollen tongue, hoarseness
- Thyroid: enlarged gland (goiter) or atrophy, tender, nodules
- Cardiac: bradycardia, decreased heart sounds, mild hypotension or diastolic hypertension, cardiomegaly
- Respiratory: dyspnea, pleural effusion
- Abdominal: hypoactive bowel sounds, ascites
- Extremities: swollen hands/feet, leg edema
- Neurological: dementia, paranoid ideation, slow/delayed reflexes, cerebellar ataxia, carpal tunnel syndrome

Diagnostic Studies
- See Table 17-3
- CBC—anemia
- Electrolytes—hyponatremia; glucose—hypoglycemia, BUN, creatinine, calcium, albumin levels, urine protein, lipid studies—hypercholesterolemia

Differential Diagnosis
- Depression
- Obesity
- Dementia
- Coronary heart disease
- Congestive heart failure
- Kidney failure
- Cirrhosis
- Nephrotic syndrome
- Chronic kidney disease
- Coexisting secondary cause

Management

Nonpharmacologic Treatment
- Education
- High-fiber diet for constipation
- Weight loss if obese

Pharmacologic Treatment
- Primary hypothyroidism
  - Levothyroxine (T_4) first-line therapy for primary hypothyroidism
  - Take on an empty stomach the first thing in morning to increase absorption
  - Drug interactions many: cholestyramine, ferrous sulfate, aluminum hydroxide antacids, sucralfate

- Concomitant use of CNS depressants, digoxin, insulin may decrease efficacy of thyroid replacement dosage
- Starting dose: 25 mcg in frail elderly or 50 mcg in healthy PO daily with increase of 25 mcg every 4–6 weeks as tolerated

When to Consult, Refer, Hospitalize
- Refer developing myxedema coma, hypothermia, decreased mentation, respiratory acidosis, hypotension, hyponatremia, hypoglycemia, hypoventilation, significant cardiac disease, secondary hypothyroidism, or radically abnormal thyroid function tests to endocrinologist

Follow-up

Expected Course
- Elderly at risk for angina as thyroid levels increase
- Measure TSH 4 to 6 weeks after initial dosage, then every 2 months until within normal limits then every 6 to 12 months (TSH levels may remain elevated for several months despite effective treatment)
- If drug dosage changed, recheck TSH levels in 2 to 3 months
- Monitor for signs and symptoms of hyperthyroidism
- Improvement within 1 month of starting medication
- Symptoms resolve within 3 to 6 months of treatment
- Annual lipid levels
- Lifelong thyroid replacement therapy: maintain lowest dosage to maintain euthyroidism

Complications
- Congestive heart failure
- Psychoses
- Thyrotoxicity
- Myxedema coma—rare
- Complication of therapy—precipitate angina

Hyperthyroidism

Description
- Clinical condition that occurs when the body tissues are exposed to an increased level of thyroid hormones

Etiology
- Autoimmune response: Graves disease (*diffuse toxic goiter*)
- Multinodular goiter (*toxic nodular goiter*)
- Solitary adenoma
- Transient thyroiditis (*viral etiology*)
- Drug induced, such as iodide and iodide-containing drugs (*amiodarone*) and contrast media

Incidence and Demographics
- Affects 2% women and 0.2% men
- Much less common in the elderly than hypothyroidism

Risk Factors
- Family history of thyroid disorders and autoimmune disorders
- Thyroid replacement hormone overdosing

Prevention and Screening
- Monitor TSH and T_4 with thyroid replacement hormone

History
- Weight changes (elderly usually lose), increased appetite, anxiety, palpitations, sweating, hypersensitivity to heat, fatigue, weakness

- Mental: confusion, severe depression, insomnia, irritability, anxiety, psychosis
- GI: increased frequency of bowel movements, diarrhea

Physical
- Adrenergic: tachycardia, nervousness, sweating, palpitations, tremor, lid lag, excitability; elderly less likely to have these symptoms
- Skin: warm, moist, diaphoresis, thin/fine hair, spider angiomas
- Eyes (Graves disease only): periorbital edema, exophthalmos, ophthalmoplegia, blurred vision, photophobia, diplopia
- Neck: goiter smooth or nodular, thyroid bruit or thrill
- Cardiac: arrhythmia, such as atrial fibrillation, sinus tachycardia, angina, congestive heart failure, systolic flow murmurs, widened pulse pressure.
- Respiratory: dyspnea on exertion, tachypnea
- Muscle: proximal myopathy, periodic paralysis, progressive wasting of muscles
- Bone: osteoporosis, hypercalcemia
- Neurologic: hyperactive reflexes, tremors

Diagnostic Studies
- See Table 17-3
- EKG

Differential Diagnosis
- Psychological disorders (e.g., anxiety, panic, psychosis)
- Pheochromocytoma
- Malignancy
- Congestive heart failure
- New onset or worsening angina
- Orbital tumors (cause exophthalmos)
- Myasthenia gravis (ophthalmoplegic changes)

Management
- Manage symptoms until patient receives definitive therapy and symptoms have abated
- Refer for definitive therapy

Nonpharmacologic Treatment
- Surgery last option due to complications of hypoparathyroidism and vocal cord paralysis

Pharmacologic Treatment
- Radioactive iodine (I^{131}) treatment choice in the elderly
  - Euthyroid in 2 to 6 months
- Antithyroid medications
  - Propylthiouracil (PTU) 100–150 mg q 8 h initially then 50–100 mg bid maintenance dose
  - Methimazole (Tapazole) 20–30 mg q 12 h initially, then 50 mg qd or bid maintenance
  - 2–3 months reach euthyroid
  - Usually remains on drug for 1–2 years, then gradually withdrawn
  - Relapses in the elderly rarely occur
  - Agranulocytosis rare side effect of drugs, order WBC before initiating antithyroid drugs
- Symptomatic therapy
  - Catecholamine symptoms: beta blocker (propranolol 10–60 mg q 6 h; atenolol 50–100 mg qd); diltiazem for patients unable to take beta blockers; gradually discontinue
  - Multivitamin, calcium replacement, and vitamin D maintain bone density
  - Ophthalmopathy: eye lubricants for mild cases

When to Consult, Refer, Hospitalize
- Endocrinologist for initial evaluation and management
- Ophthalmologist for evaluation of eye pathology

Follow-up

Expected Course
- Monitor free T_4 and TSH every 4 to 8 weeks until patient becomes euthyroid or hypothyroid
- If patient becomes hypothyroid, initiate replacement therapy
- Maintenance visits every 3 months then 6 months then annually
- After radioactive iodine therapy order TSH every 6 weeks, 12 weeks, 6 months, then annually
- Baseline CBC; LFT every 3 to 6 months while on antithyroid medications

Complications
- Thyroid storm: febrile, agitation, confusion, cardiac collapse
- Hypothyroidism due to treatment of Graves and Hashimoto diseases
- Severe depression posttreatment
- Visual disturbance from ophthalmopathy
- Atrial fibrillation and other cardiac problems
- Osteoporosis

Thyroid Nodule

Description
- Single or multiple localized enlargements within thyroid gland; may function independently of pituitary gland
- Generally found on routine thyroid examination
- Critical assessment is whether it is cancerous

Etiology
- Unknown

Incidence and Demographics
- 90% of women over 60 have a nodular thyroid gland
- 60% of men over 80 have a nodular thyroid gland
- Fewer than 10% solitary nodules are malignant
- Cysts comprise 15% to 25% of thyroid nodules

Risk Factors
- Female sex
- Increasing age; male: higher risk for malignant nodules
- Family history of thyroid cancer
- Exposure to radiation of head, neck, chest; radiation exposure patients have 25% risk developing thyroid disease
- Iodine deficiency—higher in parts of country where soil has low iodine

Assessment

History
- Hoarseness, dysphagia, obstruction, neck tenderness
- Benign or malignant nodules often asymptomatic but may have symptoms of hypo- or hyperthyroidism

Physical
- Malignant: hoarseness with cervical lymph nodes, dyspnea, tumors large, fixed, painless, hard, irregular shape, do not move with swallowing
- Benign: multiple nodules occur with Hashimoto's thyroiditis, thyroid nodule(s) tender, soft, multiple

Diagnostic Studies
- See Table 17-3

Differential Diagnosis
- Malignant nodules vs benign nodules
- Cysts

Management
- Refer

When to Consult, Refer, Hospitalize
- Refer

Follow-up

Expected Course
- Good survival rate with malignant nodules unless due to follicular carcinoma

Complications
- Tumor recurrence
- Hypo- or hyperthyroidism

CUSHING SYNDROME

Description
- Syndrome of clinical abnormalities resulting from chronic excessive amounts corticosteroids

Etiology
- In the elderly most commonly from chronic treatment with corticosteroids
- ACTH hypersecretion from pituitary gland due to benign pituitary microadenoma (most common)
- ACTH hypersecretion from adrenal adenomas or carcinomas
- Ectopic production of ACTH by malignant tumors, such as from lung

Incidence and Demographics
- Cushing's syndrome and primary adrenal tumors more common women
- Pituitary tumors 5 times more frequent in women than men

Risk Factors
- Adrenal tumor
- Pituitary tumor
- Long-term use corticosteroids

Prevention and Screening
- Limit corticosteroid use

Assessment

History
- Mental changes, emotional lability, depression, psychosis, weakness, fatigue, poor wound healing, thin skin, polyuria, polydipsia, susceptibility to infections, loss of function
- Medication use of corticosteroids

Physical
- High blood pressure
- Truncal obesity with thin extremities
- Skin: thin, atrophic, hirsutism, ecchymosis, hyperpigmentation, purple striae, poor healing
- Head: moon face
- Eyes: glaucoma, cataracts
- Abdomen: abdominal striae, protuberant
- Kidney: renal calculi
- Back: dorsal fat pad "buffalo hump"
- Musculoskeletal: weakness, atrophy of muscles, osteoporosis

Diagnostic Studies
- Urine: glycosuria, cortisol level elevated
- Plasma cortisol level: elevated evening and 24-hour levels
- Screening tests: dexamethasone overnight suppression test if diagnosis questionable
- Serum glucose elevated, hypokalemia, hypernatremia, elevated triglycerides

Differential Diagnosis
- Alcoholism
- Obesity
- Depression
- Familial cortisol resistance
- Hirsutism

Management
Nonpharmacologic Treatment
- High-protein diet

Pharmacologic Treatment
- If due to prolonged use of steroids, gradually discontinue therapy or change to alternate-day dosing schedule

When to Consult, Refer, Hospitalize
- Refer all cases to endocrinologist and coordinate primary care
- Hospitalize for acute illness as needed to hydrate and administer parenteral glucocortisol replacement

Follow-up
- If patient has recurrence of symptoms, measure urine free cortisol
- Once patients taken off corticosteroid therapy, may need to have them restarted if they get sick or stressed from any cause

Complications
- Hypertension
- Congestive heart failure
- Osteoporosis with fractures
- Diabetes mellitus
- Susceptibility to infections
- Nephrolithiasis
- Psychosis
- Peptic ulcer disease
- If untreated, morbidity and death

OBESITY

Description
- Excess of total body fat

Etiology
- Genetic predisposition; 60% risk of obesity if one parent obese, 90% risk if both
- Environmental and psychological factors
- Secondary health problems, such as adrenal problems, hypothyroid, polycystic ovarian disease occur <1% of obese patients
- Medications that can increase weight include steroids, megestrol (Megace), mirtazapine (Remeron)

Incidence and Demographics
- New onset in elderly rare, requires investigation

- Incidence and prevalence increasing in all genders and ages
- One-third of US population is obese
- Prevalence rates higher in Hispanic and black women, Asian and Pacific Islanders, Native Americans, Native Hawaiians and Alaska natives
- Over 50% Mexican American and African American women overweight

Risk Factors
- Overeating or other poor dietary habits
- Sedentary lifestyle
- Genetic predisposition

Prevention and Screening
- Balanced dietary intake throughout life span
- Exercise regularly

Assessment

History
- Obtain weight history of life span
- Obtain 24-hour diet recall
- Collect comprehensive diet history including food categories, amount servings, number of meals per day, fluid intake, snacks
- Family history of obesity, overeating, metabolic disorders, cardiovascular disease, cerebral vascular disease, hypertension, diabetes mellitus
- Exercise history
- Motivation to lose weight and prior attempts to lose weight

Physical
- Height and weight, complete physical

Diagnostic Studies
- Calculate body mass index (BMI) = [704.5 x weight in pounds divided by height squared] or go to http://www.cdc.gov/nccdphp/dnpa/bmi/bmi-adult.htm for BMI calculator
  - Healthy normal weight BMI between 18.5 and 25
  - Overweight BMI >25
  - Class I Obesity: BMI 30–34.9
  - Class II Obesity: BMI 35–39.9
  - Class III Obesity: BMI >40
- Regional fat distribution
  - Abdominal fat (visceral fat) associated with metabolic disorders (diabetes mellitus, Cushing's) and cardiovascular disease
  - Hip and thigh fat (visceral fat) more common in women and pose less medical risk than abdominal fat
  - Waist measurements >35 inches women and >40 inches men pose significant health risk for cardiovascular disease and risk of death increase with BMI >30

Differential Diagnosis
- Hypothalamic disease
- Thyroid disease
- Pituitary dysfunction
- Cushing's syndrome

Management

Nonpharmacologic Treatment
- Long-term lifestyle changes
- Comprehensive multidisciplinary approach to weight reduction includes dietary control, exercise, eating behavior modifications, psychosocial modification

DIET
- Eating behavior modification: emphasize planning, regular weights, and food diary
- Eat regular meals containing protein, control portion size
- To lose 1 pound, 500 more calories must be expended than consumed per day or 3500 fewer per week
- Calorie intake per day to maintain normal weight ranges from 900 to 1200 for adult women and 1500 to 1800 for adult men
- Limit fat to ≤30% of total calories; carbohydrate 55%–60% calories, rest from protein
- Recommend diet
  - Protein on a regular basis: meat, fish, poultry, eggs, beans, nuts
  - Fruit and vegetable groups to provide fiber and nutrients—3 to 5 servings/day
  - Carbohydrates in moderation: bread, rice, and cereals
  - Adequate calcium intake: milk, cheese, and yogurt or calcium supplement
  - Restrict consumption of sweets and fats
  - Limit or avoid alcohol

EXERCISE
- May require stress test evaluation before beginning exercise plan depending on comorbid conditions
- Exercise: for energy expenditure, exercise (walking, cycling, water walking) 4 to 5 times a week for 45 to 60 minutes, see Chapter 2 health promotion for more on exercise in the elderly
- Must plan regular exercise sessions that fit into normal routine

PSYCHOSOCIAL MODIFICATION
- Support for losing weight essential, whether from close friend, peer, therapist, or formal organization of people (such as Overeaters Anonymous, TOPS, Weight Watchers)

Pharmacologic Treatment
- Fat blocker
  - Orlistat (Xenical) 120 mg three times a day with meals only
  - May be used to help if patient has BMI >30, not recommended in the elderly due to decreased absorption of fat-soluble nutrients

Special Considerations
- Elderly at more risk from being underweight than overweight

When to Consult, Refer, Hospitalize
- Nutritional counseling
- Counselor for behavior modification
- Refer people who are morbidly obese to specialists

Follow-up
- Frequently, at least initially, to evaluate progress
- Regular monitoring and reinforcement of progress until goal weight reached
- Expected course for weight loss
  - Slow progress with expected loss of ° to 2–3 lbs per week maximum
  - Continue to monitor for obesity complications

Complications
- Cardiovascular disease: hypertension, coronary artery disease, peripheral vascular disease
- Metabolic disorders: hyperinsulinemia, type 2 diabetes, hyperlipidemia
- Cerebral vascular disease
- Pulmonary: sleep apnea syndrome, chronic respiratory infections, hypoventilation
- Degenerative joint disease, chronic orthopedic problems, impaired mobility
- Cholelithiasis

- Nephrotic syndrome
- Depression, loss self-esteem
- Psychosocial disability
- Cancers: colon, rectum, prostate, uterine, biliary tract, breast, ovarian
- Skin disorders, especially candida
- Increase perioperative morbidity and mortality

CASE STUDIES

Case 1. A 68-year-old overweight American Indian man comes to the office one afternoon with the complaint of a wound on his foot that has been there for 1 month and will not heal. Denies pain or fever. Admits to fatigue and blurred vision. Also complains of joint pain, especially in the knees and hips.
   1. What diagnostic studies would you order?
   2. Which lab test is the best for diagnosing diabetes in the elderly?
   3. What risk factors does he have for diabetes?
   4. What is your management of this patient?
   5. What complications are you worried about?

Case 2. An 82-year-old patient is brought in for geriatric assessment by her daughter. The patient is having difficulty sleeping and complains of fatigue and constipation to her family. She does not get dressed in the morning and has difficulty balancing her checkbook. She has gained 10 pounds in the last year. She is otherwise reported to be healthy and has not seen a health care provider in years. She takes Tylenol for arthritis. Her family states they think she is becoming more forgetful.
   1. What other history do you need?
   2. What physical exam would you do; what would you expect to find?
   3. What diagnostic test would be conclusive?
   4. What is your differential diagnoses. What should you rule out?

Case 3. A 74-year-old man comes to the office with a complaint of palpitations for about a month. He notices them especially at night when he is trying to sleep; he is having more trouble sleeping recently. They occur about 1 to 2 times a day. He sits and rests and they go away. He also complains of shortness of breath when walking. He has recently lost 15 pounds. Patient denies dieting.
   1. What other body systems would you inquire about?
   2. What physical exam is important?
Physical: This patient has atrial fibrillation, tachypnea, hyperactive reflexes, and a fine tremor.
   3. What is your diagnosis?
   4. What labs would confirm this diagnosis?
   5. What would you do?
   6. What is the preferred treatment?

REFERENCES

American Diabetes Association. Available at: www.diabetes.org.
American Diabetes Association. (2003) Clinical practice recommendations. *Diabetes Care*, 26(Suppl. 1), S1.
American Diabetes Association Position Statement. (2003). Diabetes nephropathy. *Diabetes Care*, 26(Suppl. 1), S94.

American Diabetes Association Position Statement. (2003). Physical activity/exercise and diabetes mellitus. *Diabetes Care, 26*(Suppl. 1), S73.

American Diabetes Association Position Statement. (2003). Preventive foot care in people with diabetes. *Diabetes Care, 26*(Suppl. 1), S78.

American Obesity Association. Available at: www.obesity.org.

Center for Disease Control BMI Calculator. Available at: http://www.cdc.gov/nccdphp/dnpa/bmi/bmi-adult.htm.

Cooper, D. S. (2001). Clinical practice. Subclinical hypothyroidism. *NEJM, 345,* 260.

Dayan, C. M. (2001). Interpretation of thyroid function tests. *Lancet, 357,* 619.

DeCoste, K. C., & Scott, L. K. (2004). Diabetes update: Promoting effective disease management. *AAPHN Journal, 52*(8), 344–353; quiz 354–355.

Doelle, G. C. (2004). The clinical picture of metabolic syndrome. An update on this complex of conditions and risk factors. *Postgraduate Medicine, 116*(1), 30–32, 35–38.

Harris, R., et al. (2003). Screening adults for type 2 diabetes: A review of the evidence for the US Preventative Services Task Force. *Ann Intern Med, 138,* 215.

Klein, I., et al. (2001). Thyroid hormone and the cardiovascular system. *NEJM, 344,* 501.

McCarren, M. (2003). American Diabetes Association Resource Guide 2003. Class action: Type 2 pills update. *Diabetes Forecast, 56*(1), 44–47.

Phillips, L. S., & Dunning, B. E. (2003). Nateglinide (Starlix): Update on a new antidiabetic agent. *International Journal Clinical Practice, 57*(6), 535–541.

UKPDS. (1998). Intensive blood glucose control with sulfonylureas or insulin compared with conventional treatment and risk of complications in patients with type 2 diabetes. *Lancet, 352,* 837.

Weetman, A. P. (2000). Graves' disease. *NEJM, 343,* 1236.

PSYCHIATRIC– MENTAL HEALTH DISORDERS 18

GERIATRIC APPROACH

Mental illnesses are common, serious brain disorders that affect thinking, motivation, emotions, and social interactions. Mental illness intrudes upon the elements of the self that define our humanity and can deprive us of the most gratifying aspects of our lives. It can prevent us from taking pleasure in everyday events and rob us of what we have achieved or become.

Normal changes of aging do not cause mental illness, although they can be a risk factor. Dementia, another disease with malfunction of the brain, must be considered when diagnosing and treating mental illness in the elderly. Whatever diagnosis is being considered, dementia must specifically be ruled out. Dementia, delirium, and associated psychotic symptoms are discussed in Chapter 4. Dementia and depression frequently present in the same manner in the elderly. They often coexist in the same patient, especially in the patient with early dementia. If you are not sure if it is depression or dementia, treat for depression and observe for improvement.

Mental disorders are greatly underdiagnosed and undertreated in the elderly, causing much needless suffering. Primary care providers have not stressed recognition and treatment of these conditions. Patients are reluctant to discuss mental illness due to social stigma. We have treatments that can greatly improve the quality of life for elders and their families.

Normal Changes of Aging
- The brain undergoes structural, neuroanatomic changes in later life; see Neurology Chapter 15 for details
  - Neuronal death
  - Decrease in neurotransmitters for acetylcholine, dopamine, and serotonin
  - Changes in short-term memory, speed of processing
  - How these changes affect psychological problems in the elderly is poorly understood.
- Personality remains stable over time, overall, with decreases in levels of impulsivity, aggression, and activity
  - Freud argued that the older mind is less able to change; many people still believe this myth.
  - Erickson discusses how people continue to change; see Chapter 3 for stages of developmental change
  - Sadavoy has identified critical age-related stresses:
    Interpersonal loss, loss of social support, such as loss of spouse, family, friends
    Physical disability, loss of strength
    Loss of youthful appearance and beauty
    Change in social role, such as children caring for parent
    Forced reliance on caregivers, other transportation
    Change in living arrangements, such as loss of house
    Confrontation with death

Clinical Implications

History
- Obtain a complete psychosocial history including mental status exam
- May need to interview family members and other caregivers to obtain history
- Typical signs and symptoms of mental illness are disturbances of attention, consciousness, emotion, affect, mood, motor activity, thought processes, disturbances in perceptions and memory
- Assessment tools are frequently helpful in the elderly. See Chapter 3.

Physical
- Observe demeanor, function, and interaction with family members or caregiver
- Are they interactive, withdrawn, or agitated
- Speech patterns
- Grooming, appearance
- Do they appear physically ill or frail as well as emotionally?

Assessment
- Distinguish between a mental disorder and a medical condition
- Many elderly have medical conditions and are on medications that can confuse the diagnosis of mental conditions

Treatment
- Most mild mental disorders can be effectively treated in a primary setting.
- Relate to patient in optimistic positive manner
- Treatment compliance is a special concern in individuals with cognitive deficits, physical problems, poor vision
- Consult, refer, or hospitalize when presenting symptoms are severe, chronic, or unresponsive to primary treatment
- Individuals with mental illness often self-medicate. Always be aware of the potential for development of tolerance, dependence, and lethality of medications when prescribing.
- Individuals who represent a clear and present danger to themselves or others, including suicidal ideation and attempt, should never be left alone and should be immediately hospitalized even when it is contrary to their wishes.

GENERAL GUIDELINES FOR PSYCHOPHARMACOLOGY IN THE ELDERLY
- Identify target symptoms to treat; failure to do so is common cause of treatment failure
- Treat systematically and change one thing at a time, allowing adequate time to evaluate the change before making another change
- Avoid using medications for their side effects only (e.g., giving sedating antidepressant to non-depressed patient with insomnia)
- Titrate dosage slowly to avoid side effects, continue to increase until therapeutic response is achieved or maximum recommended dose is reached
- Allow adequate length of time to achieve best therapeutic effects (several weeks for anti-depressants)

DEPRESSION

Description
- The predominant feature of depression is a disturbance in mood, the sustained internal emotional state of an individual who is described as sad or blue
- Loss of interest or pleasure in nearly all activities is the second major symptom; either mood disturbance or loss of interest or pleasure must be present in order to diagnose depression.
- Depression is a heterogenous disorder with much variation.

Table 18-1: DSM-IV Differential Diagnosis of Depressive Symptoms in Late Life

Disorder	Description
Mood Disorders	
Major depression	Depressed mood and/or loss of interest or pleasure, with other symptoms, present for at least 2 weeks
Dysthymia	Chronic, sustained depressed mood ongoing for a minimum of 2 years, more days than not
Bipolar disorder	Recurrent episodes of depression with episodes of mania that are characterized by lack of impulse control, excessive energy, grandiose or delusional thinking, elated mood, inappropriate behaviors, hyperactivity, pressured speech, and decreased need for sleep
Adjustment Disorders	
Adjustment disorder with depressed mood	Significant emotional or behavioral symptoms in response to a clearly identifiable psychosocial stressor(s). Symptoms develop within 3 months of the onset of the stressor(s), last no longer than 6 months and manifest themselves in a mal-adaptive response of impaired function and marked distress in excess of what would normally be expected
Uncomplicated Bereavement	
Organic mood disorders	Primary degenerative dementia with associated major depression
	Secondary to physical illness (e.g., hypothyroidism, stroke, carcinoma of the pancreas)
	Secondary to pharmacologic agents (e.g., methyldopa, propranolol)
Psychoactive substance-use disorders	Alcohol abuse and/or dependence
	Sedative, hypnotic, or anxiolytic abuse and/or dependence
Somatoform disorders	Hypochondriasis
	Somatization disorder

- Dementia frequently presents as depression.
- The Diagnostic and Statistical Manual of Mental Disorders (4th ed.) (DSM-IV) classified the types of depression. See Table 18-1.

Etiology
- Biological
  - Genetic predisposition
  - Dysregulation of chemical neurotransmitters; abnormalities in neurotransmitters in the brain, including serotonin, norepinephrine, dopamine, acetylcholine (cholinergic), epinephrine and gamma-aminobutyrate (GABA)
    - Environmental: stressful and traumatic life events, such as death of loved ones, major illness, divorce, financial difficulty, trouble with the law

Incidence and Demographics
- Depression is the most common mental illness seen in primary care practices.
- Dysthymia is more common in older adults than major depression.
- Depression occurs more frequently in women than men.
- The prevalence of depression does not differ among races.
- Statistics depend on definition used in study
- 8% to 20% of older adults in the community and 37% of older adults in primary care settings experience symptoms of depression
- 25% of older adults with chronic illness or are cognitively intact in a nursing home experience depression
- Estimated only 50% of all persons with major depression receive treatment

- NIH consensus panel found a substantial proportion of older adult patients receive no treatment or inadequate treatment for depression in primary care settings.
- Adjustment disorders
  - Common and vary widely as a function of the population and culture
- Bipolar disorder has an early onset, prior to age 30
  - Bipolar disorder persists into old age and becomes increasing difficult to treat.
  - Bipolar disorder occurs equally in both men and women.
- Suicide is a major risk of depression in older adults.
  - 15% of the individuals diagnosed with severe major depression die of suicide
  - Elderly are 12% of the population but account for 33% of suicides

Risk Factors
- Prior episodes of depression
- Family history, especially first-degree relative
- Alcohol and substance abuse
- Significant psychosocial stressors, such as divorce, death of spouse or loved ones, financial difficulty, job loss, retirement, trauma, sexual, emotional, or physical abuse
- Periods of prolonged stress
- Structural, neuroanatomic changes in later life (see Normal Changes of Aging)
- Chronic medical conditions and disabilities
- Polypharmacy

Risk Factors for Suicide
- Elderly white men who are socially isolated have the highest suicide rate.
- Social isolation
- Death or loss of spouse/loved one
- Chronic medical conditions and disabilities
- Decreased impulse control, impaired judgment
- Severe psychosocial stressors
- Prior suicide attempt(s)

Prevention and Screening
- Adequate family and social support systems
- Stress management and problem-solving techniques
- Prevention of suicide: providers must be alert to symptoms

Assessment
History
- The DSM-IV diagnostic symptoms of depression
  - Depressed mood, subjective or observed
  - Diminished interest or pleasure in activities
  - Weight loss or gain
  - Insomnia or hypersomnia
  - Psychomotor agitation or retardation
  - Fatigue or loss of energy
  - Feelings of worthlessness, or excessive or inappropriate guilt
  - Diminished ability to think or concentrate, or indecisiveness
  - Recurrent thoughts of death, recurrent suicidal ideation
- Other symptoms common in the elderly
  - Difficulty getting along with others
  - Increased social isolation and withdrawal with increased solitary behavior
  - Inattention to self-hygiene and appearance

- Increased oversensitivity to real or perceived rejections or failures
- Self-destructive behaviors
- Increased somatic complaints, such as headache, abdominal pain

ASSESSMENT TOOLS

- Mental status: MMSE, short portable rule out dementia, although depressed patients may have decreased MMSE scores due to inattention
- Depression: GDS self-report scale—the 5-item short version
  - Are you basically satisfied with your life? (no)
  - Do you often get bored? (yes)
  - Do you often feel helpless? (yes)
  - Do you prefer to stay home rather than go out and do new things? (yes)
  - Do you feel pretty worthless the way you are now? (yes)

SUICIDE ASSESSMENT

- Most patients who commit suicide have recently seen their primary care provider, usually with physical complaints or hints of depression
- Ask directly about suicidal thoughts, impulses; patient will not volunteer information but frequently will admit upon questioning
- Determine degree of risk of actual attempt
  - Plan, specificity of plan (access to method)
  - Feelings of hopelessness, helplessness
  - Giving away personal possessions
  - History of prior attempts

Physical

- A complete physical exam with a mental status and neurological exam should be performed in order to rule out organic mood disorders.
- Neurological exam gait, focal neuro signs, frontal lobe signs—structural brain abnormalities
- Weight loss or gain, psychomotor retardation—slowed movements, thinking
- Look for sad affect, anxiety, disheveled personal appearance with poor grooming, neglected hygiene

Diagnostic Studies (See Table 18-2)

- Lab to rule out medical causes
- CBC, thyroid profile, sedimentation rate, electrolytes, chemistry profile
- Serum levels of current medications if appropriate, such as TCAs, anticonvulsants, or digoxin
- Toxicology screen if appropriate
- Cortisol levels have been used to identify depression and subtypes in research but not in primary care practice.

Table 18-2: Medications That May Contribute to Depression

Class of Medication	Examples
Cardiac Medications	Digitalis, statins
Antihypertensives	Calcium channel blockers, methyldopa, thiazide diuretics
Hormones	Estrogens, progestins, corticosteroids
GI Medications	Histamine blockers, metoclopramide
Anticonvulsants	Phenytoin. barbiturates, carbamazepine, clonazepam, valproic acid
Anti-infectives	Fluoroquinolones, isoniazid, metronidazole, sulfonamides
Anxiolytics/sedatives	Benzodiazepines
Anti-inflammatory agents	NSAIDs

Differential Diagnosis
- Medical
- Illnesses
- Other mood disorders Table 18-1

ENDOCRINE DISORDERS
- Diabetes
- Hypothyroidism
- Hyperthyroidism

NEUROLOGICAL DISORDERS
- Dementia
- Stroke
- Neoplasms
- Multiple sclerosis
- Seizure disorders
- Parkinson disease
- Trauma

CARDIAC DISORDERS
- CHF
- MI

MALNUTRITION
- B$_{12}$
- Folate deficiency
- Protein/calorie deficiency

OTHER (See Table 18-2)
- Autoimmune disorder (rheumatologic disorders)
- Electrolyte imbalances
- Chronic fatigue syndrome
- COPD
- Infections
- Oncologic/hematologic disease

Management
- Most cases of depression can be safely managed by a primary practitioner
- Major depression and dysthymia have similar treatment
- Adjustment disorders are usually managed successfully with cognitive-behavioral therapy and adequate family and social support.
- Bipolar disorder should be referred for treatment.

Nonpharmacologic Treatment
- Psychosocial interventions have proved to be highly effective.
  - Pharmacological treatment should always be accompanied by some form of psychotherapy if patient accepts it; patient may be more amenable after med starts working.
  - Include patient, family, and support systems in treatment strategies and regime
  - Choose type of therapy appropriate to individual patients needs
    Cognitive-behavioral therapy with a focus on cognitive distortions
    Psychoanalysis or psychotherapy with a focus on intrapsychic phenomena
    Electroconvulsive therapy: indicated for severely depressed or suicidal patients who don't respond to pharmacological agents; main side effect is temporary memory impairment that may last up to 2 weeks
- Patient and Family Education
  - Patient and family education concerning the nature of the illness, side effects, risks and benefits of treatment, and expected outcome
  - Depression is a medical illness like any other
  - Treatment with medication replaces depleted neurotransmitters in the brain ,allowing it to function more normally

Pharmacologic Treatment (See Tables 18-3–18-5)
- Match the antidepressant and its side effects to the symptoms that are most troublesome to the patient
- In general, depressed patients can be categorized as either of two types:
  - Is the patient anxious, with insomnia and perhaps weight loss? OR
  - Patient has psychomotor retardation with hypersomnia and perhaps weight gain

Table 18-3: Medications for Target Symptoms

Symptoms	Effective Medications
Psychomotor Retardation	SRI, venlafaxine, bupropion
Anxiety	SRI* Paxil
Insomnia	Mirtazapine, trazodone
Weight Loss	Mirtazapine
Weight Gain	SRI, bupropion

*Has anxiety indication, but has been found on occasion to cause/increase anxiety in the elderly.
Paxil has some histamine effect and may be more effective for anxiety.

Table 18-4: Classification of Medications by Affected Neurotransmitter(s)

Drug Category	Serotonin	Norepinephrine	Dopamine	Others
SRIs	Yes	No	No	Epinephrine
TCAs	Yes	Yes	No	Acetylcholine, Histamine, epinephrine
Bupropion (Wellbutrin)	Yes	Yes	Yes	No
Mirtazapine (Remeron)	Yes	Yes	No	Histamine, epinephrine
Trazodone (Desyrel)	Yes	No	No	Acetylcholine, epinephrine
Venlafaxine (Effexor)	Yes	Yes	Yes	No
MAOIs	Yes	Yes	Yes	

Table 18-5: Effects According to Neurotransmitter

Neurotransmitter	Adverse Effects
Norepinephrine	Tachycardia, tremors, sexual dysfunction, augments sympathomimetics
Serotonin	Anxiety, agitation, anorexia, GI disturbances, headache, hypotension, sexual dysfunction
Dopamine	Extrapyramidal signs, increased prolactin levels, psychosis, insomnia, anorexia, psychomotor activation
Epinephrine	Orthostatic hypotension, cardiac conduction disturbance
Acetylcholine	Memory dysfunction, constipation, tachycardia, blurred vision, dry mouth, urinary retention
Histamine	Sedation, drowsiness, hypotension, weight gain

- Predicting which medication will work on which patient is difficult
- Try one medication, if not effective, change
- Older adults experience increased side effects of the medications.
- Drug interaction between antidepressants and other medications are common.
- Antidepressants or anti-anxiety agents may be given short term (1 to 3 months) for management of acute symptoms of adjustment disorder.
- Treatment with an antidepressant may precipitate a manic episode in patients with bipolar disease.

Table 18-6: SSRI Therapy

Medication	Initial Dose	Target Dose
Fluoxetine (Prozac)	10 mg qd	20–40 mg qd
Sertraline (Zoloft)	25 mg qd	50–150 mg qd
Paroxetine (Paxil)	10 mg qd	20–40 mg qd
Escitalopram (Lexapro)	5 mg qd	10–20 mg qd

SEROTONIN REUPTAKE INHIBITORS (SRIs) (See Table 18-6)

- SRIs are usually the first-line drug of choice for the treatment of major depression due to their effectiveness and safety record
- SRIs can be effective for anxiety but can cause agitation in the elderly
- All SRIs are not alike
  - Fluoxetine is very long acting (half life 36 hours), which is good if the patient forgets to take an occasional pill; however, in the elderly, it can cause agitation, which will then last for several days.
  - Sertraline (Zoloft) given in the morning can be activating.
  - Paroxetine (Paxil) also affects histamine and can cause sedation and be effective against anxiety and insomnia.
  - Citalopram (Celexa) may be less likely to cause side effects.

OTHER ANTIDEPRESSANTS (See Table 18-7)

- Some of the newer antidepressants are especially effective in the elderly.
- Bupropion (Wellbutrin XR) is activating; avoid bedtime dosing; do not use with history of seizure
- Mirtazapine (Remeron) is useful to help with insomnia, weight loss
- Venlafaxine (Effexor XR) may be activating; monitor for elevated blood pressure
- Trazodone is an older, heterocyclic medication and has been used for insomnia, now largely replaced by Mirtazapine

TRICYCLICS (See Table 18-8)

- Tricyclic antidepressants are also effective in the treatment and management of depression; however, their association with a greater incidence of side effects has reduced their use.
- Tricyclics are contraindicated in patients at risk for adverse anticholinergic effects, such as with cardiac conduction disorders, narrow angle glaucoma, and prostatic hypertrophy.
- Can also be used for pain control, especially neuropathic pain; may be especially effective in depressed patients with chronic pain
- Amitriptyline most common one used for pain but has highest side effects
- Nortriptyline fewer side effects; also effective for pain
- Tricyclic medications have a high potential for lethality in overdose

Table 18-7: Other Common Antidepressants

Medication	Initial Dose	Target Dose
Bupropion (Wellbutrin SR)	100 mg PO qd	150–400 mg PO qd
Mirtazapine (Remeron)	7.5–15 mg q hs	15–30 mg q hs
Venlafaxine (Effexor XR)	37.5 mg qd	75 mg PO bid
Trazodone (Desyrel)	50 q hs	100 mg q hs

Table 18-8: Common Tricyclic Antidepressants

Medication	Initial Dose	Target Dose
Amitriptyline (Elavil)	10–25 mg q hs	50–100 mg q hs
Desipramine (Norpramin)	25 mg q hs	50–100 mg q hs
Nortriptyline (Pamelor)	10–25 mg q hs	50–75 mg q hs

MAOIs
- Monoamine oxidase inhibitors (MAOIs), such as Nardil and Parnate, are used in the treatment of refractory or treatment-resistant depression.
- Because of the many potentially serious and lethal side effects, such as hypertensive crisis, associated with these antidepressants, patients in need of these types of medications should always be referred to a psychiatrist.

How Long to Treat
- Treatment can be divided into three phases
  - Acute: goal is symptom remission; lasts 4 to 8 weeks or more
  - Continuation: goal is stabilization when risk of relapse is high, lasts 6 to 12 months—generally requires continuation of medication for 1 year in first episodes of depression
  - Maintenance: goal is prevention of recurrences, time will vary, may be lifetime, especially in recurrent depression

Special Considerations
- Depression is a chronic illness with frequent episodes of recurrence

When to Consult, Refer, Hospitalize
- All patients who present with suicidal ideation, plan, or recent attempt should immediately be referred to an emergency room or psychiatrist for further evaluation and treatment
- Refer patients to psychiatrist or other mental health specialist if
  - Severely impaired by their symptoms
  - Psychotic symptoms, such as delusions and hallucination
  - Comorbid disorders such as obsessive-compulsive disorder, substance abuse
  - No social support
- All patients should be referred to the appropriate mental health practitioner for therapy
- Patients with symptoms attributed to adjustment disorder, lasting more then 6 months must be reevaluated and referred to a mental health specialist

Follow-up
- Patients should be followed weekly for the first 2 months while effective dosage is titrated and response to medication and side effects can be monitored
- Continue to follow monthly until stable
- Patients who are not responding to medication should be placed on another antidepressant
- When changing antidepressants, remember to first change to another class antidepressants; then refer out for TCAs or MAOIs

Expected Course
- Most patients respond to antidepressants within 2 to 3 weeks of treatment; full effect may not be seen until several months of therapy
- Recurrences are frequent
- Prognosis poorer if combined with medical illness

Complications
- Depression in older adults leads to impairments in social, mental, and physical functioning
- Major depression in older adults is associated with higher morbidity and mortality rates
- Older primary care patients with depression make more emergency room and primary care provider visits, use more medication, incur higher outpatient charges, and experience longer hospital stays
- Suicide

GRIEF/BEREAVEMENT

Description
- The emotional and physiological reaction to the death or loss of a loved one
- Grief and bereavement are the normal reaction to death or loss
- Uncomplicated grief presents as depressed mood that is situational and time limited
- Grief that lasts longer than 2 months should be evaluated for mood disorders

Etiology
- Loss

Incidence and Demographics
- Grief is a common phenomenon of the elderly
- 10% to 20% widows and widowers develop depression during the first year of bereavement

Risk Factors
- Old age

Prevention and Screening
- Ask about coping and depression in patients experiencing recent losses

Assessment
- Complete physical and neurologic exam with mental status, current medication and over-the-counter products and supplements

History
- Determine nature and occurrence of the loss
- Determine type and degree of symptom, functional impairment
- Determine social and familial support systems
- Assess for suicidal ideation, risk of lethality
- Assess cognitive state, mood, and affect

Physical
- Clinical manifestations of grief
  - Feelings of sadness and profound loss
  - Crying spells
  - Insomnia
  - Loss of appetite and weight loss
  - Survivor guilt
  - Suicidal ideation, thoughts of mortality and one's own death

Diagnostic Studies
- Laboratory and diagnostic testing as indicated by presenting individual symptoms and general medical condition
- Mini Mental Status Exam, GDS

Differential Diagnosis
- Depression
- Adjustment disorder with depressed mood

- Normal grief reaction usually begins to show marked improvement within 8 weeks
- The diagnosis of depression or adjustment disorder with depressed mood is not given unless symptoms are still present after 2 months and represent a significant change in function and impairment.

Management

Nonpharmacologic Treatment
- Encourage the expression of grief and mourning over loss
- Reassurance that grief is a normal, nonpathologic reaction to loss and is self-limited
- Encourage participation in support groups
- Provide emotional support
- Provide community resources
- Educate family and caregivers as to nature, normal course of bereavement process

Pharmacologic Treatment
- Consider mild antianxiety agents in lowest effective dose if patient is functionally impaired by grief
- Antidepressants if impaired by depression
- Short-term treatment for up to 2 months

When to Consult, Refer, Hospitalize
- Individual verbalizes suicidal ideation, plan, or desire to join deceased loved one
- Symptoms last longer than 2 months in duration
- Symptoms intensify and severely impair daily function
- Patient has a history of major depressive illness, prior suicide attempts, or other mental illness
- Suicide attempts or suicidal ideation with a plan is always a psychiatric emergency and should be immediately referred to a mental health specialist or emergency room for immediate evaluation and treatment.

Follow-up
- Patients should be followed weekly during the acute phase with consultations to a psychiatrist or mental health specialist for symptoms that last longer.

Expected Course
- The normal course of uncomplicated grief/bereavement is 2 months, frequently lasts longer
- It is common for patients to exhibit some brief, limited symptoms close to the anniversary date of the loss of a loved one
- Cognitive-behavioral therapy and social supports are associated with an improved prognosis

Complications
- Risk of depression continues to increase throughout second year of bereavement
- Older adults without adequate social/familial support are at high risk for developing major depression and suicidal ideation

ANXIETY DISORDERS

Description
- Excessive worry, feelings of apprehension, panic, or dread accompanied by symptoms of autonomic nervous system arousal (palpitations, muscle tension and restlessness, fatigue, sweating, difficulty concentrating)
- Symptoms occur more days than not, with the individual reporting little or no control, along with significant distress and impairment in social, occupational, and interpersonal areas

SUBTYPES
Generalized Anxiety Disorder—chronic free-floating anxiety for at least 1 month
- Excessive worry, irrational, pervasive anxiety without apparent etiology or cause

Phobias—massive anxiety, sudden onset, no precipitating factor
- Social phobia fear of situations in which the person is exposed to possible scrutiny by others, and fears they may do something humiliating or embarrassing
  - A severe, persistent fear of social or performance situations that provokes an immediate and intense anxiety response
  - Common examples are fear of speaking, urinating in public lavatory, saying foolish things
  - Patient then avoids social situations in which stimulus may occur
  - Patient realizes that the fear is excessive or unreasonable
- Specific phobia: persistent fear of a definite stimulus (object or situation)
  - Extreme, irrational fear of specific objects, such as elevators, snakes, or insects, that leads to avoidant behavior of that particular object
  - Exposure to the stimulus provokes an immediate anxiety response
  - Person recognizes that the fear is excessive or unreasonable

Panic Disorder—massive anxiety, sudden onset, no precipitating factor
- Discrete episodes of recurrent and intense fear that occur without apparent warning, accompanied by at least 4 symptoms of anxiety

Obsessive-Compulsive Disorder—persistent need to repeat either thoughts or behaviors
- Recurrent, repetitive, and intrusive thoughts and behaviors that are extremely difficult or impossible to control
- Thoughts and behaviors are excessive and unreasonable, resulting in significant anxiety, distress, and impairment in daily function

Post-Traumatic Stress Disorder—anxiety following a major life stressor
- Exposure to an extreme traumatic stressor, such as rape, sexual or physical abuse, natural disasters, war or other perceived or actual threat to a person's physical being or self-concept
- Results in delayed and persistent symptoms, including nightmares, flashbacks, numbing of emotion, dissociative episodes, or inability to recall specific events

Etiology
- Behavioral
  - Conditioned behavioral response to earlier interpersonal or social experiences
- Biologic
  - Genetic predisposition
  - Overstimulated autonomic nervous system, stress response
  - Abnormalities of neurotransmitter receptors in the CNS, specifically GABA receptors

Incidence and Demographics
- Anxiety disorders are one of the most common mental illness in the US
- Anxiety disorders account for 15% of the population seen in general practice settings
- Generalized anxiety disorder in older adults occurs more frequently than any other anxiety disorder
- Phobic disorders are the second most common type of anxiety in the elderly
- Panic disorder and obsessive compulsive disorder have a low incidence in older adults
- Post-traumatic stress disorder is rare in the elderly
- Anxiety disorders frequently coexist with depression in the elderly

Risk Factors
- Family history
- Exposure to traumatic events
- Genetic predisposition

Prevention and Screening
- Public, patient, and caregiver education and awareness
- Strong familial, community, and social support systems

Table 18-9: Symptoms of Anxiety Disorders

Symptom	Generalized Anxiety Disorder	Panic Attacks
Autonomic Hyperactivity	Shortness of breath, smothering sensations	
	Palpitations or tachycardia	
	Sweating or cold, clammy hands	Sweating
	Dry mouth	
	Dizziness or lightheadedness	
	Nausea, diarrhea, or other abdominal distress	Nausea or abdominal distress
	Flushes or chills	Flushes or chills
	Frequent urination	
	Trouble swallowing or "lump in throat"	Choking
Motor Tension	Trembling, twitching, or feeling shaky	Trembling or shaking
	Muscle tension, aches, or soreness	Chest pain or discomfort
	Restlessness	
	Easy fatigability	
Vigilance and Scanning	Feeling keyed up or on edge	
	Exaggerated startle response	
	Difficulty concentrating	
	Trouble falling or staying asleep	
	Irritability	
Psych Symptoms		Depersonalization or derealization
		Fear of dying
		Fear of going crazy or of doing something uncontrolled

Assessment (See Table 18-9)

History
- Determine onset, frequency, and duration and type of symptoms
- Determine degree of distress and symptom interference with daily function (work, relationships, and leisure activities)
- Elicit predisposing factors
- Obtain complete medical history, current and OTC medications, and supplements taken
- Obtain history and current patterns of use of caffeine, alcohol, and substances

Physical
- Complete physical with thorough neurologic exam to
  - Rule out medical causes of symptoms
  - Observe for signs of autonomic nervous system hyperactivity

Diagnostic Studies
- Routine diagnostic labs including CBC, metabolic panel, and thyroid function tests to rule out medical conditions that may present with anxiety
- EKG to evaluate tachyarrhythmias if indicated
- Holter monitor to evaluate episodes of palpitations to rule out arrhythmia
- Psychological testing: Mini Mental Status Exam, Hamilton Anxiety Scale

Differential Diagnosis

PSYCHOLOGICAL CONDITIONS
- Depression w/anxiety
- Schizophrenia, atypical psychosis
- Bipolar disorder with mania
- Adjustment disorder w/ anxious mood
- Substance abuse

- Neurologic disorders
  - Neoplasms
  - Trauma
  - Migraine
  - MS, seizure disorders
- Cardiac disorders
  - Arrhythmias
  - MI
  - CHF
- Endocrine Disorders
  - Cushing's Disease
  - Hyper/hypothyroidism
  - Hypoglycemia
- Pulmonary disorders
  - Hypoxia
  - COPD
  - Asthma
  - Pulmonary embolism
  - Pneumothorax
- Inflammatory
  - SLE
  - RA
  - Temporal arteritis

MEDICATIONS/SUBSTANCES INGESTED
- Medications
  - Anticholinergics
  - Antihistamines
  - Corticosteroids
  - Antihypertensives
  - Antipsychotics
  - Antidepressants
  - Bronchodilators
  - Amphetamines
  - Anesthetics
  - Sympathomimetics
  - Vasopressors
- Substance abuse
  - Stimulants
  - Cannabis (acute withdrawal or intoxication)
  - Alcohol abuse
  - Caffeine
  - Nicotine

Management
- GAD is usually responsive to medical treatment in a primary care practice setting, but should be referred for psychological therapy
- Other anxiety disorders are usually referred to a mental health specialist for management
- Patient education is essential to ensure compliance and effective treatment
- Community resources and support should be provided as possible

Nonpharmacologic Treatment
- Cognitive-behavioral therapy
- Psychotherapy and psychoanalysis
- Stress management education, courses, workshops
- Behavioral conditioning, biofeedback
- Community self-help and support groups
- Education of family members and caregivers as to behavioral techniques and interventions

Pharmacologic Treatment

ANTIDEPRESSANTS
- Antidepressants are commonly the first-line drug of choice in the treatment of anxiety disorders
- Potential for substance abuse and dependence is significantly less than with benzodiazepines
- Main therapeutic effect may take 3 to 4 weeks
- Patient education and awareness of length of time required to reach target dose and main effect of the drug is essential for greater likelihood of compliance
- Dosage is the same as for depression

Table 18-10: Anxiolytic Drug

Anxiolytic	Starting Dose	Target Dose
Buspirone (BuSpar)	5 mg/qd	15–30 mg divided tid

ANTIDEPRESSANTS WITH FDA INDICATIONS FOR ANXIETY DISORDERS (see Tables 18-6, 18-7, and 18-8 for dosing)
- Sertraline (Zoloft)—OCD, panic, post-traumatic stress disorder, social anxiety disorder
- Paroxetine (Paxil)—OCD, panic disorder, social anxiety disorder
- Fluoxetine (Prozac)—OCD
- Escitalopram (Lexapro)—GAD
- Venlafaxine (Effexor)—GAD
- Trazodone (Desyrel)—depression with or without anxiety

BUSPIRONE (BuSPAR) (See Table 18-10)
- Slower onset of action may take up to 4 weeks for antianxiety effects
- Maximum therapeutic effect may not be reached for 4 to 8 weeks
- Significant adverse reactions are found in 20% to 30% of anxious older adults
- Most frequent side effects include gastrointestinal, dizziness, headache, sleep disturbance, fatigue, nausea/vomiting.
- Less sedating than benzodiazepines
- Significant number of nonresponders

BENZODIAZEPINES (See Table 18-11)
- Use with great caution in the elderly
- Use for shortest amount of time possible until other medication has reached therapeutic level
- All benzodiazepines are effective in treating the symptoms of anxiety disorders
- Benzodiazepines have a rapid onset of action with quick symptom relief
- Benzodiazepines have a significant potential for dependence and abuse
- Patients with substance abuse histories are at high risk for abuse
- Benzodiazepine toxicity in older adults often manifests in sedation, ataxia, dysarthria, cognitive impairment, psychomotor impairment, falls, mental confusion, memory impairment
- Half-life of benzodiazepines and their metabolites may be extended significantly in older adults
- Alprazolam and lorazepam are commonly used in the elderly due to short half-time, less risk of accumulation and toxicity
- Diazepam (Valium) has long half-life and should not be used in the elderly
- Clonazepam (Klonopin) is FDA-indicated for panic disorder and may be used long term with extreme caution in the elderly (adverse reactions include CNS effects, blood dyscrasias, liver disorders)

Table 18-11: Benzodiazepine Therapy for Anxiety Disorders

Benzodiazepines	Starting Dose	Usual Dose
Alprazolam (Xanax)	0.25 mg qd bid	0.5–3 mg/day
Lorazepam (Ativan)	0.25 mg qhs	0.5 mg qd tid
Clonazepam (Klonopin)	0.25 mg qd bid	1–2 mg/day

How Long to Treat
- Length varies according to individual response and symptom management
- Mild anxiety usually resolves within 2 months

Special Considerations
- It is common for anxiety disorders to occur concomitantly with other disorders, such as depression and substance abuse
- Anxiety disorders are also commonly seen with many physical, medical disorders
- Patients with anxiety disorders need reassurance that their disorder can be effectively treated
- The establishment of a trusting, safe therapeutic relationship with the primary practitioner is essential for compliance and effective treatment

When to Consult, Refer, Hospitalize
- Chronic, disabling anxiety requires a psychiatric consultation and referral
- Severe panic attacks, intense PTSD, and disabling OCD always require a psychiatric consult or referral and usually require a combination of pharmacotherapy and cognitive-behavioral therapy

Follow-up
- Patients should be seen weekly during the acute phase of treatment
- Medications need to be monitored for effectiveness of symptom management, appropriate dose, and potential abuse

Expected Course
- Course of treatment varies according to degree of impairment and individual response

Complications
- Functional and social impairment

ALCOHOL AND OTHER SUBSTANCE ABUSE

Description
- The physiological dependence of substance as indicated by evidence of tolerance, symptoms of withdrawal, and impairment of function in social, interpersonal, and occupational areas of one's personal life
- Addiction is often characterized by a preoccupation with the substance, loss of control over the amount and frequency of use, physical and psychological dependence and tolerance
- The most common substance abuse problems are with alcohol and prescription medications, such as benzodiazepines and opioids

Etiology
- Genetic predisposition
- Social and cultural conditioning

Incidence and Demographics
- The incidence of alcoholism is about the same in elderly as it is in adults
- Prevalence of heavy drinking in older adults estimated at 3% to 9%; frequently unrecognized
- Alcoholism rates are highest in African American and Hispanic males
- Overuse of alcohol and medications is associated with psychiatric disorders and chronic pain syndrome in the elderly

Risk Factors
- Family history
- Abuse of other substances
- Cultural conditioning
- Domestic violence or abuse

- Presence of a psychiatric disorder
- Stressful events

Prevention and Screening
- Education and awareness by primary care providers of symptoms and special issues involving alcoholism and older adults
- Routinely ask questions to assess problem with alcohol

Assessment

History
- Nonspecific presentation—confusion, falls, decrease in ADLs
- History of prior substance abuse treatment
- Psychiatric history
- Current use of prescribed and OTC medications
- Affect on function and social relationships
- Any physical symptoms secondary to alcohol
  - Neurologic: confusion, seizures, tremors, agitation, paresthesias
  - Cardiac: symptoms of alcohol cardiomyopathy
  - GI: vomiting blood, reflux symptoms, melena, jaundice, hypoglycemia
- Attitudes, thoughts, feelings, and observations of family and caregivers regarding use or abuse of alcohol by older adult

Physical
- Clinical manifestations of alcoholism and alcohol abuse include:
  - Withdrawal symptoms may begin with anxiety, decreased cognition, tremulousness, then increase irritability and hyperreactivity and to tremors, hallucinations, and seizures
  - Neurological: memory impairment, hyperreflexia, ataxia, confabulation, sensory deficits
  - Cardiovascular: cardiomyopathy, hypertension, and arrhythmias, generalized edema
  - Gastrointestinal: gastric distension, ascites, enlarged liver, icterus
  - Musculoskeletal: muscle wasting, falls, fractures, other injuries
  - Generally unkempt appearance, poor personal hygiene
  - Integumentary: cushingoid appearance, flushed face, spider nevi, ecchymosis, angiomas
  - HEENT: nystagmus, smell of alcohol on breath
  - Sexual dysfunction
  - Weight loss

Assessment Tools
- CAGE
  - Have you ever felt the need to **C**ut down on drinking?
  - Have you ever felt **A**nnoyed by criticism of your drinking?
  - Have you ever felt **G**uilty about your drinking?
  - Have you ever taken a morning **E**ye opener?
- MMSE (see Chapter 4 on dementia)

Diagnostic Studies
- Blood alcohol levels
  - Limited use in primary care, more useful in acute intoxication
  - Normal level does not rule out abuse
  - Blood concentration increases disproportionately to the amount consumed
- Drug levels in opioids, not available for benzodiazepines
- CBC to rule out infection, or anemia from GI bleed or macrocytic anemia indicative of B_{12} and folate deficiency; MCV elevated in alcohol abuse

- Metabolic panel to assess kidney function, electrolytes and rule out diabetes, hypoglycemia; alk phos to rule out pancreatitis
- Liver function tests: GTT elevated early; AST twice as high as ALT is typical of alcoholic liver injury
- TSH, thyroid, T_3, T_4
- B_{12} and folate
- Prothrombin time, PTT
- Lipid panel

Differential Diagnosis
The major differential to make is whether there are underlying psychiatric problems
- Schizophrenia
- Major depressive mood disorders
- Anxiety disorders
- Bipolar disorder
- Personality disorders
- Polysubstance abuse disorder
- B_{12} and folate deficiency and malnutrition
- Endocrine disorders such as diabetes and Cushing's disease
- Neurological disorders, seizure disorders
- Cardiovascular disease

Management
Nonpharmacologic Treatment
- Substance abuse counseling
- Alcoholics Anonymous program
- Substance abuse treatment programs and halfway houses
- Cognitive-behavioral therapy
- Psychoanalysis

Pharmacologic Treatment
ALCOHOL
- Detoxification for symptoms of withdrawal done by specialist
- Commonly used agents include:
  - Maintenance therapy for alcohol abuse, NP may monitor
    Disulfiram (Antabuse) aversive treatment, causing toxic reaction to alcohol intake, even in small amounts, such as that in cough syrup
    Naltrexone 50 mg PO qd reduces cravings
    Thiamine, folic acid, and B complex supplements

PRESCRIPTION MEDICATION ABUSE
- Gradually wean patient off medication
- Decrease dosage by smallest amount possible every 2 weeks to month
- Usually requires a controlled setting as in a nursing home
- Pharmacologic and medical management of underlying medical disorders as appropriate by primary care provider

When to Consult, Refer, Hospitalize
- Patients diagnosed or suspected of alcoholism or substance abuse should always be referred to a substance abuse specialist for further evaluation and treatment
- Social issues need to be referred to a mental health specialist for long-term management

Follow-up

Expected Course
- Often chronic and relapsing

Complications
- Severe intoxication is a medical emergency and can lead to coma, respiratory depression, aspiration, and death
- Long-term use results in significant changes in brain function as well as severe impairment in social and interpersonal relations

TOBACCO USE AND SMOKING CESSATION

Description
- The repetitive use of tobacco and nicotine despite recurrent and significant adverse medical consequences
- Tobacco- and nicotine-seeking behaviors with accompanying physical dependence, tolerance, and withdrawal

Etiology
- Genetic predisposition
- Social, cultural, and behavioral influences
- Nicotine dependence

Incidence and Demographics
- Nicotine addiction is the number one health problem in the nation
- 430,000 individuals die each year of tobacco-related illnesses
- Deaths from cancer are 2 times greater for smokers than nonsmokers

Risk Factors
- Family history of use
- Polysubstance abuse
- Psychiatric disorders

Prevention and Screening
- Smoking cessation programs

Assessment

History
- History of tobacco, including past attempts to quit and techniques used; why unsuccessful
- Assess patient's desire to change behavior (see Chapter 3, Transtheoretical Model of Change)
- Perform complete medical history to rule out all underlying medical problems
- Frequent upper respiratory infections

Physical
- Hypertension
- Cigarette smell on breath, clothing, and hair
- Skin prematurely aged and wrinkled
- Stained teeth and fingers, dental caries
- Inflammation of sinuses, oropharynx, nasal cavities
- Respiratory impairment, infections
- Cardiovascular disease
- Peptic ulcer disease

Differential Diagnosis
- Polysubstance abuse
- Smokeless tobacco, snuff

Management

Nonpharmacologic Treatment

- Smoking cessation programs
- Behavioral therapy
- Hypnosis
- Reassure patient that relapses are normal, just try again
- Provide educational literature and support

Pharmacologic Treatment

- Nicotine replacement therapies
- Use with caution in patients with cardiac disease
- Must NOT smoke while using
- Taper dose gradually as craving decreases; see specific instructions with each system
- It is necessary to match the delivery system to the patient's individual needs
  - Transdermal patch—basic method of treatment
  - Nicotine gum—may be used instead of patch if chewing is satisfying to patient
  - Nicotine nasal spray—add for immediate relief of severe cravings
  - Nicotine inhaler—good for patients who are used to handling the cigarette
- Antidepressant: Bupropion sustained release (Zyban) decreases cravings
  - Stop smoking 1–2 weeks after starting medication
  - Dose 100 mg q AM for 1 week, increase as tolerated to 150 mg PO bid

How Long to Treat

- How long to treat and success rates vary with individual characteristics and motivation
- Bupropion should be given for at least 6 months, as long as patient has urge to smoke

Special Considerations

- Older adults with a history of smoking often present with severe, chronic medical problems as a consequence of chronic tobacco use
- Never too late to stop; patient and family education and support are crucial, even with older adults with a history of chronic tobacco use and their caregivers

Follow-up

- Weekly visits during attempts to quit
- Monitor withdrawal symptoms, medication compliance, and effectiveness

Expected Course

- Relapses are frequent, commonly occurring during the first 2 weeks
- Most patients have relapses before they succeed; they should be encouraged to try again at each relapse

Complications: a major cause of morbidity and mortality

- Cardiovascular disease
  - Coronary artery disease
  - Stroke
  - Hypertension
  - Peripheral artery disease
  - Elevated cholesterol levels
- Cancer: lung, mouth, throat, esophagus, larynx, pancreas, bladder, and cervical
- Respiratory: chronic obstructive pulmonary disease, asthma, pneumonia
- Peptic ulcer disease
- Death

ABUSE AND NEGLECT OF THE ELDERLY

Description
- Physical, emotional, economic, or sexual pain and injury inflicted deliberately upon an elderly person by a person who has care or custody of or stands in a position of trust, with the express goal of manipulating, intimidating, and controlling that individual within the relationship
- Includes physical abuse; neglect; sexual assault; unreasonable physical restraint; deprivation of food, water, shelter, or medical treatment; and physical abandonment

Etiology
- See Risk Factors

Incidence and Demographics
- Over 2 million elderly adults over the age of 60 are abused annually
- Greater incidence of abuse by family members than paid provider

Risk Factors
- Over age 84
- Social isolation, lack of support
- Cognitively impaired
- Physical, emotional, and financial dependency

Prevention and Screening
- Public education and awareness
- Refer families to local department of aging or social worker for assistance with in-home care, adult day care, respite care, or long-term placement or financial counseling regarding long-term care
- Social programs such as Adult Protective Services

Assessment

History
- Determine primary caregivers, living arrangements, legal custodian, and power of attorney
- History of medical treatment, accidents, fractures, physical injuries, traumas, overdose of medications
- Determine environmental, psychosocial, and financial stressors
- Any unusual or inappropriate activity in bank accounts, unpaid bills, lack of amenities, missing belongings
- Missed medical appointments
- Interview individual alone
- Mental status exam
- Document findings carefully
- Identify caregiver stress, interview caregivers and family members

Physical
- Monitor nutritional status and weight for dehydration, malnutrition
- Lacerations, bruises, wounds, burns, fractures inconsistent with explanation offered
- Delay between time of injury and treatment
- Poor skin and personal hygiene
- Fearful, evasive, guarded, depressed
- Sexually transmitted diseases, genital rash, trauma, discharge
- Rectal tissue swelling, discharge

Diagnostic Studies
- Specific to presenting symptoms
- Determine nutritional status (CBC, metabolic panel, cholesterol) (see Unintentional Weight Loss)

Differential Diagnosis

- Accidental injury
- Self-neglect due to cognitive status or physical impairment
- Depression
- Dementia

Management

- Notify Protective Services if abuse is suspected
- Manage medical conditions

When to Consult, Refer, Hospitalize

- It is mandatory by law to report all elder and disabled adult abuse and neglect to Adult Protective Service agencies
- Hospitalization or institutionalization when in the best interest of the individual

Follow-up

Expected Course

- Abuse will escalate unless there is intervention

Complications

- Death

CASE STUDIES

Case 1. A 72-year-old male presents to your office complaining of insomnia, generalized aches and pains, fatigue and a 10-pound weight loss over the past 2 months. He states he has lost interest in his hobbies, doesn't go out of the house often except to buy groceries, and spends much of his day watching television.

Medications: Advil 2–6 tabs/day for pain.

1. What additional questions would you ask?
2. What would you look for on physical examination?
3. What laboratory work would you order?
4. What treatment would you begin, assuming lab is normal?
5. What complications should you watch for?

Case 2. A 68-year-old female presents to your office complaining of difficulty swallowing, diarrhea, dizzy spells, weakness in her legs, insomnia, feelings of impending doom, and a fear of losing control.

1. What questions would you ask?
2. What would you look for on physical exam?
3. What laboratory tests would you order?
4. What treatment would you begin?
5. What complications might develop?

Case 3. Mr. Smith, 75 years old, comes for routine follow-up of diabetes. He reports his wife died 3 weeks ago. He joined AA at age 50.

Medications: Glucophage 500 mg bid

1. What questions would you ask?
2. What laboratory tests would you order?
3. What treatment would you begin?
4. What complications might develop?

REFERENCES

American Psychiatric Association. (2000). *Diagnostic and statistical manual of mental disorders* (4th ed.). Washington, DC: APA.

Dambro, M. R. (2004). *The 5 minute clinical consult.* St. Louis: Lippincott, Williams & Wilkins.

Depp, C. A., Jeste, D. V. (2004). Bipolar disorder in older adults: A critical review. *Bipolar Disorders, 6*(5), 343–367.

Depression and Bipolar Support Alliance. Available at: www.dbsalliance.

Ferri, F. F. (2003). *Ferri's clinical advisor* (6th ed.). St. Louis: Mosby.

Hoyle, M. T., et al. (1999). Development and testing of a five-item version of the geriatric depression scale. *JAGS, 47,* 873–878.

Lang, A. J., & Stein, M. B. (2001). Anxiety disorders and how to recognize and treat the medical symptoms of emotional illness. *Geriatrics, 56*(5), 24–27, 31–32, 34.

Lavretsky, H. (2000). Choosing appropriate treatment of geriatric depression. *Clinical Geriatrics, 8*(11), 99–108.

Medical Letter. (2003). Drugs for psychiatric disorders. *Treatment Guidelines, 1*(11), 69–76.

Mohlman, J., et al. (2004). Distinguishing generalized anxiety disorder, panic disorder, and mixed anxiety states in older treatment-seeking adults. *J Anxiety Disorders, 18*(3), 275–290.

Morse, J. Q., & Lynch, T. R. (2004). A preliminary investigation of self-reported personality disorders in life: Prevalence, predictors of depressive severity, and clinical correlates. *Aging Mental Health, 8*(4), 307–315.

NIH National Institutes of Mental Health. Available at: http://www.nimh.nih.gov.

Quinn, M., & Tomita, S. (1997). *Elder abuse and neglect: Cause, diagnosis and intervention strategies.* New York: Springer Pub. Co.

Parker, G., & Hadzi-Pavlovic, D. (2004). Is the female preponderance in major depression secondary to a gender difference in specific anxiety disorders? *Psychological Medicine, 34*(3), 461–470.

Sadavoy, J., & Lesczc, M. (Eds.). (1987). *Treating the elderly with psychotherapy: The scope for change in later life.* Madison, CT: International Universities Press.

Tierney, L. M., McPhee, S. J., & Papadakis, A. (2005). *Current medical diagnosis and treatment* (44th ed.). NJ: Appleton & Lange.

Unutzer, J., et al. (2002). Collaborative care management of late-life depression in the primary care setting. *JAMA, 288*(22), 2836–2845.

Williams, J. W., et al. (2000). Treatment of dysthymia and minor depression in primary care. *JAMA, 284*(12), 1519–1526.

APPENDIX A

DISCUSSION OF CASE STUDIES
Chapter 2: Dimensions of NP Role

Case 1. Your 92-year-old female patient, who lives alone at home, has fallen several times in the past few months. She refuses to have physical therapy or to move to an assisted living or nursing home. Her daughter, who has not talked to her for the past 10 years, wants you to sign a document stating her mother is not competent so she can put her in a nursing home. The daughter also wants a copy of her mother's chart.

1. What are the legal issues involved?

   Competency and confidentiality

2. Should you tell the daughter about the patient's condition or give her a copy of the chart?

   No, you would violate the patient's confidentiality, unless you got permission from the patient first.

3. Can you determine from the information given that the patient is not competent?

   No, just because the patient is making decisions that you may not agree with, does not mean that she is incompetent.

Case 2. An 82-year-old man is found to have lung cancer. This was an incidental finding on CXR for admission to assisted living. He has no symptoms. He is a widower with one son.

1. What health care documents would you ask the patient about?

   Durable power of attorney for health care and living will
   Who is named as the proxy?
   Are his finances taken care of?

2. What health care decisions would you look for on his durable power of attorney?

   CPR, mechanical respiration, and feeding tubes for artificial nutrition and hydration. Should not just say no heroic measures.

3. How would you decide how aggressively to manage this patient?

   Review durable power of attorney and explain risk/benefits of treatment options to patient and proxy. Have a conference with the patient care team, including doctor, social worker, clergy and nurse.

4. The patient becomes incompetent without writing down his wishes. You need to decide whether or not to put in a feeding tube. What question do you pose to the son?

   To the best of your knowledge, what would the patient have wanted if he were able to tell us. Not what the son wants.

Case 3. You just graduated from your nurse practitioner program.

1. What additional qualifications do you need in order to practice?

   You need a state nurse practitioner license. You must meet their requirements in order to practice. Each state has laws to establish their requirements. These vary from state to state. Most states require you are certified by a national certifying organization. Some require a

written agreement or other contract with a physician. Most have requirements for continuing education requirements.

Chapter 3: Health Care Issues

Case 1. You are asked to assess an 82-year-old man for admission to an assisted living facility.
1. What chronic conditions is he likely to have?
   Arthritis, heart disease, especially hypertension and hyperlipidemia, diabetes, stroke
2. What impairments is he likely to have?
   Hearing loss, visual impairment, decreased functional abilities, impaired nutrition, impaired safety, impaired taste
3. What kind of health insurance is he likely to have?
   Medicare (which will not pay for the assisted living)
4. What cause is he most likely to die from?
   Heart disease, cancer, stroke, COPD, pneumonia/influenza, diabetes

Case 2. A 94-year-old nursing home patient with moderate dementia has had 4 falls in the past 2 days. She had not fallen for the past year.
1. What is this an example of?
   This is a non-specific presentation of an illness.
2. How would you begin the evaluation of this problem?
   Functional assessment of patient's mobility
3. What other aspects of the functional assessment would be important in this patient?
   ADLs, medical illnesses, cognitive function, medications

Case 3. You have a new patient in the nursing home, a 78-year-old woman with moderate dementia, impaired hearing, and impaired vision.
1. Your initial approach would be
   See communicating with the demented patient.
2. How would you alter the environment to improve communication?
   See how to obtain a history.
3. How would you adjust your physical exam?
   See the physical examination of the elderly

Chapter 4: Geriatric Multisystem Syndromes

Case 1. An 82-yr-old female comes to the clinic with complaints of "nearly fainting" 3 times in the last month.

History: States that several times in past month she has had episodes when she feels like she is going to faint. The spell lasts maybe a few minutes, then she slowly feels better. If she is at home she eats something, then goes to lie down, which relieves it. She had a spell at church last Sunday and her friends insisted she come to the clinic for an evaluation.

PMH: Type 2 diabetes, osteoarthritis, hypertension, hypothyroidism, rheumatic fever as a child.

Medications: glipizide (Glucotrol XL) 10 mg PO qd, hydrochlorothiazide 25 mg qd, metoprolol (Lopressor) 100 mg qd, Synthroid 125 mg qd, naproxen (Naprosyn) 250 mg bid.
1. What part of the physical exam is appropriate?
   Complete including orthostatic blood pressures
2. Name as many possible causes and contributing factors as you can think of.
   Hypoglycemia, orthostatic hypotension secondary to BP medications, dehydration, normal changes of aging, anemia due to blood loss on NSAIDs, hypo or iatrogenic hyper thyroid, brady arrhythmia due to beta blocker, angina, cardiac valve disease, CHF, polypharmacy
3. What diagnostic tests would you order?
   EKG, glucose, CBC, BUN, creatinine, electrolytes, hemoglobin A_{1c}, TSH, fecal occult blood

Case 2. An 87-year-old man comes to your office complaining of fatigue. Patient lives in assisted living, needs help with bathing and dressing, walks with difficulty with walker, becomes SOB walking 20 feet. Feels too tired to eat. Diagnoses include COPD, CHF, Parkinson's disease. On 10 medications.

Exam shows 20-pound weight loss in past 6 months. Abdomen reveals nontender mass in left lower abdomen.

Lab tests CBC shows mild microcytic hypochromic anemia; BUN and creatinine show renal insufficiency, stool has occult blood

1. What is the most likely diagnosis?

   Cancer, probably GI

   Cancer in advanced stage

   Tests show patient has advanced colon cancer with metastasis to bone. Patient refuses treatment for the problem and starts preparing to die. He complains that the pain in his low back will not let him sleep. You determine that he is competent to make his own decisions.

2. What is your initial plan?

   Comfort measures to include:

   Start pain management—musculoskeletal pain

   For mild musculoskeletal pain, try acetaminophen or NSAIDs (with caution)

   Increase doses and start opioids as soon as needed for pain control

   Monitor closely for pain control and other symptoms

   Offer hospice

   Review advance directives

   Make sure patient is able to get his affairs in order

   Ensure that patient has someone to talk to, and feels comfortable with his caregivers

   Over the next month, the pain becomes severe and patient becomes bed bound. Because of the Parkinson disease, he is having trouble handling his secretions. He is still able to take sips of >PO liquids.

3. What is your next plan?

   Oral, personal hygiene

   Adequate opioids to avoid SOB

   Atropine or scopolamine to reduce secretions

4. What issues are likely to be the most important to this patient?

   Freedom from pain and respiratory distress

   Being kept clean

   Knowing what to expect

   Having someone he can trust

   Maintain control and dignity as much as possible

Case 3. The daughter brings her 80-year-old female with moderate Alzheimer disease for a routine check up. Her daughter reports the patient is more easily distracted, increasingly irritable, and less aware of her surroundings. Daughter is not sure how long this has been going on. She is on multiple medications for cardiac disease and Alzheimer's.

1. What part of the history would be most important?

   Complete review of systems searching for symptoms of infectious process, change in cardiac status such as MI, angina, arrhythmia, CHF, orthostasis, dehydration, bleeding or blood loss, loss of appetite or other GI symptoms, review medications for changes or missed medications, adverse reaction to med, any environmental changes, do MMSE to look for change

2. What would you look for on physical examination?

   Signs of infection, fever, clammy skin, pulmonary congestion, abdominal tenderness, cellulitis, signs of CHF, edema, arrhythmia, or signs of dehydration

3. What laboratory and diagnostic tests would you order?

EKG, CXR, urinalysis and C&S, CBC, metabolic panel, medication levels if on digoxin, TSH B$_{12}$, folate.

4. What is your differential diagnosis?

Progression of dementia versus delirium. Determine cause of delirium: change in environment, infection, any change in medication, exacerbation of heart disease such as CHF, angina, or arrhythmia.

Chapter 5: Infectious Disease

Case 1. A 96-year-old woman resides in a nursing home. She usually gets up, dresses herself, and walks to breakfast in the dining room, but today the nursing assistant reports she won't get out of bed. She is agitated, trying to hit the staff and crying out incoherently, she was incontinent of urine over night.

PMH: moderate dementia, osteoporosis, type 2 DM, CHF.

Medications: metformin (Glucophage) 500 mg PO bid, furosemide (Lasix) 20 mg PO qd, lisinopril (Zestril) 10 mg PO qd, digoxin (Lanoxin) 0.125 mg PO qod, alendronate (Fosamax) 70 mg PO q week, donepezil (Aricept) 5 mg PO qd

1. What other history or review of systems would be needed?

Pain, change in medications, any PRN medications given? change in PO intake
Review of systems to include neuro, mental status, cardiac, endocrine, musculoskeletal

2. What components of the physical exam would you perform?

Complete physical with emphasis on control of existing conditions and look for infection
Cardiac, respiratory, skin, musculoskeletal systems

3. What is your differential diagnosis?

Pneumonia, UTI, dehydration, electrolyte imbalance, acute exacerbation of CHF, hyper or hypo glycemia, medication, especially dig toxicity

4. What diagnostic tests are needed?

Glucose finger stick, CBC with differential, electrolytes, BUN, creatinine, digoxin level, urine for U/A and C&S; possibly CXR and EKG depending on physical

Case 2. A 68-year-old woman complains of diarrhea. It is soft to liquid and profuse. No nausea or vomiting. Patient was recently in the hospital for a cholecystectomy. Patient had Foley catheter during hospital stay. Was started on trimethoprim-sulfamethoxazole. Culture came back with resistant to TMP-SMZ, so was switched to Cipro. While on Cipro, she developed a pneumonia, so the Cipro was switched to Biaxin.

1. What other history or review of system would be needed?

Any change in medications or diet. Review of intake of fluids and food since diarrhea. Any abdominal pain or fever. Any odor to the stool. Review also when last large formed bowel movement was.

2. What components of the physical exam would you perform?

Abdominal and rectal, as well as cardiovascular to rule out acute changes secondary to infections. Respiratory to check for resolution of the pneumonia.

3. What is your differential diagnosis?

C *difficile*, infection versus antibiotic drug side effects

4. What diagnostic tests are needed?

CBC may reveal an elevated WBC if there is C *difficile* Stool *for* C *difficile* should be sent x 3

5. What treatment should be instituted pending diagnosis?

Adequate hydration and electrolyte replacement
Superinfections with *Clostridium difficile*—see complications of infections

Case 3. A 74-year-old female, living independently, presents with many vague complaints including: fatigue, weight loss, intermittent diarrhea, painful rash on trunk, numbness and tingling of toes, white coating in mouth. Patient's social history consists of 45 years unhappy marriage to distant husband, who died of mysterious illness in 1995 at age 80.

PE weight 108, down from 126 in past year, temporal wasting.

Rash vesicles on erythematous base in dermatome pattern on right side of trunk

Decreased reflexes to LE

White exudate that sticks to tongue in mouth, malodorous

Normal abdominal and rectal exam

1. What is your differential diagnosis?

   Herpes zoster

   Thrush

   Diarrhea

   Peripheral neuropathy

   AIDS

2. What diagnostic tests are needed?

   CBC for infection, electrolytes and BUN, for dehydration, fasting blood sugar, HIV screening, B_{12} and folate in light of neuropathy

3. What treatment would you initiate?

   Counsel regarding HIV testing and provide emotional support, refer to specialist

   Antiviral for herpes zoster

   Oral antifungal for candidiasis such as nystatin swish and swallow

   Monitor intake and output

   Pain management

Chapter 6: Dermatology

Case 1. An 86-year-old female resident of LTC facility for 2 years secondary to late stage dementia has fallen and suffered right hip fracture. She was sent to hospital for internal fixation and returned to nursing home 2 days post-op, and now has 3 x 3 cm bulla on posterior right heel. Prior to fall, she was underweight, needed assistance to ambulate, and had poor short-term memory and poor safety insight. Meds include MVI with minerals, Peri Colace, and Lovenox injection.

1. What was probable cause of right heel bulla?

   Pressure sore due to decreased mobility from impaired mobility from surgery

2. What were her risk factors for pressure ulcers pre- and post-op?

   Pre-op—age, altered nutrition and mobility

   Post-op—more limited mobility, pain, decreased alertness/cognition secondary to surgery

3. How could this heel ulcer have been prevented?

   Increased skin inspections and care, nutritional support, pressure relief of bony prominences, pain relief

4. What are basics for treatment?

   Supplement nutrition to provide adequate vitamins and minerals, extra calories and protein; provide tissue load management with repositioning and pressure relief; direct wound care to protect ulcer and avoid debridement if intact skin; adequate pain relief.

5. What are possible complications of this pressure ulcer?

   Impaired rehabilitation from fracture due to decreased mobility; wound infection/cellulitis, osteomyelitis, loss of limb

Case 2. 75-year-old blond white male, previous construction worker complains of raised lump on back of neck, which is irritated by shirt collar often, and his wife has noticed that it seems to be getting larger in color over past few months. He has no other significant medical history. Medications: Ecotrin, Lipitor, lisinopril

1. How common are skin cancers?

   Basal cell cancer most commonly seen, and Squamous cell cancer is second most common type of skin cancer

2. How does this patient follow the demographics and risk factors for skin cancer?

   See Incidence and Demographics and Risk Factors: age >40, male sex, fair skin with sun exposure

3. Does location of lesion help in assessment?

   See Risk Factors and Assessment/History: sun exposed area on back of neck

4. What diagnostic test is necessary?

   See under Assessment/Diagnostic studies: Biopsy of lesion

5. What is appropriate treatment for lesions, and what is expected outcome?

   Refer to dermatology for excision, and possibly radiation (squamous cell); resolution expected; need to monitor for new lesions

Case 3. Your 95-year-old nursing home patient has dementia and no longer ambulatory. She must be fed and she is incontinent of urine. She is obese and has diabetes mellitus, polymyalgia rheumatica, gastroesophageal reflux. Her medications arc Avandia 4 mg PO qd, prednisone 3 mg PO qd, Tylenol prn, Prilosec 20 me PO bid. The nursing assistant noticed red skin on abdomen and in perineal area when cleaning her today. You find bright red smooth macules with maceration and satellite lesions under breasts, in skin folds on abdomen and in perineal area.

1. What is your most likely diagnosis?

   Candida

2. What risk factors does she have?

   Chronic debilitation, inability to perform personal hygiene

   Diabetes

   Moisture from urine, sweat

   Obesity with redundant skin folds

   Occlusive clothing—adult diapers

   Corticosteroid use

3. What nonpharmacologic treatment would you order?

   Air exposure to affected areas

   Careful drying of skin

   Frequent changing of diapers

   Ideally weight loss, but not practical

4. What pharmacologic treatment would you order?

   Better management of diabetes

   See if you can decrease dose of prednisone

   Topical antifungal cream such as clotrimazole 1%

5. How long would it take for this to work?

   Several weeks

Chapter 7: Eyes, Ears, Nose And Throat Disorders

Case 1. 83-year-old female nursing home patient, observed to have crusting on both eyelashes in the mornings.

HPI: Patient diagnosed with Alzheimer's disease is a resident in a long-term care (LTC) facility. You are told that there have been several cases of conjunctivitis in the facility in the past week. Patient is non-verbal, but has been observed rubbing her eyes in the past few days.

PMH: Resident in LTC for several years. Her personal care is provided by nurse aides. In general good health otherwise. Under treatment for seborrheic dermatitis. No food or drug allergies.

Medication: Hydrocortisone 1% cream sparingly to affected facial area daily; multivitamin daily.

1. Which are the most likely differential diagnoses for the presenting problem?
   Conjunctivitis, blepharitis
2. Review the risk factors for the possible diagnoses.
   Conjunctivitis: acute outbreak in LTC facility, with personal care provided by staff who may be caring for others with the infection
   Blepharitis: History of seborrheic dermatitis with facial area affected
3. What further history would you obtain?
   Character of drainage, continuous or worse at morning or night
4. What key findings would you look for in the physical exam?
   Condition of conjunctiva, eyelids, and surrounding skin surfaces

Exam: Eyelids are found to be inflamed, with broken and misdirected lashes. Scaling of lids noted. Conjunctiva are mildly injected. Golden crusting is noted along lid edges; drainage is reported to be worse in the morning, staying clear through the day.

5. What treatment plan would you develop, based on these findings?
   Discuss pharmacologic and non-pharmacologic plans, including any needed staff education.
   Pharmacologic: topical ointment such as erythromycin or bacitracin ointment 1–4 x/day, depending upon severity of infection
   Nonpharmacologic: Warm soaks to remove crusts; lid hygiene bid with half and half baby shampoo and water
   With staff: review rationale for HS lid hygiene (removing bacteria which will have overgrowth through the night) which should be an ongoing part of treatment plan
6. What follow-up would you recommend?
   Maintenance of lid hygiene q HS; assess for resolution of drainage
7. Under what circumstances would you make a referral?
   Failure of infection to resolve after 1 week, or worsening of infection in the meantime, refer to Tables 7-2 and 7-5 for review

Case 2. An 82-year-old man comes to clinic accompanied by his wife. He has not been back for his routine visits for 8 months. He has no complaints, says no to every question you ask. Wife states he is driving her nuts, she thinks he is getting senile or going crazy because he has lost interest in socializing and has stopped watching TV. Chart shows patient was a construction worker. He smoked and drank heavily for many years before quitting about 15 years ago. His medical diagnoses are hypertension, osteoarthritis, and COPD; medications are atenolol (Tenormin) 50 mg PO qd, enalapril (Vasotec) 5 mg PO qd, theophylline sustained release (Theo-Dur) 100 mg PO bid, and aspirin as needed for arthritis pain.

1. What part of this history suggests hearing loss?
   Patient answer negatively to every question, denying everything, to test this rephrase a question so it requires a different answer.
   Wife thinking he is demented or mentally ill—hearing loss frequently presents as dementia or depression, loss of interest in events involving hearing
2. What risk factors for hearing loss does he have?
   Construction worker. Probable exposure to loud noises
   Aspirin ingestion
   Alcohol abuse—he drank heavily for many years
   Hypertension and COPD can contribute to hearing loss

Exam: Shows that the patient can hear sound but cannot understand many of the words.

3. What kind of hearing loss does this suggest?
   Sensory neural
4. Would a referral for a hearing aid be appropriate for this kind of hearing loss?
   Yes, can be effective for sensorineural hearing loss, may improve quality of life

Appendix A

Case 3. 65-year-old female presents with complaint of "a cold." States symptoms have been present for 6 days and include a "runny nose, cough, and just feel miserable." Has gotten worse in past 2 days. Gives history of "Allergies to pollen." No regular medications; has been taking ibuprofen and pseudo-ephedrine to control symptoms.

Exam: Patient appears mildly ill but not in distress; temp 100.2 oral; pulse 100, resp. 20, mouth breathing, but no acute respiratory distress. Ears: canals clear, TMs bilaterally dull and retracted, nasal mucosa swollen, red, with green discharge. Palpable enlarged lymph nodes tender to palpation. Chest is clear, Heart normal

1. What further history would you like?

   Ear symptoms, throat symptoms, characteristic of cough, nasal drainage, smell or taste changes; visual changes, redness or swelling of face indicating cellulitis or other severe infection; past history of allergies, sinus infections, medication allergies

2. What else is included in your physical exam?

   Facial exam, looking for edema, tenderness over sinuses, mouth, looking for dental infections, throat for purulent drainage

3. What is your diagnosis?

   Sinusitis

4. What would you do for the patient on this visit?

   Nonpharmacologic treatment—rest, and emphasize fluids, and humidification

   Prescribe an oral antibiotic: amoxicillin is first choice, followed by quinolones, cephalosporins or macrolides

   A non-sedating antihistamine may be indicated if seasonal allergies are a factor

   Consider codeine if severe night cough

   Add short course of nasal steroids if allergies an issue.

   Change pain medication to acetaminophen, as ibuprofen has been reported to be associated with hypertension.

   Schedule follow-up call in 4 days to report progress, sooner if increased pain or associated dyspnea or increased fever.

Chapter 8: Respiratory Disorders

Case 1. A 70-year-old, male comes to clinic with productive cough, shortness of breath. Denies fever, upper respiratory symptoms. Patient is a retired construction worker with history of asthma.

HPI: Medications include asthma medications: Alupent prn, Serevent 2 puffs bid, triamcinolone (Azmacort) 2 puffs bid, and Claritin prn allergies.

1. What additional history would you like?

   How much is he using his Alupent inhaler?

   How much is he coughing? What is he bringing up? Any SOB or wheezing?

Physical Exam: Vital signs stable. No acute respiratory distress, lungs without wheezes or rales (crackles), breath sounds are decreased bilaterally with prolonged expiration. Heart rate regular. Peak flow rate 300, his baseline is 350.

2. What is your assessment?

   Mild exacerbation of asthma, no evidence of infection

3. What do you think is happening?

   Forgetting to take inhalers or not using correctly

   Had a URI, exposure to his allergy trigger, exposure to environmental pollutants

   Any change in medication

4. What is your initial plan?

   Make sure he is using his inhalers correctly with spacer if needed

   Have patient use Alupent inhaler on regular basis 3–4 times a day until better.

Case 2. A 75-year-old female with complaints of productive cough, fever, chills, chest discomfort and chest congestion; fatigue and headache for 3 days.

PMH: Bronchitis. Medications: Robitussin DM and Tylenol extra strength for headache. Allergic to penicillin.

1. What additional history would you ask?

   History of bronchitis, any history of pneumonia

   Color, amount of sputum, ability to mobilize sputum

   Fluid intake; is cough keeping her awake at night

Exam: Patient appears ill; temp 100.8, tachypnea with exertion, skin warm to touch; ENT exam normal; chest splinting with fremitus and rales (crackles) in right lower lobe.

2. What diagnostic tests will you order?

   CXR, CBC with differential, pulse oximetry

3. What are the most likely diagnoses?

   The most likely differential to consider: Pneumonia, sinusitis, PE

   Pneumonia most likely due to bacteria. Streptococcus pneumoniae is the most common. Next in frequency are *Mycoplasma pneumoniae*, *Chlamydia*, and *Legionella sp*. Not likely to be caused by a Gram neg. bacilli because she is not severely ill

4. Based on your current impression, what treatment will you order?

   Best first choice is a macrolide such as clarithromycin (Biaxin) or azithromycin (Zithromax), good also because of patient's allergy to penicillin. Doxycycline would also be an acceptable choice. Fluoroquinolone not as good a choice because of low probability of gram negative bacteria

   Stop Robitussin DM use Robitussin with codeine for cough suppression, expectorant, and analgesic effect.

Case 3. A 67-year-old male complains of shortness of breath, both at rest and on exertion. Unable to perform normal activities without becoming "winded." Notes occasional cough.

PMH: hypertension. Former smoker—$1^1/_2$ ppd x 40 years. Medications: OTC cough medicine, enalapril (Vasotec) 5 mg qd for hypertension

1. What additional history would you ask?

   Timing of the worsening of the SOB, define cough in regard to daily, with activity only, with or without productive component, any hemoptysis history, number of episodes of URI

   Any peripheral edema, chest pain or pressure

   Amount of exercise, fluid intake

Exam: Vital signs—B/P 152/90; no tachypnea; ENT—normal findings; chest—increased AP diameter, hyperresonance on percussion, decreased expansion on respiration, no abnormal breath sounds; extremities—no edema, no nail clubbing

2. What diagnostic tests would you order?

   Do peak flow rate in office

   Diagnostic testing: CXR, CBC, chemistries, EKG, pulse oximetry

3. What is your differential diagnosis?

   Emphysema, COPD, CHF, Cancer, ACE inhibitor cough

4. What would you do for this patient on this visit?

   Ipratropium bromide (Atrovent) inhaler 2 inh qid

   Ensure adequate hydration

   This patient should have follow-up 1–2 weeks.

Chapter 9: Cardiovascular Disorders

Case 1. 68-year-old male is following up after consultation with an orthopedist for a recent fractured thumb. Orthopedist noted that the patient had a blood pressure of 166/104.

PMH: Chart shows that the patient had, at the last office visit, BP 144/92. Laboratory work was ordered. Review of chart shows labile blood pressure readings for the prior two years, which decreased after weight loss undertaken to treat hyperlipidemia. States he follows low salt, low fat diet and exercises 2–3 times a week. Non-smoker.

Medications include Lipitor 10 mg qd; ibuprofen (Motrin) 400 mg PO tid

FH: Diabetes type 2 and CAD

1. What cardiac risk factors does he have?
   Male sex
   Previous readings of high blood pressure
   Hyperlipidemia
   Family history of CAD
   Family history of DM

Lab findings on previous visits:

BUN 22	Cholesterol 230
Creatinine 0.8	Triglycerides 250
Na+ 136	LDL 148
K+ 4.0	HDL 32
Glucose 162	

2. What additional problem does this lab identify? Is this a significant coronary risk factor?
   Diabetes—yes

3. Is his hyperlipidemia well controlled?
   No, cholesterol is high, triglycerides are high, LDL (bad cholesterol) is high, HDL (good cholesterol) is low

Physical: Vital signs current visit: BP 160/102; pulse 98; resp 16; weight 205 lbs. height 5'9"
Cardiac: RRR, no murmur, no carotid bruits or pedal edema, no renal bruits
Resp: vesicular sounds throughout all lung fields
Funduscopic: Clear disc, obvious arteriolar narrowing with focal areas of attenuation
UA: trace glucose and protein
ECG sinus rhythm

4. What is the significance of these findings?
   Blood pressure elevated
   BP in orthopedist's office could have been elevated due to acute illness/pain. However you have two elevated readings which defines hypertension
   Urinalysis and funduscopic exam shows target organ damage
   Protein in urine may be from hypertension or diabetes
   Height and weight show patient is overweight

5. What stage hypertension does he have?
   Stage 2 hypertension with target organ damage

6. How would you manage this patient's hypertension? List steps
   Nonpharmacologic: Reinforce diet, obviously not following diet, needs low fat, low sodium and diabetic diet
   Pharmacologic: Discontinue ibuprofen
   Start on medication
   Would not start on diuretic or beta blocker because of Compelling Indication of diabetes with proteinuria
   Start on ACE inhibitor

Case 2. 73-yr-old white female complains of increasing shortness of breath and cough productive of frothy sputum over the last 24 hours. She has had trouble sleeping due to a cough she attributes to allergies, and has felt tired for the past 3 months. Two days ago she celebrated 73rd birthday.

PMH: Two years ago she had an episode of weakness and dizziness. At that time, her EKG showed changes indicative of a mild MI. She was placed on atenolol (Tenormin) 100 mg and has remained stable. Has mild hypertension, hyperlipidemia; menopause 10 yrs ago. Smoking history 20 years $1/2$ pack day; quit 5 years ago.

Lab: chest x-ray showing mild cardiomegaly, otherwise unremarkable. An echocardiogram showing EF 40%, moderate left ventricular dysfunction.

1. What is the most likely diagnosis?

   CHF

2. What factor(s) most likely to have precipitated this?

   Excess salt intake at birthday dinner—fluid overload, stress

3. What is the most likely the basic cause(s)?

   Myocardial damage

   Contributing—hypertension causing pressure overload over time.

4. What over the counter drugs should you specifically ask about?

   NSAIDs

Exam: BP 142/94, Pulse: 88; Resp: 22; Temp: 98.8; Wt: 180

Ht: 5'4" General Appearance: Appears mildly short of breath

Resp: Tachypnea, occasion non-productive cough, bi-basilar rales (crackles)

Extremities: 2+ edema extending $1/2$ way up lower legs

5. What other physical exam do you need to do and what would you look for?

   Cardiac—arrhythmias, murmur, S3, JVD

   Abdomen—ascites

   Extremities—circulation, cyanosis

Medications: Atenolol (Tenormin) 100 mg PO qd, , lovastatin (Mevacor) 20 mg qd, Aspirin 81 mg qd

6. What medications would you start today?

   Diuretic—furosemide (Lasix) 20 mg PO qd

   ACE Inhibitor—lisinopril (Zestril) 5 mg PO qd

7. What lab work would you need to check before starting these medications?

   Comprehensive lab—renal function, potassium level

8. What adverse reactions would you monitor for?

   Lasix—orthostatic hypotension, dizziness, weakness, GI upset

   Lisinopril—hyperkalemia, renal impairment, cough

Case 3. A 70-year-old Caucasian female presents for routine followup of lipids.

PMH: Her last visit she was started on a low saturated fat diet. Medical history significant for osteoporosis and hypercholesteremia. Ex-smoker with 15 pack years, quit 7 years ago. Occasional ETOH with glass of wine once a week.

Medications: Fosamax 10 mg qd; calcium and vitamin D supplements

Exam: General appearance: alert oriented, NAD; Wt. 130lbs; Height 5'5"

BP 138/82

Cardiac: RRR, no murmurs; no edema, peripheral pulses present

Resp: Vesicular breath sounds throughout all lung fields

Abdomen: soft, no hepatosplenomegaly or masses

Labs:	Last Visit	This Visit
Cholesterol, total	275	230
Triglycerides	118	104
HDL	62	56
LDL	189	140

Basic metabolic, CBC, and LFTs unremarkable

1. What is your assessment?
   Lipid panel improved significantly on lipid lowering diet in 2 months
   Borderline high blood cholesterol
   HDL remains good
   LDL borderline high risk
   No signs of coronary artery disease
2. What cardiac risk factors does this patient have?
   Hyperlipidemia
   Smoking history
   Age
3. What other risk factors should you assess?
   Sedentary life style
   Other cardiac risk factors
   Diabetes
   Family history
   History of smoking
   Stress
   Alcohol
4. What is your plan?
   Nonpharmacologic intervention exercise weight bearing for osteoporosis and to increase HDL. Continue present diet for total of 6 months before considering medications, pharmacologic treatment considered controversial in this age group.

Chapter 10: Gastrointestinal Disorders

Case 1. A 68-year-old male presents to your clinic with complaints of burning, epigastric pain after meals associated with nausea, especially when he lies down after eating. He has lost 15 lbs over the past month that he attributes to poor appetite.

HPI: The patient is a recovering alcoholic. He stopped drinking 8 months ago and has been going to AA meetings on a regular basis. The patient is also a heavy smoker and has frequent episodes of bronchitis. He continues to smoke but has cut back significantly. His past medical history includes treatment for a gastric ulcer 1 yr ago. He is not taking any medication.

1. What other questions would you ask this patient?
   Any fevers or night sweats?
   Any symptoms of cough, heartburn or regurgitation, vomiting, hematemesis, melena, rectal bleeding, or change in bowel pattern?
   Does the pain radiate anywhere; chest, back, shoulder, or to the RUQ/LUQ of the abdomen?
   Foods that may exacerbate symptoms; fatty meals, acidic foods
   NSAID use?
   What treatment did he receive for the gastric ulcer? Was he re-evaluated after treatment?
   Is there a past history of pancreatitis in this patient with history of alcoholism?

Exam: Vital signs are stable. No lymphadenopathy. Heart and lung exams are normal. Abdomen is soft, non-tender, normal bowel sounds, no hepatosplenomegaly, no masses, no abdominal bruits. Rectal exam is normal with guaiac negative stools.

2. What laboratory tests would you order?
   CBC with differential, electrolytes, BUN/CR, calcium, liver function tests, amylase and lipase
3. What other studies would you order?
   The patient has weight loss with history of gastric ulcer, alcoholism, and heavy tobacco use. A non-healing or recurrent gastric ulcer, as well as gastric cancer in this patient should be ruled out. He should have an upper endoscopy.

4. What treatment would you provide?

Referral to a gastroenterologist

Case 2. A 72-year-old male with HTN is in your office for a follow-up visit. He complains of being constipated.

HPI: The patient states that he's always had a regular bowel movement every morning. For the past month, bowel movements occur every 4 to 5 days only after he uses a laxative. Medications include a calcium channel blocker and one aspirin a day.

1. Is a new onset of constipation in a 72-year-old concerning? Or is this a normal change related to the aging process?

Constipation is more common in the elderly due to decreased colonic motility in combination with poor dietary habits and medication side effects, however any new onset of constipation would be concerning, as it could mean cancer of the colon

2. What other history would you obtain?

Character of stool, straining, incomplete evacuation, time to complete BM, manual digitations, incontinence, hemorrhoids, or other anorectal disorders?

Fevers, night sweats, anorexia, weight loss, nausea, vomiting, abdominal pain, diarrhea, melena, rectal bleeding?

Dietary intake of fiber and fluids?

Physical activity?

Change in environment?

How long has he been taking his current medications? Name and dose of laxatives?

Is there a family history of colon cancer?

Has the patient ever had a flexible sigmoidoscopy for colon cancer screening?

Exam: The patient is alert and oriented x 3. Blood pressure and other vital signs are normal. His abdomen is mildly distended but non-tender. Bowel sounds are present in all quadrants. No enlarged liver or spleen. No bruises. Rectal exam is normal, no impacted stool. The remainder of his examination is normal.

3. What laboratory tests would you order?

CBC with differential, electrolytes, calcium, BUN/CR, glucose, LFTs, alkaline phosphatase (evaluate for metastasis or increased alk phos with cancer), thyroid function tests

Stool guaiac x 3 (for 3 days prior to and during collection: no ASA, red meat, vitamin C, or raw vegetables).

4. What other studies would you order?

Flat plate and upright of the abdomen

Refer for colonoscopy to rule out cancer

5. What treatment would you provide?

Increased fiber intake with bran supplement added to diet, or with using bulk forming agents such as Metamucil or Citrucel

Increased fluid intake to 1.5–2 liters/day

Bowel training program

Regular physical activity

Re-evaluate the use of calcium channel blocker for HTN management, especially if symptoms occurred with the initiation of this medication and laboratory and diagnostic data is within normal limits.

Case 3. A 62-year-old, obese white female presents with right upper quadrant pain, nausea, and vomiting. The onset of pain was sudden and occurred after eating at a restaurant. She has had similar episodes in the past but not as severe.

1. What additional history would you like?

Quality and duration of pain, radiation of pain to chest, shoulder, back, or other area of the abdomen.

Fever, cough, heartburn, jaundice, hematemesis, diarrhea, melena, rectal bleeding
What foods precipitate symptoms? ETOH intake, NSAID use?
History of gallstones?

Exam: Temp is 99.5, with remaining vital signs normal. Abdomen is soft. Right upper quadrant pain increases when palpating the right upper quadrant during inspiration and there is localized guarding. There is no rebound tenderness. Bowel sounds are normal. No hepatosplenomegaly. There are no abdominal bruits. Rectal exam is normal with guaiac negative stool. The remainder of her exam is normal.

2. What diagnostic tests would you order?

   CBC with differential, electrolytes, BUN/CR, liver function tests, amylase and Lipase, abdominal ultrasound.

3. What is the most likely differential?

   Biliary colic, cholecystitis, pancreatitis, hepatitis, PUD, acute gastroenteritis

4. How would you treat her?

   Prompt surgical evaluation

Chapter 11: Renal And Urologic Disorders

Case 1. Your 94-year-old, demented female patient returned home from the hospital for hip surgery with a Foley catheter. She complains of hip pain but not low back or pain or suprapubic tenderness. She has been incontinent of bowel and bladder for many years. She requires total care. Patient is afebrile.

1. What lab tests would you order?

   CBC (r/o anemia-post surgical blood loss vs. due to CRF) Comprehensive metabolic—BUN, creatinine, urinalysis

   You do not order a urine C&S. Patient has risk factors for asymptomatic bacteruria and has no symptoms or signs of UTI

Lab: Her creatinine is 1.2 and her BUN is 36.
Urinalysis shows many bacteria, no WBCs

2. How do you interpret this lab work?

   They are high but may demonstrate normal changes of aging

   Urinalysis shows colonization but not infection due to lack of WBCs

   No immediate action required except to ensure adequate hydration

3. What are your initial interventions?

   You remove the Foley catheter.

   Assure adequate hydration.

   Review hygiene measures with nursing assistants.

Lab: The nurse obtains a urine culture and C&S without your order. It shows 10,000 colonies each of 3 microorganisms, which are sensitive to ciprofloxin, sulfa/trimethoprim, and Levaquin.

4. Would you treat the patient with an antibiotic?

   No, three organisms is indicative of colonization, not infection

5. What would the urinalysis show if the patient did have a UTI?

   Leukocyte esterase might be positive

   Urine would have WBCs and bacteria

   There would be minimal epithelial cells.

6. What are the possible complications of a UTI in this patient?

   Urosepsis

   Pyelonephritis

Case 2. When talking to your 74-year-old female patient you discover that she has stopped going downstairs for meals in her senior apartment building. She has also stopped going on the trips and does not have enough groceries. She denies any pain or fatigue. Seems reluctant to talk about it. Admits to urinary frequency.

History: Upon questioning, patient is afraid she might not make it to the bathroom in time, so has restricted her activities. Urinates q 1–2 hours so she won't be incontinent. Still has occasional accidents in which she looses a large amount of urine.

1. What is the significance of loss of a large amount of urine?
   Indicates urge incontinence
2. What risk factors would you inquire about?
   Estrogen deficiency
   Multiparity
   Diseases such as diabetes, MS, CVA
   Mobility
   Medications such as diuretics
3. What medications can contribute to incontinence?
   Anticholinergics
   Tricyclics
   Antispasmodics
   Opioids, beta agonists
   Calcium channel blockers
   Diuretics
   Caffeine
   Psychotropics
   Phenothiazines
   Antiparkinsonian agents
   Sedative/hypnotics
   ACE inhibitors
4. What treatment is effective for her type of incontinence?
   Bladder retraining
   Timed voiding
   Prompted voiding
   Kegels exercises
   Prevent constipation
5. What medications would you consider?
   Oxybutynin (Ditropan)
   Tolterodine (Detrol
   Hyoscyamine (Levsin)
   Propantheline (Pro-Banthine)
   Dicyclomine (Bentyl)

Case 3. An 83-year-old man has been taking ibuprofen for 20 years for DJD. He also has hypertension for which he takes hydrochlorothiazide. His blood pressure today is 160/94. He states that is what it usually is and that is fine with him. Routine screening lab shows BUN of 64 and creatinine of 1.8.

1. What is your initial assessment?
   Renal insufficiency, hypertension, not controlled. Renal insufficiency may be from long standing hypertension, exacerbated by NSAIDs
2. What other lab tests would you order? What would you look for?
   Urinalysis—proteinuria and urinary sediment
   Sodium level may be normal or low
   Potassium may be elevated

Normochromic normocytic anemia
3. Which diuretic is most effective in patients with renal insufficiency?
   Furosemide not HCTZ
4. What complications should you monitor for?
   Anemia
   CHF
   Uremia
   Infections
   Bleeding
   Death

Chapter 12: Gynecologic Disorders

Case 1. A 69-year-old female comes to your office for her annual physical exam. On exam, you note a lump in the upper outer aspect of the right breast. The lump is about 1 cm, mobile, firm, with regular borders. There is no dimpling, retraction or other breast or chest wall lesions. There is no tenderness. There is no adenopathy. The remainder of the physical exam is normal. She was not aware of this lump or other changes in her breasts. However, she does not perform regular self-breast exam. Her last mammogram was 3 years ago and last Pap smear was 1 year ago.

Breast History: The patient has no prior history of breast cancer or breast biopsies. Menarche: age 9. The patient is gravida 1, para 1, miscarriages/ abortions 0. Age at first full-term pregnancy: 36. Age at Menopause: 54. Hormones: HRT (Prempro): 10 yr

Past Medical History: Hypercholesterolemia, osteopenia

Medications: Prempro, atorvastatin (Lipitor) 20 mg, multivitamin, calcium

Habits: Diet: Generally follows low fat diet; Exercise: walks 3 times a week for $^1/_2$ hour; Alcohol: 3–4 drinks/week; Tobacco: none

1. Based on the history and physical, what is your recommendation regarding diagnostic evaluation of the breast lump?
   Since the patient has a palpable mass on clinical breast exam, a diagnostic mammogram should be ordered. This test includes an ultrasound evaluation to determine if the lesion is solid or cystic.
2. The mammogram shows a small mass in the upper outer quadrant of the right breast. The sonogram shows a cystic lesion with a small solid component in the area of the palpable mass. What would be your next recommendation for follow-up of this mass?
   Refer to a surgeon for further evaluation. Although cysts are possible in women on hormone replacement therapy, large cysts are generally uncommon in post-menopausal women. Further, this lesion does not have the classic appearance of a simple cyst on ultrasound. The cyst may be secondary to obstruction of a duct by a malignant lesion. A complex mass that has a solid component within the cyst requires biopsy.
3. What aspects of Mrs. Jones' history would be considered risk factors in assessing her risk of breast cancer?
   Age: There is an increased incidence of breast cancer in women over age 50
   Menarche age 9: Early age of menarche is associated with increased risk of breast cancer. Some studies suggest that hormone levels may be higher throughout reproductive years in women with early menarche. The cumulative exposure to higher levels of estrogen may be associated with increased risk of developing breast cancer.
   First childbirth after age 35: The first pregnancy is associated with changes in the breast epithelium and properties of breast cells. The later the age of first pregnancy, the more likely that DNA mistakes have occurred that will be propagated during pregnancy.
   Use of Hormone replacement therapy. Possibly, but remains controversial

Case 2. A 70-year-old female comes to the clinic because she thinks she is shrinking. She is 5'2", weighs 98 pounds, has smoked for 30 years, has COPD. Upon questioning, admits to having difficulty holding her urine due to frequency and urgency. She wears pads when she goes out, but she doesn't go out much because she is embarrassed.

1. What consequences of menopause does she have?
   Probable osteoporosis, vaginal atrophy with urge incontinence
2. What other consequence would you evaluate her for?
   Cardiovascular disease
3. What physical exam is indicated?
   Pelvic exam
   Cardiac exam
   Musculoskeletal exam
4. What diagnostic tests would you order?
   Routine lab optional
   Lipid profile for hyperlipidemia
   Bone densitometry (DXA scan) for osteoporosis
5. What is the single most important thing she can do to improve her health?
   Stop smoking
6. The pelvic exam shows moderate vaginal atrophy. How would you manage the vaginal atrophy?
   Vaginal Premarin or HRT

Case 3. A 78-year-old healthy female has a routine Pap results of CIN II
1. What does the CIN II mean?
   Moderate dysplasia of 2/3 of lining to full thickness
2. What counseling would you give when you told her about the results?
   This is a precancerous condition
3. What would your actions be?
   Refer all abnormal Paps to GYN
4. What would her life expectancy be if she were not treated?
   Cancer becomes invasive, and patient dies in 3–5 years
5. What followup would the patient need?
   Seek followup. Repeat cytology every 3–4 months for the first year then every 6 months for the next year then annually once a pattern of normal reading have been established

Chapter 13: Male Reproductive System Disorders

Case 1. An 83-year-old man complains of urinary hesitancy, dribbling, urinary frequency of small amounts, nocturia x 4/night. This has been gradually getting worse of past few months.
1. What is the most likely diagnosis?
   BPH, classic symptoms
   Not a UTI, no dysuria, gradual onset
   Still have to rule out prostate cancer
2. What physical exam is required?
   DRE, abdomen
3. If the symptoms are not troublesome what is the usual approach?
   Watchful waiting
4. What symptoms would require referral for treatment?
   Urinary retention, recurrent UTIs, hematuria, bladder stone, or renal insufficiency
5. What nonpharmacologic treatment may be helpful?
   Avoid medications known to worsen symptoms
   Avoid foods and caffeine and alcohol that can cause retention
   Avoid fluids at bedtime to lessen sleep interruption

6. Which medication would you consider starting the patient on? What are their main disadvantages?
   Alpha blockers: terazosin doxazosin: orthostatic hypotension
   Tamsulosin (Flomax): less risk of orthostatic hypotension
   5 alpha reductase inhibitor finasteride (Proscar): takes 6 months to take effect

Case 2. A 78-year-old black old man comes to you feeling poorly. He complains of fatigue and low back pain which has been gradually increasing for the past few months. He has had urinary symptoms which he attributed to BPH for the past 6 years, gradually worsening so that he is now having hesitancy, dribbling, and a feeling of not emptying his bladder completely. He has never sought treatment for the BPH symptoms because he thought it was an inevitable consequence of aging.
PMH: 50 packs per year smoking, COPD, osteoarthritis, hypertension, and hyperlipidemia. Medications: Combivent inhaler, Tylenol PRN pain, hydrochlorothiazide 25 mg PO qd, atorvastatin (Lipitor) 40 mg PO qd.

1. What do his urinary symptoms indicate?
   Symptoms are obstructive, could have urinary retention
2. What are the most likely possibilities for a differential diagnosis?
   BPH and prostate cancer
3. What lab work would you order?
   DRE—look for nodules, hardness
   Renal functions to assess damage to kidneys
   UA C&S to rule out hematuria, glycosuria or infection
   PSA
4. Which would be most useful to decide between the differential?
   PSA; DRE if shows hard nodule, but the cancer may not be accessible to DRE
5. What risk factors does he have?
   Race and age
6. What would you do?
   Refer to urologist
7. What follow-up is required?
   Monitor PSA

Case 3. A 68-year-old man comes to your office with the complaint of insomnia. Says he is having some problems with his wife. She is not too happy with him. Patient seems reluctant to say what is really bothering him

1. How would you approach this situation?
   Maintain an open, trustworthy, and non-judgmental approach
   Openly ask about sex. Is he having sexual relations with his wife, is it satisfactory to both of them.
   Ask specifically about his sexual function
2. What normal changes of aging affect sexual function?
   Slowed arousal, erections less firm, shorter lasting, decreased forcefulness at ejaculation, longer interval to achieve subsequent erection.

History: Patient tells you he has a gradual loss of the ability to maintain an erection for the past year or so. His wife is upset about this and has been nagging him to do something about it. The problem became worse recently, after an argument with his wife.

3. Is this ED psychological or organic?
   Probably both—gradual onset—organic, fight with wife—psychological

PMH: Patient has hypertension, diabetes, lipid disorder, osteoarthritis

4. How do these diseases affect ED?
   Hypertension—many medications can cause ED, contributes to vascular disorder
   Diabetes leads to macrovascular changes which cause decreased circulation to penis and decreased erections.

Lipid disorder contributes to vascular disorder

Arthritis causes pain which contributes to ED.

5. What would be your initial approach?

Counseling to reassure patient, discuss relationship with wife

Optimal management of diabetes

Check hypertension medications to see if you can change to one less likely to cause ED

Chapter 14: Musculoskeletal Disorders

Case 1. A thin, petite 75-year-old Asian woman comes to clinic for sudden onset of thoracic back pain 2 days ago when she coughed.

1. What pertinent history is it important to ask?

Respiratory symptoms, any other joint pain, associated symptoms, any history of malignancy

Risk factors for osteoporosis—calcium, vitamin D, protein intake

Weight bearing exercise, smoker, alcohol

Family history of osteoporosis

2. What would you expect to find on PE?

Point tenderness over thoracic spine, pain with deep respiration, kyphosis

Lateral thoracic-spine x-ray shows wedging of vertebral body

3. How would you treat this patient?

Pain relievers, start with mild, may need opioid but use with caution

Miacalcin nasal spray since patient has osteoporosis (has the risk factors, plus compression fracture is caused by osteoporosis)

4. How soon should the pain be relieved?

6 weeks

5. What follow-up?

Monitor for resolution of pain, respiratory problems due to not taking deep breaths.

Patient should have DXA scan to assess severity of osteoporosis

Case 2. A 68-year-old woman complains of hip and knee pain for many years. She is overweight and unable to walk more than a half block because of pain. She spends her day in a recliner eating snacks and watching television. She has become incontinent because she cannot make it to the toilet on time. Every once in a while she thinks her knee is going to give out from under her. She notes loud cracking noises when she stands up. Her knees are enlarged with decreased ROM.

1. What history would you expect?

Gradual, progressive onset of joint pain over years

Stiffness in morning, lasting less than $1/_2$ hour

Pain worse with activity, relieved by rest

2. Which of her symptoms are indicative of advanced disease?

Unable to walk more than $1/_2$ block because of pain

Every once in a while she thinks her knee is going to give out from under her.

Her knees are enlarged with decreased ROM

3. What is the most likely diagnosis?

Osteoarthritis

4. What nonpharmacologic treatment would you institute?

Physical activity/therapy is the cornerstone of treatment in the elderly

Occupational therapy

Social support

Help with daily activities may be needed

Arthritis self-help and water aquatics courses

Ambulation aids (canes, braces, walkers)

Weight loss programs

Glucosamine, chondroitin may be of benefit
Heat/cold to affected joint
5. What pharmacologic treatment would you order?
Simple analgesics (acetaminophen up to 4000 mg/day in divided doses is first-line therapy)
Topical analgesic creams such as capsaicin 0.025% bid to tid
NSAIDs alone or combined with analgesics (ibuprofen up to 2400 mg/day in divided doses, naproxen sodium up to 1000 mg/day in divided doses, others)
Selective COX-2 inhibitors (Celecoxib 100–200 mg/day)
6. What lab tests must be monitored if the patient is placed on a NSAID?
Renal function
7. When should you refer?
Patients with functional impairment (e.g., inability to perform normal activities of daily living) and with moderate to severe pain should be considered for joint replacement

Case 3. A 78-year-old man complains of low back pain (LBP) for past 5 days. Pain is in his lower lumbar area radiating into the left buttock. Pain is worse when sitting up in hard chair; he has not been able to go out to the park and play checkers with his friends.
PMH: Has had episodes of LBP for past 5 years. Patient worked as a truck driver, delivering packages before he retired. Has not been active recently due to COPD from smoking, gets SOB easily and cannot walk long distances.
1. What risk factors does he have for low back pain?
Physical deconditioning, poor body mechanics; cigarette smoking
2. What symptoms would prompt an emergency referral?
Bilateral leg weakness, bladder and bowel incontinence seen with large central disk herniation
3. What simple physical maneuver will be the most useful?
Straight leg raising
4. What is your most likely diagnosis?
Sciatica, (likely related to either lumbosacral strain or degenerative changes of the lumbar spine)
5. If patient is compliant with therapy, how soon can he expect to have pain resolve?
4–6 weeks

Chapter 15: Neurological Disorders

Case 1. A 72-year-old female with 3 falls in the last 2 months without serious injury. Reports difficulty getting out of chair. She feels stiff and slow. Has tremor at rest. She is otherwise healthy without significant past medical history. She takes 2 Tylenol a day for aches.
1. What other history is needed?
History surrounding the falls
Neuro for focal neuro deficits, other changes
Musculoskeletal problems
Medications
2. What assessment tools would you use?
MMSE for cognitive changes. GDS for depression. Get up and go test for mobility
3. What part of the neurologic exam should be normal?
Sensory motor, cranial nerves, reflexes
4. What abnormalities do you expect to find on neuro exam?
Rigidity, difficulty initiating movement, shuffling gait, stooped posture, cogwheeling, tremor, fixed facial expression
5. What is your most likely diagnosis?
Parkinson's disease

Case 2. A 66-year-old male presents in office for follow-up after evaluation in the emergency department for left hemiparesis lasting 30 minutes. Reported negative head CT, chemistry panel, CBC and toxicology screen. History of "borderline" hypertension. No medications except over the counter ibuprofen.

1. What was the event he had?

   Probable TIA

2. What other history do you want to obtain?

   Precipitating events, other neurologic symptoms, cardiovascular symptoms, cardiovascular risk factors, head trauma, alcohol or illicit drug use, family history of neurologic disorders and cardiovascular disease

3. What physical findings might you expect?

   May find elevated blood pressure, carotid bruit, normal neuro and cardiac exam

4. What further diagnostic tests would be indicated?

   EKG, carotid Doppler studies

5. How will you initially manage this patient?

   Start patient on aspirin 325 mg PO qd

   Counseling regarding cardiovascular risk reduction and antiplatelet therapy, alcohol use, and use of over the counter medications

Case 3. A 78-year-old female with left side headache for 2 days, no relief with 1000 mg acetaminophen every 6 hours. History of headaches since age 16. Past medical history significant for hypertension controlled with Atenolol 25 mg a day.

1. What other history is important?

   Pattern of headaches, change in headaches, neuro deficits, precipitating events, facial tenderness, rash, review of systems for other HEENT symptoms

2. What systems will you examine?

   Vital signs, HEENT, neuro

3. What diagnostic testing?

   ESR, Consider brain CT if change in headache or focal neuro exam

4. What is your differential diagnosis?

   GCA, H. Zoster, sinusitis, tension or migraine headache, trigeminal neuralgia

Chapter 16: Hematologic Disorders

Case 1. An 83-year-old white male with a chief complaint of fatigue for the past few months, which is gradually getting worse. He now is too tired to walk to the dining room in his assisted living residence.

PMH: Patient has hypertension, history of PUD with GI bleed, smoker, depression; hyperlipidemia, rheumatoid arthritis, chronic hepatitis C, renal insufficiency.

Current medications: paroxetine (Paxil) 40 mg OD; atorvastatin (Lipitor) 20 mg OD, naproxen (Naprosyn) 250 mg PO bid, amlodipine (Norvasc) 5 mg qd, omeprazole (Prilosec), and lisinopril (Zestril) 10 mg.

PE: BP 164/84; some pallor; conjunctive slightly pale

1. What types of anemia is this patient at risk for? What puts him at risk?

   Anemia of chronic disease—hepatitic C, rheumatoid arthritis

   Iron deficiency—GI bleed due to PUD, naproxen

   Anemia secondary to renal failure

Lab: CBC done one month ago, results: RBC 3.34, Hgb 10.6, Hct 31.8, MCV 95.5, MCHC 34.5, RBC morphology normal.

2. How would you classify/describe this anemia?

   Mild normocytic normochromic anemia

3. Does the lab work tell you which kind of anemia he has?
   No, Rules out iron deficiency, would be microcytic, microchromic
   Anemia of renal disease and post hemorrhagic still possibilities
4. What additional tests are needed?
   Comprehensive metabolic profile: glucose 96, BUN 46, creatinine. 1.6, albumin 3.0, total
   protein low normal at 6.2, otherwise WNL;
   Iron Studies: FE 60 (normal), TIBC 335 (normal), ferritin 37 (normal), B_{12} and folate levels
   were normal; stool guaiac for occult blood negative.
5. What is your diagnosis?
   Anemia of chronic disease
6. What treatment do you recommend?
   Optimal treatment of concurrent illnesses, no specific treatment for the anemia
7. Will an iron supplement be helpful? Why?
   Iron supplement is not helpful because the underlying defect is not iron deficiency, and could
   be harmful.

Case 2. An 88-year-old African American female is noted to have anemia on routine screening.
Last CBC was done a year ago and her H&H were 11 and 34. Patient is wheelchair bound; lives in
nursing home, a picky eater, likes sweets, eats 1–2 servings of fruit/vegetables daily. Patient recently
had an acute exacerbation of her COPD and was treated with prednisone PO for 2 weeks. Patient
was noted to have diarrhea last week.
PMH: diabetes mellitus, osteoarthritis, COPD, aortic stenosis, CHF, constipation
Medications: metformin (Glucophage) 500 mg bid, nabumetone (Relafen) 500 PO bid, Combivent
inhaler, furosemide (Lasix) 40 mg, Senokot qd
CBC: hemoglobin 9.6, hematocrit 28.9, MCV 80
Iron studies: Ferritin low with increased TIBC
1. Classify/describe the anemia
   Anemia is microcytic hypochromic
2. What anemias present as microcytic hypochromic?
   Iron deficiency anemia
PE: Pulse is 100, 20; BP 130/80 Cardiac exam shows tachycardia, murmur of atrial stenosis. Abdo-
men diffusely tender. Lungs distant lung sounds. Peripheral neuropathy present, 2 plus pedal edema
3. What do you learn from the physical exam?
   Tachycardia could have many causes—CHF, COPD, anemia
   Murmur confirms aortic stenosis. Lung sounds indicative of COPD
   Joints bony enlargement indicative of osteoarthritis
   Peripheral neuropathy can be diabetes mellitus
   Pedal edema from CHF
   Abdominal tenderness is the only physical finding not readily explained by the patient's
   known diagnoses
4. What risk factors for anemia does the patient have?
   Poor dietary intake
   History PUD, GI bleed, sudden drop indicative of post hemorrhagic
   NSAID ingestion
   Recent prednisone treatment
5. What lab tests would you order? Why?
   Iron studies because of poor diet, determine need for iron supplementation
   Stools for OB to rule out GI bleed due to Relafen and prednisone
6. The stools for occult blood come back positive. What is your diagnosis?
   Iron deficiency anemia secondary to GI bleed

Case 3. The family brings their 94-year-old mother in to clinic because she seems more confused and tired recently.

PMH: Irritable bowel syndrome, lactose intolerance, S/P cholecystitis, history asthma, macular degeneration, history of alcoholism

Current medications: dicyclomine (Bentyl) 10 mg tid, Metamucil 1 scoop qd, LactAid with meals, omeprazole (Prilosec) 20 mg qd

PE: patient confused, has peripheral neuropathy

Lab: RBC 5.23, Hgb 10.1, Hct 31.8, MCV 104.0, MCH 23.1, MCHC 29.7

1. Classify/describe this anemia

   Macrocytic anemia

2. What diagnoses are you considering?

   B_{12} deficiency, folate deficiency

3. What additional information do you need?

   B_{12} and folate levels

Lab: The B_{12} level is less than 250 and the folate level is 4 m/ng/mL

4. What is your diagnosis now?

   B_{12} deficiency

5. What risk factors does she have for B_{12} deficiency?

   Poor diet

   Malabsorption conditions, alcoholism,

   Age stomach less acidic, B_{12} needs acid to be absorbed

   Omeprazole (Prilosec) decreases stomach acid

6. Why is it necessary to screen for folate deficiency before treating B_{12} deficiency?

   See special conditions—Do not begin treatment for B_{12} deficiency without assessing for and treating folate deficiency also, as treatment of B_{12} deficiency may mask the symptoms of folate deficiency, while the damage from low folate will continue

7. What is your treatment plan?

   B_{12} injections 1000 mcg SQ q week x 4 weeks, then q month

8. Will the peripheral neuropathy resolve?

   Perhaps, not likely and damage is usually permanent unless caught early

Chapter 17: Endocrine Disorders

Case 1. A 68-year-old overweight American Indian man comes to the office one afternoon with the complaint of a wound on his foot that has been there for one month and will not heal. Denies pain, fever. Admits to fatigue, blurred vision. Also complains of joint pain especially in knees and hips.

1. What diagnostic studies would you order?

   Random glucose since patient has probably eaten today

   Order fasting glucose for morning

2. Which lab test is the best for diagnosing diabetes in the elderly?

   Fasting glucose: many elderly have impaired glucose tolerance, random glucose may be fairly high without patient having diabetes.

   Hemoglobin A_{1c} is best for monitoring for control, not diagnosis

3. What risk factors does he have for diabetes?

   Race

   Obesity

   Age

4. What is your management of this patient?

   <u>Nonpharmacologic treatment</u>

   Treat foot wound

   Foot care including good shoes

   Patient education about condition

Nutrition counseling for weight reduction, glucose control
Regular exercise
FSBS—how to do
<u>Pharmacologic treatment</u>
Which categories of medications would be appropriate as initial treatment?
Second generation sulfonylureas
Meglitinides
Biguanides
Thiazolidinediones
Alpha glucosidase inhibitors
5. What complications are you worried about?
   Infected foot with osteomyelitis, gangrene, amputation
   Coronary artery disease
   Peripheral vascular disease
   Retina blindness
   Kidney—renal insufficiency
   Peripheral neuropathy

Case 2. An 82-year-old patient is brought in for geriatric assessment by her daughter. Patient is having difficulty sleeping, complains of fatigue and constipation to her family. She does not get dressed in the morning, having difficulty balancing her checkbook. She has gained 10 pounds in the last year. She is otherwise reported to be healthy and has not seen a health care provider in years. She takes Tylenol for arthritis. Her family states they think she is becoming more forgetful.
1. What other history do you need?
   Weight history gain/loss; cold intolerance, arthralgias, myalgias, lethargy depression, weakness
   Past history of thyroid disease
   Family history of thyroid disease
2. What physical exam would you do; what would you expect to find?

Weight	gain
Face	dull expression, swollen
Skin	dry, coarse dry hair, hair loss
Thyroid	enlarged gland
Cardiac	bradycardia, cardiomegaly
Respiratory	dyspnea, pleural effusion
Abdominal	hypoactive bowel sounds
Extremities	peripheral edema
Neurological	dementia, decreased/delayed reflexes

3. What diagnostic test would be conclusive?
   TSH
4. What is your differential diagnoses. What should you rule out?
   Hypothyroidism
   Depression
   Dementia
   Diabetes
   Heart failure
   Kidney failure

Case 3. A 74-year-old man comes to office with complaint of palpitations for about a month. He notices them especially at night when he is trying to sleep; he is having more trouble sleeping recently. They occur about 1–2 times a day. He sits and rests and they go away. He also complains of shortness of breath when walking. He has recently lost 15 pounds. Patient denies dieting.

1. What other body systems would you inquire about?
   General—hypersensitivity to heat, fatigue, weakness
   Mental—anxiety, irritability, psychosis, depression
   Respiratory—cough, dyspnea
   Cardiac—chest pain, orthopnea
   GI—increased appetite, increased frequency of bowel movements, diarrhea, vomiting
2. What physical exam is important?
   Eyes
   Neck—thyroid
   Cardiac—arrhythmias exp atrial fibrillation
   Respiratory
   Musculoskeletal
   Neuro hyperactive reflexes, tremors
   Physical: This patient has atrial fibrillation, tachypnea, hyperactive reflexes, and a fine tremor
3. What is your diagnosis?
   Hyperthyroidism
4. What labs would confirm this diagnosis?
   TSH decreased or undetectable
   T_4 usually elevated, but if normal order
   T_3 elevated
5. What would you do?
   Refer to endocrinologist
   See cardiac chapter for management of the atrial fibrillation, which should resolve when hyperthyroidism is treated
   Consider adjunctive therapy to control symptoms until patient sees endocrinologist, such as beta blocker, diltiazem
6. What is the preferred treatment?
   Radioactive iodine

Chapter 18: Psychiatric-Mental Health Disorders

Case 1. A 72-year-old male presents to your office complaining of insomnia, generalized aches and pains, fatigue and a 10 pound weight loss over the past 2 months. He states he has lost interest in his hobbies, doesn't go out of the house often except to buy groceries and spends much of his day watching television.
Medications: Advil 2–6 tabs/day for pain.
1. What additional questions would you ask?
   Specifics about pain, appetite, sleep, complete review of systems to rule out physical causes including cardiopulmonary, neuro, GI, GU, prior psych history, recent losses, alcohol use, suicide intention, GDS, MMSE, current medications including OTC and herbal supplements
2. What would you look for on physical examination?
   General affect, facial expression, posture hygiene, eye contact, signs of weight loss-serial weight, lose fitting clothes, complete physical to look for clues to weight loss, fatigue such as cardiopulmonary, inflammatory, or neuromuscular disease, and cancer
3. What laboratory work would you order?
   CBC, metabolic panel, TFTs, LFTs, B_{12}, folate, possible ESR, RPR
4. What treatment would you begin, assuming lab is normal?
   Mirtazapine (Remeron) would be a good choice as it helps with sleep and stimulates appetite. An SSRI would also be acceptable choice
5. What complications should you watch for?

Increased anxiety, insomnia, GI symptoms, suicidal intent

Case 2. A 68-year-old female presents to your office complaining of difficulty swallowing, diarrhea, dizzy spells, weakness in her legs, insomnia, feelings of impending doom, and a fear of loosing control.

1. What questions would you ask?

   Length of time, previous episodes, precipitating factors, review of systems-endocrine, cardio-pulmonary, GDS, MMSE, current medications including OTC and herbal supplements, use of caffeine.

2. What would you look for on physical exam?

   Affect, cardiopulmonary-r/o arrhythmia, neurovascular, GI, neck-thyroid

3. What laboratory tests would you order?

   CBC, metabolic panel, TFTs, possible B_{12} if signs of neuropathy or macrocytosis, urinalysis r/o glycosuria, EKG, possible Holter monitor

4. What treatment would you begin?

   Paroxetine (Paxil) is the drug of first choice, consider another SSRI if patient unable to tolerate paroxetine's side effects. Use lorazepam (Ativan) only if necessary for relief of short term, until paroxetine has time to have an effect.

5. What complications might develop?

   Sedation, fatigue, confusion, falls

Case 3. Mr. Smith, 75 years old, comes for routine follow-up of diabetes. He reports his wife died 3 weeks ago. He joined AA at age 50.

Medications: Glucophage 500 mg bid

1. What questions would you ask?

   Coping skills and support systems-present and past, is hospice involved? How much alcohol is he drinking, CAGE, GDS, MMSE, appetite, sleep, and activity patterns, hypo/hyperglycemia symptoms, SI and any plan, suicide intention, plan.

2. What laboratory tests would you order?

   BUN, creatinine, glucose, electrolytes, hemoglobin A_{1c}, urinalysis

   Glucophage can cause lactic acidosis in presence of alcohol use, dehydration, and renal failure

3. What treatment would you begin?

   Grief counseling, continue hospice-bereavement care for spouse

4. What complications might develop?

   Depression, resume alcohol use which complicates diabetes management, suicide

APPENDIX B

SAMPLE GNP TEST

1. The focus of the American Nurses Association's standards and scope of Gerontological Nursing Practice (ANA, 1995) is:
   a. The requisite knowledge base
   b. The assurance of safe practice
   c. Legal guidance for practice
   d. Quality of care

2. A 76-year-old woman who has multiple chronic health problems but is fairly functional has developed an acute problem. The client is undecided about whether to proceed with the recommended treatment. The GNP's MOST appropriate initial intervention to the client would be to:
   a. Review the risks versus benefits of the proposed treatment with the patient
   b. Recommend that patient proceed with the benefit
   c. Request a formal review by an ethics or client care committee
   d. Seek a second evaluation of the situation from another health care professional

3. A 95-year-old woman in your nursing home had complained for about 3 days of pain and burning paresthesias over her right rib area. She now presents with a linear grouping of vesicles on an erythematous base along a dermatomal pathway extending from the sternum to the spine on the right side of the chest. What statement correctly describes this scenario?
   a. Probably a contact dermatitis from an incontinence diaper
   b. Evidence of Herpes Zoster from the reactivation of the Rubeola virus contracted as a child
   c. Result of untreated and repeated flea bites to trunk
   d. Signs and symptoms of Herpes Zoster, a varicella viral infection of a nerve ganglion

4. A 70-year-old man with recurrent episodes of productive cough has recently developed dyspnea with exertion. Which of the following is the most likely diagnosis?
   a. Viral respiratory infection
   b. Asthma
   c. COPD with bronchitis
   d. Allergic rhinitis

5. During cardiac auscultation, a soft S_1 with a pansystolic apical murmur that radiates to the left axilla suggests:
   a. Aortic stenosis
   b. Aortic regurgitation
   c. Mitral valve stenosis
   d. Mitral valve regurgitation

6. A 70-year-old male presents with a gnawing epigastric pain that is relieved by meals and then comes back, especially at night or when he is hungry. Abdominal exam reveals mild epigastric tenderness to deep palpation, otherwise normal. What is the best test to diagnose the cause of the patient's problem?
   a. Fasting serum gastrin level
   b. Upper endoscopy
   c. Barium upper GI series
   d. Urea breath test

7. Which of the following is a potential complication of an inadequately treated urinary tract infection?
   a. Urolithiasis
   b. Renal insufficiency
   c. Reflex incontinence
   d. Poststreptococcal glomerulonephritis

8. Which of the following postmenopausal vaginal bleeding is most likely due to cancer?
   a. Happens with cyclic HRT
   b. Happened 4 months after menopause
   c. New onset of bleeding in a woman who had not bled for 2 years
   d. Bleeding after sexual intercourse

9. Which of the following statements about sexual function in older people is true?
   a. Impotence is an inevitable consequence of aging
   b. Slower arousal and reaction times are normal signs of aging
   c. Moderate alcohol consumption can improve sexual dysfunction
   d. Hormonal replacements are necessary for sexual satisfaction

10. A previously healthy 72-year-old woman presents with a history of headache, and shoulder and hip stiffness for 2 weeks. Laboratory studies show: hemoglobin 10.7 g/dL, a normal MCV, alkaline phosphatase is 2 times normal, alanine aminotransferase (ALT) is 1.5 times normal, and ESR is 104 mm/h. Antimitochondrial antibody, liver ultrasonography, and CT of the head are all normal. What would you tell the patient to expect?
    a. Should resolve in a year with treatment, but has risk of blindness
    b. Chronic progressive course, but no acute inflammation
    c. Increased risk of fractures
    d. Episode will resolve, but expect repeated attacks

11. Which of the following is NOT recommended for primary prevention of stroke?
    a. Management of hypertension
    b. Diet counseling and exercise
    c. Warfarin
    d. Good glycemic control of diabetes

12. A 74-year-old male smokes, has indigestion, arthritis, takes ibuprofen as needed for pain. Hct 32.3 and Hgb 11.2. What type of anemia is he most likely to have?
    a. Iron deficiency
    b. Anemia of chronic disease
    c. Folate deficiency
    d. B 12 deficiency

13. A 78-year-old patient with CAD has an elevated TSH with a low T_4. What medication would you give?
    a. Cytomel 5 mcg
    b. Levothyroxine (Synthroid) 25–50 mcg

    c. Amiodarone (Cordarone) 400 mg

    d. Atenolol 50 mg

14. Which class of antidepressant medications is associated with the highest incidence of serious side effects, including possible hypertensive crisis?

    a. Selective serotonin reuptake inhibitors (SSRIs)

    b. Monoamine oxidase inhibitors (MAOIs)

    c. Tricyclics (TCAs)

    d. Atypical antidepressants such as mirtazapine (Remeron), venlafaxine (Effexor)

15. You establish a program in your health clinic for the rehabilitation of stroke patients. This program would be an example of

    a. Primary prevention

    b. Secondary prevention

    c. Tertiary prevention

    d. A screening test

16. A 65-year-old woman with end-stage, refractory metastatic breast cancer is admitted from home to the nursing home for pain management. Medications such as corticosteroids, NSAIDs have not been effective. She is now on round the clock morphine. Her private physician has turned her care over to you. Her respiratory rate is 9 per minute. Even though drowsy, she says that her pain is still 9 on a scale of 1 to 10. Which of the following would you recommend now?

    a. Do not continue to increase dosage because to do so would cause respiratory failure in the patient

    b. Reduce the dosage of morphine until her respiratory rate improves

    c. Give a bolus of 100 mg of morphine to shorten the painful dying process

    d. Continue to titrate up the morphine dosage until the patient's pain is relieved

17. Which is the most common symptom of infection in the elderly?

    a. Fever

    b. Delirium or decrease in ADLs

    c. Symptoms specific to the system that is infected

    d. Classic symptoms of that particular infection

18. A 65-year-old white male with known history of heavy social alcohol consumption, comes into the office with facial telangiectasia, rhinophyma, flushing, and many clustered erythematous papular lesions on the central area of his face. Based on these general symptoms you believe the problem is:

    a. Acne rosacea

    b. Psoriasis

    c. Xerosis

    d. Atopic dermatitis

19. Which of the following lesions frequently found on or around the eyelids of elder patient will **NOT** require antibiotic treatment?

    a. Chalazion

    b. Hordeolum

    c. Blepharitis

    d. Xanthelasma

20. A 68-year-old man with COPD has continuous symptoms. Which medication for bronchodilatation should be considered for initial treatment?

    a. Steroids

    b. Beta-agonist

    c. Antibiotics

    d. An anticholinergic

21. A 92-year-old woman comes for routine evaluation and has a blood pressure of 164/84. The chart reveals the patient's blood pressure at last visit was 158/82. What is the best advice?
   a. This is normal for the elderly, does not need treatment
   b. This is systolic hypertension, which needs to be treated
   c. Systolic BP is less important than diastolic BP in the elderly
   d. Come back in 2 weeks for recheck of BP

22. A patient with "flu-like" symptoms presents with the following lab results: transaminases: AST-1000, ALT-1500, [both highly elevated]; Alkaline phosphatase-153, [mildly elevated]; bilirubin, GGT, CBC, prothrombin time normal. The most likely diagnosis is:
   a. Acute viral hepatitis
   b. Chronic hepatitis B infection
   c. Cholestasis
   d. Alcoholic liver injury

23. Diabetes and hypertension are common etiologies for:
   a. Renal insufficiency
   b. Bacteriuria
   c. Urolithiasis
   d. Pyelonephritis

24. Which of the conditions below is an ABSOLUTE contraindication to estrogen therapy?
   a. Gallbladder disease
   b. Seizure disorder
   c. Chronic impaired liver function
   d. Unexplained genital bleeding

25. A 69-year-old man comes to the clinic complaining of difficulty starting to urinate, hesitancy during urination, and dribbling after urinating. He has nocturia 4 or 5 times per night. He denies painful urination. His current medications include atenolol, isosorbide, and diltiazem for CAD and HTN, and amitriptyline for insomnia. His residual urine volume is 100 ml. Your first action would be to:
   a. Discontinue amitriptyline
   b. Discontinue diltiazem, and replace with doxazosin to treat HTN
   c. Insert an indwelling catheter
   d. Refer the patient to a urologist for possible transurethral resection (TURP) of prostate

26. What is the first line pharmacologic treatment for osteoarthritis?
   a. Ibuprofen (Motrin)
   b. A COX-2 inhibitor such as celecoxib (Celebrex)
   c. Acetaminophen
   d. Intra-articular corticosteroid injection

27. Which of the following is **NOT** a cause of aplastic anemia?
   a. Chloramphenicol
   b. Viral
   c. Allergic
   d. Radiation

28. Which of the following procedures is most specific for confirming the diagnosis of Hashimoto's thyroiditis in a client who has clinical symptoms?
   a. Thyroid needle biopsy
   b. Thyroid stimulating hormone test
   c. Antithyroglobulin and antithyroid peroxidase antibodies
   d. Ultrasound

29. A 74-year-old female presents complaining of palpitations, tachycardia, cold clammy hands, dizziness, insomnia, generalized aches and pains, and frequent urination. EKG is normal and all lab values are within normal ranges. The most likely diagnosis is:
    a. Post Traumatic Stress Disorder
    b. Anxiety disorder
    c. Major depression
    d. Substance abuse disorder

30. The Patient Self Determination Act requires all **EXCEPT:**
    a. Health care provider to discuss end of life decision with patients
    b. Provider to train staff regarding advanced directives
    c. Patients entering health care facilities name a health care proxy.
    d. Patients entering health care facilities are informed of their right to make an advance directive

31. You have a new patient who is a 74-year-old male without major health problems. He has not consulted a health care provider for over 10 years. What screening test would you recommend MOST highly for this patient?
    a. Blood pressure
    b. PSA
    c. Cholesterol
    d. TSH

32. A 76-year-old man who says there is nothing wrong with him is brought to the clinic by his wife. She has noticed the patient getting lost when driving and getting angry when wife tries to help him. She does not think patient is managing their money correctly but patient has started hiding the checkbook from her. What is this most characteristic of?
    a. Moderate multi infarct dementia
    b. Mild Alzheimer's type dementia
    c. Delirium
    d. Normal pressure hydrocephalus

33. 73-year-old Mrs. Adams has been treated for chronic xerosis, which seems to worsen every year and be particularly bothersome in the winter. Which of the following things should be included in the patient education instructions you give to her?
    a. Do not use a humidifier in the home especially when the heat is running is important
    b. Hot water and soap for a daily bath are effective aids to decrease scaling of skin
    c. Emollient lotions should be used regularly
    d. Hydrocortisone ointment should not be used if skin is inflamed or pruritic

34. An 84-year-old man complains of pain in his right eye with red eye, tearing, blurred vision, nausea and vomiting. His IOP is 60 mmHg. He has been using Lomotil, an anticholinergic drug, for his chronic diarrhea due to short bowel syndrome. The type of glaucoma he is most likely to have would be:
    a. Open angle
    b. Angle closure glaucoma
    c. Secondary glaucoma
    d. Does not have glaucoma

35. An 85-year-old nonsmoker who has never been hospitalized develops an onset of fever and chills, productive cough, chest discomfort, and declining mental status. The physical exam shows T: 101.4° F; pulse 100; respirations 24. Lungs have rhonchi and rales (crackles) in the LLL. The most likely causative organism is:
    a. Strep pneumoniae
    b. Staph aureus

c. Moraxella catarrhalis

d. Influenza A

36. An 83-year-old man has hyperlipidemia and diabetes. He has just been diagnosed with hypertension. Which drug would you use?

a. Enalapril (Vasotec)

b. Propranolol

c. Atenolol

d. HCTZ

37. Your 70-year-old patient has gastroesophageal reflux disease (GERD). After a trial of lifestyle modifications and antacids, the patient continues to have occasional mild heartburn after meals and at night. The most appropriate next action would be to:

a. Prokinetic agents

b. H2 antagonists

c. Proton pump inhibitors

d. Sucralfate

38. When evaluating hematuria, it is crucial to rule-out:

a. Enuresis

b. Benign prostatic hypertrophy

c. Malignancy

d. Ureteral stricture

39. A 78-year-old woman comes to your office complaining of vague GI symptoms including nausea, loss of appetite, abdominal fullness, and pelvic pressure that have gradually been worsening for the past 3 years. In the past year, she has experienced fatigue and weight loss of 15 pounds without dieting. What one action would the best for you to do?

a. Discuss her diet with her

b. Treat with omeprazole (Prilosec)

c. Discuss hormone replacement therapy

d. Refer to GYN oncology

40. You discover a hard nodule when doing a digital rectal exam (DRE) on a 78 black male. You feel that the lump probably is cancerous because:

a. The lump is very painful

b. African Americans have a higher risk of prostate cancer

c. The lump is firm with hard induration

d. Patient has urinary frequency, urgency and dribbling.

41. Which patient is most likely to have osteoporosis?

a. An 80-year-old underweight male who smokes and has been on steroids for psoriasis

b. A 90-year-old female with no family history of osteoporosis who is on HRT

c. A 68-year-old overweight female who drinks 1-2 drinks alcohol/day

d. An 82-year-old female who is ideal body weight, takes calcium and vitamins, has weight bearing exercise daily

42. An 80-year-old female presents with 2 days of acute left facial weakness without any other neurologic symptoms or signs. What is the most likely diagnosis?

a. Bell palsy

b. Acoustic neuroma

c. Stroke

d. Trigeminal neuralgia

43. A patient's lab shows Hemoglobin 10.1, Hct 31.3, low MCV and MCH, with low ferritin and increased TIBC. This is characteristic of:
   a. Iron deficiency
   b. B_{12} deficiency
   c. Folate deficiency
   d. Aplastic anemia

44. 87-year-old Mrs. Black has been taking 100 mcg of Synthroid for 10 years. She comes to your office for routine follow-up, feeling well. Her heart rate is 90. Your first response is to:
   a. Increase her Synthroid
   b. Order TSH
   c. Start Atenolol
   d. Order thyroid scan

45. Which of the following psychiatric medications represents a class of drugs commonly prescribed in the older adult population that has a high incidence of abuse, misuse, and adverse reactions?
   a. Fluoxetine (Prozac)
   b. Nortriptyline (Pamelor)
   c. Risperidone (Risperdal)
   d. Lorazepam (Ativan)

46. The right of all competent patients to receive or refuse treatment is protected by:
   a. Advance directive
   b. Informed consent
   c. Standard of care
   d. Confidentiality

47. Current recommendations for exercise in older adults suggest:
   a. Only those older adults who are overweight need to exercise
   b. Exercise should be done at least daily for at least 60 minutes
   c. Exercise programs ideally should combine aerobic, resistive and stretching activities
   d. Older adults with any underlying chronic illnesses should not exercise

48. You see a 73-year-old woman with breast cancer that has recurred in the bone. Low dose oxycodone was recently added to her pain regimen of Advil 400 mg tid. Which of the following is (are) common side effect(s) of opioids that should be managed when initiating and monitoring opioid therapy?
   a. Diarrhea and vomiting
   b. Constipation and nausea
   c. Addiction or psychological dependence
   d. Anorexia

49. Which is True about HIV in the elderly?
   a. Treatment is the same as for younger adults
   b. Elderly patients have a poorer prognosis than younger adults
   c. Adverse reactions to the medications occur less frequently than with younger adults
   d. Viral burden and CD4 count do not predict prognosis

50. An elderly African American at the extended care center has had numerous problems with seborrheic dermatitis. When you go inspect him, you will be certain to examine:
   a. The fingernails
   b. The buttocks and groin
   c. The scalp, eyebrows, nasolabial folds, behind ears
   d. The palms and soles

APPENDIX C

DISCUSSION OF MULTIPLE CHOICE QUESTION/ANSWERS

1. The focus of the American Nurses Association's standards and scope of Gerontological Nursing Practice (ANA, 1995) is:
   a. The requisite knowledge base (**No, NONPF helps determine this**)
   b. The assurance of safe practice (**No, this must be the responsibility of the NP**)
   c. Legal guidance for practice (**No, the ANA cannot offer legal advice**)
   d. Quality of care (**Yes**)

2. A 76-year-old woman who has multiple chronic health problems but is fairly functional has developed an acute problem. The client is undecided about whether to proceed with the recommended treatment. The GNP's MOST appropriate initial intervention to the client would be to:
   a. Review the risks versus benefits of the proposed treatment with the patient (**Yes, the decision belongs to the patient**)
   b. Recommend that patient proceed with the benefit (**No, NP may end up doing this but first should make sure the patient understands her options**)
   c. Request a formal review by an ethics or client care committee (**No, should be reserved for difficult decisions in patient unable to make own decisions**)
   d. Seek a second evaluation of the situation from another health care professional (**No, NP should be able to handle this situation, unless it becomes complex**)

3. A 95-year-old woman in your nursing home had complained for about 3 days of pain and burning paresthesias over her right rib area. She now presents with a linear grouping of vesicles on an erythematous base along a dermatomal pathway extending from the sternum to the spine on the right side of the chest. What statement correctly describes this scenario?
   a. Probably a contact dermatitis from an incontinence diaper (**No would not be painful**)
   b. Evidence of Herpes Zoster from the reactivation of the Rubeola virus contracted as a child (**No, not the Rubeola virus**)
   c. Result of untreated and repeated flea bites to trunk (**No, would not have burning paresthesias**)
   d. Signs and symptoms of Herpes Zoster, a varicella viral infection of a nerve ganglion (**Yes, classic presentation**)

4. 70-year-old man with recurrent episodes of productive cough has recently developed dyspnea with exertion. Which of the following is the most likely diagnosis?
   a. Viral respiratory infection (**No, not recurrent**)
   b. Asthma (**No, presents with episodic shortness of breath**)
   c. COPD with bronchitis (**Yes, starts with cough, worsens over time**)
   d. Allergic rhinitis (**No, should not develop dyspnea**)

5. During cardiac auscultation, a soft S_1 with a pansystolic apical murmur that radiates to the left axilla suggests:
   a. Aortic stenosis **(No, no radiation to axilla)**
   b. Aortic regurgitation **(No, not likely to radiate)**
   c. Mitral valve stenosis **(No, not pansystolic)**
   d. Mitral valve regurgitation **(Yes)**

6. A 70-year-old male presents with a gnawing epigastric pain that is relieved by meals and then comes back, especially at night or when he is hungry. Abdominal exam reveals mild epigastric tenderness to deep palpation, otherwise normal. What is the best test to diagnose the cause of the patient's problem?
   a. Fasting serum gastrin level **(No, detects Zollinger-Ellison syndrome, patient would have more severe symptoms)**
   b. Upper endoscopy **(Yes, best test to diagnose peptic ulcer, allows for detection of malignancy and H. pylori infection)**
   c. Barium upper GI series **(No, gives less information than b.)**
   d. Urea breath test **(No, diagnoses H. pylori, used for followup more than diagnosis)**

7. Which of the following is a potential complication of an inadequately treated urinary tract infection?
   a. Urolithiasis **(No, stones may cause or aggravate UTIs, not usually the reverse)**
   b. Renal insufficiency **(Yes, early treatment of urinary tract infections in elders can prevent deterioration of renal function. Ascending infections can damage renal parenchyma irreversibly)**
   c. Reflex incontinence **(No, this type of incontinence is associated with neurologic disorders such as disk herniation or spinal cord disease)**
   d. Poststreptococcal glomerulonephritis **(No, this disorder is an immune response to a streptococcal infection; is not related to UTIs)**

8. Which of the following postmenopausal vaginal bleeding is most likely due to cancer?
   a. Happens with cyclic HRT **(No, a common problem when cyclic therapy is initiated)**
   b. Happened 4 months after menopause **(No a common occurrence)**
   c. New onset of bleeding in a woman who had not bled for 2 years **(Yes, patient should not restart bleeding without known trigger)**
   d. Bleeding after sexual intercourse **(No, most likely due to trauma to atrophic vaginitis)**

9. Which of the following statements about sexual function in older people is true?
   a. Impotence is an inevitable consequence of aging **(No, a myth and is untrue)**
   b. Slower arousal and reaction times are normal signs of aging **(Yes, this is true)**
   c. Moderate alcohol consumption can improve sexual dysfunction **(No, another myth and is untrue)**
   d. Hormonal replacements are necessary for sexual satisfaction **(No, problem is usually psychological or due to underlying condition such as diabetes)**

10. A previously healthy 72-year-old woman presents with a history of headache, and shoulder and hip stiffness for 2 weeks. Laboratory studies show: hemoglobin 10.7 g/dL, a normal MCV, alkaline phosphatase is 2 times normal, alanine aminotransferase (ALT) is 1.5 times normal, and ESR is 104 mm/h. Antimitochondrial antibody, liver ultrasonography, and CT of the head are all normal. What would you tell the patient to expect?
    a. Should resolve in a year with treatment, but has risk of blindness **(Yes, polymyalgia rheumatica)**
    b. Chronic progressive course, but no acute inflammation **(No, osteoarthritis course)**
    c. Increased risk of fractures **(No, associated with osteoporosis)**
    d. Episode will resolve, but expect repeated attacks **(No, polymyalgia rheumatica should not return)**

11. Which of the following is NOT recommended for primary prevention of stroke?
    a. Management of hypertension **(No, an important step)**
    b. Diet counseling and exercise **(No, also necessary)**
    c. Warfarin **(Yes, not primary prevention)**
    d. Good glycemic control of diabetes **(No, prevents development of plaque)**

12. A 74-year-old male smokes, has indigestion, arthritis, takes ibuprofen as needed for pain. Hct 32.3 and Hgb 11.2. What type of anemia is he most likely to have?
    a. Iron deficiency **(Yes, from chronic GI bleed)**
    b. Anemia of chronic disease **(No, does not have diagnosis of chronic disease likely to cause anemia)**
    c. Folate deficiency **(No, possible, but has more risk factors for iron deficiency)**
    d. B_{12} deficiency **(No, possible, but has more risk factors for iron deficiency)**

13. A 78-year-old patient with CAD has an elevated TSH with a low T_4. What medication would you give?
    a. Cytomel 5 mcg **(No, this T_3 medication is not recommended)**
    b. Levothyroxine (Synthroid) 25–50 mcg **(Yes, very low dose to start)**
    c. Amiodarone (Cordarone) 400 mg **(No, causes hypothyroidism)**
    d. Atenolol 50 mg **(No, used for symptoms of hyperthyroidism)**

14. Which class of antidepressant medications is associated with the highest incidence of serious side effects, including possible hypertensive crisis?
    a. Selective serotonin reuptake inhibitors (SSRIs) **(No, relatively safe)**
    b. Monoamine oxidase inhibitors (MAOIs) **(Yes)**
    c. Tricyclics (TCAs) **(No, have some serious side effects, but less than MAOIs)**
    d. Atypical antidepressants such as mirtazapine (Remeron), venlafaxine (Effexor) **(No, have side effects, but generally well tolerated)**

15. You establish a program in your health clinic for the rehabilitation of stroke patients. This program would be an example of
    a. Primary prevention **(No, prevents illness)**
    b. Secondary prevention **(No, prevents problems from an illness)**
    c. Tertiary prevention **(Yes, treatment of rehabilitation of the illness to avoid or postpone complications)**
    d. A screening test **(No, they are to detect asymptomatic illness)**

16. A 65-year-old woman with end-stage, refractory metastatic breast cancer is admitted from home to the nursing home for pain management. Medications such as corticosteroids, NSAIDs have not been effective. She is now on round the clock morphine. Her private physician has turned her care over to you. Her respiratory rate is 9 per minute. Even though drowsy, she says that her pain is still 9 on a scale of 1 to 10. Which of the following would you recommend now?
    a. Do not continue to increase dosage because to do so would cause respiratory failure in the patient **(No, not likely)**
    b. Reduce the dosage of morphine until her respiratory rate improves **(No, she is still in pain)**
    c. Give a bolus of 100 mg of morphine to shorten the painful dying process **(No, do not hasten death)**
    d. Continue to titrate up the morphine dosage until the patient's pain is relieved **(Yes, you must continue to try to control her pain)**

17. Which is the most common symptom of infection in the elderly.
    a. Fever **(No, frequently absent)**
    b. Delirium or decrease in ADLs **(Yes)**
    c. Symptoms specific to the system that is infected **(No, nonspecific)**
    d. Classic symptoms of that particular infection **(No, atypical symptoms)**

18. A 65-year-old white male with known history of heavy social alcohol consumption, comes into the office with facial telangiectasia, rhinophyma, flushing, and many clustered erythematous papular lesions on the central area of his face. Based on these general symptoms you believe the problem is:
    a. Acne rosacea **(Yes)**
    b. Psoriasis **(No, lesions with silvery scales)**
    c. Xerosis **(No, more than simple dry skin)**
    d. Atopic dermatitis **(No, does not fit description)**

19. Which of the following lesions frequently found on or around the eyelids of elder patient will NOT require antibiotic treatment?
    a. Chalazion **(No, this obstructed meibomian gland is treated with erythromycin ointment)**
    b. Hordeolum **(No, this infected Zeis/Moll gland, is often infected with S. aureus. May require ophthalmic antibiotic)**
    c. Blepharitis **(No, this inflammation of the eyelids is frequently caused by Staph infection of the follicles and is also treated with erythromycin ointment)**
    d. Xanthelasma **(Yes, this yellow plaque found along the nasal aspect of the eyelids is benign and does not require treatment)**

20. A 68-year-old man with COPD has continuous symptoms. Which medication for broncho-dilatation should be considered for initial treatment?
    a. Steroids **(No, can play a role if there is an inflammatory component to COPD)**
    b. Beta-agonist **(No, acceptable, but anticholinergic is a better choice)**
    c. Antibiotics **(No role in bronchodilatation)**
    d. An anticholinergic **(Yes, best first choice due to greater effect than beta-agonist; anticholinergics exert effect on vagal tone causing dilatation)**

21. A 92-year-old woman comes for routine evaluation and has a blood pressure of 164/84. The chart reveals the patient's blood pressure at last visit was 158/82. What is the best advice?
    a. This is normal for the elderly, does not need treatment **(No, may be common, but not normal)**
    b. This is systolic hypertension, which needs to be treated **(Yes, is a risk factor for cardiovascular disease)**
    c. Systolic BP is less important than diastolic BP in the elderly **(No, systolic more important than diastolic)**
    d. Come back in 2 weeks for recheck of BP **(No, you will ask her to come back, but first you will treat)**

22. A patient with "flu-like" symptoms presents with the following lab results: transaminases: AST-1000, ALT-1500, [both highly elevated]; Alkaline phosphatase-153, [mildly elevated]; bilirubin, GGT, CBC, prothrombin time normal. The most likely diagnosis is:
    a. Acute viral hepatitis **(Yes, classic presentation)**
    b. Chronic hepatitis B infection **(No, acute presentation)**
    c. Cholestasis **(No, Alkaline phos would be highly elevated)**
    d. Alcoholic liver injury **(No, transaminases would be mildly elevated, AST would be higher than ALT in liver injury, GGT would be elevated, CBC may show elevated MCV, also may have elevated prothrombin time)**

23. Diabetes and hypertension are common etiologies for:
    a. Renal insufficiency **(Yes, both of these conditions cause renal damage when not controlled well or present for long periods of time)**
    b. Bacteriuria **(No, bacteria in the urine is not commonly associated with these conditions)**
    c. Urolithiasis **(No, stones are not associated with these conditions)**
    d. Pyelonephritis **(No, Pyelonephritis is not associated with these conditions in the absence of urinary tract infections)**

24. Which of the conditions below is an ABSOLUTE contraindication to estrogen therapy?
    a. Gallbladder disease **(No, is a precaution)**
    b. Seizure disorder **(No, is a precaution)**
    c. Chronic impaired liver function **(No, use transdermal or vaginal instead of oral)**
    d. Unexplained genital bleeding **(Yes, could be cancer)**

25. A 69-year-old man comes to the clinic complaining of difficulty starting to urinate, hesitancy during urination, and dribbling after urinating. He has nocturia 4 or 5 times per night. He denies painful urination. His current medications include atenolol, isosorbide, and diltiazem for CAD and HTN, and amitriptyline for insomnia. His residual urine volume is 100 ml. Your first action would be to:
    a. Discontinue amitriptyline **(Yes, anticholinergic can cause urinary retention)**
    b. Discontinue diltiazem, and replace with doxazosin to treat HTN **(No, may do this later, but not first step)**
    c. Insert an indwelling catheter **(No, treatment of last resort)**
    d. Refer the patient to a urologist for possible transurethral resection (TURP) of prostate **(No, may do this later)**

26. What is the first line pharmacologic treatment for osteoarthritis?
    a. Ibuprofen (Motrin) **(No, high risk of GI side effects, including bleeding)**
    b. A COX 2 inhibitor such as celecoxib (Celebrex) **(No, used if unable to tolerate regular NSAIDs)**
    c. Acetaminophen **(Yes, effective for pain, does not cause GI side effects, but use caution if any hepatic dysfunction)**
    d. Intra-articular corticosteroid injection **(No, good for localized, single joint problems)**

27. Which of the following is NOT a cause of aplastic anemia
    a. Chloramphenicol **(No, a cause)**
    b. Viral **(No, a cause)**
    c. Allergic **(Yes, not a cause)**
    d. Radiation **(No, a cause)**

28. Which of the following procedures is most specific for confirming the diagnosis of Hashimoto's thyroiditis in a client who has clinical symptoms?
    a. Thyroid needle biopsy **(No, used to determine if nodule is cancer)**
    b. Thyroid stimulating hormone test **(No, nonspecific for cause of symptoms)**
    c. Antithyroglobulin and antithyroid peroxidase antibodies **(Yes, elevated)**
    d. Ultrasound **(No, differentiates between solid and cystic nodule)**

29. A 74-year-old female presents complaining of palpitations, tachycardia, cold clammy hands, dizziness, insomnia, generalized aches and pains, and frequent urination. EKG is normal and all lab values are within normal ranges. The most likely diagnosis is:
    a. Post Traumatic Stress Disorder **(No, would be associate with specific event)**
    b. Anxiety disorder **(Yes)**
    c. Major depression **(No, palpitations, tachycardia, dizziness, feeling of impending doom characteristic of anxiety)**
    d. Substance abuse disorder **(No, unless in withdrawal)**

30. The Patient Self Determination Act requires all EXCEPT:
    a. Health care provider to discuss end of life decision with patients **(No, requires this)**
    b. Provider to train staff regarding advanced directives **(No, requires this)**
    c. Patients entering health care facilities name a health care proxy. **(Yes, patient not forced to name someone, just be notified of their rights)**
    d. Patients entering health care facilities are informed of their right to make an advance directive **(No, this is required)**

31. You have a new patient who is a 74-year-old male without major health problems. He has not consulted a health care provider for over 10 years. What screening test would you recommend MOST highly for this patient?
    a. Blood pressure **(Yes, well documented to be beneficial)**
    b. PSA **(No, efficacy remains controversial)**
    c. Cholesterol **(No, efficacy remains controversial)**
    d. TSH **(No, low yield, especially in men)**

32. A 76-year-old man who says there is nothing wrong with him is brought to the clinic by his wife. She has noticed the patient getting lost when driving and getting angry when wife tries to help him. She does not think patient is managing their money correctly but patient has started hiding the checkbook from her. What is this most characteristic of?
    a. Moderate multi infarct dementia **(No, symptoms are of mild dementia, no risk factors for MID noted)**
    b. Mild Alzheimer's type dementia **(Yes, symptoms are of mild Alzheimer's)**
    c. Delirium **(No, not symptoms of delirium)**
    d. Normal pressure hydrocephalus **(No, that would present with early ataxia and incontinence)**

33. 73-year-old Mrs. Adams has been treated for chronic xerosis, which seems to worsen every year and be particularly bothersome in the winter. Which of the following things should be included in the patient education instructions you give to her?
    a. Do not use a humidifier in the home especially when the heat is running is important **(No, this is helpful)**
    b. Hot water and soap for a daily bath are effective aids to decrease scaling of skin **(No, hot water and soap are very drying)**
    c. Emollient lotions should be used regularly **(Yes, an important treatment)**
    d. Hydrocortisone ointment should not be used if skin is inflamed or pruritic **(No, it is useful to prevent excoriation)**

34. An 84-year-old man complains of pain in his right eye with red eye, tearing, blurred vision, nausea and vomiting. His IOP is 60 mm Hg. He has been using Lomotil, an anticholinergic drug, for his chronic diarrhea due to short bowel syndrome. The type of glaucoma he is most likely to have would be:
    a. Open angle **(No, not likely to present acutely)**
    b. Angle closure glaucoma **(Yes, sudden onset and anticholinergic drug a risk factor)**
    c. Secondary glaucoma **(No, no risk factors.)**
    d. Does not have glaucoma **(No, IOP very, high, symptoms cannot be explained by other red eye conditions)**

35. An 85-year-old nonsmoker who has never been hospitalized develops an onset of fever and chills, productive cough, chest discomfort, and declining mental status. The physical exam shows T: 101.4 F; pulse 100; respirations 24. Lungs have rhonchi and rales (crackles) in the LLL. The most likely causative organism is:
    a. Strep pneumoniae **(Yes, most prevalent cause of community acquired pneumonia)**
    b. Staph aureus **(No, less likely, can be secondary cause with viral infection)**
    c. Moraxella catarrhalis **(No, could see this in a COPD or smoking patient)**
    d. Influenza A **(No, generally would not cause mental status changes, high fever and abnormal lung sounds would not localize)**

36. An 83-year-old man has hyperlipidemia and diabetes. He has just been diagnosed with hypertension. Which drug would you use?
    a. Enalapril (Vasotec) **(Yes, ACE inhibitor has protective effect on kidney in patients with diabetes)**
    b. Propranolol **(No, nonselective beta blocker, has adverse effect on lipids, masks hypoglycemia in diabetes)**

c. Atenolol **(No, cardioselective beta blocker, safer than propranolol but still has adverse effect on lipids)**

d. HCTZ **(No, while also a first line HTN drug, enalapril is a better choice)**

37. Your 70-year-old patient has gastroesophageal reflux disease (GERD). After a trial of lifestyle modifications and antacids, the patient continues to have occasional mild heartburn after meals and at night. The most appropriate next action would be to:

a. Prokinetic agents **(No, use only as last resort, due to CNS side effects)**

b. H2 antagonists **(Yes, second line treatment of mild symptoms)**

c. Proton pump inhibitors **(No, used for moderate to severe symptoms)**

d. Sucralfate **(No, not a second line choice)**

38. When evaluating hematuria, it is crucial to rule out:

a. Enuresis **(No, not a logical answer)**

b. Benign prostatic hypertrophy **(No, not usually associated with hematuria unless infection present)**

c. Malignancy **(Yes, the provider must always rule out malignancy in an elderly patient with hematuria)**

d. Ureteral stricture **(No, possibly a cause, but not the best answer)**

39. An 78-year-old woman comes to your office complaining of vague GI symptoms including nausea, loss of appetite, abdominal fullness, and pelvic pressure that have gradually been worsening for the past 3 years. In the past year, she has experienced fatigue and weight loss of 15 pounds without dieting. What one action would the best for you to do?

a. Discuss her diet with her **(No, must first look for cancer)**

b. Treat with omeprazole (Prilosec) **(No, problem needs to evaluated first)**

c. Discuss hormone replacement therapy **(No, contraindicated)**

d. Refer to GYN oncology **(Yes, patient has signs and symptoms of ovarian cancer)**

40. You discover a hard nodule when doing a digital rectal exam (DRE) on a 78-year-old black male. You feel that the lump probably is cancerous because:

a. The lump is very painful **(No, cancer is generally painless)**

b. African Americans have a higher risk of prostate cancer **(No, true but not why you suspect cancer)**

c. The lump is firm with hard induration **(Yes, classic description of prostate cancer)**

d. Patient has urinary frequency, urgency and dribbling. **(No, these symptoms are also true of BPH)**

41. Which patient is most likely to have osteoporosis?

a. An 80-year-old underweight male who smokes and has been on steroids for psoriasis **(Yes, men get osteoporosis around age 70, has risk factors)**

b. A 90-year-old female with no family history of osteoporosis who is on HRT **(No, is on preventive therapy)**

c. A 68-year-old overweight female who drinks 1-2 drinks alcohol/day **(No, moderate overweight not associated with increased risk, must be heavy alcohol intake to increase risk)**

d. A 82-year-old female who is ideal body weight, takes calcium and vitamins, has weight bearing exercise daily **(No, doing nonpharmacologic prevention)**

42. An 80-year-old female presents with 2 days of acute left facial weakness without any other neurologic symptoms or signs. What is the most likely diagnosis?

a. Bell's palsy **(Yes, typical presentation)**

b. Acoustic neuroma **(No, affects hearing)**

c. Stroke **(No, causes more extensive damage)**

d. Trigeminal neuralgia **(No, causes pain, not weakness)**

43. A patient's lab shows Hemoglobin 10.1, Hct 31.3, low MCV and MCH, with low ferritin and increased TIBC. This is characteristic of:
   a. Iron deficiency **(Yes, microcytic hypochromic anemia)**
   b. B_{12} deficiency **(No, macrocytic anemia)**
   c. Folate deficiency **(No, macrocytic anemia)**
   d. Aplastic anemia **(No, pancytopenia)**

44. 87-year-old Mrs. Black has been taking 100 mcg of Synthroid for 10 years. She comes to your office for routine follow-up, feeling well. Her heart rate is 90. Your first response is to:
   a. Increase her Synthroid **(No, must diagnose problem first)**
   b. Order TSH **(Yes, to determine if she is on right dose of Synthroid)**
   c. Start Atenolol **(No, you may do this if she has trouble tolerating the increased heart rate)**
   d. Order thyroid scan **(No, used for nodule)**

45. Which of the following psychiatric medications represents a class of drugs commonly prescribed in the older adult population that has a high incidence of abuse, misuse, and adverse reactions?
   a. Fluoxetine (Prozac) **(No, generally safe and effective)**
   b. Nortriptyline (Pamelor) **(No, many adverse reactions but low abuse potential)**
   c. Risperidone (Risperdal) **(No, potentially serious adverse reactions but no abuse potential)**
   d. Lorazepam (Ativan) **(Yes, use with caution)**

46. The right of all competent patients to receive or refuse treatment is protected by:
   a. Advance directive **(No, this provides for decision making when patient becomes incompetent)**
   b. Informed consent **(Yes)**
   c. Standard of care **(No, relates to the level of care given)**
   d. Confidentiality **(No, provides for privacy)**

47. Current recommendations for exercise in older adults suggest:
   a. Only those older adults who are overweight need to exercise **(No, benefits everyone)**
   b. Exercise should be done at least daily for at least 60 minutes **(No, 30 minutes is enough to get benefit)**
   c. Exercise programs ideally should combine aerobic, resistive and stretching activities **(Yes, a variety of exercises is very beneficial in the elderly, should be individualized according to their ability)**
   d. Older adults with any underlying chronic illnesses should not exercise **(No, benefits them too)**

48. You see a 73-year-old woman with breast cancer that has recurred in the bone. Low dose oxycodone was recently added to her pain regimen of Advil 400 mg tid. Which of the following is (are) common side effect(s) of opioids that should be managed when initiating and monitoring opioid therapy?
   a. Diarrhea and vomiting **(No, does not cause diarrhea)**
   b. Constipation and nausea **(Yes, the most common and bothersome)**
   c. Addiction or psychological dependence **(No, not concern in cancer patients)**
   d. Anorexia **(No, can be a problem, but less likely than constipation)**

49. Which is TRUE about HIV in the elderly?
   a. Treatment is the same as for younger adults **(No, this is untrue)**
   b. Elderly patients have a poorer prognosis than younger adults **(Yes, have a much poorer prognosis)**
   c. Adverse reactions to the medications occur less frequently than with younger adults **(No, this is untrue)**
   d. Viral burden and CD4 count do not predict prognosis **(No, viral burden and CD4 count do predict prognosis)**

50. An elderly African American at the extended care center has had numerous problems with seborrheic dermatitis. When you go inspect him, you will be certain to examine:
   a. The fingernails **(No, certain other fungal infections located here)**
   b. The buttocks and groin **(No, frequent location of candida)**
   c. The scalp, eyebrows, nasolabial folds, behind ears **(Yes)**
   d. The palms and soles **(No, uncommon to have rash here)**

BIBLIOGRAPHY

GENERAL BIBLIOGRAPHY

American Geriatric Society (2002). *Geriatrics Review Syllabus* (ed 4). New York, NY: Kendall/Hunt.

Aldelman A and Daley M (2001) *Twenty Common Problems in Geriatrics*. New York, NY: McGraw-Hill.

Barker LR, Burton JR, Zieve PD (2002). *Principles of Ambulatory Medicine* (ed 6). Baltimore, MD: Lippincott, Williams & Wilkins.

Bates B (2004). *A Guide to Physical Examination and History Taking* (ed 8). Philadelphia, PA: J. B, Lippincott, Williams & Wilkins.

Beers MH and Berkow R (2000) *The Merck Manual of Geriatrics* (ed 3). Whitehouse Station, NJ: Merck Research Laboratories

Burke MM & Laramie JA (2004). *Primary Care of the Older Adult* (ed 2). St. Louis, MO: Mosby.

Dambro MR (2004). *The 5 Minute Clinical Consult* (ed 12). St. Louis: Lippincott, Williams & Wilkins.

Edmunds MW, Mayhew MS (2004). *Pharmacology for the Primary Care Provider* (ed 2). St. Louis: Mosby.

Fauci AS et al. (2002). *Harrison's Principles of Internal Medicine*. New York: McGraw-Hill Health Professions Division.

Ferri FF (2004). *Ferri's Clinical Advisor* (ed 6). St. Louis , MO: Mosby.

Edmunds MW, Mayhew MS (2004). *Pharmacology for the Primary Care Provider* (ed 2) St. Louis, MO: Mosby.

Gallo JJ et al. (2000). *Handbook of Geriatric Assessment* (ed 3). MD: Aspen.

Goroll AH, May LA, Mulley AG (2000). *Primary Care Medicine: Office Evaluation and Management of the Adult Patient* (ed 4). Philadelphia, PA: J.B. Lippincott Company.

Hazzard WR, Bierman, EL, Blass, JP et al. (2003). *Principles of Geriatric Medicine and Gerontology* (ed 54). New York, NY: McGraw-Hill.

Meredith PV Horan, NM (2000). *Adult Primary Care*. Philadelphia, PA: WB Saunders.

Rakel RE (2004). *Conn's Current Therapy 2004*. Philadelphia: WB Saunders Company.

Tierney LM, McPhee SJ, Papadakis A (2005). *Current Medical Diagnosis and Treatment* (ed 44). NJ: Appleton & Lange.

United States Preventive Services Task Force (USPSTF) (2002). *Guide to Clinical Preventive Services* (ed 3). McLean, VA: International Medical Publishing

WEB SITES
Government Web Sites

Agency for Health Care Research and Quality www.ahcpr.gov Clinical information on evidence based practice, outcomes and effectiveness, technology assessment, preventive services

Centers for Disease Control and Prevention www.cdc.gov, includes the MMWR (Morbidity and Mortality Weekly Report)

Centers for Medicare and Medicaid Services www.cms.hhs.gov The CMS Quarterly Provider Update source of National Medicare Provider Information, information for professionals and consumers

Combined Health Information Database http://chid.nih.gov This is a bibliographic database produced by health-related agencies of the Federal Government providing titles, abstracts, and availability information for health information and health eduction resources

Government Web Portal www.health.gov A portal to the Web sites of a number of multi-agency health initiatives and activities of the US Department of Heath and Human Services and other Federal departments and agencies

Medicare Part B www.partbnews.com newsletter reporting on the changes in Medicare Part B coverage, coding, billing and reimbursement rules for physician services

National Guideline Clearinghouse www.guideline.gov a public resource for evidence-based clinical practice guidelines, sponsored by the Agency for Healthcare Research and Quality, US Department of Health and Human Services.

NIH www.nih.gov The national Institutes of Health home page with health information and access to the institutes, centers and offices of the NIH

NIH national Library of Medicine www.medlineplus.gov with many resources including searching MedlinePlus.

NIH Office of Dietary Supplements http://dietary-supplements.info.nih.gov

NIH Heart, Lung and Blood Institute www.nhlbi.nih.gov

NIH National Center for Complementary and Alternative Medicine www.nccam.nih.gov with health information and clinical trials

NIH National Institute on Aging www.nih.gov/nia

NIH National Institute of Diabetes and Digestive and Kidney Disease www.niddk.nih.gov

Office of the Surgeon General www.surgeongeneral.gov has publications and information on health topics for consumers

PubMed www.ncbi.nlm.nih.gov/PubMed Entrez is the text-based search and retrieval system used at NCBI (National Center for Biotechnology Information) for the major databases, including PubMed, Nucleotide and Protein Sequences, Protein Structures, Complete Genomes, Taxonomy, and others.

US Department of Agriculture (USDA) Food and Nutrition Information Center www.nal.usda.gov/fnic/index.html

USDA National Nutrient Database www.nal.usda.gov/fnic/foodcomp/index.html

US Food and Drug Administration Center for Food Safety and Applied Nutrition www.fda.gov

US Government Printing Office www.gpoaccess.gov/index.html disseminates official information from all three branches of the Federal Government

Web site for consumers www.healthfinder.gov a resource for finding government and nonprofit heath and human services information, with links to over 1,700 sites

Organizations

www.ama-assn.org   American Medical Association
www.aafp.org   American Association of Family Physicians
www.mayoclinic.com   Mayo Clinic general info for patients
www.acponline.org   American College of Physicians

Commercial Web Resources

Medscape at www.medscape.com Click on "other specialties" then on "nurses" to find nursing pages.
www.freemedicaljournals.com—source for journals with complete articles on line
www.merckmedicus.com—good general source, includes Cecils, Harrisons, and Merck Manual textbooks

INDEX